2023

T0075369

Changes | An Insider's View

cpt®

current procedural
terminology

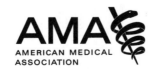

AMA
AMERICAN MEDICAL
ASSOCIATION

Executive Vice President, Chief Executive Officer: James L. Madara, MD

Senior Vice President, Health Solutions: Lori Prestesater

Vice President, Coding and Reimbursement Policy and Strategy: Jay Ahlman

Director, CPT Editorial and Regulatory Services: Zachary Hochstetler

Director, CPT Content Management and Development: Leslie W. Prellwitz

Manager, CPT Editorial Panel Processes: Desiree Rozell

Manager, CPT Content Management and Development: Karen E. O'Hara

Healthcare Coding Analysts/Senior Healthcare Coding Analysts: Thilani Attale; Kemi Borokini; Jennifer Bell; Martha Espronceda; Desiree Evans; Dehandro Hayden; Charniece Martin; Sara Nakira; Lianne Stancik; Keisha Sutton-Asaya

Senior Clinical Content Manager: Kerri Fei

Program Manager, CPT Editorial Processes: Caitlin Mora

Vice President, Operations: Denise Foy

Senior Manager, Publishing Operations: Elizabeth Goodman Duke

Manager, Developmental Editor: Lisa Chin-Johnson

Editorial Assistant: Paige Downie

Production Specialist: Julia Enamorado

Vice President, Sales and Marketing: Sue Wilson

Director, Print, Digital and Guides: Erin Kalitowski

Director, CPT Operations and Infrastructure: Barbara Benstead

Director, Product Management, CPT Infrastructure: Julio Rodriguez

Marketing Manager II: Vanessa Prieto

Copyright © 2022 by the American Medical Association. All rights reserved.
CPT® is a registered trademark of the American Medical Association

Printed in the United States of America. 22 23 24/ BD-Quad / 9 8 7 6 5 4 3 2 1
Additional copies of this book may be ordered by calling (800) 621-8335 or visit the AMA Store at amastore.com. Refer to product number OP512923.

No part of this publication may be reproduced, stored in a retrieval system, transmitted in any form, or by any means, electronic, mechanical, photo-copying, recording, or otherwise, without prior written permission of the publisher.

Current Procedural Terminology (CPT®) is copyright 1966, 1970, 1973, 1977, 1981, 1983–2022 by the American Medical Association. All rights reserved.

The AMA does not directly or indirectly practice medicine or dispense medical services. This publication does not replace the AMA's Current Proce-dural Terminology codebook or other appropriate coding authority. The coding information in this publication should be used only as a guide.

Internet address: www.ama-assn.org

To request a license for distribution of products containing or reprinting CPT codes and/or guidelines, please see our website at www.ama-assn.org/go/cpt, or contact the American Medical Association CPT/DBP Intellectual Property Services, 330 North Wabash Avenue, Suite 39300, Chicago, IL 60611, 312 464-5022.

ISBN: 978-1-64016-218-1

Contents

Foreword. viii

Using This Book ix
    The Symbols ix
    The Rationale ix
    Reading the Clinical Examples x
    Summary of Additions, Deletions, and Revisions and Indexes x
    CPT Codebook Conventions and Styles x

Introduction 1
    Instructions for Use of the
    CPT Codebook 1
        Add-on Codes 2
        Code Symbols 2

Evaluation and Management 3
    Summary of Additions, Deletions, and Revisions 3

Evaluation and Management (E/M) Services Guidelines 20
    E/M Guidelines Overview 20
    Classification of Evaluation and Management (E/M) Services 20
        New and Established Patients 20
        ►Initial and Subsequent Services◄ 21
        Services Reported Separately 21
        History and/or Examination 22
    ►Levels of E/M Services◄ 22
        ►Guidelines for Selecting Level of Service Based on Medical Decision Making◄ 23
        Number and Complexity of Problems Addressed at the Encounter 23
        ►Amount and/or Complexity of Data to Be Reviewed and Analyzed◄ 26
        ►Risk of Complications and/or Morbidity or Mortality of Patient Management◄ 27
        ►Guidelines for Selecting Level of Service Based on Time◄ 28
    Unlisted Service 29
    Special Report 29
    Office or Other Outpatient Services 31
    Hospital Observation Services 31
        Observation Care Discharge Services 31
        Initial Observation Care 31
        Subsequent Observation Care 31
    ►Hospital Inpatient and Observation Care Services◄ 31
        ►Initial Hospital Inpatient or Observation Care◄ 32
        ►Subsequent Hospital Inpatient or Observation Care◄ 34
        ►Hospital Inpatient or Observation Care Services (Including Admission
        and Discharge Services)◄ 35
        ►Hospital Inpatient or Observation Discharge Services◄ 37
    Consultations 38
        Office or Other Outpatient Consultations 38
        ►Inpatient or Observation Consultations◄ 40
    Emergency Department Services 42
        New or Established Patient 42

Nursing Facility Services 44

    Initial Nursing Facility Care 45

    Subsequent Nursing Facility Care 47

    Nursing Facility Discharge Services 48

    Other Nursing Facility Services 48

Domiciliary, Rest Home (eg, Boarding Home), or Custodial Care Services 48

    New Patient 48

    Established Patient 48

Domiciliary, Rest Home (eg, Assisted Living Facility), or Home Care Plan Oversight Services 49

    ►Home or Residence Services◄ 49

    New Patient 49

    Established Patient 51

Prolonged Services 52

    Prolonged Service With Direct Patient Contact (Except with Office or Other
    Outpatient Services) 52

    ►Prolonged Service on Date Other Than the Face-to-Face Evaluation and Management
    Service Without Direct Patient Contact◄ 52

    Prolonged Clinical Staff Services With Physician or Other Qualified Health Care
    Professional Supervision 53

    ►Prolonged Service With or Without Direct Patient Contact on the Date of an Evaluation
    and Management Service◄ 54

Case Management Services 56

    Medical Team Conferences 56

Care Plan Oversight Services 57

Preventive Medicine Services 57

    Counseling Risk Factor Reduction and Behavior Change Intervention 58

Non-Face-to-Face Services 58

    Telephone Services 58

    Online Digital Evaluation and Management Services 58

    Interprofessional Telephone/Internet/Electronic Health Record Consultations 59

    Digitally Stored Data Services/Remote Physiologic Monitoring 60

    Remote Physiologic Monitoring Treatment Management Services 61

Newborn Care Services 62

Delivery/Birthing Room Attendance and Resuscitation Services 62

Inpatient Neonatal Intensive Care Services and Pediatric and Neonatal Critical Care Services . . . 63

    Pediatric Critical Care Patient Transport 63

    Inpatient Neonatal and Pediatric Critical Care 64

    Initial and Continuing Intensive Care Services 65

Cognitive Assessment and Care Plan Services 66

Care Management Services 68

    Chronic Care Management Services 68

    Complex Chronic Care Management Services 68

    Principal Care Management Services 69

Transitional Care Management Services 70

Advance Care Planning 72

Surgery **73**

Summary of Additions, Deletions, and Revisions 73

Integumentary System 76

Skin, Subcutaneous, and Accessory Structures. 76
    Repair (Closure). 76
Musculoskeletal System. 78
    General 78
    Spine (Vertebral Column) 81
    Pelvis and Hip Joint 82
    Femur (Thigh Region) and Knee Joint 83
Respiratory System. 83
    Nose 83
    Trachea and Bronchi 84
Cardiovascular System 84
    Heart and Pericardium 85
    Arteries and Veins 93
Hemic and Lymphatic Systems. 99
    Transplantation and Post-Transplantation Cellular Infusions 99
Digestive System 100
    Esophagus. 100
    Intestines (Except Rectum). 102
    Biliary Tract. 102
    Abdomen, Peritoneum, and Omentum 103
Urinary System 112
    Kidney 112
    Bladder 114
Male Genital System 114
    Prostate. 114
Maternity Care and Delivery 115
Nervous System 116
    Extracranial Nerves, Peripheral Nerves, and Autonomic Nervous System. 116
Eye and Ocular Adnexa. 121
    Anterior Segment 121
Auditory System 121
    External Ear. 121
    Middle Ear. 122
    Inner Ear 125

Radiology **127**
Summary of Additions, Deletions, and Revisions 127
Diagnostic Radiology (Diagnostic Imaging) 128
    Vascular Procedures 128
Diagnostic Ultrasound 130
    Extremities 130
    Ultrasonic Guidance Procedures. 131
Radiologic Guidance. 132
    Fluoroscopic Guidance 132
Radiation Oncology. 132
    Hyperthermia 132
Nuclear Medicine 133
    Diagnostic. 133

Contents

Pathology and Laboratory **135**

    Summary of Additions, Deletions, and Revisions 135

    Pathology Clinical Consultations 139

    Genomic Sequencing Procedures and Other Molecular Multianalyte Assays 139

    Chemistry 143

    Microbiology 143

    Surgical Pathology 146

    Proprietary Laboratory Analyses 151

Medicine **167**

    Summary of Additions, Deletions, and Revisions 167

    Immunization Administration for Vaccines/Toxoids 169

    Vaccines, Toxoids 176

    Psychiatry 180

        Psychiatric Diagnostic Procedures 181

    Dialysis 183

        Hemodialysis 183

        Miscellaneous Dialysis Procedures 183

    Gastroenterology 184

        Other Procedures 184

    Ophthalmology 184

        Special Ophthalmological Services 184

    Special Otorhinolaryngologic Services 186

        Vestibular Function Tests, Without Electrical Recording 186

        Evaluative and Therapeutic Services 186

    Cardiovascular 187

        Therapeutic Services and Procedures 187

        Cardiography 189

        Cardiovascular Monitoring Services 190

        Cardiac Catheterization 190

        Intracardiac Electrophysiological Procedures/Studies 197

        Peripheral Arterial Disease Rehabilitation 197

        Home and Outpatient International Normalized Ratio (INR) Monitoring Services 197

    Pulmonary 198

        Ventilator Management 198

        Pulmonary Diagnostic Testing, Rehabilitation, and Therapies 198

    Allergy and Clinical Immunology 198

    Neurology and Neuromuscular Procedures 199

        Electromyography 199

        Nerve Conduction Tests 200

        Autonomic Function Tests 200

    Health Behavior Assessment and Intervention 200

    ▶Behavior Management Services◀ 201

    Hydration, Therapeutic, Prophylactic, Diagnostic Injections and Infusions, and Chemotherapy
    and Other Highly Complex Drug or Highly Complex Biologic Agent Administration 203

        Therapeutic, Prophylactic, and Diagnostic Injections and Infusions (Excludes
        Chemotherapy and Other Highly Complex Drug or Highly Complex Biologic
        Agent Administration) 203

Physical Medicine and Rehabilitation 204

    Modalities. 204

    Therapeutic Procedures 204

Acupuncture 205

Osteopathic Manipulative Treatment. 205

Chiropractic Manipulative Treatment. 206

Education and Training for Patient Self-Management. 206

Non-Face-to-Face Nonphysician Services 207

    Qualified Nonphysician Health Care Professional Online Digital Assessment
and Management Service. 207

    Remote Therapeutic Monitoring Services 207

    Remote Therapeutic Monitoring Treatment Management Services 208

Home Health Procedures/Services. 209

Category III Codes. 211

Summary of Additions, Deletions, and Revisions 211

Appendix A. 251

Summary of Additions, Deletions, and Revisions 251

Modifiers. 252

Appendix C. 253

Clinical Examples 253

Appendix O. 255

Summary of Additions, Deletions, and Revisions 255

Multianalyte Assays with Algorithmic Analyses and Proprietary Laboratory Analyses. 259

Appendix P. 303

Summary of Additions, Deletions, and Revisions 303

CPT Codes That May Be Used For Synchronous Telemedicine Services 304

Appendix Q. 305

Severe Acute Respiratory Syndrome Coronavirus 2 (SARS-CoV-2) (coronavirus disease
[COVID-19]) Vaccines 305

Appendix R. 309

Digital Medicine–Services Taxonomy 309

Appendix S. 315

    ▶Artificial Intelligence Taxonomy for Medical Services and Procedures◀ 315

▶Appendix T◀ 317

Summary of Additions, Deletions, and Revisions 317

    ▶CPT Codes That May Be Used For Synchronous Real-Time Interactive Audio-Only
Telemedicine Services◀ 319

Indexes 320

Instructions for the Use of the Changes Indexes. 320

    Index of Coding Changes 321

    Index of Modifiers. 334

Foreword

The American Medical Association (AMA) is pleased to offer *CPT® Changes 2023: An Insider's View (CPT Changes)*. Since this book was first published in 2000, it has served as the definitive text on additions, revisions, and deletions to the CPT code set.

In developing this book, our intention was to provide CPT users with a glimpse of the logic, rationale, and proposed function of the changes in the CPT code set that resulted from the decisions of the CPT Editorial Panel and the yearly update process. The AMA staff members have the unique perspective of being both participants in the CPT editorial process and users of the CPT code set.

CPT Changes is intended to bridge understanding between clinical decisions made by the CPT Editorial Panel regarding appropriate service or procedure descriptions with functional interpretations of coding guidelines, code intent, and code combinations, which are necessary for users of the CPT code set. A new edition of this book, like the codebook, is published annually.

To assist CPT users in applying the new and revised CPT codes, this book includes clinical examples that describe the typical patient who might undergo the procedure and detailed descriptions of the procedure. Both of these are required as a part of the CPT code change proposal process, which are used by the CPT Editorial Panel in crafting language, guidelines, and parenthetical notes associated with the new or revised codes. In addition, many of the clinical examples and descriptions of the procedures are used in the AMA/Specialty Society Relative Value Scale (RVS) Update (RUC) process to conduct surveys on physician work and to develop work relative value recommendations to the Centers for Medicare & Medicaid Services (CMS) as part of the Medicare physician fee schedule (MPFS).

We are confident that the information provided in *CPT Changes* will prove to be a valuable resource to CPT users, not only as they apply changes for the year of publication, but also as a resource for frequent reference as they continue their education in CPT coding. The AMA makes every effort to be a voice of clarity and consistency in an otherwise confusing system of health care claims and payment, and *CPT Changes 2023: An Insider's View* demonstrates our continued commitment to assist users of the CPT code set.

Using This Book

This book is designed to serve as a reference guide to understanding the changes contained in the Current Procedural Terminology (CPT®) 2023 code set and is not intended to replace the CPT codebook. Every effort is made to ensure accuracy; however, if differences exist, you should always defer to the information in the *CPT® 2023* codebook.

The Symbols

This book uses the same coding conventions as those used in the CPT nomenclature.

● Indicates a new procedure number was added to the CPT nomenclature

▲ Indicates a code revision has resulted in a substantially altered procedure descriptor

✚ Indicates a CPT add-on code

⊘ Indicates a code that is exempt from the use of modifier 51 but is not designated as a CPT add-on procedure or service

►◄ Indicates revised guidelines, cross-references, and/or explanatory text

✗ Indicates a code for a vaccine that is pending FDA approval

\# Indicates a resequenced code. Note that rather than deleting and renumbering, resequencing allows existing codes to be relocated to an appropriate location for the code concept, regardless of the numeric sequence. Numerically placed references (ie, Code is out of numerical sequence. See...) are used as navigational alerts in the CPT codebook to direct the user to the location of an out-of-sequence code. Therefore, remember to refer to the CPT codebook for these references.

★ Indicates a telemedicine code

⌘ Indicates a duplicate PLA test

⇅ Indicates a Category I PLA

◀ Indicates Audio-only Telemedicine Services

Whenever possible, complete segments of text from the CPT codebook are provided; however, in some instances, only pertinent text is included.

The Rationale

After listing each change or series of changes from the CPT codebook, a rationale is provided. The rationale is intended to provide a brief clarification and explanation of the changes. Nevertheless, it is important to note that they may not address every question that may arise as a result of the changes.

Reading the Clinical Examples

The clinical examples and their procedural descriptions, which reflect typical clinical situations found in the healthcare setting, are included in this text with many of the codes to provide practical situations for which the new and/or revised codes in the CPT 2023 code set would be appropriately reported. It is important to note that these examples do not suggest limiting the use of a code; instead, they are meant to represent the typical patient and service or procedure, as previously stated. In addition, they do not describe the universe of patients for whom the service or procedure would be appropriate. It is important to also note that third-party payer reporting policies may differ.

Summary of Additions, Deletions, and Revisions and Indexes

A **summary of additions, deletions, and revisions** for the section is presented in a tabular format at the beginning of each section. This table provides readers with the ability to quickly search and have an overview of all of the new, revised, and deleted codes for 2023. In addition to the tabular review of changes, the coding index individually lists all of the new, revised, and deleted codes with each code's status (new, revised, deleted) in parentheses. For more information about these indexes, please read the Instructions for the **Use of the Changes Indexes** on page 320.

CPT Codebook Conventions and Styles

Similar to the CPT codebook, the guidelines and revised and new CPT code descriptors and parenthetical notes in *CPT Changes 2023* are set in green type. Any revised text, guidelines, and/or headings are indicated with the ▶ ◀ symbols. To match the style used in the codebook, the revised or new text symbol is placed at the beginning and end of a paragraph or section that contains revisions, and the use of green text visually indicates new and/or revised content. Similarly, each section's and subsections' (Surgery) complete code range are listed in the tabs, regardless if these codes are discussed in this book. In addition, all of the different level of headings in the codebook are also picked up, as appropriate, and set in the same style and color. Besides matching the convention and style used in the CPT codebook, the Rationales are placed within a shaded box to distinguish them from the rest of the content for quick and easy reference.

Introduction

Current Procedural Terminology (CPT®), Fourth Edition, is a set of codes, descriptions, and guidelines intended to describe procedures and services performed by physicians and other qualified health care professionals, or entities. Each procedure or service is identified with a five-digit code. The use of CPT codes simplifies the reporting of procedures and services. In the CPT code set, the term "procedure" is used to describe services, including diagnostic tests.

Inclusion of a descriptor and its associated five-digit code number in the CPT Category I code set is based on whether the procedure or service is consistent with contemporary medical practice and is performed by many practitioners in clinical practice in multiple locations. Inclusion in the CPT code set of a procedure or service, or proprietary name, does not represent endorsement by the American Medical Association (AMA) of any particular diagnostic or therapeutic procedure or service or proprietary test or manufacturer. Inclusion or exclusion of a procedure or service, or proprietary name, does not imply any health insurance coverage or reimbursement policy.

The main body of the Category I section is listed in six sections. Each section is divided into subsections with anatomic, procedural, condition, or descriptor subheadings. The procedures and services with their identifying codes are presented in numeric order with the exception of the resequenced codes and the entire **Evaluation and Management** section (99202-99499), which appears at the beginning of the listed procedures. The evaluation and management codes are used by most physicians in reporting a significant portion of their services.

Instructions for Use of the CPT Codebook

Select the name of the procedure or service that accurately identifies the service performed. Do not select a CPT code that merely approximates the service provided. If no such specific code exists, then report the service using the appropriate unlisted procedure or service code. In surgery, it may be an operation; in medicine, a diagnostic or therapeutic procedure; in radiology, a radiograph. Other additional procedures performed or pertinent special services are also listed. When necessary, any modifying or extenuating circumstances are added. Any service or procedure should be adequately documented in the medical record.

It is equally important to recognize that as techniques in medicine and surgery have evolved, new types of services, including minimally invasive surgery, as well as endovascular, percutaneous, and endoscopic interventions have challenged the traditional distinction of Surgery vs Medicine. Thus, the listing of a service or procedure in a specific section of this book should not be interpreted as strictly classifying the service or procedure as "surgery" or "not surgery" for insurance or other purposes. The placement of a given service in a specific section of the book may reflect historical or other considerations (eg, placement of the percutaneous peripheral vascular endovascular interventions in the Surgery/Cardiovascular System section, while the percutaneous coronary interventions appear in the Medicine/Cardiovascular section).

▶When advanced practice nurses and physician assistants are working with physicians, they are considered as working in the exact same specialty and subspecialty as the physician. A "physician or other qualified health care professional" is an individual who is qualified by education, training, licensure/regulation (when applicable), and facility privileging (when applicable) who performs a professional service within his/her scope of practice and independently reports that professional service. These professionals are distinct from "clinical staff." A clinical staff member is a person who works under the supervision of a physician or other qualified health care professional and who is allowed by law, regulation, and facility policy to perform or assist in the performance of a specified professional service but who does not individually report that professional service. Other policies may also affect who may report specific services.◀

Throughout the CPT code set the use of terms such as "physician," "qualified health care professional," or "individual" is not intended to indicate that other entities may not report the service. In selected instances, specific instructions may define a service as limited to professionals or limited to other entities (eg, hospital or home health agency).

Instructions, typically included as parenthetical notes with selected codes, indicate that a code should not be reported with another code or codes. These instructions are intended to prevent errors of significant probability and are not all inclusive. For example, the code with such instructions may be a component of another code and therefore it would be incorrect to report both codes even when the component service is performed. These instructions are not intended as a listing of all possible code combinations that should not be reported, nor do they indicate all possible code combinations that are appropriately reported. When reporting codes for services provided, it is important to assure the accuracy and quality of coding through verification of the intent of the code by use of the related guidelines, parenthetical instructions, and coding resources, including *CPT Assistant* and other publications resulting from collaborative efforts of the American Medical Association with the medical specialty societies (ie, *Clinical Examples in Radiology*).

Rationale

In accordance with the changes in the evaluation and management (E/M) guidelines, the **Instructions for Use of the CPT Codebook** in the Introduction section have been revised to reflect these changes. Refer to the codebook and the Rationale for the E/M Services guidelines for a full discussion of these changes.

Add-on Codes

Some of the listed procedures are commonly carried out in addition to the primary procedure performed. These additional or supplemental procedures are designated as add-on codes with the ✚ symbol and they are listed in **Appendix D** of the CPT codebook. Add-on codes in CPT 2023 can be readily identified by specific descriptor nomenclature that includes phrases such as "each additional" or "(List separately in addition to primary procedure)."

The add-on code concept in CPT 2023 applies only to add-on procedures or services performed by the same physician. Add-on codes describe additional intra-service work associated with the primary procedure, eg, additional digit(s), lesion(s), neurorrhaphy(s), vertebral segment(s), tendon(s), joint(s).

▶Add-on codes are always performed in addition to the primary service or procedure and must never be reported as a stand-alone code. The inclusionary parenthetical notes following the add-on codes are designed to include the typical base code(s) and not every possible reportable code combination. When the add-on procedure can be reported bilaterally and is performed bilaterally, the appropriate add-on code is reported twice, unless the code descriptor, guidelines, or parenthetical instructions for that particular add-on code instructs otherwise. Do not report modifier 50, *Bilateral Procedures*, in conjunction with add-on codes. All add-on codes in the CPT code set are exempt from the multiple procedure concept. See the definitions of modifier 50 and 51 in **Appendix A.**◀

Rationale

The Add-On Codes subsection guidelines in the Introduction section of the CPT codebook have been revised to clarify that inclusionary parenthetical notes following add-on codes are designed to include the typical base code(s) of a service or procedure. It is important to note that not every possible, reportable combination of codes (ie, base code[s] and add-on code[s]) will be included in inclusionary parenthetical notes following add-on codes.

Code Symbols

A summary listing of additions, deletions, and revisions applicable to the CPT codebook is found in **Appendix B**. New procedure numbers added to the CPT codebook are identified throughout the text with the ● symbol placed before the code number. In instances where a code revision has resulted in a substantially altered procedure descriptor, the ▲ symbol is placed before the code number. The ▶◀ symbols are used to indicate new and revised text other than the procedure descriptors. These symbols indicate CPT Editorial Panel actions. The AMA reserves the right to correct typographical errors and make stylistic improvements.

▶CPT add-on codes are annotated by the ✚ symbol and are listed in **Appendix D**. The symbol ⦰ is used to identify codes that are exempt from the use of modifier 51 but have not been designated as CPT add-on procedures or services. A list of codes exempt from modifier 51 usage is included in **Appendix E**. The ⊬ symbol is used to identify codes for vaccines that are pending FDA approval (see **Appendix K**). The # symbol is used to identify codes that are listed out of numerical sequence (see **Appendix N**). The ★ symbol is used to identify codes that may be used to report telemedicine services when appended by modifier 95 (see **Appendix P**). The ◀ symbol is used to identify codes that may be used to report audio-only telemedicine services when appended by modifier 93 (see **Appendix T**).◀

Rationale

The Code Symbols subsection, which lists and explains the different definitions of all of the CPT code symbols, has been revised because a new symbol (◀) has been created for the CPT 2023 code set to identify codes that may be used to report audio-only telemedicine services when appended by modifier 93 (see Appendix T).

Evaluation and Management

Summary of Additions, Deletions, and Revisions

The summary of changes shows the actual changes that have been made to the code descriptors.

New codes appear with a bullet (●) and are indicated as "Code added." Revised codes are preceded with a triangle (▲). Within revised codes, or if a code symbol has been deleted, the deleted language and code symbol appear with a ~~strikethrough~~, while new text appears <u>underlined</u>.

The ⚡ symbol is used to identify codes for vaccines that are pending FDA approval. The # symbol is used to identify codes that have been resequenced. CPT add-on codes are annotated by the ✚ symbol. The ⊘ symbol is used to identify codes that are exempt from the use of modifier 51. The ★ symbol is used to identify codes that may be used for reporting telemedicine services. The ✕ symbol is used to identify a proprietary laboratory analyses (PLA) test that has an identical descriptor as another PLA test. A PLA code that satisfies Category I code criteria and has been accepted by the CPT Editorial Panel is annotated with the ↕ symbol. The ◀ symbol is used to identify codes that may be used to report audio-only telemedicine services when appended by modifier 93 (see Appendix T).

Code	Description
99217	~~Observation care discharge~~ day management (This code is to be utilized to report all services provided to a patient on discharge from outpatient hospital "observation status" if the discharge is on other than the initial date of "observation status." To report services to a patient designated as "observation status" or "inpatient status" and discharged on the same date, use the codes for Observation or Inpatient Care Services (including Admission and Discharge Services, 99234-99236 as appropriate.)~~
99218	~~Initial observation care,~~ per day, for the evaluation and management of a patient which requires these 3 key components: ■ ~~A detailed or comprehensive history;~~ ■ ~~A detailed or comprehensive examination; and~~ ■ ~~Medical decision making that is straightforward or of low complexity.~~ ~~Counseling and/or coordination of care with other physicians, other qualified health care professionals, or agencies are provided consistent with the nature of the problem(s) and the patient's and/or family's needs.~~ ~~Usually, the problem(s) requiring admission to outpatient hospital "observation status" are of low severity. Typically, 30 minutes are spent at the bedside and on the patient's hospital floor or unit.~~
99219	~~Initial observation care,~~ per day, for the evaluation and management of a patient, which requires these 3 key components: ■ ~~A comprehensive history;~~ ■ ~~A comprehensive examination; and~~ ■ ~~Medical decision making of moderate complexity.~~ ~~Counseling and/or coordination of care with other physicians, other qualified health care professionals, or agencies are provided consistent with the nature of the problem(s) and the patient's and/or family's needs.~~ ~~Usually, the problem(s) requiring admission to outpatient hospital "observation status" are of moderate severity. Typically, 50 minutes are spent at the bedside and on the patient's hospital floor or unit.~~

Code	Description
99220	**Initial observation care,** per day, for the evaluation and management of a patient, which requires these 3 key components: ■ **A comprehensive history;** ■ **A comprehensive examination; and** ■ **Medical decision making of high complexity.** Counseling and/or coordination of care with other physicians, other qualified health care professionals, or agencies are provided consistent with the nature of the problem(s) and the patient's and/or family's needs. Usually, the problem(s) requiring admission to outpatient hospital "observation status" are of high severity. Typically, 70 minutes are spent at the bedside and on the patient's hospital floor or unit.
99224	**Subsequent observation care,** per day, for the evaluation and management of a patient, which requires at least 2 of these 3 key components: ■ **Problem focused interval history;** ■ **Problem focused examination;** ■ **Medical decision making that is straightforward or of low complexity.** Counseling and/or coordination of care with other physicians, other qualified health care professionals, or agencies are provided consistent with the nature of the problem(s) and the patient's and/or family's needs. Usually, the patient is stable, recovering, or improving. Typically, 15 minutes are spent at the bedside and on the patient's hospital floor or unit.
99225	**Subsequent observation care,** per day, for the evaluation and management of a patient, which requires at least 2 of these 3 key components: ■ **An expanded problem focused interval history;** ■ **An expanded problem focused examination;** ■ **Medical decision making of moderate complexity.** Counseling and/or coordination of care with other physicians, other qualified health care professionals, or agencies are provided consistent with the nature of the problem(s) and the patient's and/or family's needs. Usually, the patient is responding inadequately to therapy or has developed a minor complication. Typically, 25 minutes are spent at the bedside and on the patient's hospital floor or unit.
99226	**Subsequent observation care,** per day, for the evaluation and management of a patient, which requires at least 2 of these 3 key components: ■ **A detailed interval history;** ■ **A detailed examination;** ■ **Medical decision making of high complexity.** Counseling and/or coordination of care with other physicians, other qualified health care professionals, or agencies are provided consistent with the nature of the problem(s) and the patient's and/or family's needs. Usually, the patient is unstable or has developed a significant complication or a significant new problem. Typically, 35 minutes are spent at the bedside and on the patient's hospital floor or unit.

★ = Telemedicine   ◀ = Audio-only   ✚ = Add-on code   ⊬ = FDA approval pending   # = Resequenced code   ⦸ = Modifier 51 exempt

Code	Description
▲99221	**Initial hospital <u>inpatient or observation</u> care,** per day, for the evaluation and management of a patient, which requires <u>a medically appropriate history and/or examination and straightforward or low level medical decision making.</u> ~~these 3 key components:~~ ■ ~~A detailed or comprehensive history;~~ ■ ~~A detailed or comprehensive examination; and~~ ■ ~~Medical decision making that is straightforward or of low complexity.~~ ~~Counseling and/or coordination of care with other physicians, other qualified health care professionals, or agencies are provided consistent with the nature of the problem(s) and the patient's and/or family's needs.~~ ~~Usually, the problem(s) requiring admission are of low severity. Typically, 30 minutes are spent at the bedside and on the patient's hospital floor or unit.~~ <u>When using total time on the date of the encounter for code selection, 40 minutes must be met or exceeded.</u>
▲99222	**Initial hospital <u>inpatient or observation</u> care,** per day, for the evaluation and management of a patient, which requires <u>a medically appropriate history and/or examination and moderate level of medical decision making.</u> ~~these 3 key components:~~ ■ ~~A comprehensive history;~~ ■ ~~A comprehensive examination; and~~ ■ ~~Medical decision making of moderate complexity.~~ ~~Counseling and/or coordination of care with other physicians, other qualified health care professionals, or agencies are provided consistent with the nature of the problem(s) and the patient's and/or family's needs.~~ ~~Usually, the problem(s) requiring admission are of moderate severity. Typically, 50 minutes are spent at the bedside and on the patient's hospital floor or unit.~~ <u>When using total time on the date of the encounter for code selection, 55 minutes must be met or exceeded.</u>
▲99223	**Initial hospital <u>inpatient or observation</u> care,** per day, for the evaluation and management of a patient, which requires <u>a medically appropriate history and/or examination and high level of medical decision making.</u> ~~these 3 key components:~~ ■ ~~A comprehensive history;~~ ■ ~~A comprehensive examination; and~~ ■ ~~Medical decision making of high complexity.~~ ~~Counseling and/or coordination of care with other physicians, other qualified health care professionals, or agencies are provided consistent with the nature of the problem(s) and the patient's and/or family's needs.~~ ~~Usually, the problem(s) requiring admission are of high severity. Typically, 70 minutes are spent at the bedside and on the patient's hospital floor or unit.~~ <u>When using total time on the date of the encounter for code selection, 75 minutes must be met or exceeded.</u>

Code	Description
★▲99231	**Subsequent hospital <u>inpatient or observation</u> care,** per day, for the evaluation and management of a patient, which requires <u>a medically appropriate history and/or examination and straightforward or low level of medical decision making.</u> ~~at least 2 of these 3 key components:~~ ■ ~~A problem focused interval history;~~ ■ ~~A problem focused examination;~~ ■ ~~Medical decision making that is straightforward or of low complexity.~~ ~~Counseling and/or coordination of care with other physicians, other qualified health care professionals, or agencies are provided consistent with the nature of the problem(s) and the patient's and/or family's needs.~~ ~~Usually, the patient is stable, recovering or improving. Typically, 15 minutes are spent at the bedside and on the patient's hospital floor or unit.~~ <u>When using total time on the date of the encounter for code selection, 25 minutes must be met or exceeded.</u>
★▲99232	**Subsequent hospital <u>inpatient or observation</u> care,** per day, for the evaluation and management of a patient, which requires <u>a medically appropriate history and/or examination and moderate level of medical decision making.</u> ~~at least 2 of these 3 key components:~~ ■ ~~An expanded problem focused interval history;~~ ■ ~~An expanded problem focused examination;~~ ■ ~~Medical decision making of moderate complexity.~~ ~~Counseling and/or coordination of care with other physicians, other qualified health care professionals, or agencies are provided consistent with the nature of the problem(s) and the patient's and/or family's needs.~~ ~~Usually, the patient is responding inadequately to therapy or has developed a minor complication. Typically, 25 minutes are spent at the bedside and on the patient's hospital floor or unit.~~ <u>When using total time on the date of the encounter for code selection, 35 minutes must be met or exceeded.</u>
★▲99233	**Subsequent hospital <u>inpatient or observation</u> care,** per day, for the evaluation and management of a patient, which requires <u>a medically appropriate history and/or examination and high level of medical decision making.</u> ~~at least 2 of these 3 key components:~~ ■ ~~A detailed interval history;~~ ■ ~~A detailed examination;~~ ■ ~~Medical decision making of high complexity.~~ ~~Counseling and/or coordination of care with other physicians, other qualified health care professionals, or agencies are provided consistent with the nature of the problem(s) and the patient's and/or family's needs.~~ ~~Usually, the patient is unstable or has developed a significant complication or a significant new problem. Typically, 35 minutes are spent at the bedside and on the patient's hospital floor or unit.~~ <u>When using total time on the date of the encounter for code selection, 50 minutes must be met or exceeded.</u>

★=Telemedicine ◀=Audio-only ✚=Add-on code ✕=FDA approval pending #=Resequenced code ⊘=Modifier 51 exempt

Code	Description
▲99234	**Hospital inpatient or ~~O~~observation ~~or inpatient hospital~~ care,** for the evaluation and management of a patient including admission and discharge on the same date, which requires a medically appropriate history and/or examination and straightforward or low level of medical decision making.~~these 3 key components:~~ ■ ~~A detailed or comprehensive history;~~ ■ ~~A detailed or comprehensive examination; and~~ ■ ~~Medical decision making that is straightforward or of low complexity.~~ ~~Counseling and/or coordination of care with other physicians, other qualified health care professionals, or agencies are provided consistent with the nature of the problem(s) and the patient's and/or family's needs.~~ ~~Usually the presenting problem(s) requiring admission are of low severity. Typically, 40 minutes are spent at the bedside and on the patient's hospital floor or unit.~~ When using total time on the date of the encounter for code selection, 45 minutes must be met or exceeded.
▲99235	**Hospital inpatient or ~~O~~observation ~~or inpatient hospital~~ care,** for the evaluation and management of a patient including admission and discharge on the same date, which requires a medically appropriate history and/or examination and moderate level of medical decision making.~~these 3 key components:~~ ■ ~~A comprehensive history;~~ ■ ~~A comprehensive examination; and~~ ■ ~~Medical decision making of moderate complexity.~~ ~~Counseling and/or coordination of care with other physicians, other qualified health care professionals, or agencies are provided consistent with the nature of the problem(s) and the patient's and/or family's needs.~~ ~~Usually the presenting problem(s) requiring admission are of moderate severity. Typically, 50 minutes are spent at the bedside and on the patient's hospital floor or unit.~~ When using total time on the date of the encounter for code selection, 70 minutes must be met or exceeded.
▲99236	**Hospital inpatient or ~~O~~observation ~~or inpatient hospital~~ care,** for the evaluation and management of a patient including admission and discharge on the same date, which requires a medically appropriate history and/or examination and high level of medical decision making.~~these 3 key components:~~ ■ ~~A comprehensive history;~~ ■ ~~A comprehensive examination; and~~ ■ ~~Medical decision making of high complexity.~~ ~~Counseling and/or coordination of care with other physicians, other qualified health care professionals, or agencies are provided consistent with the nature of the problem(s) and the patient's and/or family's needs.~~ ~~Usually the presenting problem(s) requiring admission are of high severity. Typically, 55 minutes are spent at the bedside and on the patient's hospital floor or unit.~~ When using total time on the date of the encounter for code selection, 85 minutes must be met or exceeded.
▲99238	**Hospital inpatient or observation discharge day management**; 30 minutes or less on the date of the encounter
▲99239	more than 30 minutes on the date of the encounter

Evaluation / Management 99202-99499

Code	Description
99241	**Office consultation** for a new or established patient, which requires these 3 key components: ■ **A problem focused history;** ■ **A problem focused examination; and** ■ **Straightforward medical decision making.** Counseling and/or coordination of care with other physicians, other qualified health care professionals, or agencies are provided consistent with the nature of the problem(s) and the patient's and/or family's needs. Usually, the presenting problem(s) are self limited or minor. Typically, 15 minutes are spent face-to-face with the patient and/or family.
★▲99242	**Office <u>or other outpatient</u> consultation** for a new or established patient, which requires <u>a medically appropriate history and/or examination and straightforward medical decision making.</u>these 3 key components: ■ An expanded problem focused history; ■ An expanded problem focused examination; and ■ Straightforward medical decision making. Counseling and/or coordination of care with other physicians, other qualified health care professionals, or agencies are provided consistent with the nature of the problem(s) and the patient's and/or family's needs. Usually, the presenting problem(s) are of low severity. Typically, 30 minutes are spent face-to-face with the patient and/or family. <u>When using total time on the date of the encounter for code selection, 20 minutes must be met or exceeded.</u>
★▲99243	**Office <u>or other outpatient</u> consultation** for a new or established patient, which requires <u>a medically appropriate history and/or examination and low level of medical decision making.</u>these 3 key components: ■ A detailed history; ■ A detailed examination; and ■ Medical decision making of low complexity. Counseling and/or coordination of care with other physicians, other qualified health care professionals, or agencies are provided consistent with the nature of the problem(s) and the patient's and/or family's needs. Usually, the presenting problem(s) are of moderate severity. Typically, 40 minutes are spent face-to-face with the patient and/or family. <u>When using total time on the date of the encounter for code selection, 30 minutes must be met or exceeded.</u>
★▲99244	**Office <u>or other outpatient</u> consultation** for a new or established patient, which requires <u>a medically appropriate history and/or examination and moderate level of medical decision making.</u>these 3 key components: ■ A comprehensive history; ■ A comprehensive examination; and ■ Medical decision making of moderate complexity. Counseling and/or coordination of care with other physicians, other qualified health care professionals, or agencies are provided consistent with the nature of the problem(s) and the patient's and/or family's needs. Usually, the presenting problem(s) are of moderate to high severity. Typically, 60 minutes are spent face-to-face with the patient and/or family. <u>When using total time on the date of the encounter for code selection, 40 minutes must be met or exceeded.</u>

★=Telemedicine   ◀=Audio-only   ✚=Add-on code   ✗=FDA approval pending   #=Resequenced code   ⊘=Modifier 51 exempt

Code	Description
★▲99245	**Office or other outpatient consultation** for a new or established patient, which requires a medically appropriate history and/or examination and high level of medical decision making.~~these 3 key components:~~ ■ ~~A comprehensive history;~~ ■ ~~A comprehensive examination; and~~ ■ ~~Medical decision making of high complexity.~~ ~~Counseling and/or coordination of care with other physicians, other qualified health care professionals, or agencies are provided consistent with the nature of the problem(s) and the patient's and/or family's needs.~~ ~~Usually, the presenting problem(s) are of moderate to high severity. Typically, 80 minutes are spent face-to-face with the patient and/or family.~~ When using total time on the date of the encounter for code selection, 55 minutes must be met or exceeded.
99251	~~**Inpatient consultation** for a new or established patient, which requires these 3 key components:~~ ■ ~~**A problem focused history;**~~ ■ ~~**A problem focused examination; and**~~ ■ ~~**Straightforward medical decision making.**~~ ~~Counseling and/or coordination of care with other physicians, other qualified health care professionals, or agencies are provided consistent with the nature of the problem(s) and the patient's and/or family's needs.~~ ~~Usually, the presenting problem(s) are self limited or minor. Typically, 20 minutes are spent at the bedside and on the patient's hospital floor or unit.~~
★▲99252	**Inpatient or observation consultation** for a new or established patient, which requires a medically appropriate history and/or examination and straightforward medical decision making.~~these 3 key components:~~ ■ ~~An expanded problem focused history;~~ ■ ~~An expanded problem focused examination; and~~ ■ ~~Straightforward medical decision making.~~ ~~Counseling and/or coordination of care with other physicians, other qualified health care professionals, or agencies are provided consistent with the nature of the problem(s) and the patient's and/or family's needs.~~ ~~Usually, the presenting problem(s) are of low severity. Typically, 40 minutes are spent at the bedside and on the patient's hospital floor or unit.~~ When using total time on the date of the encounter for code selection, 35 minutes must be met or exceeded.
★▲99253	**Inpatient or observation consultation** for a new or established patient, which requires a medically appropriate history and/or examination and low level of medical decision making.~~these 3 key components:~~ ■ ~~A detailed history;~~ ■ ~~A detailed examination; and~~ ■ ~~Medical decision making of low complexity.~~ ~~Counseling and/or coordination of care with other physicians, other qualified health care professionals, or agencies are provided consistent with the nature of the problem(s) and the patient's and/or family's needs.~~ ~~Usually, the presenting problem(s) are of moderate severity. Typically, 55 minutes are spent at the bedside and on the patient's hospital floor or unit.~~ When using total time on the date of the encounter for code selection, 45 minutes must be met or exceeded.

Code	Description
★▲99254	**Inpatient or observation consultation** for a new or established patient, which requires <u>a medically appropriate history and/or examination and moderate level of medical decision making.</u>~~these 3 key components:~~ ■ ~~A comprehensive history;~~ ■ ~~A comprehensive examination; and~~ ■ ~~Medical decision making of moderate complexity.~~ ~~Counseling and/or coordination of care with other physicians, other qualified health care professionals, or agencies are provided consistent with the nature of the problem(s) and the patient's and/or family's needs. Usually, the presenting problem(s) are of moderate to high severity. Typically, 80 minutes are spent at the bedside and on the patient's hospital floor or unit.~~ <u>When using total time on the date of the encounter for code selection, 60 minutes must be met or exceeded.</u>
★▲99255	**Inpatient or observation consultation** for a new or established patient, which requires <u>a medically appropriate history and/or examination and high level of medical decision making.</u>~~these 3 key components:~~ ■ ~~A comprehensive history;~~ ■ ~~A comprehensive examination; and~~ ■ ~~Medical decision making of high complexity.~~ ~~Counseling and/or coordination of care with other physicians, other qualified health care professionals, or agencies are provided consistent with the nature of the problem(s) and the patient's and/or family's needs. Usually, the presenting problem(s) are of moderate to high severity. Typically, 110 minutes are spent at the bedside and on the patient's hospital floor or unit.~~ <u>When using total time on the date of the encounter for code selection, 80 minutes must be met or exceeded.</u>
▲99281	**Emergency department visit** for the evaluation and management of a patient~~, which requires these 3 key components:~~ <u>that may not require the presence of a physician or other qualified health care professional</u> ■ ~~A problem focused history;~~ ■ ~~A problem focused examination; and~~ ■ ~~Straightforward medical decision making.~~ ~~Counseling and/or coordination of care with other physicians, other qualified health care professionals, or agencies are provided consistent with the nature of the problem(s) and the patient's and/or family's needs.~~ ~~Usually, the presenting problem(s) are self limited or minor.~~
▲99282	**Emergency department visit** for the evaluation and management of a patient, <u>which requires a medically appropriate history and/or examination and straightforward medical decision making</u>~~which requires these 3 key components:~~ ■ ~~An expanded problem focused history;~~ ■ ~~An expanded problem focused examination; and~~ ■ ~~Medical decision making of low complexity.~~ ~~Counseling and/or coordination of care with other physicians, other qualified health care professionals, or agencies are provided consistent with the nature of the problem(s) and the patient's and/or family's needs.~~ ~~Usually, the presenting problem(s) are of low to moderate severity.~~

★=Telemedicine ◀=Audio-only ✚=Add-on code ✗=FDA approval pending #=Resequenced code ⊘=Modifier 51 exempt

Code	Description
▲99283	**Emergency department visit** for the evaluation and management of a patient, <u>which requires a medically appropriate history and/or examination and low level of medical decision making</u>~~which requires these 3 key components~~: ■ ~~An expanded problem focused history;~~ ■ ~~An expanded problem focused examination; and~~ ■ ~~Medical decision making of moderate complexity.~~ ~~Counseling and/or coordination of care with other physicians, other qualified health care professionals, or agencies are provided consistent with the nature of the problem(s) and the patient's and/or family's needs.~~ ~~Usually, the presenting problem(s) are of moderate severity.~~
▲99284	**Emergency department visit** for the evaluation and management of a patient, <u>which requires a medically appropriate history and/or examination and moderate level of medical decision making</u>~~which requires these 3 key components~~: ■ ~~A detailed history;~~ ■ ~~A detailed examination; and~~ ■ ~~Medical decision making of moderate complexity.~~ ~~Counseling and/or coordination of care with other physicians, other qualified health care professionals, or agencies are provided consistent with the nature of the problem(s) and the patient's and/or family's needs.~~ ~~Usually, the presenting problem(s) are of high severity, and require urgent evaluation by the physician, or other qualified health care professionals but do not pose an immediate significant threat to life or physiologic function.~~
▲99285	**Emergency department visit** for the evaluation and management of a patient, <u>which requires a medically appropriate history and/or examination and high level of medical decision making</u>~~which requires these 3 key components within the constraints imposed by the urgency of the patient's clinical condition and/or mental status~~: ■ ~~A comprehensive history;~~ ■ ~~A comprehensive examination; and~~ ■ ~~Medical decision making of high complexity.~~ ~~Counseling and/or coordination of care with other physicians, other qualified health care professionals, or agencies are provided consistent with the nature of the problem(s) and the patient's and/or family's needs.~~ ~~Usually, the presenting problem(s) are of high severity and pose an immediate significant threat to life or physiologic function.~~
▲99304	Initial nursing facility care, per day, for the evaluation and management of a patient, which requires <u>a medically appropriate history and/or examination and straightforward or low level of medical decision making.</u>~~these 3 key components~~: ■ ~~A detailed or comprehensive history;~~ ■ ~~A detailed or comprehensive examination; and~~ ■ ~~Medical decision making that is straightforward or of low complexity.~~ ~~Counseling and/or coordination of care with other physicians, other qualified health care professionals, or agencies are provided consistent with the nature of the problem(s) and the patient's and/or family's needs.~~ ~~Usually, the problem(s) requiring admission are of low severity. Typically, 25 minutes are spent at the bedside and on the patient's facility floor or unit.~~ <u>When using total time on the date of the encounter for code selection, 25 minutes must be met or exceeded.</u>

Evaluation / Management 99202-99499

Code	Description
▲99305	Initial nursing facility care, per day, for the evaluation and management of a patient, which requires <u>a medically appropriate history and/or examination and moderate level of medical decision making.</u>these 3 key components:
	■ A comprehensive history;
	■ A comprehensive examination; and
	■ Medical decision making of moderate complexity.
	Counseling and/or coordination of care with other physicians, other qualified health care professionals, or agencies are provided consistent with the nature of the problem(s) and the patient's and/or family's needs.
	Usually, the problem(s) requiring admission are of moderate severity. Typically, 35 minutes are spent at the bedside and on the patient's facility floor or unit.
	<u>When using total time on the date of the encounter for code selection, 35 minutes must be met or exceeded.</u>
▲99306	Initial nursing facility care, per day, for the evaluation and management of a patient, which requires <u>a medically appropriate history and/or examination and high level of medical decision making.</u>these 3 key components:
	■ A comprehensive history;
	■ A comprehensive examination; and
	■ Medical decision making of high complexity.
	Counseling and/or coordination of care with other physicians, other qualified health care professionals, or agencies are provided consistent with the nature of the problem(s) and the patient's and/or family's needs.
	Usually, the problem(s) requiring admission are of high severity. Typically, 45 minutes are spent at the bedside and on the patient's facility floor or unit.
	<u>When using total time on the date of the encounter for code selection, 45 minutes must be met or exceeded.</u>
★▲99307	Subsequent nursing facility care, per day, for the evaluation and management of a patient, which requires <u>a medically appropriate history and/or examination and straightforward medical decision making.</u>at least 2 of these 3 key components:
	■ A problem focused interval history;
	■ A problem focused examination;
	■ Straightforward medical decision making.
	Counseling and/or coordination of care with other physicians, other qualified health care professionals, or agencies are provided consistent with the nature of the problem(s) and the patient's and/or family's needs.
	Usually, the patient is stable, recovering, or improving. Typically, 10 minutes are spent at the bedside and on the patient's facility floor or unit.
	<u>When using total time on the date of the encounter for code selection, 10 minutes must be met or exceeded.</u>
★▲99308	Subsequent nursing facility care, per day, for the evaluation and management of a patient, which requires <u>a medically appropriate history and/or examination and low level of medical decision making.</u>at least 2 of these 3 key components:
	■ An expanded problem focused interval history;
	■ An expanded problem focused examination;
	■ Medical decision making of low complexity.
	Counseling and/or coordination of care with other physicians, other qualified health care professionals, or agencies are provided consistent with the nature of the problem(s) and the patient's and/or family's needs.
	Usually, the patient is responding inadequately to therapy or has developed a minor complication. Typically, 15 minutes are spent at the bedside and on the patient's facility floor or unit.
	<u>When using total time on the date of the encounter for code selection, 15 minutes must be met or exceeded.</u>

★ = Telemedicine   ◀ = Audio-only   ✛ = Add-on code   ⁄ = FDA approval pending   # = Resequenced code   ⦸ = Modifier 51 exempt

Code	Description
★▲**99309**	Subsequent nursing facility care, per day, for the evaluation and management of a patient, which requires <u>a medically appropriate history and/or examination and moderate level of medical decision making.</u>at least 2 of these 3 key components:
	■ A detailed interval history;
	■ A detailed examination;
	■ Medical decision making of moderate complexity.
	Counseling and/or coordination of care with other physicians, other qualified health care professionals, or agencies are provided consistent with the nature of the problem(s) and the patient's and/or family's needs.
	Usually, the patient has developed a significant complication or a significant new problem. Typically, 25 minutes are spent at the bedside and on the patient's facility floor or unit.
	<u>When using total time on the date of the encounter for code selection, 30 minutes must be met or exceeded.</u>
★▲**99310**	Subsequent nursing facility care, per day, for the evaluation and management of a patient, which requires <u>a medically appropriate history and/or examination and high level of medical decision making.</u>at least 2 of these 3 key components:
	■ A comprehensive interval history;
	■ A comprehensive examination;
	■ Medical decision making of high complexity.
	Counseling and/or coordination of care with other physicians, other qualified health care professionals, or agencies are provided consistent with the nature of the problem(s) and the patient's and/or family's needs. The patient may be unstable or may have developed a significant new problem requiring immediate physician attention. Typically, 35 minutes are spent at the bedside and on the patient's facility floor or unit.
	<u>When using total time on the date of the encounter for code selection, 45 minutes must be met or exceeded.</u>
▲**99315**	Nursing facility discharge day management; 30 minutes or less <u>total time on the date of the encounter</u>
▲**99316**	more than 30 minutes <u>total time on the date of the encounter</u>
99318	Evaluation and management of a patient involving an annual nursing facility assessment, which requires these 3 key components:
	■ **A detailed interval history;**
	■ **A comprehensive examination; and**
	■ **Medical decision making that is of low to moderate complexity.**
	Counseling and/or coordination of care with other physicians, other qualified health care professionals, or agencies are provided consistent with the nature of the problem(s) and the patient's and/or family's needs.
	Usually, the patient is stable, recovering, or improving. Typically, 30 minutes are spent at the bedside and on the patient's facility floor or unit.
99324	Domiciliary or rest home visit for the evaluation and management of a new patient, which requires these 3 key components:
	■ **A problem focused history;**
	■ **A problem focused examination; and**
	■ **Straightforward medical decision making.**
	Counseling and/or coordination of care with other physicians, other qualified health care professionals, or agencies are provided consistent with the nature of the problem(s) and the patient's and/or family's needs.
	Usually, the presenting problem(s) are of low severity. Typically, 20 minutes are spent with the patient and/or family or caregiver.

Code	Description
99325	~~Domiciliary or rest home visit for the evaluation and management of a new patient, which requires these 3 key components:~~ ■ ~~An expanded problem focused history;~~ ■ ~~An expanded problem focused examination; and~~ ■ ~~Medical decision making of low complexity.~~ ~~Counseling and/or coordination of care with other physicians, other qualified health care professionals, or agencies are provided consistent with the nature of the problem(s) and the patient's and/or family's needs.~~ ~~Usually, the presenting problem(s) are of moderate severity. Typically, 30 minutes are spent with the patient and/or family or caregiver.~~
99326	~~Domiciliary or rest home visit for the evaluation and management of a new patient, which requires these 3 key components:~~ ■ ~~A detailed history;~~ ■ ~~A detailed examination; and~~ ■ ~~Medical decision making of moderate complexity.~~ ~~Counseling and/or coordination of care with other physicians, other qualified health care professionals, or agencies are provided consistent with the nature of the problem(s) and the patient's and/or family's needs.~~ ~~Usually, the presenting problem(s) are of moderate to high severity. Typically, 45 minutes are spent with the patient and/or family or caregiver.~~
99327	~~Domiciliary or rest home visit for the evaluation and management of a new patient, which requires these 3 key components:~~ ■ ~~A comprehensive history;~~ ■ ~~A comprehensive examination; and~~ ■ ~~Medical decision making of moderate complexity.~~ ~~Counseling and/or coordination of care with other physicians, other qualified health care professionals, or agencies are provided consistent with the nature of the problem(s) and the patient's and/or family's needs.~~ ~~Usually, the presenting problem(s) are of high severity. Typically, 60 minutes are spent with the patient and/or family or caregiver.~~
99328	~~Domiciliary or rest home visit for the evaluation and management of a new patient, which requires these 3 key components:~~ ■ ~~A comprehensive history;~~ ■ ~~A comprehensive examination; and~~ ■ ~~Medical decision making of high complexity.~~ ~~Counseling and/or coordination of care with other physicians, other qualified health care professionals, or agencies are provided consistent with the nature of the problem(s) and the patient's and/or family's needs.~~ ~~Usually, the patient is unstable or has developed a significant new problem requiring immediate physician attention. Typically, 75 minutes are spent with the patient and/or family or caregiver.~~

Code	Description
99334	Domiciliary or rest home visit for the evaluation and management of an established patient, which requires at least 2 of these 3 key components: ■ A problem focused interval history; ■ A problem focused examination; ■ Straightforward medical decision making. Counseling and/or coordination of care with other physicians, other qualified health care professionals, or agencies are provided consistent with the nature of the problem(s) and the patient's and/or family's needs. Usually, the presenting problem(s) are self-limited or minor. Typically, 15 minutes are spent with the patient and/or family or caregiver.
99335	Domiciliary or rest home visit for the evaluation and management of an established patient, which requires at least 2 of these 3 key components: ■ An expanded problem focused interval history; ■ An expanded problem focused examination; ■ Medical decision making of low complexity. Counseling and/or coordination of care with other physicians, other qualified health care professionals, or agencies are provided consistent with the nature of the problem(s) and the patient's and/or family's needs. Usually, the presenting problem(s) are of low to moderate severity. Typically, 25 minutes are spent with the patient and/or family or caregiver.
99336	Domiciliary or rest home visit for the evaluation and management of an established patient, which requires at least 2 of these 3 key components: ■ A detailed interval history; ■ A detailed examination; ■ Medical decision making of moderate complexity. Counseling and/or coordination of care with other physicians, other qualified health care professionals, or agencies are provided consistent with the nature of the problem(s) and the patient's and/or family's needs. Usually, the presenting problem(s) are of moderate to high severity. Typically, 40 minutes are spent with the patient and/or family or caregiver.
99337	Domiciliary or rest home visit for the evaluation and management of an established patient, which requires at least 2 of these 3 key components: ■ A comprehensive interval history; ■ A comprehensive examination; ■ Medical decision making of moderate to high complexity. Counseling and/or coordination of care with other physicians, other qualified health care professionals, or agencies are provided consistent with the nature of the problem(s) and the patient's and/or family's needs. Usually, the presenting problem(s) are of moderate to high severity. The patient may be unstable or may have developed a significant new problem requiring immediate physician attention. Typically, 60 minutes are spent with the patient and/or family or caregiver.
99339	Individual physician supervision of a patient (patient not present) in home, domiciliary or rest home (eg, assisted living facility) requiring complex and multidisciplinary care modalities involving regular physician development and/or revision of care plans, review of subsequent reports of patient status, review of related laboratory and other studies, communication (including telephone calls) for purposes of assessment or care decisions with health care professional(s), family member(s), surrogate decision maker(s) (eg, legal guardian) and/or key caregiver(s) involved in patient's care, integration of new information into the medical treatment plan and/or adjustment of medical therapy, within a calendar month; 15-29 minutes

Evaluation / Management 99202-99499

Code	Description
99340	~~30 minutes or more~~
▲**99341**	**Home or residence visit** for the evaluation and management of a new patient, which requires <u>a medically appropriate history and/or examination and straightforward medical decision making.</u>~~these 3 key components:~~ ~~A problem focused history;~~ ~~A problem focused examination; and~~ ~~Straightforward medical decision making.~~ ~~Counseling and/or coordination of care with other physicians, other qualified health care professionals, or agencies are provided consistent with the nature of the problem(s) and the patient's and/or family's needs.~~ ~~Usually, the presenting problem(s) are of low severity. Typically, 20 minutes are spent face-to-face with the patient and/or family.~~ <u>When using total time on the date of the encounter for code selection, 15 minutes must be met or exceeded.</u>
▲**99342**	**Home or residence visit** for the evaluation and management of a new patient, which requires <u>a medically appropriate history and/or examination and low level of medical decision making.</u>~~these 3 key components:~~ ~~■ An expanded problem focused history;~~ ~~■ An expanded problem focused examination; and~~ ~~■ Medical decision making of low complexity.~~ ~~Counseling and/or coordination of care with other physicians, other qualified health care professionals, or agencies are provided consistent with the nature of the problem(s) and the patient's and/or family's needs.~~ ~~Usually, the presenting problem(s) are of moderate severity. Typically, 30 minutes are spent face-to-face with the patient and/or family.~~ <u>When using total time on the date of the encounter for code selection, 30 minutes must be met or exceeded.</u>
99343	~~**Home visit** for the evaluation and management of a new patient, which requires these 3 key components:~~ ~~■ **A detailed history;**~~ ~~■ **A detailed examination; and**~~ ~~■ **Medical decision making of moderate complexity.**~~ ~~Counseling and/or coordination of care with other physicians, other qualified health care professionals, or agencies are provided consistent with the nature of the problem(s) and the patient's and/or family's needs.~~ ~~Usually, the presenting problem(s) are of moderate to high severity. Typically, 45 minutes are spent face-to-face with the patient and/or family.~~
▲**99344**	**Home or residence visit** for the evaluation and management of a new patient, which requires <u>a medically appropriate history and/or examination and moderate level of medical decision making.</u>~~these 3 key components:~~ ~~■ A comprehensive history;~~ ~~■ A comprehensive examination; and~~ ~~■ Medical decision making of moderate complexity.~~ ~~Counseling and/or coordination of care with other physicians, other qualified health care professionals, or agencies are provided consistent with the nature of the problem(s) and the patient's and/or family's needs.~~ ~~Usually, the presenting problem(s) are of high severity. Typically, 60 minutes are spent face-to-face with the patient and/or family.~~ <u>When using total time on the date of the encounter for code selection, 60 minutes must be met or exceeded.</u>

★ = Telemedicine   ◀ = Audio-only   ✛ = Add-on code   ⋏ = FDA approval pending   # = Resequenced code   ⊘ = Modifier 51 exempt

Code	Description
▲99345	**Home or residence visit** for the evaluation and management of a new patient, which requires <u>a medically appropriate history and/or examination and high level of medical decision making.</u>~~these 3 key components:~~ ■ ~~A comprehensive history;~~ ■ ~~A comprehensive examination; and~~ ■ ~~Medical decision making of high complexity.~~ ~~Counseling and/or coordination of care with other physicians, other qualified health care professionals, or agencies are provided consistent with the nature of the problem(s) and the patient's and/or family's needs.~~ ~~Usually, the patient is unstable or has developed a significant new problem requiring immediate physician attention. Typically, 75 minutes are spent face-to-face with the patient and/or family.~~ <u>When using total time on the date of the encounter for code selection, 75 minutes must be met or exceeded.</u>
▲99347	**Home or residence visit** for the evaluation and management of an established patient, which requires <u>a medically appropriate history and/or examination and straightforward medical decision making.</u>~~at least 2 of these 3 key components:~~ ■ ~~A problem focused interval history;~~ ■ ~~A problem focused examination;~~ ■ ~~Straightforward medical decision making.~~ ~~Counseling and/or coordination of care with other physicians, other qualified health care professionals, or agencies are provided consistent with the nature of the problem(s) and the patient's and/or family's needs.~~ ~~Usually, the presenting problem(s) are self limited or minor. Typically, 15 minutes are spent face-to-face with the patient and/or family.~~ <u>When using total time on the date of the encounter for code selection, 20 minutes must be met or exceeded.</u>
▲99348	**Home or residence visit** for the evaluation and management of an established patient, which requires <u>a medically appropriate history and/or examination and low level of medical decision making.</u>~~at least 2 of these 3 key components:~~ ■ ~~An expanded problem focused interval history;~~ ■ ~~An expanded problem focused examination;~~ ■ ~~Medical decision making of low complexity.~~ ~~Counseling and/or coordination of care with other physicians, other qualified health care professionals, or agencies are provided consistent with the nature of the problem(s) and the patient's and/or family's needs.~~ ~~Usually, the presenting problem(s) are of low to moderate severity. Typically, 25 minutes are spent face-to-face with the patient and/or family.~~ <u>When using total time on the date of the encounter for code selection, 30 minutes must be met or exceeded.</u>
▲99349	**Home or residence visit** for the evaluation and management of an established patient, which requires <u>a medically appropriate history and/or examination and moderate level of medical decision making.</u>~~at least 2 of these 3 key components:~~ ~~A detailed interval history;~~ ~~A detailed examination;~~ ~~Medical decision making of moderate complexity.~~ ~~Counseling and/or coordination of care with other physicians, other qualified health care professionals, or agencies are provided consistent with the nature of the problem(s) and the patient's and/or family's needs.~~ ~~Usually, the presenting problem(s) are moderate to high severity. Typically, 40 minutes are spent face-to-face with the patient and/or family.~~ <u>When using total time on the date of the encounter for code selection, 40 minutes must be met or exceeded.</u>

Evaluation / Management   99202-99499

Code	Description
▲99350	**Home or residence visit** for the evaluation and management of an established patient, which requires a medically appropriate history and/or examination and high level of medical decision making. ~~at least 2 of these 3 key components:~~ ■ ~~A comprehensive interval history;~~ ■ ~~A comprehensive examination;~~ ■ ~~Medical decision making of moderate to high complexity.~~ ~~Counseling and/or coordination of care with other physicians, other qualified health care professionals, or agencies are provided consistent with the nature of the problem(s) and the patient's and/or family's needs.~~ ~~Usually, the presenting problem(s) are of moderate to high severity. The patient may be unstable or may have developed a significant new problem requiring immediate physician attention. Typically, 60 minutes are spent face-to-face with the patient and/or family.~~ When using total time on the date of the encounter for code selection, 60 minutes must be met or exceeded.
~~99354~~	~~Prolonged service(s) in the outpatient setting requiring direct patient contact beyond the time of the usual service; first hour (List separately in addition to code for outpatient **Evaluation and Management** or psychotherapy service, except with office or other outpatient services [99202, 99203, 99204, 99205, 99212, 99213, 99214, 99215])~~
~~99355~~	~~each additional 30 minutes (List separately in addition to code for prolonged service)~~
~~99356~~	~~Prolonged service in the inpatient or observation setting, requiring unit/floor time beyond the usual service; first hour (List separately in addition to code for inpatient or observation **Evaluation and Management** service)~~
~~99357~~	~~each additional 30 minutes (List separately in addition to code for prolonged service)~~
#★✚▲99417	Prolonged ~~office or other~~ outpatient evaluation and management service(s) time with or without direct patient contact beyond the ~~minimum~~ required time of the primary ~~service procedure which~~ when the primary service level has been selected using total time, ~~requiring total time with or without direct patient contact beyond the usual service, on the date of the primary service,~~ each 15 minutes of total time (List separately in addition to ~~codes 99205, 99215 for office or other~~ the code of the outpatient **Evaluation and Management** services)
#★✚●99418	Code added
▲99446	Interprofessional telephone/Internet/electronic health record assessment and management service provided by a consultative physician or other qualified health care professional, including a verbal and written report to the patient's treating/requesting physician or other qualified health care professional; 5-10 minutes of medical consultative discussion and review
▲99447	11-20 minutes of medical consultative discussion and review
▲99448	21-30 minutes of medical consultative discussion and review
▲99449	31 minutes or more of medical consultative discussion and review
#▲99451	Interprofessional telephone/Internet/electronic health record assessment and management service provided by a consultative physician or other qualified health care professional, including a written report to the patient's treating/requesting physician or other qualified health care professional, 5 minutes or more of medical consultative time

★=Telemedicine   ◀=Audio-only   ✚=Add-on code   ⊁=FDA approval pending   #=Resequenced code   ⊘=Modifier 51 exempt

Code	Description
▲ **99483**	Assessment of and care planning for a patient with cognitive impairment, requiring an independent historian, in the office or other outpatient, home or domiciliary or rest home, with all of the following required elements: ■ Cognition-focused evaluation including a pertinent history and examination, ■ Medical decision making of moderate or high complexity, ■ Functional assessment (eg, basic and instrumental activities of daily living), including decision-making capacity, ■ Use of standardized instruments for staging of dementia (eg, functional assessment staging test [FAST], clinical dementia rating [CDR]), ■ Medication reconciliation and review for high-risk medications, ■ Evaluation for neuropsychiatric and behavioral symptoms, including depression, including use of standardized screening instrument(s), ■ Evaluation of safety (eg, home), including motor vehicle operation, ■ Identification of caregiver(s), caregiver knowledge, caregiver needs, social supports, and the willingness of caregiver to take on caregiving tasks, ■ Development, updating or revision, or review of an Advance Care Plan, ■ Creation of a written care plan, including initial plans to address any neuropsychiatric symptoms, neuro-cognitive symptoms, functional limitations, and referral to community resources as needed (eg, rehabilitation services, adult day programs, support groups) shared with the patient and/or caregiver with initial education and support Typically, ~~50~~60 minutes of total time is ~~are~~ spent on the date of the encounter.~~face-to-face with the patient and/or family or caregiver.~~
★ ▲ **99495**	**Transitional ~~C~~care ~~M~~management ~~S~~services** with the following required elements: ■ Communication (direct contact, telephone, electronic) with the patient and/or caregiver within 2 business days of discharge ■ ~~Medical decision making of a~~At least moderate ~~level of complexity~~ medical decision making during the service period ■ Face-to-face visit, within 14 calendar days of discharge
★ ▲ **99496**	**Transitional ~~C~~care ~~M~~management ~~S~~services** with the following required elements: ■ Communication (direct contact, telephone, electronic) with the patient and/or caregiver within 2 business days of discharge ■ ~~Medical decision making of h~~High ~~level of complexity~~ medical decision making during the service period ■ Face-to-face visit, within 7 calendar days of discharge

Evaluation / Management   99202-99499

Evaluation and Management (E/M) Services Guidelines

In addition to the information presented in the Introduction, several other items unique to this section are defined or identified here.

E/M Guidelines Overview

▶The E/M guidelines have sections that are common to all E/M categories and sections that are category specific. Most of the categories and many of the subcategories of service have special guidelines or instructions unique to that category or subcategory. Where these are indicated, eg, "Hospital Inpatient and Observation Care," special instructions are presented before the listing of the specific E/M services codes. It is important to review the instructions for each category or subcategory. These guidelines are to be used by the reporting physician or other qualified health care professional to select the appropriate level of service. These guidelines do not establish documentation requirements or standards of care. The main purpose of documentation is to support care of the patient by current and future health care team(s). These guidelines are for services that require a face-to-face encounter with the patient and/or family/caregiver. (For 99211 and 99281, the face-to-face services may be performed by clinical staff.)

In the **Evaluation and Management** section (99202-99499), there are many code categories. Each category may have specific guidelines, or the codes may include specific details. These E/M guidelines are written for the following categories:

- Office or Other Outpatient Services
- Hospital Inpatient and Observation Care Services
- Consultations
- Emergency Department Services
- Nursing Facility Services
- Home or Residence Services
- Prolonged Service With or Without Direct Patient Contact on the Date of an Evaluation and Management Service◀

Classification of Evaluation and Management (E/M) Services

▶The E/M section is divided into broad categories, such as office visits, hospital inpatient or observation care visits, and consultations. Most of the categories are further divided into two or more subcategories of E/M services. For example, there are two subcategories of office visits (new patient and established patient) and there are two subcategories of hospital inpatient and observation care visits (initial and subsequent). The subcategories of E/M services are further classified into levels of E/M services that are identified by specific codes.

The basic format of codes with levels of E/M services based on medical decision making (MDM) or time is the same. First, a unique code number is listed. Second, the place and/or type of service is specified (eg, office or other outpatient visit). Third, the content of the service is defined. Fourth, time is specified. (A detailed discussion of time is provided in the Guidelines for Selecting Level of Service Based on Time.)

The place of service and service type are defined by the location where the face-to-face encounter with the patient and/or family/caregiver occurs. For example, service provided to a nursing facility resident brought to the office is reported with an office or other outpatient code.◀

New and Established Patients

▶Solely for the purposes of distinguishing between new and established patients, **professional services** are those face-to-face services rendered by physicians and other qualified health care professionals who may report evaluation and management services. A new patient is one who has not received any professional services from the physician or other qualified health care professional or another physician or other qualified health care professional of the **exact** same specialty **and subspecialty** who belongs to the same group practice, within the past three years.

An established patient is one who has received professional services from the physician or other qualified health care professional or another physician or other qualified health care professional of the **exact** same specialty **and subspecialty** who belongs to the same group practice, within the past three years. See Decision Tree for New vs Established Patients.

In the instance where a physician or other qualified health care professional is on call for or covering for another physician or other qualified health care professional, the patient's encounter will be classified as it would have been by the physician or other qualified

★ = Telemedicine   ◀ = Audio-only   ✛ = Add-on code   ✗ = FDA approval pending   # = Resequenced code   ⦰ = Modifier 51 exempt

health care professional who is not available. When advanced practice nurses and physician assistants are working with physicians, they are considered as working in the **exact** same specialty **and subspecialty** as the physician.◄

No distinction is made between new and established patients in the emergency department. E/M services in the emergency department category may be reported for any new or established patient who presents for treatment in the emergency department.

The Decision Tree for New vs Established Patients is provided to aid in determining whether to report the E/M service provided as a new or an established patient encounter.

—— *Coding Tip* ——

Instructions for Use of the CPT Codebook

When advanced practice nurses and physician assistants are working with physicians, they are considered as working in the exact same specialty and subspecialty as the physician. A "physician or other qualified health care professional" is an individual who is qualified by education, training, licensure/regulation (when applicable), and facility privileging (when applicable) who performs a professional service within his or her scope of practice and independently reports that professional service. These professionals are distinct from "clinical staff." A clinical staff member is a person who works under the supervision of a physician or other qualified health care professional, and who is allowed by law, regulation and facility policy to perform or assist in the performance of a specific professional service but does not individually report that professional service. Other policies may also affect who may report specific services.

CPT Coding Guidelines, Introduction, Instructions for Use of the CPT Codebook

►Initial and Subsequent Services◄

►Some categories apply to both new and established patients (eg, hospital inpatient or observation care). These categories differentiate services by whether the service is the initial service or a subsequent service. For the purpose of distinguishing between initial or subsequent visits, professional services are those face-to-face services rendered by physicians and other qualified health care professionals who may report evaluation and management services. An initial service is when the patient has not received any professional services from the physician or other qualified health care professional or another physician or other qualified health care professional of the exact same specialty and subspecialty

who belongs to the same group practice, during the inpatient, observation, or nursing facility admission and stay.

A subsequent service is when the patient has received professional service(s) from the physician or other qualified health care professional or another physician or other qualified health care professional of the exact same specialty and subspecialty who belongs to the same group practice, during the admission and stay.

In the instance when a physician or other qualified health care professional is on call for or covering for another physician or other qualified health care professional, the patient's encounter will be classified as it would have been by the physician or other qualified health care professional who is not available. When advanced practice nurses and physician assistants are working with physicians, they are considered as working in the exact same specialty and subspecialty as the physician.

For reporting hospital inpatient or observation care services, a stay that includes a transition from observation to inpatient is a single stay. For reporting nursing facility services, a stay that includes transition(s) between skilled nursing facility and nursing facility level of care is the same stay.◄

Services Reported Separately

Any specifically identifiable procedure or service (ie, identified with a specific CPT code) performed on the date of E/M services may be reported separately.

►The ordering and actual performance and/or interpretation of diagnostic tests/studies during a patient encounter are not included in determining the levels of E/M services when the professional interpretation of those tests/studies is reported separately by the physician or other qualified health care professional reporting the E/M service. Tests that do not require separate interpretation (eg, tests that are results only) and are analyzed as part of MDM do not count as an independent interpretation, but may be counted as ordered or reviewed for selecting an MDM level. The performance of diagnostic tests/studies for which specific CPT codes are available may be reported separately, in addition to the appropriate E/M code. The interpretation of the results of diagnostic tests/studies (ie, professional component) with preparation of a separate distinctly identifiable signed written report may also be reported separately, using the appropriate CPT code and, if required, with modifier 26 appended.◄

The physician or other qualified health care professional may need to indicate that on the day a procedure or service identified by a CPT code was performed, the patient's condition required a significant separately identifiable E/M service. The E/M service may be caused or prompted by the symptoms or condition for which the procedure and/or service was provided. This circumstance

Decision Tree for New vs Established Patients

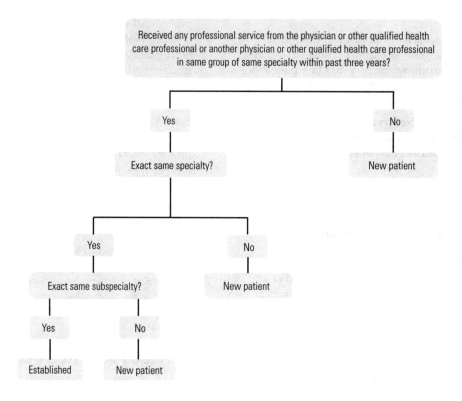

may be reported by adding modifier 25 to the appropriate level of E/M service. As such, different diagnoses are not required for reporting of the procedure and the E/M services on the same date.

History and/or Examination

►E/M codes that have levels of services include a medically appropriate history and/or physical examination, when performed. The nature and extent of the history and/or physical examination are determined by the treating physician or other qualified health care professional reporting the service. The care team may collect information, and the patient or caregiver may supply information directly (eg, by electronic health record [EHR] portal or questionnaire) that is reviewed by the reporting physician or other qualified health care professional. The extent of history and physical examination is not an element in selection of the level of these E/M service codes.◄

►Levels of E/M Services◄

Select the appropriate level of E/M services based on the following:

1. The level of the MDM as defined for each service, **or**

2. The total time for E/M services performed on the date of the encounter.

►Within each category or subcategory of E/M service based on MDM or time, there are three to five levels of E/M services available for reporting purposes. Levels of E/M services are **not** interchangeable among the different categories or subcategories of service. For example, the first level of E/M services in the subcategory of office visit, new patient, does not have the same definition as the first level of E/M services in the subcategory of office visit, established patient. Each level of E/M services may be used by all physicians or other qualified health care professionals.◄

★=Telemedicine ◄=Audio-only ✚=Add-on code ✚=FDA approval pending #=Resequenced code ⊘=Modifier 51 exempt

▶Guidelines for Selecting Level of Service Based on Medical Decision Making◀

▶Four types of MDM are recognized: straightforward, low, moderate, and high. The concept of the level of MDM does not apply to 99211, 99281.

MDM includes establishing diagnoses, assessing the status of a condition, and/or selecting a management option. MDM is defined by three elements. The elements are:

- *The number and complexity of problem(s) that are addressed during the encounter.*
- *The amount and/or complexity of data to be reviewed and analyzed.* These data include medical records, tests, and/or other information that must be obtained, ordered, reviewed, and analyzed for the encounter. This includes information obtained from multiple sources or interprofessional communications that are not reported separately and interpretation of tests that are not reported separately. Ordering a test is included in the category of test result(s) and the review of the test result is part of the encounter and not a subsequent encounter. Ordering a test may include those considered but not selected after shared decision making. For example, a patient may request diagnostic imaging that is not necessary for their condition and discussion of the lack of benefit may be required. Alternatively, a test may normally be performed, but due to the risk for a specific patient it is not ordered. These considerations must be documented. Data are divided into three categories:

- Tests, documents, orders, or independent historian(s). (Each unique test, order, or document is counted to meet a threshold number.)
- Independent interpretation of tests (not separately reported).
- Discussion of management or test interpretation with external physician or other qualified health care professional or appropriate source (not separately reported).

- *The risk of complications and/or morbidity or mortality of patient management.* This includes decisions made at the encounter associated with diagnostic procedure(s) and treatment(s). This includes the possible management options selected and those considered but not selected after shared decision making with the patient and/or family. For example, a decision about hospitalization includes consideration of alternative levels of care. Examples may include a psychiatric patient with a sufficient degree of support in the outpatient setting or the decision to not hospitalize a patient with advanced dementia with an acute condition that would generally warrant inpatient care, but for whom the goal is palliative treatment.

Shared decision making involves eliciting patient and/or family preferences, patient and/or family education, and explaining risks and benefits of management options.◀

MDM may be impacted by role and management responsibility.

▶When the physician or other qualified health care professional is reporting a separate CPT code that includes interpretation and/or report, the interpretation and/or report is not counted toward the MDM when selecting a level of E/M services. When the physician or other qualified health care professional is reporting a separate service for discussion of management with a physician or another qualified health care professional, the discussion is not counted toward the MDM when selecting a level of E/M services.

The Levels of Medical Decision Making (MDM) table (Table 1) is a guide to assist in selecting the level of MDM for reporting an E/M services code. The table includes the four levels of MDM (ie, straightforward, low, moderate, high) and the three elements of MDM (ie, number and complexity of problems addressed at the encounter, amount and/or complexity of data reviewed and analyzed, and risk of complications and/or morbidity or mortality of patient management). To qualify for a particular level of MDM, two of the three elements for that level of MDM must be met or exceeded.

Examples in the table may be more or less applicable to specific settings of care. For example, the decision to hospitalize applies to the outpatient or nursing facility encounters, whereas the decision to escalate hospital level of care (eg, transfer to ICU) applies to the hospitalized or observation care patient. See also the introductory guidelines of each code family section.◀

Number and Complexity of Problems Addressed at the Encounter

▶One element used in selecting the level of service is the number and complexity of the problems that are addressed at the encounter. Multiple new or established conditions may be addressed at the same time and may affect MDM. Symptoms may cluster around a specific diagnosis and each symptom is not necessarily a unique condition. Comorbidities and underlying diseases, in and of themselves, are not considered in selecting a level of E/M services **unless** they are addressed, and their presence increases the amount and/or complexity of data to be reviewed and analyzed or the risk of complications and/or morbidity or mortality of patient management. The final diagnosis for a condition does not, in and of itself, determine the complexity or risk, as extensive evaluation may be required to reach the conclusion that the signs or symptoms do not represent a highly morbid condition. Therefore, presenting symptoms that are likely

(continued on page 25)

Table 1: Levels of Medical Decision Making (MDM)

	►Elements of Medical Decision Making		
Level of MDM (Based on 2 out of 3 Elements of MDM)	Number and Complexity of Problems Addressed at the Encounter	Amount and/or Complexity of Data to Be Reviewed and Analyzed *Each unique test, order, or document contributes to the combination of 2 or combination of 3 in Category 1 below.*	Risk of Complications and/or Morbidity or Mortality of Patient Management
Straightforward	Minimal ■ **1** self-limited or minor problem	Minimal or none	Minimal risk of morbidity from additional diagnostic testing or treatment
Low	Low ■ **2** or more self-limited or minor problems; or ■ **1** stable, chronic illness; or ■ **1** acute, uncomplicated illness or injury; or ■ **1** stable, acute illness; or ■ **1** acute, uncomplicated illness or injury requiring hospital inpatient or observation level of care	Limited *(Must meet the requirements of at least 1 out of 2 categories)* **Category 1: Tests and documents** ■ **Any combination of 2 from the following:** • Review of prior external note(s) from each unique source*; • Review of the result(s) of each unique test*; • Ordering of each unique test* **or** **Category 2: Assessment requiring an independent historian(s)** *(For the categories of independent interpretation of tests and discussion of management or test interpretation, see moderate or high)*	Low risk of morbidity from additional diagnostic testing or treatment
Moderate	Moderate ■ **1** or more chronic illnesses with exacerbation, progression, or side effects of treatment; or ■ **2** or more stable, chronic illnesses; or ■ **1** undiagnosed new problem with uncertain prognosis; or ■ **1** acute illness with systemic symptoms; or ■ **1** acute, complicated injury	Moderate *(Must meet the requirements of at least 1 out of 3 categories)* **Category 1: Tests, documents, or independent historian(s)** ■ **Any combination of 3 from the following:** • Review of prior external note(s) from each unique source*; • Review of the result(s) of each unique test*; • Ordering of each unique test*; • Assessment requiring an independent historian(s) **or** **Category 2: Independent interpretation of tests** ■ Independent interpretation of a test performed by another physician/other qualified health care professional (not separately reported); **or** **Category 3: Discussion of management or test interpretation** ■ Discussion of management or test interpretation with external physician/other qualified health care professional/appropriate source (not separately reported)	Moderate risk of morbidity from additional diagnostic testing or treatment *Examples only:* ■ Prescription drug management ■ Decision regarding minor surgery with identified patient or procedure risk factors ■ Decision regarding elective major surgery without identified patient or procedure risk factors ■ Diagnosis or treatment significantly limited by social determinants of health

(continued)

★ = Telemedicine   ◀ = Audio-only   ✚ = Add-on code   𝒩 = FDA approval pending   # = Resequenced code   ⊘ = Modifier 51 exempt

Elements of Medical Decision Making

Level of MDM (Based on 2 out of 3 Elements of MDM)	Number and Complexity of Problems Addressed at the Encounter	Amount and/or Complexity of Data to Be Reviewed and Analyzed *Each unique test, order, or document contributes to the combination of 2 or combination of 3 in Category 1 below.*	Risk of Complications and/or Morbidity or Mortality of Patient Management
High	**High** ■ **1** or more chronic illnesses with severe exacerbation, progression, or side effects of treatment; **or** ■ **1** acute or chronic illness or injury that poses a threat to life or bodily function	**Extensive** *(Must meet the requirements of at least 2 out of 3 categories)* **Category 1: Tests, documents or independent historian(s)** ■ **Any combination of 3 from the following:** • Review of prior external note(s) from each unique source*; • Review of the result(s) of each unique test*; • Ordering of each unique test*; • Assessment requiring an independent historian(s) **or** **Category 2: Independent interpretation of tests** ■ Independent interpretation of a test performed by another physician/other qualified health care professional (not separately reported); **or** **Category 3: Discussion of management or test interpretation** ■ Discussion of management or test interpretation with external physician/other qualified health care professional/appropriate source (not separately reported)	**High risk of morbidity from additional diagnostic testing or treatment** *Examples only:* ■ Drug therapy requiring intensive monitoring for toxicity ■ Decision regarding elective major surgery with identified patient or procedure risk factors ■ Decision regarding emergency major surgery ■ Decision regarding hospitalization or escalation of hospital-level care ■ Decision not to resuscitate or to de-escalate care because of poor prognosis ■ Parenteral controlled substances◄

(continued from page 23)

to represent a highly morbid condition may "drive" MDM even when the ultimate diagnosis is not highly morbid. The evaluation and/or treatment should be consistent with the likely nature of the condition. Multiple problems of a lower severity may, in the aggregate, create higher risk due to interaction.◄

The term "risk" as used in these definitions relates to risk from the condition. While condition risk and management risk may often correlate, the risk from the condition is distinct from the risk of the management.

►Definitions for the elements of MDM (see Table 1, Levels of Medical Decision Making) are:◄

Problem: A problem is a disease, condition, illness, injury, symptom, sign, finding, complaint, or other matter addressed at the encounter, with or without a diagnosis being established at the time of the encounter.

►*Problem addressed:* A problem is addressed or managed when it is evaluated or treated at the encounter by the physician or other qualified health care professional reporting the service. This includes consideration of further testing or treatment that may not be elected by virtue of risk/benefit analysis or patient/parent/guardian/surrogate choice. Notation in the patient's medical record that another professional is

managing the problem without additional assessment or care coordination documented does not qualify as being addressed or managed by the physician or other qualified health care professional reporting the service. Referral without evaluation (by history, examination, or diagnostic study[ies]) or consideration of treatment does not qualify as being addressed or managed by the physician or other qualified health care professional reporting the service. For hospital inpatient and observation care services, the problem addressed is the problem status on the date of the encounter, which may be significantly different than on admission. It is the problem being managed or co-managed by the reporting physician or other qualified health care professional and may not be the cause of admission or continued stay.

Minimal problem: A problem that may not require the presence of the physician or other qualified health care professional, but the service is provided under the physician's or other qualified health care professional's supervision (see 99211, 99281).◄

Self-limited or minor problem: A problem that runs a definite and prescribed course, is transient in nature, and is not likely to permanently alter health status.

▶*Stable, chronic illness:* A problem with an expected duration of at least one year or until the death of the patient. For the purpose of defining chronicity, conditions are treated as chronic whether or not stage or severity changes (eg, uncontrolled diabetes and controlled diabetes are a single chronic condition). "Stable" for the purposes of categorizing MDM is defined by the specific treatment goals for an individual patient. A patient who is not at his or her treatment goal is not stable, even if the condition has not changed and there is no short-term threat to life or function. For example, a patient with persistently poorly controlled blood pressure for whom better control is a goal is not stable, even if the pressures are not changing and the patient is asymptomatic. The risk of morbidity **without** treatment is significant.

Acute, uncomplicated illness or injury: A recent or new short-term problem with low risk of morbidity for which treatment is considered. There is little to no risk of mortality with treatment, and full recovery without functional impairment is expected. A problem that is normally self-limited or minor but is not resolving consistent with a definite and prescribed course is an acute, uncomplicated illness.

Acute, uncomplicated illness or injury requiring hospital inpatient or observation level care: A recent or new short-term problem with low risk of morbidity for which treatment is required. There is little to no risk of mortality with treatment, and full recovery without functional impairment is expected. The treatment required is delivered in a hospital inpatient or observation level setting.

Stable, acute illness: A problem that is new or recent for which treatment has been initiated. The patient is improved and, while resolution may not be complete, is stable with respect to this condition.

Chronic illness with exacerbation, progression, or side effects of treatment: A chronic illness that is acutely worsening, poorly controlled, or progressing with an intent to control progression and requiring additional supportive care or requiring attention to treatment for side effects.

Undiagnosed new problem with uncertain prognosis: A problem in the differential diagnosis that represents a condition likely to result in a high risk of morbidity without treatment.

Acute illness with systemic symptoms: An illness that causes systemic symptoms and has a high risk of morbidity without treatment. For systemic general symptoms, such as fever, body aches, or fatigue in a minor illness that may be treated to alleviate symptoms, see the definitions for *self-limited or minor problem* or *acute, uncomplicated illness or injury.* Systemic symptoms may not be general but may be single system.

Acute, complicated injury: An injury which requires treatment that includes evaluation of body systems that are not directly part of the injured organ, the injury is extensive, or the treatment options are multiple and/or associated with risk of morbidity.

Chronic illness with severe exacerbation, progression, or side effects of treatment: The severe exacerbation or progression of a chronic illness or severe side effects of treatment that have significant risk of morbidity and may require escalation in level of care.

Acute or chronic illness or injury that poses a threat to life or bodily function: An acute illness with systemic symptoms, an acute complicated injury, or a chronic illness or injury with exacerbation and/or progression or side effects of treatment, that poses a threat to life or bodily function in the near term without treatment. Some symptoms may represent a condition that is significantly probable and poses a potential threat to life or bodily function. These may be included in this category when the evaluation and treatment are consistent with this degree of potential severity.◀

▶Amount and/or Complexity of Data to Be Reviewed and Analyzed◀

▶One element used in selecting the level of services is the amount and/or complexity of data to be reviewed or analyzed at an encounter.◀

Analyzed: The process of using the data as part of the MDM. The data element itself may not be subject to analysis (eg, glucose), but it is instead included in the thought processes for diagnosis, evaluation, or treatment. Tests ordered are presumed to be analyzed when the results are reported. Therefore, when they are ordered during an encounter, they are counted in that encounter. Tests that are ordered outside of an encounter may be counted in the encounter in which they are analyzed. In the case of a recurring order, each new result may be counted in the encounter in which it is analyzed. For example, an encounter that includes an order for monthly prothrombin times would count for one prothrombin time ordered and reviewed. Additional future results, if analyzed in a subsequent encounter, may be counted as a single test in that subsequent encounter. Any service for which the professional component is separately reported by the physician or other qualified health care professional reporting the E/M services is not counted as a data element ordered, reviewed, analyzed, or independently interpreted for the purposes of determining the level of MDM.

Test: Tests are imaging, laboratory, psychometric, or physiologic data. A clinical laboratory panel (eg, basic metabolic panel [80047]) is a single test. The differentiation between single or multiple tests is defined in accordance with the CPT code set. For the purpose of data reviewed and analyzed, pulse oximetry is not a test.

Unique: A unique test is defined by the CPT code set. When multiple results of the same unique test (eg, serial blood glucose values) are compared during an E/M service, count it as one unique test. Tests that have overlapping elements are not unique, even if they are identified with distinct CPT codes. For example, a CBC with differential would incorporate the set of hemoglobin, CBC without differential, and platelet count. A unique source is defined as a physician or other qualified health care professional in a distinct group or different specialty or subspecialty, or a unique entity. Review of all materials from any unique source counts as one element toward MDM.

Combination of Data Elements: A combination of different data elements, for example, a combination of notes reviewed, tests ordered, tests reviewed, or independent historian, allows these elements to be summed. It does not require each item type or category to be represented. A unique test ordered, plus a note reviewed and an independent historian would be a combination of three elements.

External: External records, communications and/or test results are from an external physician, other qualified health care professional, facility, or health care organization.

External physician or other qualified health care professional: An external physician or other qualified health care professional who is not in the same group practice or is of a different specialty or subspecialty. This includes licensed professionals who are practicing independently. The individual may also be a facility or organizational provider such as from a hospital, nursing facility, or home health care agency.

Discussion: Discussion requires an interactive exchange. The exchange must be direct and not through intermediaries (eg, clinical staff or trainees). Sending chart notes or written exchanges that are within progress notes does not qualify as an interactive exchange. The discussion does not need to be on the date of the encounter, but it is counted only once and only when it is used in the decision making of the encounter. It may be asynchronous (ie, does not need to be in person), but it must be initiated and completed within a short time period (eg, within a day or two).

▶**Independent historian(s):** An individual (eg, parent, guardian, surrogate, spouse, witness) who provides a history in addition to a history provided by the patient who is unable to provide a complete or reliable history (eg, due to developmental stage, dementia, or psychosis) or because a confirmatory history is judged to be necessary. In the case where there may be conflict or poor communication between multiple historians and more than one historian is needed, the independent historian requirement is met. It does not include translation services. The independent history does not need to be

obtained in person but does need to be obtained directly from the historian providing the independent information.

Independent interpretation: The interpretation of a test for which there is a CPT code, and an interpretation or report is customary. This does not apply when the physician or other qualified health care professional who reports the E/M service is reporting or has previously reported the test. A form of interpretation should be documented but need not conform to the usual standards of a complete report for the test.◀

Appropriate source: For the purpose of the **discussion of management** data element (see Table 1, Levels of Medical Decision Making), an appropriate source includes professionals who are not health care professionals but may be involved in the management of the patient (eg, lawyer, parole officer, case manager, teacher). It does not include discussion with family or informal caregivers.

▶Risk of Complications and/or Morbidity or Mortality of Patient Management◀

One element used in selecting the level of service is the risk of complications and/or morbidity or mortality of patient management at an encounter. This is distinct from the risk of the condition itself.

▶**Risk:** The probability and/or consequences of an event. The assessment of the level of risk is affected by the nature of the event under consideration. For example, a low probability of death may be high risk, whereas a high chance of a minor, self-limited adverse effect of treatment may be low risk. Definitions of risk are based upon the usual behavior and thought processes of a physician or other qualified health care professional in the same specialty. Trained clinicians apply common language usage meanings to terms such as *high, medium, low,* or *minimal* risk and do not require quantification for these definitions (though quantification may be provided when evidence-based medicine has established probabilities). For the purpose of MDM, level of risk is based upon consequences of the problem(s) addressed at the encounter when appropriately treated. Risk also includes MDM related to the need to initiate or forego further testing, treatment, and/or hospitalization. The risk of patient management criteria applies to the patient management decisions made by the reporting physician or other qualified health care professional as part of the reported encounter.◀

Morbidity: A state of illness or functional impairment that is expected to be of substantial duration during which function is limited, quality of life is impaired, or there is organ damage that may not be transient despite treatment.

Evaluation / Management 99202-99499

Social determinants of health: Economic and social conditions that influence the health of people and communities. Examples may include food or housing insecurity.

Surgery (minor or major, elective, emergency, procedure or patient risk):

Surgery—Minor or Major: The classification of surgery into minor or major is based on the common meaning of such terms when used by trained clinicians, similar to the use of the term "risk." These terms are not defined by a surgical package classification.

Surgery—Elective or Emergency: Elective procedures and emergent or urgent procedures describe the timing of a procedure when the timing is related to the patient's condition. An elective procedure is typically planned in advance (eg, scheduled for weeks later), while an emergent procedure is typically performed immediately or with minimal delay to allow for patient stabilization. Both elective and emergent procedures may be minor or major procedures.

Surgery—Risk Factors, Patient or Procedure: Risk factors are those that are relevant to the patient and procedure. Evidence-based risk calculators may be used, but are not required, in assessing patient and procedure risk.

▶**Drug therapy requiring intensive monitoring for toxicity:** A drug that requires intensive monitoring is a therapeutic agent that has the potential to cause serious morbidity or death. The monitoring is performed for assessment of these adverse effects and not primarily for assessment of therapeutic efficacy. The monitoring should be that which is generally accepted practice for the agent but may be patient-specific in some cases. Intensive monitoring may be long-term or short-term. Long-term intensive monitoring is not performed less than quarterly. The monitoring may be performed with a laboratory test, a physiologic test, or imaging. Monitoring by history or examination does not qualify. The monitoring affects the level of MDM in an encounter in which it is considered in the management of the patient. An example may be monitoring for cytopenia in the use of an antineoplastic agent between dose cycles. Examples of monitoring that do not qualify include monitoring glucose levels during insulin therapy, as the primary reason is the therapeutic effect (unless severe hypoglycemia is a current, significant concern); or annual electrolytes and renal function for a patient on a diuretic, as the frequency does not meet the threshold.◀

▶Guidelines for Selecting Level of Service Based on Time◀

▶Certain categories of time-based E/M codes that do not have levels of services based on MDM (eg, Critical Care Services) in the E/M section use time differently. It is important to review the instructions for each category.

Time is **not** a descriptive component for the emergency department levels of E/M services because emergency department services are typically provided on a variable intensity basis, often involving multiple encounters with several patients over an extended period of time.

When time is used for reporting E/M services codes, the time defined in the service descriptors is used for selecting the appropriate level of services. The E/M services for which these guidelines apply require a face-to-face encounter with the physician or other qualified health care professional and the patient and/or family/caregiver. For office or other outpatient services, if the physician's or other qualified health care professional's time is spent in the supervision of clinical staff who perform the face-to-face services of the encounter, use 99211.

For coding purposes, time for these services is the total time on the date of the encounter. It includes both the face-to-face time with the patient and/or family/caregiver and non-face-to-face time personally spent by the physician and/or other qualified health care professional(s) on the day of the encounter (includes time in activities that require the physician or other qualified health care professional and does not include time in activities normally performed by clinical staff). It includes time regardless of the location of the physician or other qualified health care professional (eg, whether on or off the inpatient unit or in or out of the outpatient office). It does not include any time spent in the performance of other separately reported service(s).

A shared or split visit is defined as a visit in which a physician and other qualified health care professional(s) both provide the face-to-face and non-face-to-face work related to the visit. When time is being used to select the appropriate level of services for which time-based reporting of shared or split visits is allowed, the time personally spent by the physician and other qualified health care professional(s) assessing and managing the patient and/or counseling, educating, communicating results to the patient/family/caregiver on the date of the encounter is summed to define total time. Only distinct time should be summed for shared or split visits (ie, when two or more individuals jointly meet with or discuss the patient, only the time of one individual should be counted).

★ = Telemedicine   ◀ = Audio-only   ✛ = Add-on code   ✗ = FDA approval pending   # = Resequenced code   ⊘ = Modifier 51 exempt

When prolonged time occurs, the appropriate prolonged services code may be reported. The total time on the date of the encounter spent caring for the patient should be documented in the medical record when it is used as the basis for code selection.

Physician or other qualified health care professional time includes the following activities, when performed:

- preparing to see the patient (eg, review of tests)
- obtaining and/or reviewing separately obtained history
- performing a medically appropriate examination and/or evaluation
- counseling and educating the patient/family/caregiver
- ordering medications, tests, or procedures
- referring and communicating with other health care professionals (when not separately reported)
- documenting clinical information in the electronic or other health record
- independently interpreting results (not separately reported) and communicating results to the patient/family/caregiver
- care coordination (not separately reported)◄

Do not count time spent on the following:

- the performance of other services that are reported separately
- travel
- teaching that is general and not limited to discussion that is required for the management of a specific patient

Unlisted Service

An E/M service may be provided that is not listed in this section of the CPT codebook. When reporting such a service, the appropriate unlisted code may be used to indicate the service, identifying it by "Special Report," as discussed in the following paragraph. The "Unlisted Services" and accompanying codes for the E/M section are as follows:

Special Report

An unlisted service or one that is unusual, variable, or new may require a special report demonstrating the medical appropriateness of the service. Pertinent information should include an adequate definition or description of the nature, extent, and need for the procedure and the time, effort, and equipment necessary

to provide the service. Additional items that may be included are complexity of symptoms, final diagnosis, pertinent physical findings, diagnostic and therapeutic procedures, concurrent problems, and follow-up care.

Rationale

In 2021, only the evaluation and management (E/M) office or other outpatient codes' (99202-99215) code structure underwent significant changes. Rather than requiring fulfillment of the key components of history, examination, and medical decision making (MDM) for code-level selection, which was the requirement prior to 2021, reporting these services were restructured to require a medically appropriate history and/or examination, and code selection was based on the level of MDM or time. The rest of the E/M services codes (ie, hospital observation, hospital inpatient, consultations, emergency department [ED], nursing facility, domiciliary, rest home, or custodial care, and home E/M services), which were also based on levels, remained unchanged at that time. The E/M introductory guidelines were reorganized to accommodate the changes, because two sets of guidelines were needed: one set for the office or other outpatient E/M codes and another for the remaining E/M codes.

For 2023, to standardize the coding of all level-based E/M services, the remaining level-based E/M services codes have been revised to match the changes that were made to the office or other outpatient codes to standardize these codes for consistency. The E/M introductory guidelines have also been revised for 2023 to reflect this standardization of the level-based codes, thereby further reducing the administrative burden for users of the E/M codes, because they no longer need to refer to two separate sets of guidelines for level-based E/M services. Refer to the codebook and the Rationale for hospital inpatient and observation care, consultations, ED, nursing facility, and home or residence services for a full discussion of these changes.

The Classification of Evaluation and Management (E/M) Service subsection guidelines has been revised to clarify that the place of service (POS) and type of service are defined by the location where the face-to-face encounter occurs (eg, if a nursing facility resident is brought to the office for an E/M service, the appropriate code from the office or other outpatient service codes would be reported).

A new subsection, ie, Initial and Subsequent Services, has been added to the E/M introductory guidelines to distinguish initial vs subsequent services in terms of how they relate to new vs established patients.

The title of the "Time" heading in the E/M Services Guidelines has been revised to "Guidelines for Selecting Level of Service Based on Time," and the guidelines regarding time have been revised. The guidelines now clarify that time used in the level-based codes is the total time personally spent by the physician and/or other qualified health care professional (QHP) on the day of the encounter. This is regardless of the location (eg, inpatient unit, outpatient office) of the physician or other QHP. Total time includes time spent with the patient and/or family/caregiver and time spent performing activities that require the physician or other QHP. Total time does not include time in activities performed by clinical staff. In addition, total time of the E/M service does not include the time spent performing other separately reported service(s).

It is important to note that the guidelines specify that although certain E/M codes are time-based, they are not based on MDM (eg, critical care services codes 99291, 99292). Time is used differently for these codes; therefore, it is important to review the instructions for each category of E/M codes for the correct use of time when reporting the codes.

Prior to 2023, definitions for problems addressed, data analyzed, and risk of complications were all listed under the "Number and Complexity of Problems Addressed at the Encounter" heading of the E/M Services Guidelines. However, in order to more accurately delineate these different categories, two additional headings have been added (Amount and/or Complexity of Data to Be Reviewed and Analyzed, and Risk of Complications and/or Morbidity or Mortality of Patient Management), and these definitions are now placed under these subheadings, as appropriate.

In addition, the definitions for the number and complexity of problems addressed at the encounter have been revised. The definition of "problem addressed" has been revised to clarify that for hospital inpatient and observation care services, the problem addressed refers to the problem status on the date of the encounter, which may be different than the problem status on the day of admission. The definition for "minimal problem" has been revised by the inclusion of code 99281 as one of the codes, whose services may not require the presence of a physician or other QHP. Furthermore, the definition for acute or chronic illness or injury that poses a threat to life or bodily function has been revised with an additional statement that some symptoms may represent a condition that is significantly probable and poses a potential threat to life or bodily function and may be included in this definition when the evaluation and treatment are consistent with this degree of potential severity. Two new definitions have also been added to the guidelines. The

first is for acute, uncomplicated illness or injury requiring hospital inpatient or observation level care, which is a recent or new short-term problem with low risk of morbidity for which treatment is delivered in a hospital inpatient or observation level setting. The second is for stable, acute illness, which is a problem that is new or recent for which treatment has been initiated.

Evaluation and Management

Office or Other Outpatient Services

The following codes are used to report evaluation and management services provided in the office or in an outpatient or other ambulatory facility. A patient is considered an outpatient until inpatient admission to a health care facility occurs.

▶To report services provided to a patient who is admitted to a hospital or nursing facility in the course of an encounter in the office or other ambulatory facility, see the notes for initial hospital inpatient or observation care or initial nursing facility care.◀

For services provided in the emergency department, see 99281-99285.

▶For observation care, see 99221-99239.◀

▶For hospital inpatient or observation care services (including admission and discharge services), see 99234-99236.◀

— *Coding Tip* —

Determination of Patient Status as New or Established Patient

Solely for the purposes of distinguishing between new and established patients, **professional services** are those face-to-face services rendered by physicians and other qualified health care professionals who may report evaluation and management services. A new patient is one who has not received any professional services from the physician or other qualified health care professional or another physician or other qualified health care professional of the **exact** same specialty and subspecialty who belongs to the same group practice, within the past three years.

An established patient is one who has received professional services from the physician or other qualified health care professional or another physician or other qualified health care professional of the **exact** same specialty **and subspecialty** who belongs to the same group practice, within the past three years.

In the instance where a physician or other qualified health care professional is on call for or covering for another physician or other qualified health care professional, the patient's encounter will be classified as it would have been by the physician or other qualified

health care professional who is not available. When advanced practice nurses and physician assistants are working with physicians they are considered as working in the **exact** same specialty and **subspecialty** as the physician.

CPT Coding Guidelines, Evaluation and Management, Classification of Evaluation and Management (E/M) Services, New and Established Patients

Rationale

In accordance with the revision of codes 99221-99239 to include observation care services, the office or other outpatient services guidelines have been revised to reflect these changes.

Refer to the codebook and the Rationale for codes 99221-99239 for a full discussion of these changes.

Hospital Observation Services

Observation Care Discharge Services

▶(99217 has been deleted. To report observation care discharge services, see 99238, 99239)◀

Initial Observation Care

New or Established Patient

▶(99218, 99219, 99220 have been deleted. To report initial observation care, new or established patient, see 99221, 99222, 99223)◀

Subsequent Observation Care

▶(99224, 99225, 99226 have been deleted. To report subsequent observation care, see 99231, 99232, 99233)◀

▶Hospital Inpatient and Observation Care Services◀

▶The following codes are used to report initial and subsequent evaluation and management services provided to hospital inpatients and to patients designated as hospital outpatient "observation status." Hospital inpatient or observation care codes are also used to report partial hospitalization services.

For patients designated/admitted as "observation status" in a hospital, it is not necessary that the patient be located in an observation area designated by the hospital. If such an area does exist in a hospital (as a separate unit in the hospital, in the emergency department, etc), these codes may be utilized if the patient is placed in such an area.

For a patient admitted and discharged from hospital inpatient or observation status on the same date, report 99234, 99235, 99236, as appropriate.

Total time on the date of the encounter is by calendar date. When using MDM or total time for code selection, a continuous service that spans the transition of two calendar dates is a single service and is reported on one calendar date. If the service is continuous before and through midnight, all the time may be applied to the reported date of the service. ◄

►Initial Hospital Inpatient or Observation Care◄

New or Established Patient

►The following codes are used to report the first hospital inpatient or observation status encounter with the patient.

An initial service may be reported when the patient has not received any professional services from the physician or other qualified health care professional or another physician or other qualified health care professional of the exact same specialty and subspecialty who belongs to the same group practice during the stay. When advanced practice nurses and physician assistants are working with physicians, they are considered as working in the exact same specialty and subspecialty as the physician. ◄

For admission services for the neonate (28 days of age or younger) requiring intensive observation, frequent interventions, and other intensive care services, see 99477.

►When the patient is admitted to the hospital as an inpatient or to observation status in the course of an encounter in another site of service (eg, hospital emergency department, office, nursing facility), the services in the initial site may be separately reported. Modifier 25 may be added to the other evaluation and management service to indicate a significant, separately identifiable service by the same physician or other qualified health care professional was performed on the same date.

In the case when the services in a separate site are reported and the initial inpatient or observation care service is a consultation service, do not report 99221, 99222, 99223, 99252, 99253, 99254, 99255. The consultant reports the subsequent hospital inpatient or observation care codes 99231, 99232, 99233 for the second service on the same date.

If a consultation is performed in anticipation of, or related to, an admission by another physician or other qualified health care professional, and then the same consultant performs an encounter once the patient is admitted by the other physician or other qualified health care professional, report the consultant's inpatient encounter with the appropriate subsequent care code (99231, 99232, 99233). This instruction applies whether the consultation occurred on the date of the admission or a date previous to the admission. It also applies for consultations reported with any appropriate code (eg, office or other outpatient visit or office or other outpatient consultation).

For a patient admitted and discharged from hospital inpatient or observation status on the same date, report 99234, 99235, 99236, as appropriate.

For the purpose of reporting an initial hospital inpatient or observation care service, a transition from observation level to inpatient does not constitute a new stay. ◄

Rationale

Observation care codes 99217, 99218-99220, and 99224-99226 have been deleted, and the hospital inpatient codes 99221-99239 and inpatient consultation codes 99252-99255 have been revised to include observation care. The title of the Hospital Inpatient Services subsection has been revised to "Hospital Inpatient and Observation Care Services" because of the common confusion about inpatient and observation services. These code families have been combined to directly address the administration burden in the current code structure. The "Initial Hospital Care" and "Subsequent Hospital Care" headings have also been revised accordingly. The Inpatient Consultations subsection has been revised to "Inpatient or Observation Consultations."

In addition to the inclusion of observation care services, the hospital inpatient services codes 99221-99223 and 99231-99233, office or other outpatient consultation codes 99242-99245, and inpatient consultation codes 99252-99255 have been revised to be reported based on either total time or MDM level, and require a medically appropriate history and/or examination. Each code indicates the total time that must be met or exceeded in order to be reported. Office or other outpatient consultation code 99241 and inpatient consultation code 99251 have been deleted.

The guidelines have been revised to provide guidance on the appropriate reporting of these codes. It is important to review these guidelines before reporting the codes.

Refer to the codebook and the Rationale for the E/M introductory guidelines for a full discussion of these changes.

★=Telemedicine   ◄=Audio-only   ✛=Add-on code   ✗=FDA approval pending   #=Resequenced code   ⊘=Modifier 51 exempt

▲ **99221** **Initial hospital inpatient or observation care,** per day, for the evaluation and management of a patient, which requires a medically appropriate history and/or examination and straightforward or low level medical decision making.

When using total time on the date of the encounter for code selection, 40 minutes must be met or exceeded.

▲ **99222** **Initial hospital inpatient or observation care,** per day, for the evaluation and management of a patient, which requires a medically appropriate history and/or examination and moderate level of medical decision making.

When using total time on the date of the encounter for code selection, 55 minutes must be met or exceeded.

▲ **99223** **Initial hospital inpatient or observation care,** per day, for the evaluation and management of a patient, which requires a medically appropriate history and/or examination and high level of medical decision making.

When using total time on the date of the encounter for code selection, 75 minutes must be met or exceeded.

▶(For services of 90 minutes or longer, use prolonged services code 99418)◀

Clinical Example (99221)

A patient with an acute uncomplicated illness or injury is admitted for either initial inpatient or observation care services.

Description of Procedure (99221)

Review available prior medical records and data, place requests for other records and data as necessary for the new patient visit/observation/admission service. Coordinate with other members of the health care team regarding the observation/admission service. Visit patient location (eg, floor, observation area, unit) and confirm patient's identity. Review the medical history with patient and/or family/caregiver. Review vital signs obtained by clinical staff. Obtain a medically appropriate history. Synthesize all the information, including the relevant history and physical examination, to formulate a differential diagnosis and treatment plan (requiring straightforward or low medical decision making [MDM]). Consider patient's discharge needs. Discuss treatment plan with patient and/or family/caregiver. Provide patient education and respond to questions from patient and/or family/caregiver. Write and/or review observation or inpatient admission orders, including arranging for necessary diagnostic testing, consultation(s), and therapeutic intervention(s). Document the encounters throughout the calendar day in the medical record. Address interval data obtained and reported changes in condition. Communicate results and additional care plans to other health care

professionals and to the patient and/or family/caregivers throughout the calendar day. Perform electronic data capture and reporting to comply with quality payment program and other electronic mandates. Answer follow-up questions from patient and/or family/caregiver that may occur within the calendar day and respond to treatment failures.

Clinical Example (99222)

A patient with an acute illness with systemic symptoms or acute complicated injury is admitted for either initial inpatient or observation care services.

Description of Procedure (99222)

Review available prior medical records and data, place requests for other records and data as necessary for the new patient visit/observation/admission service. Coordinate with other members of the health care team regarding the observation/admission service. Visit patient location (eg, floor, observation area, unit) and confirm patient's identity. Review the medical history with patient and/or family/caregiver. Review vital signs obtained by clinical staff. Obtain a medically appropriate history. Synthesize all the information, including the relevant history and physical examination, to formulate a differential diagnosis and treatment plan (requiring moderate MDM). Consider patient's discharge needs. Discuss treatment plan with patient and/or family/caregiver. Provide patient education and respond to questions from the patient and/or family/caregiver. Write and/or review observation or inpatient admission orders, including arranging for necessary diagnostic testing, consultation(s), and therapeutic intervention(s). Document the encounters throughout the calendar day in the medical record. Address interval data obtained and reported changes in condition. Communicate results and additional care plans to other health care professionals and to the patient and/or family/caregivers throughout the calendar day. Perform electronic data capture and reporting to comply with quality payment program and other electronic mandates. Answer follow-up questions from patient and/or family/caregiver that may occur within the calendar day and respond to treatment failures.

Clinical Example (99223)

A patient with a chronic illness with severe exacerbation, or an acute illness/injury that poses a threat to life or bodily function, is admitted for either initial inpatient or observation care services.

Description of Procedure (99223)

Review available prior medical records and data, place requests for other records and data as necessary for the new patient visit/observation/admission service. Coordinate with other members of the health care team regarding the observation/admission service. Visit patient location (eg, floor, observation area, unit) and confirm patient's identity. Review the medical history with patient and/or family/caregiver. Review vital signs obtained by clinical staff. Obtain a medically appropriate history. Synthesize all the information, including the relevant history and physical examination, to formulate a differential diagnosis and treatment plan (requiring high MDM). Consider patient's discharge needs. Discuss treatment plan with patient and family/caregiver. Provide patient education and respond to questions from the patient and/or family/caregiver. Write and/or review observation or inpatient admission orders, including arranging for necessary diagnostic testing, consultation(s), and therapeutic intervention(s). Document the encounters throughout the calendar day in the medical record. Address interval data obtained and reported changes in condition. Communicate results and additional care plans to other health care professionals and to patient and/or family/caregivers throughout the calendar day. Perform electronic data capture and reporting to comply with quality payment program and other electronic mandates. Answer follow-up questions from patient and/or family/caregiver that may occur within the calendar day and respond to treatment failures.

▶Subsequent Hospital Inpatient or Observation Care◀

★▲ 99231   **Subsequent hospital inpatient or observation care,** per day, for the evaluation and management of a patient, which requires a medically appropriate history and/or examination and straightforward or low level of medical decision making.

When using total time on the date of the encounter for code selection, 25 minutes must be met or exceeded.

★▲ 99232   **Subsequent hospital inpatient or observation care,** per day, for the evaluation and management of a patient, which requires a medically appropriate history and/or examination and moderate level of medical decision making.

When using total time on the date of the encounter for code selection, 35 minutes must be met or exceeded.

★▲ 99233   **Subsequent hospital inpatient or observation care,** per day, for the evaluation and management of a patient, which requires a medically appropriate history and/or examination and high level of medical decision making.

When using total time on the date of the encounter for code selection, 50 minutes must be met or exceeded.

▶(For services of 65 minutes or longer, use prolonged services code 99418)◀

Clinical Example (99231)

A patient with an acute illness or injury whose condition is improving or is stable receives subsequent hospital inpatient or observation care.

Description of Procedure (99231)

If necessary, review interval correspondence, referral notes, and medical records generated since the last visit/observation/admission service. Coordinate with other members of the health care team regarding the observation/admission service. Visit patient location (eg, floor, observation area, unit) and confirm patient's identity. Review the medical history with the patient as well as the prior clinical notes. Review vital signs obtained by clinical staff. Obtain a medically appropriate history. Update pertinent components of history of present illness (HPI), review of systems, social history, family history, and allergies, and reconcile the patient's medications. Perform a medically appropriate examination. Synthesize all the information, including the relevant history and physical examination, to formulate a differential diagnosis and treatment plan (requiring straightforward or low MDM). Consider patient's discharge needs. Discuss treatment plan with patient and family/caregiver. Provide patient education and respond to questions from the patient and/or family/caregiver. Write and/or review observation or inpatient admission orders, including arranging for necessary diagnostic testing, consultation(s), and therapeutic intervention(s). Document the encounters throughout the calendar day in the medical record. Address interval data obtained and reported changes in condition. Communicate results and additional care plans to other health care professionals and to the patient and/or family and/or caregivers throughout the calendar day. Perform electronic data capture and reporting to comply with quality payment program and other electronic mandates. Answer follow-up questions from patient and/or family/caregiver that may occur within the calendar day and respond to treatment failures.

Clinical Example (99232)

A patient with an illness or acute injury that is progressing or requires ongoing diagnostic evaluation, medical management, or potential surgical treatment receives subsequent hospital inpatient or observation care.

Description of Procedure (99232)

If necessary, review interval correspondence, referral notes, and medical records generated since the last visit/observation/admission service. Coordinate with other members of the health care team regarding the observation/admission service. Visit patient location (eg, floor, observation area, unit) and confirm patient's identity. Review the medical history with the patient as well as the prior clinical notes. Review vital signs obtained by clinical staff. Obtain a medically appropriate history. Update pertinent components of HPI, review of systems, social history, family history, and allergies and reconcile the patient's medications. Perform a medically appropriate examination. Synthesize all the information, including the relevant history and physical examination, to formulate a differential diagnosis and treatment plan (requiring moderate MDM). Consider patient's discharge needs. Discuss treatment plan with patient and/or family/caregiver. Provide patient education and respond to questions from the patient and/or family/caregiver. Write and/or review observation or inpatient admission orders, including arranging for necessary diagnostic testing, consultation(s), and therapeutic intervention(s). Document the encounters throughout the calendar day in the medical record. Address interval data obtained and reported changes in condition. Communicate results and additional care plans to other health care professionals and to the patient and/or family/caregivers throughout the calendar day. Perform electronic data capture and reporting to comply with quality payment program and other electronic mandates. Answer follow-up questions from patient and/or family/caregiver that may occur within the calendar day and respond to treatment failures.

Clinical Example (99233)

A patient who is unstable or has developed a significant complication or a significant new problem receives subsequent hospital inpatient or observation care encounter.

Description of Procedure (99233)

If necessary, review interval correspondence, referral notes, and medical records generated since the last visit/observation/admission service. Coordinate with other members of the health care team regarding the observation/admission service. Visit patient location (eg,

floor, observation area, unit) and confirm patient's identity. Review the medical history with the patient as well as the prior clinical notes. Review vital signs obtained by clinical staff. Obtain a medically appropriate history. Update pertinent components of HPI, review of systems, social history, family history, and allergies and reconcile the patient's medications. Perform a medically appropriate examination. Synthesize all the information, including the relevant history and physical examination, to formulate a differential diagnosis and treatment plan (requiring high MDM). Consider patient's discharge needs. Discuss treatment plan with patient and/or family/caregiver. Provide patient education and respond to questions from the patient and/or family/caregiver. Write and/or review observation or inpatient admission orders, including arranging for necessary diagnostic testing, consultation(s), and therapeutic intervention(s). Document the encounters throughout the calendar day in the medical record. Address interval data obtained and reported changes in condition. Communicate results and additional care plans to other health care professionals and to the patient and/or family/caregivers throughout the calendar day. Perform electronic data capture and reporting to comply with quality payment program and other electronic mandates. Answer follow-up questions from patient and/or family/caregiver that may occur within the calendar day and respond to treatment failures.

▶Hospital Inpatient or Observation Care Services (Including Admission and Discharge Services)◀

▶The following codes are used to report hospital inpatient or observation care services provided to patients admitted and discharged on the same date of service.

For patients admitted to hospital inpatient or observation care and discharged on a different date, see 99221, 99222, 99223, 99231, 99232, 99233, 99238, 99239.

Codes 99234, 99235, 99236 require two or more encounters on the same date of which one of these encounters is an initial admission encounter and another encounter being a discharge encounter. For a patient admitted and discharged at the same encounter (ie, one encounter), see 99221, 99222, 99223. Do not report 99238, 99239 in conjunction with 99221, 99222, 99223 for admission and discharge services performed on the same date.◀

▶(For discharge services provided to newborns admitted and discharged on the same date, use 99463)◀

▲ **99234** **Hospital inpatient or observation care,** for the evaluation and management of a patient including admission and discharge on the same date, which requires a medically appropriate history and/or examination and straightforward or low level of medical decision making.

When using total time on the date of the encounter for code selection, 45 minutes must be met or exceeded.

▲ **99235** **Hospital inpatient or observation care,** for the evaluation and management of a patient including admission and discharge on the same date, which requires a medically appropriate history and/or examination and moderate level of medical decision making.

When using total time on the date of the encounter for code selection, 70 minutes must be met or exceeded.

▲ **99236** **Hospital inpatient or observation care,** for the evaluation and management of a patient including admission and discharge on the same date, which requires a medically appropriate history and/or examination and high level of medical decision making.

When using total time on the date of the encounter for code selection, 85 minutes must be met or exceeded.

▶(For services of 100 minutes or longer, use prolonged services code 99418)◀

Clinical Example (99234)

A patient with an acute, uncomplicated illness or injury is admitted for either initial inpatient or observation care services. The patient is discharged later that same day. (This service includes two or more encounters on the same date, one of which one is an initial admission encounter and the other is a discharge encounter.)

Description of Procedure (99234)

Review available prior medical records and data, place requests for other records and data as necessary for the new patient visit/observation/admission service. Coordinate with other members of the health care team regarding the observation/admission service. Visit patient location (eg, floor, observation area, unit) and confirm patient's identity. Review the medical history with the patient and/or family/caregiver. Review vital signs obtained by clinical staff. Obtain a medically appropriate history. Synthesize all the information, including the relevant history and physical examination, to formulate a differential diagnosis and treatment plan (requiring straightforward or low MDM). Consider patient's discharge needs. Discuss treatment plan with patient and family/caregiver. Provide patient education and respond to questions from the patient and/or family/caregiver. Write and/or review observation or inpatient admission

orders, including arranging for necessary diagnostic testing, consultation(s), and therapeutic intervention(s). Document the encounters throughout the calendar day in the medical record. Address interval data obtained and reported changes in condition. Communicate results and additional care plans to other health care professionals and to the patient and/or family/caregivers throughout the calendar day. Provide care coordination for the transition, including instructions to caregivers for aftercare. Arrange for post-discharge follow-up professional services and testing. Reconcile patient's medications with attention to pre-admission therapy, observation therapy, and outpatient formulary; write prescriptions as necessary. Perform electronic data capture and reporting to comply with quality payment program and other electronic mandates. Answer follow-up questions from patient and/or family/caregiver that may occur within the calendar day, and prior to discharge, respond to treatment failures during the admission.

Clinical Example (99235)

A patient with an acute illness with systemic symptoms or a patient with an acute complicated injury that requires medical management or potential surgical treatment is admitted for either initial inpatient or observation care services. The patient is discharged later that same day. (This service includes two or more encounters on the same date, one of which is an initial admission encounter and the other is a discharge encounter.)

Description of Procedure (99235)

Review available prior medical records and data, place requests for other records and data as necessary for the new patient visit/observation/admission service. Coordinate with other members of the health care team regarding the observation/admission service. Visit patient location (eg, floor, observation area, unit) and confirm patient's identity. Review the medical history with the patient and/or family/caregiver. Review vital signs obtained by clinical staff. Obtain a medically appropriate history. Synthesize all the information, including the relevant history and physical examination, to formulate a differential diagnosis and treatment plan (requiring moderate MDM). Consider patient's discharge needs. Discuss treatment plan with patient and/or family/caregiver. Provide patient education and respond to questions from the patient and/or family/caregiver. Write and/or review observation or inpatient admission orders, including arranging for necessary diagnostic testing, consultation(s), and therapeutic intervention(s).

★ = Telemedicine ◀ = Audio-only ✚ = Add-on code 🗲 = FDA approval pending # = Resequenced code ⊘ = Modifier 51 exempt

Document the encounters throughout the calendar day in the medical record. Address interval data obtained and reported changes in condition. Communicate results and additional care plans to other health care professionals and to the patient and/or family/caregivers throughout the calendar day. Provide care coordination for the transition, including instructions to caregivers for aftercare. Arrange for post-discharge follow-up professional services and testing. Reconcile patient's medications with attention to pre-admission therapy, observation therapy, and outpatient formulary; write prescriptions as necessary. Perform electronic data capture and reporting to comply with quality payment program and other electronic mandates. Answer follow-up questions from patient and/or family/caregiver that may occur within the calendar day, and prior to discharge, respond to treatment failures during the admission.

Clinical Example (99236)

A patient with a severe exacerbation of a chronic illness or an acute illness/injury that poses a threat to life or bodily function is admitted for either initial inpatient or observation care services. The patient is discharged later that same day. (This service includes two or more encounters on the same date, one of which is an initial admission encounter and the other is a discharge encounter.)

Description of Procedure (99236)

Review available prior medical records and data, place requests for other records and data as necessary for the new patient visit/observation/admission service. Coordinate with other members of the health care team regarding the observation/admission service. Visit patient location (eg, floor, observation area, unit) and confirm patient's identity. Review the medical history with the patient and/or family/caregiver. Review vital signs obtained by clinical staff. Obtain a medically appropriate history. Synthesize all the information, including the relevant history and physical examination, to formulate a differential diagnosis and treatment plan (requiring high MDM). Consider patient's discharge needs. Discuss treatment plan with patient and/or family/caregiver. Provide patient education and respond to questions from the patient and/or family/caregiver. Write and/or review observation or inpatient admission orders, including arranging for necessary diagnostic testing, consultation(s), and therapeutic intervention(s). Document the encounters throughout the calendar day in the medical record. Address interval data obtained and reported changes in condition. Communicate results and additional care plans to other health care professionals and to the patient and/or family/caregivers throughout the calendar day. Provide care coordination for the transition, including instructions to caregivers for

aftercare. Arrange for post-discharge follow-up professional services and testing. Reconcile patient's medications with attention to pre-admission therapy, observation therapy, and outpatient formulary; write prescriptions as necessary. Perform electronic data capture and reporting to comply with quality payment program and other electronic mandates. Answer follow-up questions from patient and/or family/caregiver that may occur within the calendar day, and prior to discharge, respond to treatment failures during the admission.

▶Hospital Inpatient or Observation Discharge Services◀

▶The hospital inpatient or observation discharge day management codes are to be used to report the total duration of time on the date of the encounter spent by a physician or other qualified health care professional for final hospital or observation discharge of a patient, even if the time spent by the physician or other qualified health care professional on that date is not continuous. The codes include, as appropriate, final examination of the patient, discussion of the hospital stay, instructions for continuing care to all relevant caregivers, and preparation of discharge records, prescriptions, and referral forms. These codes are to be utilized to report all services provided to a patient on the date of discharge, if other than the initial date of inpatient or observation status. For a patient admitted and discharged from hospital inpatient or observation status on the same date, report 99234, 99235, 99236, as appropriate.

Codes 99238, 99239 are to be used by the physician or other qualified health care professional who is responsible for discharge services. Services by other physicians or other qualified health care professionals that may include instructions to the patient and/or family/caregiver and coordination of post-discharge services may be reported with 99231, 99232, 99233.◀

▲ 99238 **Hospital inpatient or observation discharge day management**; 30 minutes or less on the date of the encounter

▲ 99239 more than 30 minutes on the date of the encounter

▶(For hospital inpatient or observation care including the admission and discharge of the patient on the same date, see 99234, 99235, 99236)◀

(For discharge services provided to newborns admitted and discharged on the same date, use 99463)

Clinical Example (99238)

A patient receives hospital inpatient or observation discharge day management services requiring 30 minutes or less of total time.

Description of Procedure (99238)

Review medical records and other available data. Obtain an interval history and perform a physical examination. Formulate and/or revise diagnosis and treatment plan(s), including making the decision for discharge. Review information regarding availability, safety, and adequacy of post-discharge support systems. Discuss aftercare treatment with patient, family, and/or caregivers and other health care professionals. Provide care coordination for transition that includes instructions to patient and/or family/caregivers for aftercare. Write orders for post-discharge follow-up professional services and testing as necessary. Reconcile patient's medications with attention to pre-admission therapy, inpatient/observation therapy, and outpatient formulary. Write prescriptions as necessary. Complete discharge and aftercare forms. Inform referring physician of discharge plans. Complete medical record documentation.

Clinical Example (99239)

A patient receives hospital inpatient or observation discharge day management services requiring greater than 30 minutes of total time.

Description of Procedure (99239)

Review medical records and other available data. Obtain an interval history and perform a physical examination. Formulate and/or revise diagnosis and treatment plan(s), including making the decision for discharge. Review information regarding availability, safety, and adequacy of post-discharge support systems. Discuss aftercare treatment with patient and/or family/caregiver and other health care professionals. Provide care coordination for transition that includes instructions to patient and/or family/caregivers for aftercare. Write orders for post-discharge follow-up professional services and testing as necessary. Reconcile patient's medications with attention to pre-admission therapy, inpatient/observation therapy, and outpatient formulary. Write prescriptions as necessary. Complete discharge and aftercare forms. Inform referring physician of discharge plans. Complete medical record documentation.

Consultations

▶A consultation is a type of evaluation and management service provided at the request of another physician, other qualified health care professional, or appropriate source to recommend care for a specific condition or problem.

A physician or other qualified health care professional consultant may initiate diagnostic and/or therapeutic services at the same or subsequent visit.

A "consultation" initiated by a patient and/or family, and not requested by a physician, other qualified health care professional, or other appropriate source (eg, non-clinical social worker, educator, lawyer, or insurance company), is not reported using the consultation codes.

The consultant's opinion and any services that were ordered or performed must also be communicated by written report to the requesting physician, other qualified health care professional, or other appropriate source.◀

If a consultation is mandated (eg, by a third-party payer) modifier 32 should also be reported.

▶To report services when a patient is admitted to hospital inpatient, or observation status, or to a nursing facility in the course of an encounter in another setting, see **Initial Hospital Inpatient or Observation Care** or **Initial Nursing Facility Care.**◀

Office or Other Outpatient Consultations

New or Established Patient

▶The following codes may be used to report consultations that are provided in the office or other outpatient site, including the home or residence, or emergency department. Follow-up visits in the consultant's office or other outpatient facility that are initiated by the consultant or patient are reported using the appropriate codes for established patients in the office (99212, 99213, 99214, 99215) or home or residence (99347, 99348, 99349, 99350). Services that constitute transfer of care (ie, are provided for the management of the patient's entire care or for the care of a specific condition or problem) are reported with the appropriate new or established patient codes for office or other outpatient visits or home or residence services.◀

> ▶(For an outpatient consultation requiring prolonged services, use 99417)◀
>
> ▶(99241 has been deleted. To report, use 99242)◀

★▲ **99242** **Office or other outpatient consultation** for a new or established patient, which requires a medically appropriate history and/or examination and straightforward medical decision making.

When using total time on the date of the encounter for code selection, 20 minutes must be met or exceeded.

★▲ **99243** **Office or other outpatient consultation** for a new or established patient, which requires a medically appropriate history and/or examination and low level of medical decision making.

When using total time on the date of the encounter for code selection, 30 minutes must be met or exceeded.

★ = Telemedicine   ◀ = Audio-only   ✚ = Add-on code   ✚ = FDA approval pending   # = Resequenced code   ⊘ = Modifier 51 exempt

★▲ **99244** **Office or other outpatient consultation** for a new or established patient, which requires a medically appropriate history and/or examination and moderate level of medical decision making.

When using total time on the date of the encounter for code selection, 40 minutes must be met or exceeded.

★▲ **99245** **Office or other outpatient consultation** for a new or established patient, which requires a medically appropriate history and/or examination and high level of medical decision making.

When using total time on the date of the encounter for code selection, 55 minutes must be met or exceeded.

▶(For services 70 minutes or longer, use prolonged services code 99417)◀

Clinical Example (99242)

A requested office consultation, which includes review of relevant data and a medically appropriate history and/or examination, is performed. The problem is determined to be self-limited. A report is generated and sent to the requesting provider.

Description of Procedure (99242)

Physician or other qualified health care professional (QHP) typical activities performed within 3 calendar days prior to the office or outpatient consultation and within 7 calendar days after the day of the consultation include the following: Review the referring physician or other QHP request for the consultant's expert opinion regarding evaluation and/or management of a specific medical problem. Document the request for the consultation in the medical record. Obtain and review prior medical records, including laboratory test results and imaging, if available. Order and review additional diagnostic laboratory tests, imaging, and/or other tests, as needed. Incorporate pertinent information into the medical record. Review the medical history forms completed by the patient. Review vital signs obtained by clinical staff. Obtain a medically appropriate history. Perform a medically appropriate examination. Synthesize the relevant history, physical examination, and test results to formulate a differential diagnosis requiring straightforward MDM. Discuss the findings with the patient and/or family/caregiver and respond to their questions. Document the encounter in the medical record. Perform electronic data capture and reporting to comply with quality payment program and other electronic mandates. Generate a written report that identifies additional laboratory tests, imaging, and/or tests ordered and reviewed, test findings, and expert opinion for management of the patient to the requesting provider. Document the report in the medical record. Communicate with other members of the health care team regarding the visit. Respond to follow-up questions

from the requesting physician or other QHP and patient/family/caregiver.

Clinical Example (99243)

A requested office consultation, which includes review of the relevant data and a medically appropriate history and/or examination, is performed. The problem is determined to be an acute uncomplicated illness or injury. A report is generated and sent to the requesting provider.

Description of Procedure (99243)

Physician or other QHP typical activities performed within 3 calendar days prior to the office or outpatient consultation and within 7 calendar days after the day of the consultation include the following: Review the referring physician or other QHP request for the consultant's expert opinion regarding evaluation and/or management of a specific medical problem. Document the request for the consultation in the medical record. Obtain and review prior medical records, including laboratory test results and imaging, if available. Order and review additional diagnostic laboratory tests, imaging, and/or other tests, as needed. Incorporate pertinent information into the medical record. Review the medical history forms completed by the patient. Review vital signs obtained by clinical staff. Obtain a medically appropriate history. Perform a medically appropriate examination. Synthesize the relevant history, physical examination, and tests to formulate a differential diagnosis requiring low MDM. Discuss the findings with the patient and/or family/caregiver and respond to their questions. Document the encounter in the medical record. Perform electronic data capture and reporting to comply with quality payment program and other electronic mandates. Generate a written report that identifies additional laboratory tests, imaging, and/or tests ordered and reviewed, test findings, and expert opinion for management of the patient to the requesting provider. Document the report in the medical record. Communicate with other members of the health care team regarding the visit. Respond to follow-up questions from the requesting physician or other QHP and patient/family/caregiver.

Clinical Example (99244)

A requested office consultation, which includes review of the relevant data and a medically appropriate history and/or examination, is performed. The problem is determined to be an undiagnosed new problem with uncertain prognosis or chronic illness with progression. A report is generated and sent to the requesting provider.

Description of Procedure (99244)

Physician or other QHP typical activities performed within 3 calendar days prior to the office or outpatient consultation and within 7 calendar days after the day of the consultation include the following: Review the referring physician or other QHP request for the consultant's expert opinion regarding evaluation and/or management of a specific medical problem. Document the request for the consultation in the medical record. Obtain and review prior medical records, including laboratory test results and imaging, if available. Order and review additional diagnostic laboratory results, imaging, and/or other tests, as needed. Incorporate pertinent information into the medical record. Review the medical history forms completed by the patient. Review vital signs obtained by clinical staff. Obtain a medically appropriate history. Perform a medically appropriate examination. Synthesize the relevant history, physical examination, and tests to formulate a differential diagnosis requiring moderate MDM. Discuss the findings with the patient and/or family/caregiver and respond to their questions. Document the encounter in the medical record. Perform electronic data capture and reporting to comply with quality payment program and other electronic mandates. Generate a written report that identifies additional laboratory tests, imaging, and/or tests ordered and reviewed, test findings, and expert opinion for management of the patient to the requesting provider. Document the report in the medical record. Communicate with other members of the health care team regarding the visit. Respond to follow-up questions from the requesting physician or other QHP and patient/family/caregiver.

Clinical Example (99245)

A requested office consultation, which includes review of the relevant data and a medically appropriate history and/or examination, is performed. The problem is determined to be a chronic illness with severe exacerbation, progression, or side effects of treatment. A report is generated and sent to the requesting provider.

Description of Procedure (99245)

Physician or other QHP typical activities performed within 3 calendar days prior to the office or outpatient consultation and within 7 calendar days after the day of the consultation include the following: Review the referring physician or other QHP request for the consultant's expert opinion regarding evaluation and/or management of a specific medical problem. Document the request for the consultation in the medical record. Obtain and review prior medical records, including laboratory test results and imaging, if available. Order and review additional diagnostic laboratory tests, imaging, and/or other tests, as needed. Incorporate

pertinent information into the medical record. Review the medical history forms completed by the patient. Review vital signs obtained by clinical staff. Obtain a medically appropriate history. Perform a medically appropriate examination. Synthesize the relevant history, physical examination, and tests to formulate a differential diagnosis requiring high MDM. Discuss the findings with the patient and/or family/caregiver and respond to their questions. Document the encounter in the medical record. Perform electronic data capture and reporting to comply with quality payment program and other electronic mandates. Generate a written report that identifies additional laboratory tests, imaging, and/or tests ordered and reviewed, test findings, and expert opinion for management of the patient to the requesting provider. Document the report in the medical record. Communicate with other members of the health care team regarding the visit. Respond to follow-up questions from the requesting physician or other QHP and patient/family/caregiver.

►Inpatient or Observation Consultations◄

New or Established Patient

►Codes 99252, 99253, 99254, 99255 are used to report physician or other qualified health care professional consultations provided to hospital inpatients, observation-level patients, residents of nursing facilities, or patients in a partial hospital setting, and when the patient has not received any face-to-face professional services from the physician or other qualified health care professional or another physician or other qualified health care professional of the exact same specialty and subspecialty who belongs to the same group practice during the stay. When advanced practice nurses and physician assistants are working with physicians, they are considered as working in the exact same specialty and subspecialty as the physician. Only one consultation may be reported by a consultant per admission. Subsequent consultation services during the same admission are reported using subsequent inpatient or observation hospital care codes (99231-99233) or subsequent nursing facility care codes (99307-99310).◄

►(For an inpatient or observation consultation requiring prolonged services, use 99418)◄

►(99251 has been deleted. To report, use 99252)◄

★▲ **99252** **Inpatient or observation consultation** for a new or established patient, which requires a medically appropriate history and/or examination and straightforward medical decision making.

When using total time on the date of the encounter for code selection, 35 minutes must be met or exceeded.

★=Telemedicine   ◄=Audio-only   ✚=Add-on code   ✗=FDA approval pending   #=Resequenced code   ⊘=Modifier 51 exempt

★▲ **99253**   **Inpatient or observation consultation** for a new or established patient, which requires a medically appropriate history and/or examination and low level of medical decision making.

> When using total time on the date of the encounter for code selection, 45 minutes must be met or exceeded.

★▲ **99254**   **Inpatient or observation consultation** for a new or established patient, which requires a medically appropriate history and/or examination and moderate level of medical decision making.

> When using total time on the date of the encounter for code selection, 60 minutes must be met or exceeded.

★▲ **99255**   **Inpatient or observation consultation** for a new or established patient, which requires a medically appropriate history and/or examination and high level of medical decision making.

> When using total time on the date of the encounter for code selection, 80 minutes must be met or exceeded.

▶(For services 95 minutes or longer, use prolonged services code 99418)◀

Clinical Example (99252)

A requested inpatient consultation, which includes review of the relevant data and a medically appropriate history and/or examination, is performed. The problem is determined to be self-limited. A report is generated and sent to the requesting provider.

Description of Procedure (99252)

Review the referring physician or other QHP request for the consultant's expert opinion for management of a specific medical problem. Review available prior medical records, including laboratory test results and imaging, if available. Order and review additional diagnostic laboratory tests, as necessary for the consultation. Incorporate pertinent information into the medical record. Coordinate with other members of the health care team. Visit patient location (eg, floor, observation area, unit) and confirm patient's identity. Review the medical history with the patient and/or family/caregiver. Review vital signs obtained by clinical staff. Obtain a medically appropriate history. Synthesize all the information, including the relevant history and physical examination, to formulate a differential diagnosis requiring straightforward MDM. Discuss the findings with the patient and/or family/caregiver. Provide patient education and respond to questions from the patient and/or family/caregiver. Document the encounter in the medical record. Perform electronic data capture and reporting to comply with quality payment program and other electronic mandates. Generate a written report that identifies additional laboratory tests, imaging, and/or tests ordered and reviewed, test findings, and expert

opinion for management of the patient to the requesting provider. Document the report in the medical record. Communicate with other members of the health care team regarding the consultation. Respond to follow-up questions from the requesting physician or other QHP and patient/family/caregiver.

Clinical Example (99253)

A requested inpatient consultation, which includes review of the relevant data and a medically appropriate history and/or examination, is performed. The problem is determined to be an acute uncomplicated illness or injury. A report is generated and sent to the requesting provider.

Description of Procedure (99253)

Review the referring physician or other QHP request for the consultant's expert opinion for management of a specific medical problem. Review available prior medical records, including laboratory test results and imaging, if available. Order and review additional diagnostic laboratory tests, as necessary for the consultation. Incorporate pertinent information into the medical record. Coordinate with other members of the health care team. Visit patient location (eg, floor, observation area, unit) and confirm patient's identity. Review the medical history with the patient and/or family/caregiver. Review vital signs obtained by clinical staff. Obtain a medically appropriate history. Synthesize all the information, including the relevant history and physical examination, to formulate a differential diagnosis requiring low MDM. Discuss the findings with the patient and/or family/caregiver. Provide patient education and respond to questions from the patient and/or family/caregiver. Document the encounter in the medical record. Perform electronic data capture and reporting to comply with quality payment program and other electronic mandates. Generate a written report that identifies additional laboratory tests, imaging, and/or tests ordered and reviewed, test findings, and expert opinion for management of the patient to the requesting provider. Document the report in the medical record. Communicate with other members of the health care team regarding the consultation. Respond to follow-up questions from the requesting physician or other QHP and patient/family/caregiver.

Clinical Example (99254)

A requested inpatient consultation, which includes review of the relevant data and a medically appropriate history and/or examination, is performed. The problem is determined to be an undiagnosed new problem with uncertain prognosis or chronic illness with progression. A report is generated and sent to the requesting provider.

Description of Procedure (99254)

Review the referring physician or other QHP request for the consultant's expert opinion for management of a specific medical problem. Review available prior medical records, including laboratory test results and imaging, if available. Order and review additional diagnostic laboratory tests, as necessary for the consultation. Incorporate pertinent information into the medical record. Coordinate with other members of the health care team. Visit patient location (eg, floor, observation area, unit) and confirm patient's identity. Review the medical history with the patient and/or family/caregiver. Review vital signs obtained by clinical staff. Obtain a medically appropriate history. Synthesize all the information, including the relevant history and physical examination, to formulate a differential diagnosis requiring moderate MDM. Discuss the findings with the patient and/or family/caregiver. Provide patient education and respond to questions from the patient and/or family/caregiver. Document the encounter in the medical record. Perform electronic data capture and reporting to comply with quality payment program and other electronic mandates. Generate a written report that identifies additional laboratory tests, imaging, and/or tests ordered and reviewed, test findings, and expert opinion for management of the patient to the requesting provider. Document the report in the medical record. Communicate with other members of the health care team regarding the consultation. Respond to follow-up questions from the requesting physician or other QHP and patient/family/caregiver.

Clinical Example (99255)

A requested inpatient consultation, which includes review of the relevant data and a medically appropriate history and/or examination, is performed. The problem is determined to be a chronic illness with severe exacerbation, progression, or side effects of treatment. A report is generated and sent to the requesting provider.

Description of Procedure (99255)

Review the referring physician or other QHP request for the consultant's expert opinion for management of a specific medical problem. Review available prior medical records, including laboratory test results and imaging, if available. Order and review additional diagnostic laboratory tests, as necessary for the consultation. Incorporate pertinent information into the medical record. Coordinate with other members of the health care team. Visit patient location (eg, floor, observation area, unit) and confirm patient's identity. Review the medical history with the patient and/or family/caregiver. Review vital signs obtained by clinical staff. Obtain a medically appropriate history. Synthesize all the information, including the relevant history and physical

examination, to formulate a differential diagnosis requiring high MDM. Discuss the findings with the patient and/or family/caregiver. Provide patient education and respond to questions from the patient and/or family/caregiver. Document the encounter in the medical record. Perform electronic data capture and reporting to comply with quality payment program and other electronic mandates. Generate a written report that identifies additional laboratory tests, imaging, and/or tests ordered and reviewed, test findings, and expert opinion for management of the patient to the requesting provider. Document the report in the medical record. Communicate with other members of the health care team regarding the consultation. Respond to follow-up questions from the requesting physician or other QHP and patient/family/caregiver.

Emergency Department Services

New or Established Patient

The following codes are used to report evaluation and management services provided in the emergency department. No distinction is made between new and established patients in the emergency department.

An emergency department is defined as an organized hospital-based facility for the provision of unscheduled episodic services to patients who present for immediate medical attention. The facility must be available 24 hours a day.

▶For critical care services provided in the emergency department, see Critical Care guidelines and 99291, 99292. Critical care and emergency department services may both be reported on the same day when after completion of the emergency department service, the condition of the patient changes and critical care services are provided.

For evaluation and management services provided to a patient in observation status, see 99221, 99222, 99223 for the initial observation encounter and 99231, 99232, 99233, 99238, 99239 for subsequent or discharge hospital inpatient or observation encounters.

For hospital inpatient or observation care services (including admission and discharge services), see 99234, 99235, 99236.

To report services when a patient is admitted to hospital inpatient or observation status, or to a nursing facility in the course of an encounter in another setting, see **Initial Hospital Inpatient or Observation Care** or **Initial Nursing Facility Care**.

For procedures or services identified by a CPT code that may be separately reported on the same date, use the appropriate CPT code. Use the appropriate modifier(s) to report separately identifiable evaluation and management services and the extent of services provided in a surgical package.

If a patient is seen in the emergency department for the convenience of a physician or other qualified health care professional, use office or other outpatient services codes (99202-99215).◄

Coding Tip

Time as a Factor in the Emergency Department Setting

Time is **not** a descriptive component for the emergency department levels of E/M services because emergency department services are typically provided on a variable intensity basis, often involving multiple encounters with several patients over an extended period of time.

CPT Coding Guidelines, Evaluation and Management, Guidelines for Selecting Level of Service Based on Time

▲ **99281**   **Emergency department visit** for the evaluation and management of a patient that may not require the presence of a physician or other qualified health care professional

▲ **99282**   **Emergency department visit** for the evaluation and management of a patient, which requires a medically appropriate history and/or examination and straightforward medical decision making

▲ **99283**   **Emergency department visit** for the evaluation and management of a patient, which requires a medically appropriate history and/or examination and low level of medical decision making

▲ **99284**   **Emergency department visit** for the evaluation and management of a patient, which requires a medically appropriate history and/or examination and moderate level of medical decision making

▲ **99285**   **Emergency department visit** for the evaluation and management of a patient, which requires a medically appropriate history and/or examination and high level of medical decision making

Coding Tip

Emergency Department Classification of New vs Established Patient

No distinction is made between new and established patients in the emergency department. E/M services in the emergency department category may be reported for any new or established patient who presents for treatment in the emergency department.

CPT Coding Guidelines, Evaluation and Management, Classification of E/M Services, New and Established Patients

Rationale

In accordance with the standardization of level-based E/M codes, ED services codes 99281-99285 have been revised to be reported based on MDM level and require a medically appropriate history and/or examination. It is important to note that the code selection for these codes will remain the same, ie, they should not be reported based on total time on the date of the encounter.

The guidelines have been revised to provide guidance on the appropriate reporting of these codes. It is important to review these guidelines before reporting the codes.

Refer to the codebook and the Rationale for the E/M introductory guidelines for a full discussion of these changes.

Clinical Example (99281)

A patient presents to the emergency department (ED) for suture removal after repair of a forearm laceration by a different provider in another location. There are no complaints, and the wound appears well healed.

Description of Procedure (99281)

Obtain a medically appropriate history, including interviews with patient, prehospital personnel, family members, and caregivers in person or by phone as needed, and perform a medically appropriate physical examination. Formulate a diagnosis and develop a treatment plan (MDM is not a component). Enter orders in the electronic health record (EHR) during the evaluation of the patient and begin the documentation. Formulate a discharge plan. Discuss follow-up and reasons for return to the emergency department. Explain any prescriptions or other treatments and work, school, or activity restrictions. Answer patient and/or family/caregiver questions.

Clinical Example (99282)

A patient presents to the ED with a self-limited or minor problem.

Description of Procedure (99282)

Obtain a medically appropriate history, including interviews with patient, prehospital personnel, and family members in person or by phone as needed. Perform a medically appropriate examination; formulate a diagnosis and develop a treatment plan (straightforward MDM). Enter orders in the EHR during the evaluation of the patient and begin the medical record. Explain any prescriptions required along with discharge instructions and any follow-up care required, including reasons to return to the ED. Answer patient and/or family/caregiver questions.

Clinical Example (99283)

A patient presents to the ED with a stable chronic illness or acute uncomplicated injury.

Description of Procedure (99283)

Obtain a medically appropriate history, including interviews with patient, physician office, nursing home, or emergency medical services (EMS) personnel, and family members in person or by phone as needed, and perform a medically appropriate examination. Formulate a diagnosis and treatment plan (low MDM). Enter orders in the EHR during the evaluation of the patient and begin the medical record. Communicate with other health care professionals as necessary during the encounter. Evaluate response to therapy, review data from diagnostic testing, and reassess the patient. Formulate a discharge plan, including medication and other treatments as well as follow-up planning. Explain any prescriptions or other therapies required along with discharge instructions, activity limitations, and any follow-up care required, including reasons to return to the ED. Answer patient and/or family/caregiver questions.

Clinical Example (99284)

A patient presents to the ED with a progressing illness or acute injury that requires medical management or potential surgical treatment.

Description of Procedure (99284)

Obtain a medically appropriate history, including interviews with patient, physician office, nursing home, or EMS personnel, and family members and caregivers present or by phone as needed. Perform a medically appropriate physical examination. Formulate a diagnosis and treatment plan (moderate MDM). Enter orders in the EHR during the evaluation of the patient and begin the medical record. Communicate with other health care professionals as necessary during the encounter. Review data from diagnostic testing and evaluate response to therapy by reassessing the patient and then adjusting the treatment plan accordingly. Formulate a discharge plan, included needed medications, therapies, and work or activity restrictions and recommendations. Arrange and review follow-up. Explain any prescriptions and treatments required along with discharge instructions and any follow-up care required, including reasons to return to the ED. Answer patient and/or family/caregiver questions.

Clinical Example (99285)

A patient presents to the ED with a chronic illness with severe exacerbation that poses a threat to life or bodily function, or an acute illness/injury that poses a threat to life or bodily function.

Description of Procedure (99285)

Obtain a medically appropriate history, including interviews with patient, physician office, nursing home, or EMS personnel, and family members and caregivers present or by phone. Perform a medically appropriate physical examination. Formulate a diagnosis and treatment plan (high MDM). Enter orders in the EHR during the evaluation of the patient and begin the medical record. Review data from diagnostic testing, including laboratory tests, imaging, and imaging interpretation. Reassess the patient multiple times, order additional diagnostic tests as indicated, and adjust treatment plan accordingly. Communicate with other health care professionals as necessary for consultation or care coordination during the encounter. Formulate a disposition plan, including communication to and coordination with an inpatient team if appropriate, or more typically, prepare a discharge plan, with prescriptions and additional therapies, work or activity restrictions, and arrange follow-up appointments or testing as needed. Explain any prescriptions or other therapies as required along with discharge instructions, expected course, and any follow-up care required, including reasons to return to the ED. Answer patient and/or family/caregiver questions.

Nursing Facility Services

▶The following codes are used to report evaluation and management services to patients in nursing facilities and skilled nursing facilities. These codes should also be used to report evaluation and management services provided to a patient in a psychiatric residential treatment center and immediate care facility for individuals with intellectual disabilities.

Regulations pertaining to the care of nursing facility residents govern the nature and minimum frequency of assessments and visits. These regulations also govern who may perform the initial comprehensive visit.

These services are performed by the principal physician(s) and other qualified health care professional(s) overseeing the care of the patient in the facility. The principal physician is sometimes referred to as the admitting physician and is the physician who oversees the patient's care as opposed to other physicians or other qualified health care professionals who may be furnishing specialty care. These services are also performed by physicians or other qualified health care professionals in the role of a specialist performing a consultation or concurrent care. Modifiers may be required to identify the role of the individual performing the service.◀

Two major subcategories of nursing facility services are recognized: Initial Nursing Facility Care and Subsequent Nursing Facility Care. Both subcategories apply to new or established patients.

▶The types of care (eg, skilled nursing facility and nursing facility care) are reported with the same codes. Place of service codes should be reported to specify the type of facility (and care) where the service(s) is performed.

When selecting a level of medical decision making (MDM) for nursing facility services, the number and complexity of problems addressed at the encounter is considered. For this determination, a high-level MDM-type specific to initial nursing facility care by the principal physician or other qualified health care professional is recognized. This type is:

Multiple morbidities requiring intensive management: A set of conditions, syndromes, or functional impairments that are likely to require frequent medication changes or other treatment changes and/or re-evaluations. The patient is at significant risk of worsening medical (including behavioral) status and risk for (re)admission to a hospital.

The definitions and requirements related to the amount and/or complexity of data to be reviewed and analyzed and the risk of complications and/or morbidity or mortality of patient management are unchanged.◀

Initial Nursing Facility Care

New or Established Patient

▶When the patient is admitted to the nursing facility in the course of an encounter in another site of service (eg, hospital emergency department, office), the services in the initial site may be separately reported. Modifier 25 may be added to the other evaluation and management

service to indicate a significant, separately identifiable service by the same physician or other qualified health care professional was performed on the same date.

In the case when services in a separate site are reported and the initial nursing facility care service is a consultation service performed by the same physician or other qualified health care professional and reported on the same date, do not report 99252, 99253, 99254, 99255, 99304, 99305, 99306. The consultant reports the subsequent nursing facility care codes 99307, 99308, 99309, 99310 for the second service on the same date.

Hospital inpatient or observation discharge services performed on the same date of nursing facility admission or readmission may be reported separately. For a patient discharged from inpatient or observation status on the same date of nursing facility admission or readmission, the hospital or observation discharge services may be reported with codes 99238, 99239, as appropriate. For a patient admitted and discharged from hospital inpatient or observation status on the same date, see 99234, 99235, 99236. Time related to hospital inpatient or observation care services may not be used for code selection of any nursing facility service.

Initial nursing facility care codes 99304, 99305, 99306 may be used once per admission, per physician or other qualified health care professional, regardless of length of stay. They may be used for the initial comprehensive visit performed by the principal physician or other qualified health care professional. Skilled nursing facility initial comprehensive visits must be performed by a physician. Qualified health care professionals may report initial comprehensive nursing facility visits for nursing facility level of care patients, if allowed by state law or regulation. The principal physician or other qualified health care professional may work with others (who may not always be in the same group) but are overseeing the overall medical care of the patient, in order to provide timely care to the patient. Medically necessary assessments conducted by these professionals prior to the initial comprehensive visit are reported using subsequent care codes (99307, 99308, 99309, 99310).

Initial services by other physicians and other qualified health care professionals who are performing consultations may be reported using initial nursing facility care codes (99304, 99305, 99306) or inpatient or observation consultation codes (99252, 99253, 99254, 99255). This is not dependent upon the principal care professional's completion of the initial comprehensive services first.

An initial service may be reported when the patient has not received any face-to-face professional services from the physician or other qualified health care professional or another physician or other qualified health care professional of the exact same specialty and subspecialty who belongs to the same group practice during the stay.

When advanced practice nurses or physician assistants are working with physicians, they are considered as working in the exact same specialty and subspecialty as the physician. An initial service may also be reported if the patient is a new patient as defined in the Evaluation and Management Guidelines.

For reporting initial nursing facility care, transitions between skilled nursing facility level of care and nursing facility level of care do not constitute a new stay.◄

Rationale

In accordance with the standardization of level-based E/M codes, initial nursing facility care codes 99304-99306 and subsequent nursing facility care codes 99307-99310 have been revised to be reported based on either total time on the date of the encounter or MDM level and require a medically appropriate history and/or examination. Each code indicates the total time that must be met or exceeded in order to be reported. The guidelines have been revised to provide guidance on the appropriate reporting of these codes. It is important to review these guidelines before reporting the codes.

The guidelines for nursing facility discharge services codes 99315 and 99316 have been revised to clarify that the face-to-face encounter with the patient and/or family/caregiver may be performed on a date prior to the date of discharge, and that the total time of the face-to-face encounter should be used to report the service.

Other nursing facility services code 99318 has been deleted. These services will be reported with subsequent nursing facility care codes 99307-99310.

Refer to the codebook and the Rationale for the E/M introductory guidelines for a full discussion of these changes.

▲ 99304 Initial nursing facility care, per day, for the evaluation and management of a patient, which requires a medically appropriate history and/or examination and straightforward or low level of medical decision making.

When using total time on the date of the encounter for code selection, 25 minutes must be met or exceeded.

▲ 99305 Initial nursing facility care, per day, for the evaluation and management of a patient, which requires a medically appropriate history and/or examination and moderate level of medical decision making.

When using total time on the date of the encounter for code selection, 35 minutes must be met or exceeded.

▲ 99306 Initial nursing facility care, per day, for the evaluation and management of a patient, which requires a medically appropriate history and/or examination and high level of medical decision making.

When using total time on the date of the encounter for code selection, 45 minutes must be met or exceeded.

►(For services 60 minutes or longer, use prolonged services code 99418)◄

Clinical Example (99304)

Initial nursing facility visit for a patient with limited support at home receiving post-acute care for an operative procedure that was uncomplicated.

Description of Procedure (99304)

Obtain a detailed history and fluid intake and other health conditions from patient's family, assisted living staff, and other health care professionals as necessary. Note vital signs. Perform a comprehensive physical examination that includes inspecting skin for pre-ulcerations and ulcerations; evaluating patient's oral hygiene; cardiovascular, pulmonary, abdominal, and genitourinary (GU) examinations for evidence of obstructive urinary retention and fecal impaction; evaluating patient's ability to communicate; and assessing safety of patient's gait.

Clinical Example (99305)

Initial nursing facility visit for a patient recovering from an illness or acute injury that requires ongoing medical management of their multiple stable problems.

Description of Procedure (99305)

Obtain a comprehensive history and perform a comprehensive physical examination. Review patient's intake and hydration status, postoperative condition, initial rehabilitation results, and status of recent urosepsis and pressure ulcer. Evaluate status of patient's multiple chronic health problems. Examine patient's vision and hearing and neurological examination. Develop a multidisciplinary plan of care that includes physical therapy (PT) and occupational therapy (OT) services, initiation of a pressure wound care program, adjustments in diet, weaning off catheter, retitration of medications, evaluation of dietary and fluid intake, and monitoring for mental status changes due to changes in environment.

Clinical Example (99306)

Initial nursing facility visit for a patient with multiple morbidities requiring intensive management.

Description of Procedure (99306)

Obtain a comprehensive history and perform a comprehensive physical examination. Review patient's intake and hydration status and sliding scale insulin and psychotropic regimen. Discuss patient's multiple, still

★=Telemedicine ◀=Audio-only ✚=Add-on code ✗=FDA approval pending #=Resequenced code ⊘=Modifier 51 exempt

unstable, health problems with health care professionals. Assess current status of cardiopulmonary function, swallowing and mobility function, and cognitive function. Review laboratory test findings including oxygenation, hydration, white blood cell count (WBC), cardiac rhythm, and glucose level trends. Initiate orders for oxygen, intravenous (IV) fluids, antibiotics, pain control, rehabilitation, and diagnostic testing to assess status. Develop a multidisciplinary care plan that includes PT, respiratory therapy (RT), and speech services; titration off insulin sliding scale; adjustments in diet and hydration; retitration of psychotropic and analgesic medications; and monitoring for mental status changes.

Subsequent Nursing Facility Care

★▲ **99307** Subsequent nursing facility care, per day, for the evaluation and management of a patient, which requires a medically appropriate history and/or examination and straightforward medical decision making.

When using total time on the date of the encounter for code selection, 10 minutes must be met or exceeded.

★▲ **99308** Subsequent nursing facility care, per day, for the evaluation and management of a patient, which requires a medically appropriate history and/or examination and low level of medical decision making.

When using total time on the date of the encounter for code selection, 15 minutes must be met or exceeded.

★▲ **99309** Subsequent nursing facility care, per day, for the evaluation and management of a patient, which requires a medically appropriate history and/or examination and moderate level of medical decision making.

When using total time on the date of the encounter for code selection, 30 minutes must be met or exceeded.

★▲ **99310** Subsequent nursing facility care, per day, for the evaluation and management of a patient, which requires a medically appropriate history and/or examination and high level of medical decision making.

When using total time on the date of the encounter for code selection, 45 minutes must be met or exceeded.

▶(For services 60 minutes or longer, use prolonged services code 99418)◀

Clinical Example (99307)

Subsequent nursing facility visit for a patient with a self-limited or minor problem.

Description of Procedure (99307)

Obtain an interval history that reveals ongoing poor dietary intake and urinary incontinence in a patient who

cannot participate in pressure relief activities because of cognitive impairment. Perform a focused physical examination that reveals an improving lesion with no peripheral inflammation and no evidence of systemic involvement. As a result, alter patient's topical regimen, order a new nutritional program, and authorize a support surface.

Clinical Example (99308)

Subsequent nursing facility visit for a patient with a stable chronic illness or recovering from an acute uncomplicated injury.

Description of Procedure (99308)

Obtain an expanded history that includes intake and hydration information, discussion of the suprapubic-localized discomfort, muscle spasm, and psychosocial review of patient's coping ability with underlying disease. Perform an expanded physical examination, which reveals no evidence of dehydration, additional gross hematuria, or focal neurological findings; however, increased patient depression is observed. After necessary laboratory tests are ordered, patient is treated for urinary tract infection (UTI) and started on antidepressant medication.

Clinical Example (99309)

Subsequent nursing facility visit for a patient with a new or progressing illness or acute injury that requires diagnostic evaluation, medical management, or possible surgical treatment.

Description of Procedure (99309)

Obtain a detailed interval history of each organ system that has an acute or active medical problem, including review of patient's multiple medications and recent laboratory and diagnostic testing ordered to evaluate patient's compromised respiratory condition. Perform a detailed physical examination and update the nursing plan of care.

Clinical Example (99310)

Subsequent nursing facility visit for a patient with a chronic illness with severe exacerbation that poses a threat to life or bodily function, or an acute illness/injury that poses a threat to life or bodily function.

Description of Procedure (99310)

Obtain a comprehensive history. Perform a comprehensive physical examination. Formulate a multidisciplinary treatment plan that includes IV hydration and antibiotic therapy; nursing instructions regarding monitoring of respiratory, mental, functional, and diabetic status; respiratory and physical therapy assessments with treatment as indicated; and additional laboratory monitoring to track effectiveness of treatment.

Nursing Facility Discharge Services

▶The nursing facility discharge management codes are to be used to report the total duration of time spent by a physician or other qualified health care professional for the final nursing facility discharge of a patient. The codes include, as appropriate, final examination of the patient, discussion of the nursing facility stay, even if the time spent on that date is not continuous. Instructions are given for continuing care to all relevant caregivers, and preparation of discharge records, prescriptions, and referral forms. These services require a face-to-face encounter with the patient and/or family/caregiver that may be performed on a date prior to the date the patient leaves the facility. Code selection is based on the total time on the date of the discharge management face-to-face encounter.◀

▲ **99315** Nursing facility discharge management; 30 minutes or less total time on the date of the encounter

▲ **99316** more than 30 minutes total time on the date of the encounter

Clinical Example (99315)

Final nursing facility day visit for a 72-year-old male with congestive heart failure and multiple comorbidities, who is being discharged home on diet and oral medications.

Description of Procedure (99315)

Review medical records and other available data. Obtain an interval history and perform a physical examination. Formulate and/or revise diagnosis and treatment plan(s), including making the decision for discharge. Review information regarding availability, safety, and adequacy of post-discharge support systems. Discuss aftercare treatment with patient, family, and/or caregivers and other health care professionals. Provide care coordination for transition that includes instructions to caregivers for aftercare. Arrange for post-discharge follow-up professional services and testing as necessary. Reconcile patient's medications with attention to pre-admission therapy, inpatient therapy, and outpatient formulary. Write prescriptions as necessary. Complete discharge and aftercare forms. Inform referring physician of discharge plans. Complete medical record documentation.

Clinical Example (99316)

Final nursing facility day visit for an 84-year-old male who suffered a cerebrovascular accident with hemiparesis

and who has congestive heart failure, peripheral vascular disease, and diabetes. The patient needs help transferring and is unable to administer his own insulin but has adequate support at home to be discharged to the community.

Description of Procedure (99316)

Review medical records and other available data. Obtain an interval history and perform a physical examination. Consider relevant data, options, and risks and formulate and/or revise diagnosis and treatment plan(s), including making the decision for discharge. Review information regarding the availability, adequacy, and safety of post-discharge support systems. Discuss aftercare treatment with patient and/or family/caregivers and other health care professionals. Provide care coordination for the transition, including instructions to caregivers for aftercare. Arrange for post-discharge follow-up professional services and testing. Reconcile patient's medications with attention to pre-admission therapy, inpatient therapy, and outpatient formulary. Write prescriptions as necessary. Complete discharge and aftercare forms. Inform the referring physician of discharge plans. Complete medical record documentation.

Other Nursing Facility Services

▶(99318 has been deleted. To report, see 99307, 99308, 99309, 99310)◀

Domiciliary, Rest Home (eg, Boarding Home), or Custodial Care Services

New Patient

▶(99324, 99325, 99326, 99327, 99328 have been deleted. For domiciliary, rest home [eg, boarding home], or custodial care services, new patient, see home or residence services codes 99341, 99342, 99344, 99345)◀

Established Patient

▶(99334, 99335, 99336, 99337 have been deleted. For domiciliary, rest home [eg, boarding home], or custodial care services, established patient, see home or residence services codes 99347, 99348, 99349, 99350)◀

★=Telemedicine   ◀=Audio-only   ✚=Add-on code   ⅄=FDA approval pending   #=Resequenced code   ⊘=Modifier 51 exempt

Domiciliary, Rest Home (eg, Assisted Living Facility), or Home Care Plan Oversight Services

▶(99339, 99340 have been deleted. For domiciliary, rest home [eg, assisted living facility], or home care plan oversight services, see care management services codes 99437, 99491, or principal care management codes 99424, 99425)◀

▶Home or Residence Services◀

▶The following codes are used to report evaluation and management services provided in a home or residence. Home may be defined as a private residence, temporary lodging, or short-term accommodation (eg, hotel, campground, hostel, or cruise ship).

These codes are also used when the residence is an assisted living facility, group home (that is not licensed as an intermediate care facility for individuals with intellectual disabilities), custodial care facility, or residential substance abuse treatment facility.

For services in an intermediate care facility for individuals with intellectual disabilities and services provided in a psychiatric residential treatment center, see **Nursing Facility Services**.

When selecting code level using time, do not count any travel time.

To report services when a patient is admitted to hospital inpatient, observation status, or to a nursing facility in the course of an encounter in another setting, see **Initial Hospital Inpatient and Observation Care** or **Initial Nursing Facility Care**.◀

Rationale

Domiciliary, rest home (eg, boarding home), or custodial care services codes 99324-99328 and 99334-99337 have been deleted. For 2023, care provided in the domiciliary, rest home (eg, boarding home), or custodial setting will be reported with codes 99341, 99342, 99344, 99345, and 99347-99350. The Home Services subsection, which includes codes 99341, 99342, 99344, 99345, and 99347-99350, has been revised to "Home or Residence Services" to accurately reflect the inclusion of services provided in these settings. These code families have been combined to provide efficiencies as the code families are all highly analogous. The Home or Residence Services subsection guidelines have been revised to define "residence" in

reference to codes 99341-99350 and to provide instruction on the appropriate use of these codes. Home or residence services new patient code 99343 has been deleted.

In accordance with the standardization of level-based E/M codes, codes 99341, 99342, 99344, 99345, and 99347-99350 have been revised to be reported based on either total time on the date of the encounter or MDM level and require a medically appropriate history and/or examination. Each code indicates the total time that must be met or exceeded in order to be reported. The guidelines have been revised to provide guidance on the appropriate reporting of these codes. It is important to review these guidelines before reporting the codes.

For 2023, codes 99339-99340 (domiciliary, rest home [eg, assisted living facility], or home care plan oversight services) have been deleted. A parenthetical note has been added directing users to codes 99437 and 99491 (care management services) or codes 99424 and 99425 (principal care management).

Refer to the codebook and the Rationale for the E/M introductory guidelines for a full discussion of these changes.

New Patient

▲ **99341** **Home or residence visit** for the evaluation and management of a new patient, which requires a medically appropriate history and/or examination and straightforward medical decision making.

When using total time on the date of the encounter for code selection, 15 minutes must be met or exceeded.

▲ **99342** **Home or residence visit** for the evaluation and management of a new patient, which requires a medically appropriate history and/or examination and low level of medical decision making.

When using total time on the date of the encounter for code selection, 30 minutes must be met or exceeded.

▶(99343 has been deleted. To report, see 99341, 99342, 99344, 99345)◀

▲ **99344** **Home or residence visit** for the evaluation and management of a new patient, which requires a medically appropriate history and/or examination and moderate level of medical decision making.

When using total time on the date of the encounter for code selection, 60 minutes must be met or exceeded.

▲ **99345** **Home or residence visit** for the evaluation and management of a new patient, which requires a medically appropriate history and/or examination and high level of medical decision making.

When using total time on the date of the encounter for code selection, 75 minutes must be met or exceeded.

▶(For services 90 minutes or longer, see prolonged services code 99417)◀

Clinical Example (99341)

Home or residence visit for a new patient with a self-limited problem.

Description of Procedure (99341)

Confirm patient's identity. Obtain vital signs and a medically appropriate history. Update pertinent components of HPI, review of systems, social history, family history, and allergies, and reconcile patient's medications. Perform a medically appropriate examination. Synthesize all the information, including the relevant history and physical examination, to formulate a differential diagnosis and treatment plan requiring straightforward MDM. Discuss treatment plan with patient and/or family/caregiver. Provide patient education and respond to questions from the patient and/or family/caregiver. Write orders, as necessary, for diagnostic imaging, laboratory tests, tests, and/or therapeutic intervention(s). [**Note:** This service is provided in a home or residence. Home may be defined as a private residence, temporary lodging, or short-term accommodation {eg, hotel, campground, hostel, or cruise ship}. A residence is an assisted living facility, group home {ie, not licensed as an intermediate care facility for individuals with intellectual disabilities}, custodial care facility, or residential substance abuse treatment facility.]

Clinical Example (99342)

Home or residence visit for a new patient with an acute uncomplicated illness or injury.

Description of Procedure (99342)

Confirm patient's identity. Obtain vital signs and a medically appropriate history. Update pertinent components of HPI, review of systems, social history, family history, and allergies, and reconcile the patient's medications. Perform a medically appropriate examination. Synthesize all the information, including the relevant history and physical examination, to formulate a differential diagnosis and treatment plan requiring low MDM. Discuss treatment plan with patient and/or family/caregiver. Provide patient education and respond to questions from the patient and/or family/caregiver. Write orders, as necessary, for diagnostic imaging, laboratory tests, tests, and/or therapeutic intervention(s). [**Note:** This service is provided in a home or residence. Home may be defined as a private residence, temporary lodging, or short-term accommodation {eg, hotel, campground, hostel, or cruise

ship}. A residence is an assisted living facility, group home {ie, not licensed as an intermediate care facility for individuals with intellectual disabilities}, custodial care facility, or residential substance abuse treatment facility.]

Clinical Example (99344)

Home or residence visit for a new patient with a progressing illness or acute injury that requires diagnostic evaluation, medical management, or potential surgical treatment.

Description of Procedure (99344)

Confirm patient's identity. Obtain vital signs and a medically appropriate history. Update pertinent components of HPI, review of systems, social history, family history, and allergies, and reconcile the patient's medications. Perform a medically appropriate examination. Synthesize all the information, including the relevant history and physical examination, to formulate a differential diagnosis and treatment plan requiring moderate MDM. Discuss the treatment plan with patient and/or family/caregiver. Provide patient education and respond to questions from the patient and/or family/caregiver. Write orders, as necessary, for diagnostic imaging, laboratory tests, tests, and/or therapeutic intervention(s). [**Note:** This service is provided in a home or residence. Home may be defined as a private residence, temporary lodging, or short-term accommodation {eg, hotel, campground, hostel, or cruise ship}. A residence is an assisted living facility, group home {ie, not licensed as an intermediate care facility for individuals with intellectual disabilities}, custodial care facility, or residential substance abuse treatment facility.]

Clinical Example (99345)

Home or residence visit for a new patient with a chronic illness with severe exacerbation that poses a threat to life or bodily function, or an acute illness/injury that poses a threat to life or bodily function.

Description of Procedure (99345)

Confirm patient's identity. Obtain vital signs and a medically appropriate history. Update pertinent components of HPI, review of systems, social history, family history, and allergies, and reconcile the patient's medications. Perform a medically appropriate examination. Synthesize all the information, including the relevant history and physical examination, to formulate a differential diagnosis and treatment plan requiring high MDM. Discuss treatment plan with patient and/or family/caregiver. Provide patient education and respond to questions from the patient and/or family/caregiver. Write orders, as necessary, for diagnostic imaging, laboratory tests, tests, and/or therapeutic intervention(s). [**Note:** This service is provided in a home or residence. Home may be defined as a private residence, temporary lodging, or short-term accommodation {eg, hotel, campground, hostel, or cruise ship}. A residence is an assisted living facility, group home {ie, not licensed as an intermediate care facility for individuals with intellectual disabilities}, custodial care facility, or residential substance abuse treatment facility.]

Established Patient

▲ **99347**   **Home or residence visit** for the evaluation and management of an established patient, which requires a medically appropriate history and/or examination and straightforward medical decision making.

         When using total time on the date of the encounter for code selection, 20 minutes must be met or exceeded.

▲ **99348**   **Home or residence visit** for the evaluation and management of an established patient, which requires a medically appropriate history and/or examination and low level of medical decision making.

         When using total time on the date of the encounter for code selection, 30 minutes must be met or exceeded.

▲ **99349**   **Home or residence visit** for the evaluation and management of an established patient, which requires a medically appropriate history and/or examination and moderate level of medical decision making.

         When using total time on the date of the encounter for code selection, 40 minutes must be met or exceeded.

▲ **99350**   **Home or residence visit** for the evaluation and management of an established patient, which requires a medically appropriate history and/or examination and high level of medical decision making.

         When using total time on the date of the encounter for code selection, 60 minutes must be met or exceeded.

       ▶(For services 75 minutes or longer, see prolonged services code 99417)◀

Clinical Example (99347)

Home or residence visit for an established patient with a self-limited problem.

Description of Procedure (99347)

Confirm patient's identity. Review prior clinical notes. Obtain vital signs and a medically appropriate history. Update pertinent components of HPI, review of systems, social history, family history, and allergies, and reconcile the patient's medications. Perform a medically appropriate examination. Synthesize all the information, including the relevant history and physical examination, to formulate a differential diagnosis and treatment plan

requiring straightforward MDM. Discuss treatment plan with patient and/or family/caregiver. Provide patient education and respond to questions from the patient and/or family/caregiver. Write orders, as necessary, for diagnostic imaging, laboratory tests, tests, and/or therapeutic intervention(s). [**Note:** This service is provided in a home or residence. Home may be defined as a private residence, temporary lodging, or short-term accommodation {eg, hotel, campground, hostel, or cruise ship}. A residence is an assisted living facility, group home {ie, not licensed as an intermediate care facility for individuals with intellectual disabilities}, custodial care facility, or residential substance abuse treatment facility.]

Clinical Example (99348)

Home or residence visit for an established patient with a stable chronic illness or acute uncomplicated injury.

Description of Procedure (99348)

Confirm patient's identity. Review prior clinical notes. Obtain vital signs and a medically appropriate history. Update pertinent components of HPI, review of systems, social history, family history, and allergies, and reconcile the patient's medications. Perform a medically appropriate examination. Synthesize all the information, including the relevant history and physical examination, to formulate a differential diagnosis and treatment plan requiring low MDM. Discuss the treatment plan with patient and/or family/caregiver. Provide patient education and respond to questions from the patient and/or family/caregiver. Write orders, as necessary, for diagnostic imaging, laboratory tests, tests, and/or therapeutic intervention(s). [**Note:** This service is provided in a home or residence. Home may be defined as a private residence, temporary lodging, or short-term accommodation {eg, hotel, campground, hostel, or cruise ship}. A residence is an assisted living facility, group home {ie, not licensed as an intermediate care facility for individuals with intellectual disabilities}, custodial care facility, or residential substance abuse treatment facility.]

Clinical Example (99349)

Home or residence visit for an established patient with a progressing illness or acute injury that requires medical management or potential surgical treatment.

Description of Procedure (99349)

Confirm patient's identity. Review prior clinical notes. Obtain vital signs and a medically appropriate history. Update pertinent components of HPI, review of systems, social history, family history, and allergies, and reconcile the patient's medications. Perform a medically appropriate examination. Synthesize all the information, including the relevant history and physical examination, to formulate a differential diagnosis and treatment plan requiring moderate MDM. Discuss treatment plan with patient and/or family/caregiver. Provide patient education and respond to questions from the patient and/or family/caregiver. Write orders, as necessary, for diagnostic imaging, laboratory tests, tests, and/or therapeutic intervention(s). [**Note:** This service is provided in a home or residence. Home may be defined as a private residence, temporary lodging, or short-term accommodation {eg, hotel, campground, hostel, or cruise ship}. A residence is an assisted living facility, group home {ie, not licensed as an intermediate care facility for individuals with intellectual disabilities}, custodial care facility, or residential substance abuse treatment facility.]

Clinical Example (99350)

Home or residence visit for an established patient with a chronic illness with severe exacerbation that poses a threat to life or bodily function, or an acute illness/injury that poses a threat to life or bodily function.

Description of Procedure (99350)

Confirm patient's identity. Review prior clinical notes. Obtain vital signs and a medically appropriate history. Update pertinent components of HPI, review of systems, social history, family history, and allergies, and reconcile the patient's medications. Perform a medically appropriate examination. Synthesize all the information, including the relevant history and physical examination, to formulate a differential diagnosis and treatment plan requiring high MDM. Discuss treatment plan with patient and/or family/caregiver. Provide patient education and respond to questions from the patient and/or family/caregiver. Write orders, as necessary, for diagnostic imaging, laboratory tests, tests, and/or therapeutic intervention(s). [**Note:** This service is provided in a home or residence. Home may be defined as a private residence, temporary lodging, or short-term accommodation {eg, hotel, campground, hostel, or cruise ship}. A residence is an assisted living facility, group home {ie, not licensed as an intermediate care facility for individuals with intellectual disabilities}, custodial care facility, or residential substance abuse treatment facility.]

Prolonged Services

Prolonged Service With Direct Patient Contact (Except with Office or Other Outpatient Services)

▶(99354, 99355 have been deleted. For prolonged evaluation and management services on the date of an outpatient service, home or residence service, or cognitive assessment and care plan, use 99417)◀

▶(99356, 99357 have been deleted. For prolonged evaluation and management services on the date of an inpatient or observation or nursing facility service, use 99418)◀

▶Prolonged Service on Date Other Than the Face-to-Face Evaluation and Management Service Without Direct Patient Contact◀

▶Codes 99358 and 99359 are used when a prolonged service is provided on a date other than the date of a face-to-face evaluation and management encounter with the patient and/or family/caregiver. Codes 99358, 99359 may be reported for prolonged services in relation to any evaluation and management service on a date other than the face-to-face service, whether or not time was used to select the level of the face-to-face service.

This service is to be reported in relation to other physician or other qualified health care professional services, including evaluation and management services at any level, on a date other than the face-to-face service to which it is related. Prolonged service without direct patient contact may only be reported when it occurs on a **date other than** the date of the evaluation and management service. For example, extensive record review may relate to a previous evaluation and management service performed at an earlier date. However, it must relate to a service or patient in which (face-to-face) patient care has occurred or will occur and relate to ongoing patient management.◀

Codes 99358 and 99359 are used to report the total duration of non-face-to-face time spent by a physician or other qualified health care professional on a given date providing prolonged service, even if the time spent by the physician or other qualified health care professional on that date is not continuous. Code 99358 is used to report the first hour of prolonged service on a given date regardless of the place of service. It should be used only once per date.

Prolonged service of less than 30 minutes total duration on a given date is not separately reported.

★ = Telemedicine   ◀ = Audio-only   ✛ = Add-on code   ✗ = FDA approval pending   # = Resequenced code   ⊘ = Modifier 51 exempt

Code 99359 is used to report each additional 30 minutes beyond the first hour. It may also be used to report the final 15 to 30 minutes of prolonged service on a given date.

Prolonged service of less than 15 minutes beyond the first hour or less than 15 minutes beyond the final 30 minutes is not reported separately.

▶Do not report 99358, 99359 for time without direct patient contact reported in other services, such as care plan oversight services (99374-99380), chronic care management by a physician or other qualified health care professional (99437, 99491), principal care management by a physician or other qualified health care professional (99424, 99425, 99426, 99427), home and outpatient INR monitoring (93792, 93793), medical team conferences (99366-99368), interprofessional telephone/Internet/electronic health record consultations (99446, 99447, 99448, 99449, 99451, 99452), or online digital evaluation and management services (99421, 99422, 99423).◀

99358 **Prolonged evaluation and management service** before and/or after direct patient care; first hour

+ 99359 each additional 30 minutes (List separately in addition to code for prolonged service)

(Use 99359 in conjunction with 99358)

▶(Do not report 99358, 99359 on the same date of service as 99202, 99203, 99204, 99205, 99212, 99213, 99214, 99215, 99221, 99222, 99223, 99231, 99232, 99233, 99234, 99235, 99236, 99242, 99243, 99244, 99245, 99252, 99253, 99254, 99255, 99281, 99282, 99283, 99284, 99285, 99304, 99305, 99306, 99307, 99308, 99309, 99310, 99341, 99342, 99344, 99345, 99347, 99348, 99349, 99350, 99417, 99418, 99483)◀

Total Duration of Prolonged Services Without Direct Face-to-Face Contact	Code(s)
less than 30 minutes	Not reported separately
30-74 minutes (30 minutes - 1 hr. 14 min.)	99358 X 1
75-104 minutes (1 hr. 15 min. - 1 hr. 44 min.)	99358 X 1 AND 99359 X 1
105 minutes or more (1 hr. 45 min. or more)	99358 X 1 AND 99359 X 2 or more for each additional 30 minutes

Prolonged Clinical Staff Services With Physician or Other Qualified Health Care Professional Supervision

▶Codes 99415, 99416 are used when an evaluation and management (E/M) service is provided in the office or outpatient setting that involves prolonged clinical staff face-to-face time with the patient and/or family/caregiver. The physician or other qualified health care professional is present to provide direct supervision of the clinical staff. This service is reported in addition to the designated E/M services and any other services provided at the same session as E/M services.

Codes 99415, 99416 are used to report the total duration of face-to-face time with the patient and/or family/caregiver spent by clinical staff on a given date providing prolonged service in the office or other outpatient setting, even if the time spent by the clinical staff on that date is not continuous. Time spent performing separately reported services other than the E/M service is not counted toward the prolonged services time.

Code 99415 is used to report the first hour of prolonged clinical staff service on a given date. Code 99415 should be used only once per date, even if the time spent by the clinical staff is not continuous on that date. Prolonged service of less than 30 minutes total duration on a given date is not separately reported. When face-to-face time is noncontinuous, use only the face-to-face time provided to the patient and/or family/caregiver by the clinical staff.◀

Code 99416 is used to report each additional 30 minutes of prolonged clinical staff service beyond the first hour. Code 99416 may also be used to report the final 15-30 minutes of prolonged service on a given date. Prolonged service of less than 15 minutes beyond the first hour or less than 15 minutes beyond the final 30 minutes is not reported separately.

▶Codes 99415, 99416 may be reported for no more than two simultaneous patients and the time reported is the time devoted only to a single patient.

For prolonged services by the physician or other qualified health care professional on the date of an office or other outpatient evaluation and management service (with or without direct patient contact), use 99417. Do not report 99415, 99416 in conjunction with 99417.◀

Facilities may not report 99415, 99416.

#+ 99415 Prolonged clinical staff service (the service beyond the highest time in the range of total time of the service) during an evaluation and management service in the office or outpatient setting, direct patient contact with physician supervision; first hour (List separately in addition to code for outpatient **Evaluation and Management** service)

(Use 99415 in conjunction with 99202, 99203, 99204, 99205, 99212, 99213, 99214, 99215)

▶(Do not report 99415 in conjunction with 99417)◀

#✛ **99416**   each additional 30 minutes (List separately in addition to code for prolonged service)

(Use 99416 in conjunction with 99415)

▶(Do not report 99416 in conjunction with 99417)◀

▶The starting point for 99415 is 30 minutes beyond the typical clinical staff time for ongoing assessment of the patient during the office visit. The Reporting Prolonged Clinical Staff Time table provides the typical clinical staff times for the office or other outpatient primary codes, the range of time beyond the clinical staff time for which 99415 may be reported, and the starting point at which 99416 may be reported.◀

▶**Reporting Prolonged Clinical Staff Time**

Code	Typical Clinical Staff Time	99415 Time Range (Minutes)	99416 Start Point (Minutes)
99202	29	59-103	104
99203	34	64-108	109
99204	41	71-115	116
99205	46	76-120	121
99211	16	46-90	91
99212	24	54-98	99
99213	27	57-101	102
99214	40	70-114	115
99215	45	75-119	120◀

▶Prolonged Service With or Without Direct Patient Contact on the Date of an Evaluation and Management Service◀

▶Code 99417 is used to report prolonged total time (ie, combined time with and without direct patient contact) provided by the physician or other qualified health care professional on the date of office or other outpatient services, office consultation, or other outpatient evaluation and management services (ie, 99205, 99215, 99245, 99345, 99350, 99483). Code 99418 is used to report prolonged total time (ie, combined time with and without direct patient contact) provided by the physician or other qualified health care professional on the date of an inpatient evaluation and management service (ie, 99223, 99233, 99236, 99255, 99306, 99310). Prolonged total time is time that is 15 minutes beyond the time

required to report the highest-level primary service. Codes 99417, 99418 are only used when the primary service has been selected using time alone as the basis and only after the time required to report the highest-level service has been exceeded by 15 minutes. To report a unit of 99417, 99418, 15 minutes of time must have been attained. Do not report 99417, 99418 for any time increment of less than 15 minutes.

When reporting 99417, 99418, the initial time unit of 15 minutes should be added once the time in the primary E/M code has been surpassed by 15 minutes. For example, to report the initial unit of 99417 for a new patient encounter (99205), do not report 99417 until at least 15 minutes of time has been accumulated beyond 60 minutes (ie, 75 minutes) on the date of the encounter. For an established patient encounter (99215), do not report 99417 until at least 15 minutes of time has been accumulated beyond 40 minutes (ie, 55 minutes) on the date of the encounter.

Time spent performing separately reported services other than the primary E/M service and prolonged E/M service is not counted toward the primary E/M and prolonged services time.

For prolonged services on a date other than the date of a face-to-face evaluation and management encounter with the patient and/or family/caregiver, see 99358, 99359. For E/M services that require prolonged clinical staff time and may include face-to-face services by the physician or other qualified health care professional, see 99415, 99416. Do not report 99417, 99418 in conjunction with 99358, 99359, 99415, 99416.◀

#★✛▲ **99417**   Prolonged outpatient evaluation and management service(s) time with or without direct patient contact beyond the required time of the primary service when the primary service level has been selected using total time, each 15 minutes of total time (List separately in addition to the code of the outpatient **Evaluation and Management** service)

▶(Use 99417 in conjunction with 99205, 99215, 99245, 99345, 99350, 99483)◀

▶(Do not report 99417 on the same date of service as 90833, 90836, 90838, 99358, 99359, 99415, 99416)◀

(Do not report 99417 for any time unit less than 15 minutes)

#★✛● **99418**   Prolonged inpatient or observation evaluation and management service(s) time with or without direct patient contact beyond the required time of the primary service when the primary service level has been selected using total time, each 15 minutes of total time (List separately in addition to the code of the inpatient and observation **Evaluation and Management** service)

▶(Use 99418 in conjunction with 99223, 99233, 99236, 99255, 99306, 99310)◀

★=Telemedicine   ◀=Audio-only   ✛=Add-on code   ⱄ=FDA approval pending   #=Resequenced code   ⊘=Modifier 51 exempt

▶(Do not report 99418 on the same date of service as 90833, 90836, 90838, 99358, 99359)◀

▶(Do not report 99418 for any time unit less than 15 minutes)◀

▶Total Duration of New Patient Office or Other Outpatient Services (use with 99205)	Code(s)
less than 75 minutes	Not reported separately
75-89 minutes	99205 X 1 and 99417 X 1
90-104 minutes	99205 X 1 and 99417 X 2
105 minutes or more	99205 X 1 and 99417 X 3 or more for each additional 15 minutes

Total Duration of Established Patient Office or Other Outpatient Services (use with 99215)	Code(s)
less than 55 minutes	Not reported separately
55-69 minutes	99215 X 1 and 99417 X 1
70-84 minutes	99215 X 1 and 99417 X 2
85 minutes or more	99215 X 1 and 99417 X 3 or more for each additional 15 minutes

Total Duration of Office or Other Outpatient Consultation Services (use with 99245)	Code(s)
less than 70 minutes	Not reported separately
70-84 minutes	99245 X 1 and 99417 X 1
80-99 minutes	99245 X 1 and 99417 X 2
100 minutes or more	99245 X 1 and 99417 X 3 or more for each additional 15 minutes◀

Rationale

Many changes have been made to the Prolonged Services subsection for 2023. Prolonged service with direct patient contact (except with office or other outpatient services) codes 99354-99357 have been deleted. For 2023, prolonged E/M services on the date of an outpatient service, home or residence service, or cognitive assessment and care plan will be reported with outpatient prolonged services code 99417. Guidelines and parenthetical notes throughout the Prolonged Services subsection have been revised to reflect the deletion of codes 99354-99357.

The heading and guidelines for prolonged service without direct patient contact codes 99358 and 99359 have been revised to clarify that codes 99358 and 99359 describe prolonged services provided on a date other than the face-to-face E/M service to which they are related. The guidelines also have been revised to clarify that these codes are used to report prolonged service provided to the patient and/or family/caregiver and may be reported in relation to any E/M service whether or not time was used to select the level of service. An exclusionary parenthetical note has been added listing the specific E/M codes with which codes 99358 and 99359 should not be reported on the same date.

The guidelines for Prolonged Clinical Staff Services With Physician or Other Qualified Health Care Professional Supervision codes 99415 and 99416 have been revised to clarify that they describe prolonged clinical staff time with the patient and/or family/caregiver. Codes 99415 and 99416 may be reported for no more than two simultaneous patients. The guidelines have been revised to clarify that the time reported is the time devoted to a single patient.

The Prolonged Service With or Without Direct Patient Contact on the Date of an Office or Other Outpatient Service subsection has been revised to include prolonged E/M services provided in the inpatient, as well as the outpatient setting. Code 99417 has been revised with the replacement of the phrase "office or other outpatient" with "outpatient," because code 99417 may now be reported for prolonged services provided beyond the required time of any of the highest level outpatient E/M services (ie, 99205, 99215, 99245, 99345, 99350, 99483) when time is used for code selection. Code 99417 is not reported on the same date of service with code 90833, 90836, 90838, 99358, 99359, 99415, or 99416. Code 99418 has been added to describe prolonged services provided on the date of an inpatient or observation or nursing facility service beyond the required time of the highest level primary service (ie, 99223, 99233, 99236, 99255, 99306, 99310) when time is used for code selection. Code 99418 is not reported on the same date of service with codes 90833, 90836, 90838, 99358, or 99359. The subsection heading has been revised so it no longer refers specifically to office or other outpatient services. The guidelines have been revised to clearly distinguish the differences between codes 99417 and 99418, and to indicate that the prolonged total time is time that is 15 minutes beyond the time required to report the highest-level primary service. Codes 99417 and 99418 are not reported for any time unit less than 15 minutes.

Clinical Example (99417)

Office visit for a patient with a chronic illness with severe exacerbation that poses a threat to life or bodily function, or an acute illness/injury that poses a threat to life or bodily function.

Description of Procedure (99417)

Continue the work of evaluation and management lasting 15 minutes beyond the time of the usual service, either face-to-face or non-face-to-face. Includes tasks such as formulating a treatment plan; discussing the diagnoses, workup, and treatment options with patient and/or family/caregiver; providing additional patient education and responding to questions; analyzing test results; documenting the encounter in the medical record and additional discussions with other physicians or other QHPs; coordinating additional care with other physicians or members of the health care team as necessary for additional work.

Clinical Example (99418)

Hospital visit for a patient with a chronic illness with severe exacerbation that poses a threat to life or bodily function, or an acute illness/injury that poses a threat to life or bodily function.

Description of Procedure (99418)

Continue the work of evaluation and management lasting 15 minutes beyond the time of the usual service, either face-to-face or non-face-to-face. Includes tasks such as formulating a treatment plan; discussing the diagnoses, workup, and treatment options with patient and family; providing additional patient education and responding to questions; analyzing test results; documenting the encounter in the medical record and additional discussions with other physicians and other QHPs; coordinating additional care with other physicians or members of the health care team necessary for additional work.

Case Management Services

Medical Team Conferences

Medical team conferences include face-to-face participation by a minimum of three qualified health care professionals from different specialties or disciplines (each of whom provide direct care to the patient), with or without the presence of the patient, family member(s), community agencies, surrogate decision maker(s) (eg, legal guardian), and/or caregiver(s). The participants are actively involved in the development, revision, coordination, and implementation of health care services needed by the patient. Reporting participants shall have performed face-to-face evaluations or treatments of the patient, independent of any team conference, within the previous 60 days.

▶Physicians or other qualified health care professionals who may report evaluation and management services should report their time spent in a team conference with the patient and/or family/caregiver present using evaluation and management (E/M) codes. These introductory guidelines do not apply to services reported using E/M codes (see E/M Services Guidelines). However, the individual must be directly involved with the patient, providing face-to-face services outside of the conference visit with other physicians, and qualified health care professionals, or agencies.◀

Reporting participants shall document their participation in the team conference as well as their contributed information and subsequent treatment recommendations.

No more than one individual from the same specialty may report 99366-99368 at the same encounter.

Individuals should not report 99366-99368 when their participation in the medical team conference is part of a facility or organizational service contractually provided by the organization or facility.

▶The team conference starts at the beginning of the review of an individual patient and ends at the conclusion of the review. Time related to record keeping and report generation is not reported. The reporting participant shall be present for all time reported. The time reported is not limited to the time that the participant is communicating to the other team members or patient and/or family/caregiver. Time reported for medical team conferences may not be used in the determination of time for other services such as care plan oversight (99374-99380), prolonged services (99358, 99359), psychotherapy, or any E/M service. For team conferences where the patient is present for any part of the duration of the conference, nonphysician qualified health care professionals (eg, speech-language pathologists, physical therapists, occupational therapists, social workers, dietitians) report the team conference face-to-face code 99366.◀

Rationale

In accordance with the deletion of codes 99339, 99340, and 99354-99357, the Medical Team Conferences subsection guidelines have been revised to reflect these changes.

Refer to the codebook and the Rationale for codes 99339, 99340, and 99354-99357 for a full discussion of these changes.

★ = Telemedicine　◀ = Audio-only　✦ = Add-on code　✒ = FDA approval pending　# = Resequenced code　⊘ = Modifier 51 exempt

Medical Team Conference, Without Direct (Face-to-Face) Contact With Patient and/or Family

99367 **Medical team conference** with interdisciplinary team of health care professionals, patient and/or family not present, 30 minutes or more; participation by physician

99368 participation by nonphysician qualified health care professional

(Team conference services of less than 30 minutes duration are not reported separately)

▶(Do not report 99367, 99368 during the same month with 99437, 99439, 99487, 99489, 99490, 99491)◀

Rationale

Parenthetical notes listed for use of principal care management (PCM) services in conjunction with medical team conference services have been revised to provide instructions regarding appropriate reporting when these services are performed together.

Refer to the codebook and the Rationale for changes to the PCM services codes (99424-99427) for a full discussion of these changes.

Care Plan Oversight Services

▶Care plan oversight services are reported separately from codes for office/outpatient, hospital, home or residence (including assisted living facility, group home, custodial care facility, residential substance abuse treatment facility, rest home), nursing facility, or non-face-to-face services. The complexity and approximate time of the care plan oversight services provided within a 30-day period determine code selection. Only one individual may report services for a given period of time to reflect the sole or predominant supervisory role with a particular patient. These codes should not be reported for supervision of patients in nursing facilities or under the care of home health agencies, unless they require recurrent supervision of therapy.◀

The work involved in providing very low intensity or infrequent supervision services is included in the pre- and post-encounter work for home, office/outpatient and nursing facility or domiciliary visit codes.

▶(For care plan oversight services provided in rest home [eg, assisted living facility] or home, see care management services codes 99437, 99491, or principal care management codes 99424, 99425, and for hospice agency, see 99377, 99378)◀

(Do not report 99374-99380 for time reported with 98966, 98967, 98968, 99421, 99422, 99423, 99441, 99442, 99443)

(Do not report 99374-99378 during the same month with 99487, 99489)

99374 **Supervision** of a patient under care of home health agency (patient not present) in home, domiciliary or equivalent environment (eg, Alzheimer's facility) requiring complex and multidisciplinary care modalities involving regular development and/or revision of care plans by that individual, review of subsequent reports of patient status, review of related laboratory and other studies, communication (including telephone calls) for purposes of assessment or care decisions with health care professional(s), family member(s), surrogate decision maker(s) (eg, legal guardian) and/or key caregiver(s) involved in patient's care, integration of new information into the medical treatment plan and/or adjustment of medical therapy, within a calendar month; 15-29 minutes

99375 30 minutes or more

Rationale

In accordance with the deletion of codes 99339, 99340, and 99354-99357, the Care Plan Oversight Services sub-section guidelines have been revised to reflect these changes.

Refer to the codebook and the Rationale for codes 99339, 99340, and 99354-99357 for a full discussion of these changes.

Preventive Medicine Services

Codes 99381-99397 include counseling/anticipatory guidance/risk factor reduction interventions which are provided at the time of the initial or periodic comprehensive preventive medicine examination. (Refer to 99401, 99402, 99403, 99404, 99411, and 99412 for reporting those counseling/anticipatory guidance/risk factor reduction interventions that are provided at an encounter separate from the preventive medicine examination.)

(For behavior change intervention, see 99406, 99407, 99408, 99409)

▶Vaccine/toxoid products, immunization administrations, ancillary studies involving laboratory, radiology, other procedures, or screening tests (eg, vision, hearing, developmental) identified with a specific CPT code are reported separately. For immunization administration and vaccine risk/benefit counseling, see 90460, 90461, 90471-90474, 0001A, 0002A, 0003A,

0004A, 0011A, 0012A, 0013A, 0021A, 0022A, 0031A, 0034A, 0041A, 0042A, 0051A, 0052A, 0053A, 0054A, 0064A, 0071A, 0072A, 0073A, 0074A, 0081A, 0082A, 0083A, 0094A, 0104A, 0111A, 0112A. For vaccine/toxoid products, see 90476-90759, 91300-91311.◄

Rationale

In accommodation of the new codes that have been added to the code set for COVID-19 vaccination products and administrations, codes 0003A, 0004A, 0013A, 0034A, 0051A-0054A, 0064A, 0071A-0074A, 0081A-0083A, 0094A, 0104A, 0111A, and 0112A have been added to the Preventive Services subsection's introductory guidelines that direct users to these codes.

Refer to the codebook and the Rationale for codes 0003A-0112A for a full discussion of these changes.

Counseling Risk Factor Reduction and Behavior Change Intervention

New or Established Patient

Preventive Medicine, Group Counseling

99417   Code is out of numerical sequence. See 99358-99366

99418   Code is out of numerical sequence. See 99358-99366

Non-Face-to-Face Services

Telephone Services

99441   Telephone evaluation and management service by a physician or other qualified health care professional who may report evaluation and management services provided to an established patient, parent, or guardian not originating from a related E/M service provided within the previous 7 days nor leading to an E/M service or procedure within the next 24 hours or soonest available appointment; 5-10 minutes of medical discussion

99442   11-20 minutes of medical discussion

99443   21-30 minutes of medical discussion

►(Do not report 99441-99443 when using 99374-99380 for the same call[s])◄

(Do not report 99441-99443 for home and outpatient INR monitoring when reporting 93792, 93793)

(Do not report 99441-99443 during the same month with 99487-99489)

(Do not report 99441-99443 when performed during the service time of codes 99495 or 99496)

Rationale

In accordance with the deletion of codes 99339 and 99340, the exclusionary parenthetical note following codes 99441-99443 has been revised to reflect these changes.

Refer to the codebook and the Rationale for codes 99339 and 99340 for a full discussion of these changes.

Online Digital Evaluation and Management Services

 # 99421   Online digital evaluation and management service, for an established patient, for up to 7 days, cumulative time during the 7 days; 5-10 minutes

 # 99422   11-20 minutes

 # 99423   21 or more minutes

(Report 99421, 99422, 99423 once per 7-day period)

(Clinical staff time is not calculated as part of cumulative time for 99421, 99422, 99423)

(Do not report online digital E/M services for cumulative service time less than 5 minutes)

(Do not count 99421, 99422, 99423 time otherwise reported with other services)

►(Do not report 99421, 99422, 99423 on a day when the physician or other qualified health care professional reports E/M services [99202, 99203, 99204, 99205, 99212, 99213, 99214, 99215, 99242, 99243, 99244, 99245])◄

►(Do not report 99421, 99422, 99423 when using 99091, 99374, 99375, 99377, 99378, 99379, 99380, 99424, 99425, 99426, 99427, 99437, 99487, 99489, 99491, 99495, 99496, for the same communication[s])◄

(Do not report 99421, 99422, 99423 for home and outpatient INR monitoring when reporting 93792, 93793)

Rationale

In accordance with the deletion of codes 99241, 99339, and 99340, two exclusionary parenthetical notes following codes 99421-99423 have been revised to reflect these changes.

Refer to the codebook and the Rationale for codes 99241, 99339, and 99340 for a full discussion of these changes.

Interprofessional Telephone/ Internet/Electronic Health Record Consultations

▶The consultant should use codes 99446, 99447, 99448, 99449, 99451 to report interprofessional telephone/ Internet/electronic health record consultations. An interprofessional telephone/Internet/electronic health record consultation is an assessment and management service in which a patient's treating (eg, attending or primary) physician or other qualified health care professional requests the opinion and/or treatment advice of a physician or other qualified health care professional with specific specialty expertise (the consultant) to assist the treating physician or other qualified health care professional in the diagnosis and/or management of the patient's problem without patient face-to-face contact with the consultant.◀

The patient for whom the interprofessional telephone/ Internet/electronic health record consultation is requested may be either a new patient to the consultant or an established patient with a new problem or an exacerbation of an existing problem. However, the consultant should not have seen the patient in a face-to-face encounter within the last 14 days. When the telephone/Internet/electronic health record consultation leads to a transfer of care or other face-to-face service (eg, a surgery, a hospital visit, or a scheduled office evaluation of the patient) within the next 14 days or next available appointment date of the consultant, these codes are not reported.

Review of pertinent medical records, laboratory studies, imaging studies, medication profile, pathology specimens, etc is included in the telephone/Internet/electronic health record consultation service and should not be reported separately when reporting 99446, 99447, 99448, 99449, 99451. The majority of the service time reported (greater than 50%) must be devoted to the medical consultative verbal or Internet discussion. If greater than 50% of the time for the service is devoted to data review and/or analysis, 99446, 99447, 99448, 99449 should not be reported. However, the service time for 99451 is based on total review and interprofessional-communication time.

If more than one telephone/Internet/electronic health record contact(s) is required to complete the consultation request (eg, discussion of test results), the entirety of the service and the cumulative discussion and information review time should be reported with a single code. Codes 99446, 99447, 99448, 99449, 99451 should not be reported more than once within a seven-day interval.

The written or verbal request for telephone/Internet/ electronic health record advice by the treating/requesting physician or other qualified health care professional should be documented in the patient's medical record,

including the reason for the request. Codes 99446, 99447, 99448, 99449 conclude with a verbal opinion report and written report from the consultant to the treating/requesting physician or other qualified health care professional. Code 99451 concludes with only a written report.

Telephone/Internet/electronic health record consultations of less than five minutes should not be reported. Consultant communications with the patient and/or family may be reported using 98966, 98967, 98968, 99421, 99422, 99423, 99441, 99442, 99443, and the time related to these services is not used in reporting 99446, 99447, 99448, 99449. Do not report 99358, 99359 for any time within the service period, if reporting 99446, 99447, 99448, 99449, 99451.

When the sole purpose of the telephone/Internet/ electronic health record communication is to arrange a transfer of care or other face-to-face service, these codes are not reported.

▶The treating/requesting physician or other qualified health care professional may report 99452, if spending 16-30 minutes in a service day preparing for the referral and/or communicating with the consultant. Do not report 99452 more than once in a 14-day period. The treating/requesting physician or other qualified health care professional may report the prolonged service codes 99417, 99418 for the time spent on the interprofessional telephone/Internet/electronic health record discussion with the consultant (eg, specialist), if the time **exceeds 30 minutes** beyond the typical time of the appropriate E/M service performed and the patient is present (on-site) and accessible to the treating/requesting physician or other qualified health care professional. If the interprofessional telephone/Internet/electronic health record assessment and management service occurs when the patient is not present and the time spent in a day **exceeds 30 minutes,** then the non-face-to-face prolonged service codes 99358, 99359 may be reported by the treating/requesting physician or other qualified health care professional.◀

> ▶(For telephone services provided by a physician or other qualified health care professional to a patient, see 99441, 99442, 99443)◀

> ▶(For telephone services provided by a qualified nonphysician health care professional who may not report evaluation and management services [eg, speech-language pathologists, physical therapists, occupational therapists, social workers, dietitians], see 98966, 98967, 98968)◀

> (For online digital E/M services provided by a physician or other qualified health care professional to a patient, see 99421, 99422, 99423)

Rationale

In accordance with the revisions to codes 99446-99449 and 99451, the Interprofessional Telephone/Internet/Electronic Health Record Consultations subsection's introductory guidelines have been revised to include "or other qualified health care professional."

The guidelines have also been revised in accordance with the deletion of codes 99354-99357, the revision of code 99417, and the establishment of code 99418.

Refer to the codebook and the Rationale for codes 99354-99357, 99417-99418, 99446-99449, and 99451 for a full discussion of these changes.

▲ **99446** Interprofessional telephone/Internet/electronic health record assessment and management service provided by a consultative physician or other qualified health care professional, including a verbal and written report to the patient's treating/requesting physician or other qualified health care professional; 5-10 minutes of medical consultative discussion and review

▲ **99447** 11-20 minutes of medical consultative discussion and review

▲ **99448** 21-30 minutes of medical consultative discussion and review

▲ **99449** 31 minutes or more of medical consultative discussion and review

#▲ **99451** Interprofessional telephone/Internet/electronic health record assessment and management service provided by a consultative physician or other qualified health care professional, including a written report to the patient's treating/requesting physician or other qualified health care professional, 5 minutes or more of medical consultative time

Rationale

Codes 99446-99449 and 99451 have been revised to include "other qualified health care professional." The original code descriptor only specified "physician" and did not directly identify "or other qualified health care professional." Therefore, to provide clarity on the reporting of these services, the wording "or other qualified health care professional" has been added.

Digitally Stored Data Services/ Remote Physiologic Monitoring

Codes 99453 and 99454 are used to report remote physiologic monitoring services (eg, weight, blood pressure, pulse oximetry) during a 30-day period. To report 99453, 99454, the device used must be a medical device as defined by the FDA, and the service must be ordered by a physician or other qualified health care professional. Code 99453 may be used to report the set-up and patient education on use of the device(s). Code 99454 may be used to report supply of the device for daily recording or programmed alert transmissions. Codes 99453, 99454 are not reported if monitoring is less than 16 days. Do not report 99453, 99454 when these services are included in other codes for the duration of time of the physiologic monitoring service (eg, 95250 for continuous glucose monitoring requires a minimum of 72 hours of monitoring).

Code 99091 should be reported no more than once in a 30-day period to include the physician or other qualified health care professional time involved with data accession, review and interpretation, modification of care plan as necessary (including communication to patient and/or caregiver), and associated documentation.

If the services described by 99091 or 99474 are provided on the same day the patient presents for an evaluation and management (E/M) service to the same provider, these services should be considered part of the E/M service and not reported separately.

▶Do not report 99091 for time in the same calendar month when used to meet the criteria for care plan oversight services (99374, 99375, 99377, 99378, 99379, 99380), remote physiologic monitoring services (99457, 99458), or personally performed chronic or principal care management (99424, 99425, 99426, 99427, 99437, 99491). Do not report 99091 if other more specific codes exist (eg, 93227, 93272 for cardiographic services; 95250 for continuous glucose monitoring). Do not report 99091 for transfer and interpretation of data from hospital or clinical laboratory computers.◀

Code 99453 is reported for each episode of care. For coding remote monitoring of physiologic parameters, an episode of care is defined as beginning when the remote monitoring physiologic service is initiated, and ends with attainment of targeted treatment goals.

Rationale

In accordance with the deletion of codes 99324-99328, 99334-99337, 99339, and 99340, the Digitally Stored Data Services/Remote Physiologic Monitoring subsection guidelines have been revised to reflect these changes.

Refer to the codebook and the Rationale for codes 99324-99328, 99334-99337, 99339, and 99340 for a full discussion of these changes.

★=Telemedicine   ◀=Audio-only   ✚=Add-on code   ✒=FDA approval pending   #=Resequenced code   ⊘=Modifier 51 exempt

99453

Remote monitoring of physiologic parameter(s) (eg, weight, blood pressure, pulse oximetry, respiratory flow rate), initial; set-up and patient education on use of equipment

(Do not report 99453 more than once per episode of care)

(Do not report 99453 for monitoring of less than 16 days)

99454

device(s) supply with daily recording(s) or programmed alert(s) transmission, each 30 days

(For physiologic monitoring treatment management services, use 99457)

(Do not report 99454 for monitoring of less than 16 days)

(Do not report 99453, 99454 in conjunction with codes for more specific physiologic parameters [eg, 93296, 94760])

▶(For remote therapeutic monitoring, see 98975, 98976, 98977, 98978)◀

(For self-measured blood pressure monitoring, see 99473, 99474)

Rationale

In accordance with the establishment of code 98978, the instructional parenthetical note following code 99454 has been revised to reflect this addition.

Refer to the codebook and the Rationale for code 98978 for a full discussion of these changes.

99091

Collection and interpretation of physiologic data (eg, ECG, blood pressure, glucose monitoring) digitally stored and/or transmitted by the patient and/or caregiver to the physician or other qualified health care professional, qualified by education, training, licensure/regulation (when applicable) requiring a minimum of 30 minutes of time, each 30 days

(Do not report 99091 in conjunction with 99457, 99458)

▶(Do not report 99091 for time in a calendar month when used to meet the criteria for 99374, 99375, 99377, 99378, 99379, 99380, 99424, 99425, 99426, 99427, 99437, 99457, 99487, 99491)◀

Rationale

In accordance with the deletion of codes 99339 and 99340, an exclusionary parenthetical note has been revised to reflect these changes.

Refer to the codebook and the Rationale for codes 99339 and 99340 for a full discussion of these changes.

Remote Physiologic Monitoring Treatment Management Services

Remote physiologic monitoring treatment management services are provided when clinical staff/physician/other qualified health care professional use the results of remote physiological monitoring to manage a patient under a specific treatment plan. To report remote physiological monitoring, the device used must be a medical device as defined by the FDA, and the service must be ordered by a physician or other qualified health care professional. Do not use 99457, 99458 for time that can be reported using codes for more specific monitoring services. Codes 99457, 99458 may be reported during the same service period as chronic care management services (99437, 99439, 99487, 99489, 99490, 99491), principal care management services (99424, 99425, 99426, 99427), transitional care management services (99495, 99496), and behavioral health integration services (99484, 99492, 99493, 99494). However, time spent performing these services should remain separate and no time should be counted twice toward the required time for any services in a single month. Codes 99457, 99458 require a live, interactive communication with the patient/caregiver. The interactive communication contributes to the total time, but it does not need to represent the entire cumulative reported time of the treatment management service. For the first completed 20 minutes of clinical staff/physician/other qualified health care professional time in a calendar month report 99457, and report 99458 for each additional completed 20 minutes. Do not report 99457, 99458 for services of less than 20 minutes. Report 99457 one time regardless of the number of physiologic monitoring modalities performed in a given calendar month.

To report remote therapeutic monitoring treatment management services provided by physician or other qualified health care professional, see 98980, 98981.

▶Do not count any time on a day when the physician or other qualified health care professional reports an E/M service (office or other outpatient services 99202, 99203, 99204, 99205, 99211, 99212, 99213, 99214, 99215, home or residence services 99341, 99342, 99344, 99345, 99347, 99348, 99349, 99350, initial or subsequent hospital inpatient or observation services 99221, 99222, 99223, 99231, 99232, 99233, inpatient or observation consultations 99252, 99253, 99254, 99255). Do not count any time related to other reported services (eg, 93290, 93793, 99291, 99292).◀

Rationale

In accordance with the deletion of codes 99251, 99324-99328, 99334-99337, 99339, 99340, and 99343, the Remote Physiologic Monitoring Treatment Management Services subsection guidelines have been revised to reflect these changes.

Refer to the codebook and the Rationale for codes 99251, 99324-99328, 99334-99337, 99339, 99340, and 99343 for a full discussion of these changes.

Newborn Care Services

The following codes are used to report the services provided to newborns (birth through the first 28 days) in several different settings. Use of the normal newborn codes is limited to the initial care of the newborn in the first days after birth prior to home discharge.

Evaluation and Management (E/M) services for the newborn include maternal and/or fetal and newborn history, newborn physical examination(s), ordering of diagnostic tests and treatments, meetings with the family, and documentation in the medical record.

When delivery room attendance services (99464) or delivery room resuscitation services (99465) are required, report these in addition to normal newborn services Evaluation and Management codes.

▶For E/M services provided to newborns who are other than normal, see codes for hospital inpatient or observation services (99221-99233) and neonatal intensive and critical care services (99466-99469, 99477-99480). When normal newborn services are provided by the same individual on the same date that the newborn later becomes ill and receives additional intensive or critical care services, report the appropriate E/M code with modifier 25 for these services in addition to the normal newborn code.◀

Procedures (eg, 54150, newborn circumcision) are not included with the normal newborn codes, and when performed, should be reported in addition to the newborn services.

▶When newborns are seen in follow-up after the date of discharge in the office or other outpatient setting, see 99202-99215, 99381, 99391, as appropriate.◀

Rationale

In accordance with the revision of codes 99221-99223 to include observation care, the Newborn Care Services guidelines have been revised to reflect these changes.

Refer to the codebook and the Rationale for codes 99221-99223 for a full discussion of these changes.

Delivery/Birthing Room Attendance and Resuscitation Services

99464   Attendance at delivery (when requested by the delivering physician or other qualified health care professional) and initial stabilization of newborn

▶(99464 may be reported in conjunction with 99221, 99222, 99223, 99291, 99460, 99468, 99477)◀

(Do not report 99464 in conjunction with 99465)

99465   Delivery/birthing room resuscitation, provision of positive pressure ventilation and/or chest compressions in the presence of acute inadequate ventilation and/or cardiac output

▶(99465 may be reported in conjunction with 99221, 99222, 99223, 99291, 99460, 99468, 99477)◀

(Do not report 99465 in conjunction with 99464)

(Procedures that are performed as a necessary part of the resuscitation [eg, intubation, vascular lines] are reported separately in addition to 99465. In order to report these procedures, they must be performed as a necessary component of the resuscitation and not as a convenience before admission to the neonatal intensive care unit)

Rationale

The parenthetical notes following codes 99464 and 99465 have been editorially revised to include initial day hospital care services codes 99221-99223, and critical care code 99291.

A newborn is typically a unique patient in the hospital setting because various levels of care may need to be provided. A physician may be asked to attend the delivery because of a known or suspected problem. Oftentimes, the newborn can transition from delivery to normal status with little more than the typical newborn service. More often though, these newborns will require medical interventions to deal with concerns that led the physician to be called to the delivery room in the first place. Because of the varying degrees of issues a newborn may present with, the initial day hospital care services codes 99221-99223 and critical care code 99291 have been added to the parenthetical notes following codes 99464 and 99465.

Inpatient Neonatal Intensive Care Services and Pediatric and Neonatal Critical Care Services

Pediatric Critical Care Patient Transport

Codes 99466, 99467 are used to report the physical attendance and direct face-to-face care by a physician during the interfacility transport of a critically ill or critically injured pediatric patient 24 months of age or younger. Codes 99485, 99486 are used to report the control physician's non-face-to-face supervision of interfacility transport of a critically ill or critically injured pediatric patient 24 months of age or younger. These codes are not reported together for the same patient by the same physician. For the purpose of reporting 99466 and 99467, face-to-face care begins when the physician assumes primary responsibility of the pediatric patient at the referring facility, and ends when the receiving facility accepts responsibility for the pediatric patient's care. Only the time the physician spends in direct face-to-face contact with the patient during the transport should be reported. Pediatric patient transport services involving less than 30 minutes of face-to-face physician care should not be reported using 99466, 99467. Procedure(s) or service(s) performed by other members of the transporting team may not be reported by the supervising physician.

Codes 99485, 99486 may be used to report control physician's non-face-to-face supervision of interfacility pediatric critical care transport, which includes all two-way communication between the control physician and the specialized transport team prior to transport, at the referring facility and during transport of the patient back to the receiving facility. The "control" physician is the physician directing transport services. These codes do not include pretransport communication between the control physician and the referring facility before or following patient transport. These codes may only be reported for patients 24 months of age or younger who are critically ill or critically injured. The control physician provides treatment advice to a specialized transport team who are present and delivering the hands-on patient care. The control physician does not report any services provided by the specialized transport team. The control physician's non-face-to-face time begins with the first contact by the control physician with the specialized transport team and ends when the patient's care is handed over to the receiving facility team. Refer to 99466 and 99467 for face-to-face transport care of the critically ill/injured

patient. Time spent with the individual patient's transport team and reviewing data submissions should be recorded. Code 99485 is used to report the first 16-45 minutes of direction on a given date and should only be used once even if time spent by the physician is discontinuous. Do not report services of 15 minutes or less or any time when another physician is reporting 99466, 99467. Do not report 99485 or 99486 in conjunction with 99466, 99467 when performed by the same physician.

For the definition of the critically injured pediatric patient, see the **Neonatal and Pediatric Critical Care Services** section.

The non-face-to-face direction of emergency care to a patient's transporting staff by a physician located in a hospital or other facility by two-way communication is not considered direct face-to-face care and should not be reported with 99466, 99467. Physician-directed non-face-to-face emergency care through outside voice communication to transporting staff personnel is reported with 99288 or 99485, 99486 based upon the age and clinical condition of the patient.

►Emergency department services (99281-99285), initial hospital inpatient or observation care (99221-99223), critical care (99291, 99292), initial date neonatal intensive (99477), or critical care (99468) may only be reported after the patient has been admitted to the emergency department, the hospital inpatient or observation floor, or the critical care unit of the receiving facility. If inpatient critical care services are reported in the referring facility prior to transfer to the receiving hospital, use the critical care codes (99291, 99292).◄

The following services are included when performed during the pediatric patient transport by the physician providing critical care and may not be reported separately: routine monitoring evaluations (eg, heart rate, respiratory rate, blood pressure, and pulse oximetry), the interpretation of cardiac output measurements (93598), chest X rays (71045, 71046), pulse oximetry (94760, 94761, 94762), blood gases and information data stored in computers (eg, ECGs, blood pressures, hematologic data), gastric intubation (43752, 43753), temporary transcutaneous pacing (92953), ventilatory management (94002, 94003, 94660, 94662), and vascular access procedures (36000, 36400, 36405, 36406, 36415, 36591, 36600). Any services performed which are not listed above should be reported separately.

Inpatient Neonatal and Pediatric Critical Care

The same definitions for critical care services apply for the adult, child, and neonate.

Codes 99468, 99469 may be used to report the services of directing the inpatient care of a critically ill neonate or infant 28 days of age or younger. They represent care starting with the date of admission (99468) for critical care services and all subsequent day(s) (99469) that the neonate remains in critical care. These codes may be reported only by a single individual and only once per calendar day, per patient. Initial inpatient neonatal critical care (99468) may only be reported once per hospital admission. If readmitted for neonatal critical care services during the same hospital stay, then report the subsequent inpatient neonatal critical care code (99469) for the first day of readmission to critical care, and 99469 for each day of critical care following readmission.

The initial inpatient neonatal critical care code (99468) can be used in addition to 99464 or 99465 as appropriate, when the physician or other qualified health care professional is present for the delivery (99464) or resuscitation (99465) is required. Other procedures performed as a necessary part of the resuscitation (eg, endotracheal intubation [31500]) may also be reported separately, when performed as part of the pre-admission delivery room care. In order to report these procedures separately, they must be performed as a necessary component of the resuscitation and not simply as a convenience before admission to the neonatal intensive care unit.

Codes 99471-99476 may be used to report the services of directing the inpatient care of a critically ill infant or young child from 29 days of postnatal age through 5 years of age. They represent care starting with the date of admission (99471, 99475) for pediatric critical care services and all subsequent day(s) (99472, 99476) that the infant or child remains in critical condition. These codes may only be reported by a single individual and only once per calendar day, per patient. Services for the critically ill or critically injured child 6 years of age or older would be reported with the time-based critical care codes (99291, 99292). Initial inpatient critical care (99471, 99475) may only be reported once per hospital admission. If readmitted to the pediatric critical care unit during the same hospital stay, then report the subsequent inpatient pediatric critical care code 99472 or 99476 for the first day of readmission to critical care and 99472 or 99476 for each day of critical care following readmission.

The pediatric and neonatal critical care codes include those procedures listed for the critical care codes (99291, 99292). In addition, the following procedures are also included (and are not separately reported by professionals,

but may be reported by facilities) in the pediatric and neonatal critical care service codes (99468-99472, 99475, 99476) and the intensive care services codes (99477-99480).

Any services performed that are not included in these listings may be reported separately. For initiation of selective head or total body hypothermia in the critically ill neonate, report 99184. Facilities may report the included services separately.

Invasive or non-invasive electronic monitoring of vital signs

Vascular access procedures

    Peripheral vessel catheterization (36000)

    Other arterial catheters (36140, 36620)

    Umbilical venous catheters (36510)

    Central vessel catheterization (36555)

    Vascular access procedures (36400, 36405, 36406)

    Vascular punctures (36420, 36600)

    Umbilical arterial catheters (36660)

Airway and ventilation management

    Endotracheal intubation (31500)

    Ventilatory management (94002-94004)

    Bedside pulmonary function testing (94375)

    Surfactant administration (94610)

    Continuous positive airway pressure (CPAP) (94660)

Monitoring or interpretation of blood gases or oxygen saturation (94760-94762)

Car Seat Evaluation (94780-94781)

Transfusion of blood components (36430, 36440)

Oral or nasogastric tube placement (43752)

Suprapubic bladder aspiration (51100)

Bladder catheterization (51701, 51702)

Lumbar puncture (62270)

Any services performed which are not listed above may be reported separately.

When a neonate or infant is not critically ill but requires intensive observation, frequent interventions, and other intensive care services, the Continuing Intensive Care Services codes (99477-99480) should be used to report these services.

To report critical care services provided in the outpatient setting (eg, emergency department or office) for neonates and pediatric patients of any age, see the Critical Care codes 99291, 99292. If the same individual provides critical care services for a neonatal or pediatric patient less than 6 years of age in both the outpatient and inpatient settings on the same day, report only the appropriate

Neonatal or Pediatric Critical Care codes 99468-99476 for all critical care services provided on that day. Critical care services provided by a second individual of a different specialty not reporting a per-day neonatal or pediatric critical care code can be reported with 99291, 99292.

When critical care services are provided to neonates or pediatric patients less than 6 years of age at two separate institutions by an individual from a different group on the same date of service, the individual from the referring institution should report their critical care services with the time-based critical care codes (99291, 99292) and the receiving institution should report the appropriate initial day of care code 99468, 99471, 99475 for the same date of service.

Critical care services to a pediatric patient 6 years of age or older are reported with the time based critical care codes 99291, 99292.

►When the critically ill neonate or pediatric patient improves and is transferred to a lower level of care to another individual in another group within the same facility, the transferring individual does not report a per day critical care service. Subsequent hospital inpatient or observation care (99231-99233) or time-based critical care services (99291-99292) is reported, as appropriate, based upon the condition of the neonate or child. The receiving individual reports subsequent intensive care (99478-99480) or subsequent hospital inpatient or observation care (99231-99233) services, as appropriate, based upon the condition of the neonate or child.

When the neonate or infant becomes critically ill on a day when initial or subsequent intensive care services (99477-99480), hospital inpatient or observation services (99221-99233), or normal newborn services (99460, 99461, 99462) have been performed by one individual and is transferred to a critical care level of care provided by a different individual in a different group, the transferring individual reports either the time-based critical care services (99291, 99292) performed for the time spent providing critical care to the patient, the intensive care service (99477-99480), hospital inpatient or observation care services (99221-99233), or normal newborn service (99460, 99461, 99462) performed, but only one service. The receiving individual reports initial or subsequent inpatient neonatal or pediatric critical care (99468-99476), as appropriate, based upon the patient's age and whether this is the first or subsequent admission to the critical care unit for the hospital stay.◄

When a newborn becomes critically ill on the same day they have already received normal newborn care (99460, 99461, 99462), and the same individual or group assumes critical care, report initial critical care service (99468) with modifier 25 in addition to the normal newborn code.

When a neonate, infant, or child requires initial critical care services on the same day the patient already has received hospital care or intensive care services by the same individual or group, only the initial critical care service code (99468, 99471, 99475) is reported.

Time-based critical care services (99291, 99292) are not reportable by the same individual or different individual of the same specialty and same group, when neonatal or pediatric critical care services (99468-99476) may be reported for the same patient on the same day. Time-based critical care services (99291, 99292) may be reported by an individual of a different specialty from either the same or different group on the same day that neonatal or pediatric critical care services are reported. Critical care interfacility transport face-to-face (99466, 99467) or supervisory (99485, 99486) services may be reported by the same or different individual of the same specialty and same group, when neonatal or pediatric critical care services (99468-99476) are reported for the same patient on the same day.

Initial and Continuing Intensive Care Services

Code 99477 represents the initial day of inpatient care for the child who is not critically ill but requires intensive observation, frequent interventions, and other intensive care services. Codes 99478-99480 are used to report the subsequent day services of directing the continuing intensive care of the low birth weight (LBW 1500-2500 grams) present body weight infant, very low birth weight (VLBW less than 1500 grams) present body weight infant, or normal (2501-5000 grams) present body weight newborn who does not meet the definition of critically ill but continues to require intensive observation, frequent interventions, and other intensive care services. These services are for infants and neonates who are not critically ill but continue to require intensive cardiac and respiratory monitoring, continuous and/or frequent vital sign monitoring, heat maintenance, enteral and/or parenteral nutritional adjustments, laboratory and oxygen monitoring, and constant observation by the health care team under direct supervision of the physician or other qualified health care professional. Codes 99477-99480 may be reported by a single individual and only once per day, per patient in a given facility. If readmitted to the intensive care unit during the same hospital stay, report 99478-99480 for the first day of intensive care and for each successive day that the child requires intensive care services.

These codes include the same procedures that are outlined in the **Neonatal and Pediatric Critical Care Services** section and these services should not be separately reported.

The initial day neonatal intensive care code (99477) can be used in addition to 99464 or 99465 as appropriate, when the physician or other qualified health care professional is present for the delivery (99464) or resuscitation (99465) is required. In this situation, report 99477 with modifier 25. Other procedures performed as a necessary part of the resuscitation (eg, endotracheal intubation [31500]) are also reported separately when performed as part of the pre-admission delivery room care. In order to report these procedures separately, they must be performed as a necessary component of the resuscitation and not simply as a convenience before admission to the neonatal intensive care unit.

The same procedures are included as bundled services with the neonatal intensive care codes as those listed for the neonatal (99468, 99469) and pediatric (99471-99476) critical care codes.

►When the neonate or infant improves after the initial day and no longer requires intensive care services and is transferred to a lower level of care, the transferring individual does not report a per day intensive care service. Subsequent hospital inpatient or observation care (99231-99233) or subsequent normal newborn care (99460, 99462) is reported, as appropriate, based upon the condition of the neonate or infant. If the transfer to a lower level of care occurs on the same day as initial intensive care services were provided by the transferring individual, 99477 may be reported.

When the neonate or infant is transferred after the initial day within the same facility to the care of another individual in a different group, both individuals report subsequent hospital inpatient or observation care (99231-99233) services. The receiving individual reports subsequent hospital inpatient or observation care (99231-99233) or subsequent normal newborn care (99462).◄

When the neonate or infant becomes critically ill on a day when initial or subsequent intensive care services (99477-99480) have been reported by one individual and is transferred to a critical care level of care provided by a different individual from a different group, the transferring individual reports either the time-based critical care services performed (99291, 99292) for the time spent providing critical care to the patient or the initial or subsequent intensive care (99477-99480) service, but not both. The receiving individual reports initial or subsequent inpatient neonatal or pediatric critical care (99468-99476) based upon the patient's age and whether this is the first or subsequent admission to critical care for the same hospital stay.

When the neonate or infant becomes critically ill on a day when initial or subsequent intensive care services (99477-99480) have been performed by the same individual or group, report only initial or subsequent inpatient neonatal or pediatric critical care (99468-99476) based upon the patient's age and whether this is the first or subsequent admission to critical care for the same hospital stay.

For the subsequent care of the sick neonate younger than 28 days of age but more than 5000 grams who does not require intensive or critical care services, use codes 99231-99233.

99477   **Initial hospital care,** per day, for the evaluation and management of the neonate, 28 days of age or younger, who requires intensive observation, frequent interventions, and other intensive care services

(For the initiation of inpatient care of the normal newborn, use 99460)

(For the initiation of care of the critically ill neonate, use 99468)

►(For initiation of hospital inpatient or observation care of the ill neonate not requiring intensive observation, frequent interventions, and other intensive care services, see 99221-99223)◄

Rationale

In accordance with the revision of codes 99221-99223 to include observation care, guidelines and parenthetical notes throughout the Inpatient Neonatal Intensive Care Services and Pediatric and Neonatal Critical Care Services subsection have been revised to reflect these changes.

Refer to the codebook and the Rationale for codes 99221-99223 for a full discussion of these changes.

Cognitive Assessment and Care Plan Services

▲ **99483**   Assessment of and care planning for a patient with cognitive impairment, requiring an independent historian, in the office or other outpatient, home or domiciliary or rest home, with all of the following required elements:

- Cognition-focused evaluation including a pertinent history and examination,
- Medical decision making of moderate or high complexity,
- Functional assessment (eg, basic and instrumental activities of daily living), including decision-making capacity,
- Use of standardized instruments for staging of dementia (eg, functional assessment staging test [FAST], clinical dementia rating [CDR]),
- Medication reconciliation and review for high-risk medications,

- Evaluation for neuropsychiatric and behavioral symptoms, including depression, including use of standardized screening instrument(s),

- Evaluation of safety (eg, home), including motor vehicle operation,

- Identification of caregiver(s), caregiver knowledge, caregiver needs, social supports, and the willingness of caregiver to take on caregiving tasks,

- Development, updating or revision, or review of an Advance Care Plan,

- Creation of a written care plan, including initial plans to address any neuropsychiatric symptoms, neuro-cognitive symptoms, functional limitations, and referral to community resources as needed (eg, rehabilitation services, adult day programs, support groups) shared with the patient and/or caregiver with initial education and support.

Typically, 60 minutes of total time is spent on the date of the encounter.

▶(For services of 75 minutes or longer, use 99417)◀

▶(Do not report 99483 in conjunction with E/M services [99202, 99203, 99204, 99205, 99211, 99212, 99213, 99214, 99215, 99242, 99243, 99244, 99245, 99341, 99342, 99344, 99345, 99347, 99348, 99349, 99350, 99366, 99367, 99368, 99497, 99498]; psychiatric diagnostic procedures [90785, 90791, 90792]; brief emotional/behavioral assessment [96127]; psychological or neuropsychological test administration [96146]; health risk assessment administration [96160, 96161]; medication therapy management services [99605, 99606, 99607])◀

Rationale

Cognitive assessment and care plan services code 99483 has been revised. Prior to 2023, code 99483 described 50 minutes spent face-to-face with the patient and/or family/caregiver. For 2023, the time has been revised to 60 minutes of total time spent on the date of the encounter. When total time is 75 minutes or longer, prolonged services code 99417 should be reported. An instructional parenthetical note has been added directing users to prolonged services code 99417 for services of 75 minutes or longer.

In accordance with the deletion of codes 99241, 99324-99328, 99334-99337, and 99343, the exclusionary parenthetical note following code 99483 has been revised to reflect these changes.

Refer to the codebook and the Rationale for codes 99241, 99324-99328, 99334-99337, and 99343 for a full discussion of these changes.

Clinical Example (99483)

An 83-year-old female with hypertension, diabetes, arthritis, and coronary artery disease presents with confusion, weight loss, and failure to maintain her house, where she lives alone.

Description of Procedure (99483)

Obtain a complete history, including a focus on the patient's decline, from the patient and/or family/caregiver to include identification of potential symptoms that may indicate confounding underlying disease. Review vital signs. Perform a pertinent physical examination and assessment of affect, cognition, and functional status (basic activities of daily living and instrumental activities of daily living), including decision-making capacity, mobility, balance, vision, hearing, psychosocial function, and safety (ie, at home and/or driving). Evaluate the patient for neuropsychiatric and behavioral symptoms, including depression, mood instability, psychotic symptoms, aggression, apathy, and other behavioral disturbance. Assess the stage of dementia using standardized instruments. Reconcile medications and perform a review for high-risk medications that may affect cognition (separate from rating scales noted in preservice). Discuss the values and preferences of the patient and family/caregiver for care and goals of care (eg, quality of life, advance care planning). Evaluate and discuss the caregiver's relationship to the patient, availability, knowledge, general capability (eg, any physical limitation), and ability and willingness to implement a care plan. Consider relevant data, options, and risks. Formulate a diagnosis and develop a care plan (moderate to high MDM). Meet with clinical care team to review findings and develop a care plan. Based on medication reconciliation, write prescription(s) and arrange for diagnostic testing or referrals as necessary. Create a written care plan and provide a copy to the patient and/or family/caregiver. Review findings and the care plan with the patient and/or family/caregiver, to include the etiology and severity of the cognitive impairment, goals of treatment, changes in medication, and recommendations for PT and/or OT. Address safety issues, discuss caregiving issues, and make recommendations for appropriate community services (eg, rehabilitation services, adult day programs, support groups).

Evaluation / Management 99202-99499

Care Management Services

Chronic Care Management Services

 # 99490 Chronic care management services with the following required elements:

- multiple (two or more) chronic conditions expected to last at least 12 months, or until the death of the patient,
- chronic conditions that place the patient at significant risk of death, acute exacerbation/decompensation, or functional decline,
- comprehensive care plan established, implemented, revised, or monitored;

first 20 minutes of clinical staff time directed by a physician or other qualified health care professional, per calendar month.

#+ 99439 each additional 20 minutes of clinical staff time directed by a physician or other qualified health care professional, per calendar month (List separately in addition to code for primary procedure)

(Use 99439 in conjunction with 99490)

(Chronic care management services of less than 20 minutes duration in a calendar month are not reported separately)

(Chronic care management services of 60 minutes or more and requiring moderate or high complexity medical decision making may be reported using 99487, 99489)

(Do not report 99439 more than twice per calendar month)

▶(Do not report 99439, 99490 in the same calendar month with 90951-90970, 99374, 99375, 99377, 99378, 99379, 99380, 99424, 99425, 99426, 99427, 99437, 99487, 99489, 99491, 99605, 99606, 99607)◀

(Do not report 99439, 99490 for service time reported with 93792, 93793, 98960, 98961, 98962, 98966, 98967, 98968, 98970, 98971, 98972, 99071, 99078, 99080, 99091, 99358, 99359, 99366, 99367, 99368, 99421, 99422, 99423, 99441, 99442, 99443, 99605, 99606, 99607)

 # 99491 Chronic care management services with the following required elements:

- multiple (two or more) chronic conditions expected to last at least 12 months, or until the death of the patient,
- chronic conditions that place the patient at significant risk of death, acute exacerbation/decompensation, or functional decline,
- comprehensive care plan established, implemented, revised, or monitored;

first 30 minutes provided personally by a physician or other qualified health care professional, per calendar month.

#+ 99437 each additional 30 minutes by a physician or other qualified health care professional, per calendar month (List separately in addition to code for primary procedure)

(Use 99437 in conjunction with 99491)

(Do not report 99437 for less than 30 minutes)

▶(Do not report 99437, 99491 in the same calendar month with 90951-90970, 99374, 99375, 99377, 99378, 99379, 99380, 99424, 99425, 99426, 99427, 99439, 99487, 99489, 99490, 99605, 99606, 99607)◀

(Do not report 99437, 99491 for service time reported with 93792, 93793, 98960, 98961, 98962, 98966, 98967, 98968, 98970, 98971, 98972, 99071, 99078, 99080, 99091, 99358, 99359, 99366, 99367, 99368, 99421, 99422, 99423, 99441, 99442, 99443, 99495, 99496, 99605, 99606, 99607)

Rationale

In accordance with the deletion of codes 99339 and 99340, exclusionary parenthetical notes following codes 99437 and 99439 have been revised to reflect these changes.

Refer to the codebook and the Rationale for codes 99339 and 99340 for a full discussion of these changes.

Complex Chronic Care Management Services

99487 Complex chronic care management services with the following required elements:

- multiple (two or more) chronic conditions expected to last at least 12 months, or until the death of the patient,
- chronic conditions that place the patient at significant risk of death, acute exacerbation/decompensation, or functional decline,
- comprehensive care plan established, implemented, revised, or monitored,
- moderate or high complexity medical decision making;

first 60 minutes of clinical staff time directed by a physician or other qualified health care professional, per calendar month.

(Complex chronic care management services of less than 60 minutes duration in a calendar month are not reported separately)

★=Telemedicine   ◀=Audio-only   +=Add-on code   𝗡=FDA approval pending   #=Resequenced code   ⊘=Modifier 51 exempt

+ **99489**　each additional 30 minutes of clinical staff time directed by a physician or other qualified health care professional, per calendar month (List separately in addition to code for primary procedure)

(Report 99489 in conjunction with 99487)

(Do not report 99489 for care management service of less than 30 minutes)

▶(Do not report 99487, 99489 during the same calendar month with 90951-90970, 99374, 99375, 99377, 99378, 99379, 99380, 99424, 99425, 99426, 99427, 99437, 99439, 99490, 99491)◀

(Do not report 99487, 99489 for service time reported with 93792, 93793, 98960, 98961, 98962, 98966, 98967, 98968, 98970, 98971, 98972, 99071, 99078, 99080, 99091, 99358, 99359, 99366, 99367, 99368, 99421, 99422, 99423, 99441, 99442, 99443, 99605, 99606, 99607)

Rationale

In accordance with the deletion of codes 99339 and 99340, an exclusionary parenthetical note following code 99489 has been revised to reflect these changes.

Refer to the codebook and the Rationale for codes 99339 and 99340 for a full discussion of these changes.

Principal Care Management Services

\# **99424**　Principal care management services, for a single high-risk disease, with the following required elements:

- one complex chronic condition expected to last at least 3 months, and that places the patient at significant risk of hospitalization, acute exacerbation/decompensation, functional decline, or death,
- the condition requires development, monitoring, or revision of disease-specific care plan,
- the condition requires frequent adjustments in the medication regimen and/or the management of the condition is unusually complex due to comorbidities,
- ongoing communication and care coordination between relevant practitioners furnishing care;

first 30 minutes provided personally by a physician or other qualified health care professional, per calendar month.

\#+ **99425**　each additional 30 minutes provided personally by a physician or other qualified health care professional, per calendar month (List separately in addition to code for primary procedure)

(Use 99425 in conjunction with 99424)

(Principal care management services of less than 30 minutes duration in a calendar month are not reported separately)

▶(Do not report 99424, 99425 in the same calendar month with 90951-90970, 99374, 99375, 99377, 99378, 99379, 99380, 99426, 99427, 99437, 99439, 99473, 99474, 99487, 99489, 99490, 99491)◀

(Do not report 99424, 99425 for service time reported with 93792, 93793, 98960, 98961, 98962, 98966, 98967, 98968, 98970, 98971, 98972, 99071, 99078, 99080, 99091, 99358, 99359, 99366, 99367, 99368, 99421, 99422, 99423, 99441, 99442, 99443, 99605, 99606, 99607)

\# **99426**　Principal care management services, for a single high-risk disease, with the following required elements:

- one complex chronic condition expected to last at least 3 months, and that places the patient at significant risk of hospitalization, acute exacerbation/decompensation, functional decline, or death,
- the condition requires development, monitoring, or revision of disease-specific care plan,
- the condition requires frequent adjustments in the medication regimen and/or the management of the condition is unusually complex due to comorbidities,
- ongoing communication and care coordination between relevant practitioners furnishing care;

first 30 minutes of clinical staff time directed by physician or other qualified health care professional, per calendar month.

\#+ **99427**　each additional 30 minutes of clinical staff time directed by a physician or other qualified health care professional, per calendar month (List separately in addition to code for primary procedure)

(Use 99427 in conjunction with 99426)

(Principal care management services of less than 30 minutes duration in a calendar month are not reported separately)

(Do not report 99427 more than twice per calendar month)

▶(Do not report 99426, 99427 in the same calendar month with 90951-90970, 99374, 99375, 99377, 99378, 99379, 99380, 99424, 99425, 99437, 99439, 99473, 99474, 99487, 99489, 99490, 99491)◀

(Do not report 99426, 99427 for service time reported with 93792, 93793, 98960, 98961, 98962, 98966, 98967, 98968, 98970, 98971, 98972, 99071, 99078, 99080, 99091, 99358, 99359, 99366, 99367, 99368, 99421, 99422, 99423, 99441, 99442, 99443, 99605, 99606, 99607)

Rationale

Parenthetical notes listed for use of principal care management (PCM) services in conjunction with medical therapy management services and medical team conference services have been revised to provide instructions regarding appropriate reporting when these services are performed together. In addition, these parenthetical notes have been revised to reflect the deletion of codes 99339 and 99340, and to restrict reporting PCM codes 99424-99427 in conjunction with self-measured blood pressure.

Parenthetical notes included within the PCM section following codes 99425 and 99427 have been revised to allow reporting of medical therapy management services when separate time is performed for each service. Although PCM services inherently include management of medication during the time when principal care is provided, the parenthetical note following the noted PCM codes has been revised to acknowledge separate reporting for the effort of providing medication management of a different condition than the condition being addressed by the PCM service. As a result, the management of that separate condition may be separately reported, as long as the time spent performing the medication management of that additional condition is different from the time spent managing the condition at issue for the principal care service. (**Note:** Time spent for the same condition being addressed by the PCM service is considered as part of the time for the reported PCM code.) As a result, codes 99605-99607 have been removed from the exclusionary parenthetical notes following codes 99425 and 99427 within the PCM section.

Codes 99473 and 99474 have also been added to the exclusionary parenthetical notes following codes 99425 and 99427 that restrict reporting when performed in conjunction with PCM. This acknowledges nonreporting of self-measured BP services when performed within the period when PCM is performed.

In alignment with separate reportability of time provided for PCM when performed with medication therapy management for a different condition or separately provided time, the exclusionary parenthetical note following medical team conference code 99368 has been revised by deleting PCM codes 99424-99427 from the parenthetical note. This allows separate reporting for medical team conferences without direct (face-to-face) contact with the patient and/or family/caregiver when separate time is provided for both the PCM and medical team conference of a different condition from that addressed for the PCM.

Transitional Care Management Services

▶Codes 99495 and 99496 are used to report transitional care management services (TCM). These services are for a new or established patient whose medical and/or psychosocial problems require a moderate or high level of medical decision making during transitions in care from an inpatient hospital setting (including acute hospital, rehabilitation hospital, long-term acute care hospital), partial hospital, observation status in a hospital, or skilled nursing facility/nursing facility to the patient's community setting (eg, home, rest home, or assisted living). Home may be defined as a private residence, temporary lodging, or short-term accommodation (eg, hotel, campground, hostel, or cruise ship).

These codes are also used when the residence is an assisted living facility, group home (that is not licensed as an intermediate care facility for individuals with intellectual disabilities), custodial care facility, or residential substance abuse treatment facility.◀

TCM commences upon the date of discharge and continues for the next 29 days.

TCM is comprised of one face-to-face visit within the specified timeframes, in combination with non-face-to-face services that may be performed by the physician or other qualified health care professional and/or licensed clinical staff under his/her direction.

Non-face-to-face services provided by clinical staff, under the direction of the physician or other qualified health care professional, may include:

- communication (with patient, family members, guardian or caretaker, surrogate decision makers, and/or other professionals) regarding aspects of care,
- communication with home health agencies and other community services utilized by the patient,
- patient and/or family/caretaker education to support self-management, independent living, and activities of daily living,
- assessment and support for treatment regimen adherence and medication management,
- identification of available community and health resources,
- facilitating access to care and services needed by the patient and/or family

Non-face-to-face services provided by the physician or other qualified health care provider may include:

- obtaining and reviewing the discharge information (eg, discharge summary, as available, or continuity of care documents);

- reviewing need for or follow-up on pending diagnostic tests and treatments;

- interaction with other qualified health care professionals who will assume or reassume care of the patient's system-specific problems;

- education of patient, family, guardian, and/or caregiver;

- establishment or reestablishment of referrals and arranging for needed community resources;

- assistance in scheduling any required follow-up with community providers and services.

TCM requires a face-to-face visit, initial patient contact, and medication reconciliation within specified time frames. The first face-to-face visit is part of the TCM service and not reported separately. Additional E/M services provided on subsequent dates after the first face-to-face visit may be reported separately. TCM requires an interactive contact with the patient or caregiver, as appropriate, within two business days of discharge. The contact may be direct (face-to-face), telephonic, or by electronic means. Medication reconciliation and management must occur no later than the date of the face-to-face visit.

These services address any needed coordination of care performed by multiple disciplines and community service agencies. The reporting individual provides or oversees the management and/or coordination of services, as needed, for all medical conditions, psychosocial needs and activity of daily living support by providing first contact and continuous access.

▶Medical decision making and the date of the first face-to-face visit are used to select and report the appropriate TCM code. For 99496, the face-to-face visit must occur within 7 calendar days of the date of discharge and there must be a high level of medical decision making. For 99495, the face-to-face visit must occur within 14 calendar days of the date of discharge and there must be at least a moderate level of medical decision making.

Level of Medical Decision Making	Face-to-Face Visit Within 7 Days	Face-to-Face Visit Within 8 to 14 Days
Moderate	99495	99495
High	99496	99495

Medical decision making is defined by the E/M Services Guidelines. The medical decision making over the service period reported is used to define the medical decision making of TCM. Documentation includes the timing of the initial post-discharge communication with the patient or caregivers, date of the face-to-face visit, and the level of medical decision making.◀

Only one individual may report these services and only once per patient within 30 days of discharge. Another TCM may not be reported by the same individual or group for any subsequent discharge(s) within the 30 days. The same individual may report hospital or observation discharge services and TCM. However, the discharge service may not constitute the required face-to-face visit. The same individual should not report TCM services provided in the postoperative period of a service that the individual reported.

★▲ **99495** **Transitional care management services** with the following required elements:

- Communication (direct contact, telephone, electronic) with the patient and/or caregiver within 2 business days of discharge

- At least moderate level of medical decision making during the service period

- Face-to-face visit, within 14 calendar days of discharge

★▲ **99496** **Transitional care management services** with the following required elements:

- Communication (direct contact, telephone, electronic) with the patient and/or caregiver within 2 business days of discharge

- High level of medical decision making during the service period

- Face-to-face visit, within 7 calendar days of discharge

Rationale

In accordance with the revisions to the E/M MDM guidelines, the term "complexity" has been changed to "level" in the Transitional Care Management Services subsection guidelines and code descriptors. The guidelines have also been revised in accordance with the revisions to the home or residence services codes 99341-99350.

Refer to the codebook and the Rationale for the E/M introductory guidelines and home or residence services codes 99341-99350 for a full discussion of these changes.

Evaluation / Management 99202-99499

Advance Care Planning

Codes 99497, 99498 are used to report the face-to-face service between a physician or other qualified health care professional and a patient, family member, or surrogate in counseling and discussing advance directives, with or without completing relevant legal forms. An advance directive is a document appointing an agent and/or recording the wishes of a patient pertaining to his/her medical treatment at a future time should he/she lack decisional capacity at that time. Examples of written advance directives include, but are not limited to, Health Care Proxy, Durable Power of Attorney for Health Care, Living Will, and Medical Orders for Life-Sustaining Treatment (MOLST).

When using codes 99497, 99498, no active management of the problem(s) is undertaken during the time period reported.

►Codes 99497, 99498 may be reported separately if these services are performed on the same day as another evaluation and management service (99202-99215, 99221, 99222, 99223, 99231, 99232, 99233, 99234, 99235, 99236, 99238, 99239, 99242, 99243, 99244, 99245, 99252, 99253, 99254, 99255, 99281, 99282, 99283, 99284, 99285, 99304, 99305, 99306, 99307, 99308, 99309, 99310, 99315, 99316, 99341, 99342, 99344, 99345, 99347, 99348, 99349, 99350, 99381-99397, 99495, 99496).◄

★◀ **99497** Advance care planning including the explanation and discussion of advance directives such as standard forms (with completion of such forms, when performed), by the physician or other qualified health care professional; first 30 minutes, face-to-face with the patient, family member(s), and/or surrogate

★+◀ **99498** each additional 30 minutes (List separately in addition to code for primary procedure)

(Use 99498 in conjunction with 99497)

(Do not report 99497 and 99498 on the same date of service as 99291, 99292, 99468, 99469, 99471, 99472, 99475, 99476, 99477, 99478, 99479, 99480, 99483)

Rationale

In accordance with the deletion of codes 99217-99219, 99220, 99224-99226, 99241, 99251, 99318, 99324-99328, 99334-99337, and 99343, the Advanced Care Planning subsection guidelines have been revised to reflect these changes.

Refer to the codebook and the Rationale for codes 99217-99220, 99224-99226, 99241, 99251, 99318, 99324-99328, 99334-99337, and 99343 for a full discussion of these changes.

★=Telemedicine ◀=Audio-only +=Add-on code ✎=FDA approval pending #=Resequenced code ⦸=Modifier 51 exempt

Surgery

Summary of Additions, Deletions, and Revisions

The summary of changes shows the actual changes that have been made to the code descriptors.

New codes appear with a bullet (●) and are indicated as "Code added." Revised codes are preceded with a triangle (▲). Within revised codes, or if a code symbol has been deleted, the deleted language and code symbol appear with a ~~strikethrough~~, while new text appears underlined.

The ⟋ symbol is used to identify codes for vaccines that are pending FDA approval. The # symbol is used to identify codes that have been resequenced. CPT add-on codes are annotated by the ✚ symbol. The ⊘ symbol is used to identify codes that are exempt from the use of modifier 51. The ★ symbol is used to identify codes that may be used for reporting telemedicine services. The ✤ symbol is used to identify a proprietary laboratory analyses (PLA) test that has an identical descriptor as another PLA test. A PLA code that satisfies Category I code criteria and has been accepted by the CPT Editorial Panel is annotated with the ↕ symbol. The ◀ symbol is used to identify codes that may be used to report audio-only telemedicine services when appended by modifier 93 **(see Appendix T)**.

Code	Description
●**15778**	Code added
15850	~~Removal of sutures under anesthesia (other than local), same surgeon~~
▲**15851**	Removal of sutures or staples ~~under~~ requiring anesthesia (ie, general anesthesia, moderate sedation)~~(other than local), other surgeon~~
#✚●**15853**	Code added
#✚●**15854**	Code added
▲**22857**	Total disc arthroplasty (artificial disc), anterior approach, including discectomy to prepare interspace (other than for decompression)~~;~~; single interspace, lumbar
✚●**22860**	Code added
▲**27280**	Arthrodesis, ~~open,~~ sacroiliac joint, open, ~~including~~ includes obtaining bone graft, including instrumentation, when performed
●**30469**	Code added
●**33900**	Code added
●**33901**	Code added
●**33902**	Code added
●**33903**	Code added
✚●**33904**	Code added
▲**35883**	Revision, femoral anastomosis of synthetic arterial bypass graft in groin, open; with nonautogenous patch graft (eg, ~~Dacron~~ polyester, ePTFE, bovine pericardium)
#●**36836**	Code added
#●**36837**	Code added

Code	Description
#●**43290**	Code added
#●**43291**	Code added
49560	~~Repair initial incisional or ventral hernia; reducible~~
49561	~~incarcerated or strangulated~~
49565	~~Repair recurrent incisional or ventral hernia; reducible~~
49566	~~incarcerated or strangulated~~
49568	~~Implantation of mesh or other prosthesis for open incisional or ventral hernia repair or mesh for closure of debridement for necrotizing soft tissue infection (List separately in addition to code for the incisional or ventral hernia repair)~~
49570	~~Repair epigastric hernia (eg, preperitoneal fat); reducible (separate procedure)~~
49572	~~incarcerated or strangulated~~
49580	~~Repair umbilical hernia, younger than age 5 years; reducible~~
49582	~~incarcerated or strangulated~~
49585	~~Repair umbilical hernia, age 5 years or older; reducible~~
49587	~~incarcerated or strangulated~~
49590	~~Repair spigelian hernia~~
●**49591**	Code added
●**49592**	Code added
●**49593**	Code added
●**49594**	Code added
●**49595**	Code added
●**49596**	Code added
#●**49613**	Code added
#●**49614**	Code added
#●**49615**	Code added
#●**49616**	Code added
#●**49617**	Code added
#●**49618**	Code added
#●**49621**	Code added
#●**49622**	Code added
#✚●**49623**	Code added
49652	~~Laparoscopy, surgical, repair, ventral, umbilical, spigelian or epigastric hernia (includes mesh insertion, when performed); reducible~~
49653	~~incarcerated or strangulated~~

★=Telemedicine　◀=Audio-only　✚=Add-on code　✔=FDA approval pending　#=Resequenced code　⊘=Modifier 51 exempt

Code	Description
49654	~~Laparoscopy, surgical, repair, incisional hernia (includes mesh insertion, when performed); reducible~~
49655	~~incarcerated or strangulated~~
49656	~~Laparoscopy, surgical, repair, recurrent incisional hernia (includes mesh insertion, when performed); reducible~~
49657	~~incarcerated or strangulated~~
▲**50080**	Percutaneous nephrolithotomy~~nephrostolithotomy~~ or pyelolithotomy~~pyelostolithotomy~~, ~~with or without dilation, endoscopy,~~ lithotripsy, ~~stenting, or~~ stone ~~basket~~ extraction, antegrade ureteroscopy, antegrade stent placement and nephrostomy tube placement, when performed, including imaging guidance; simple (eg, stone[s] up to 2 cm in single location of kidney or renal pelvis, nonbranching stones)
▲**50081**	complex (eg, stone[s] > 2 cm, branching stones, stones in multiple locations, ureter stones, complicated anatomy) ~~over 2 cm~~
●**55867**	Code added
▲**64415**	brachial plexus, including imaging guidance, when performed
▲**64416**	brachial plexus, continuous infusion by catheter (including catheter placement), including imaging guidance, when performed
▲**64417**	axillary nerve, including imaging guidance, when performed
▲**64445**	sciatic nerve, including imaging guidance, when performed
▲**64446**	sciatic nerve, continuous infusion by catheter (including catheter placement), including imaging guidance, when performed
▲**64447**	femoral nerve, including imaging guidance, when performed
▲**64448**	femoral nerve, continuous infusion by catheter (including catheter placement), including imaging guidance, when performed
▲**66174**	Transluminal dilation of aqueous outflow canal (eg, canaloplasty); without retention of device or stent
▲**66175**	with retention of device or stent
#▲**69716**	with magnetic transcutaneous attachment to external speech processor, within the mastoid and/or resulting in removal of less than 100 sq mm surface area of bone deep to the outer cranial cortex
#●**69729**	Code added
#▲**69717**	~~Revision or r~~Replacement (including removal of existing device), osseointegrated implant, skull; with percutaneous attachment to external speech processor
#▲**69719**	with magnetic transcutaneous attachment to external speech processor, within the mastoid and/or involving a bony defect less than 100 sq mm surface area of bone deep to the outer cranial cortex
#●**69730**	Code added
#▲**69726**	Removal, entire osseointegrated implant, skull; with percutaneous attachment to external speech processor
#▲**69727**	with magnetic transcutaneous attachment to external speech processor, within the mastoid and/or involving a bony defect less than 100 sq mm surface area of bone deep to the outer cranial cortex
#●**69728**	Code added

Surgery

Integumentary System

Skin, Subcutaneous, and Accessory Structures

Debridement

+ **11008** Removal of prosthetic material or mesh, abdominal wall for infection (eg, for chronic or recurrent mesh infection or necrotizing soft tissue infection) (List separately in addition to code for primary procedure)

(Use 11008 in conjunction with 10180, 11004-11006)

(Report skin grafts or flaps separately when performed for closure at the same session as 11004-11008)

▶(For implantation of absorbable mesh or other prosthesis for delayed closure of external genitalia, perineum, and/or abdominal wall defect[s] due to soft tissue infection or trauma, use 15778)◀

Rationale

In accordance with the deletion of codes 49560-49590 and 49652-49657 and the establishment of new hernia repair codes 49591-49622 and add-on code 49623, a parenthetical note has been established instructing the use of new code 15778 for implantation of absorbable mesh or other prosthesis for delayed closure of defect(s) due to soft tissue infection or trauma.

Refer to the codebook and the Rationale for codes 49591-49622 for a full discussion of these changes.

Repair (Closure)

Other Flaps and Grafts

+ **15777** Implantation of biologic implant (eg, acellular dermal matrix) for soft tissue reinforcement (ie, breast, trunk) (List separately in addition to code for primary procedure)

(For implantation of biologic implants for soft tissue reinforcement in tissues other than breast and trunk, use 17999)

(For bilateral breast procedure, report 15777 twice. Do not report modifier 50 in conjunction with 15777)

(For topical application of skin substitute graft to a wound surface, see 15271-15278)

(The supply of biologic implant should be reported separately in conjunction with 15777)

● **15778** Implantation of absorbable mesh or other prosthesis for delayed closure of defect(s) (ie, external genitalia, perineum, abdominal wall) due to soft tissue infection or trauma

▶(For repair of anorectal fistula with plug [eg, porcine small intestine submucosa {SIS}], use 46707)◀

▶(For implantation of mesh or other prosthesis for anterior abdominal hernia repair or parastomal hernia repair, see 49591-49622)◀

▶(For insertion of mesh or other prosthesis for repair of pelvic floor defect, use 57267)◀

▶(For implantation of non-biologic or synthetic implant for fascial reinforcement of the abdominal wall, use 0437T)◀

Rationale

In accordance with the deletion of codes 49560-49590 and 49652-49657 and the establishment of new hernia repair codes 49591-49622 and add-on code 49623, code 15778 has been established to report implantation of absorbable mesh or other prosthesis for delayed closure of defect.

In addition, four new parenthetical notes have been established to direct users to the appropriate codes for repair using a plug, mesh, or other prosthesis, or non-biologic or synthetic implant.

Refer to the codebook and the Rationale for codes 49591-49622 for a full discussion of these changes.

Clinical Example (15778)

A 60-year-old obese male with a large abdominal wall defect because of necrotizing infection and extensive debridement of all involved skin, subcutaneous tissue, fascia, and muscle undergoes delayed closure with implantation of absorbable mesh.

Description of Procedure (15778)

Examine the extent of the open wound including assessment of adherence of intestine and intra-abdominal contents to the fascia. Perform adhesiolysis, separating these contents from the fascial boundaries to allow for mesh fixation. Take care during the lysis of adhesions to avoid injury to inflamed, exposed intra-abdominal contents including small intestine and colon. Drape omentum across the exposed intestine. Measure the abdominal wall defect resulting from the surgical debridement. Size an absorbable mesh to allow for closure of the abdominal wall defect and re-establishment of abdominal wall integrity. Suture the mesh to the fascial edges circumferentially, avoiding errant placement of sutures injuring the inflamed, exposed intra-abdominal contents.

Other Procedures

+ 15847 Excision, excessive skin and subcutaneous tissue (includes lipectomy), abdomen (eg, abdominoplasty) (includes umbilical transposition and fascial plication) (List separately in addition to code for primary procedure)

(Use 15847 in conjunction with 15830)

(For other abdominoplasty, use 17999)

▶(For inguinal hernia repair, see 49491-49525)◀

▶(For anterior abdominal hernia[s] repair, see 49591-49618)◀

▶(15850 has been deleted. To report, use 15851)◀

Rationale

In accordance with the deletion of codes 49560-49590 and 49652-49657 and the establishment of new hernia repair codes 49591-49622 and add-on code 49623, a parenthetical note following 15847 has been revised to reflect these changes. A new parenthetical note has also been established to instruct users to report new codes 49591-49618 for anterior abdominal hernia repair.

Refer to the codebook and the Rationale for codes 49591-49622 for a full discussion of these changes.

▲ 15851 Removal of sutures **or** staples requiring anesthesia (ie, general anesthesia, moderate sedation)

▶(Do not report 15851 for suture and/or staple removal to re-open a wound prior to performing another procedure through the same incision)◀

#+● 15853 Removal of sutures **or** staples not requiring anesthesia (List separately in addition to E/M code)

▶(Use 15853 in conjunction with 99202, 99203, 99204, 99205, 99211, 99212, 99213, 99214, 99215, 99281, 99282, 99283, 99284, 99285, 99341, 99342, 99344, 99345, 99347, 99348, 99349, 99350)◀

▶(Do not report 15853 in conjunction with 15854)◀

#+● 15854 Removal of sutures **and** staples not requiring anesthesia (List separately in addition to E/M code)

▶(Use 15854 in conjunction with 99202, 99203, 99204, 99205, 99211, 99212, 99213, 99214, 99215, 99281, 99282, 99283, 99284, 99285, 99341, 99342, 99344, 99345, 99347, 99348, 99349, 99350)◀

▶(Do not report 15854 in conjunction with 15853)◀

15852 Dressing change (for other than burns) under anesthesia (other than local)

15853 Code is out of numerical sequence. See 15851-15860

15854 Code is out of numerical sequence. See 15851-15860

Rationale

Changes have been made to the reporting of suture removal procedures. Code 15850 has been deleted and code 15851 has been revised. Add-on codes 15853 and 15854 have been established.

Prior to 2023, codes 15850 and 15851 made a distinction between suture removal by the same surgeon who performed the primary procedure (15850) and suture removal performed by a different surgeon. However, whether the surgeon who performed the primary procedure or another surgeon performed the suture removal is not relevant to the reporting of suture removal. Also, code 15850 described suture removal under anesthesia other than local anesthesia, but did not specify general anesthesia or moderate sedation. There was no coding mechanism to identify the removal of sutures that did not require anesthesia.

Effective in 2023, code 15850 has been deleted, and code 15851 has been revised with the removal of the reference to "other surgeon." Additional revisions to code 15851 include clarification that it describes suture or staple removal requiring general anesthesia or moderate sedation. It is important to note that code 15851 is not intended to report suture and/or staple removal to re-open a wound prior to performing another procedure through the same incision. An instructional parenthetical note has been added to clarify this.

Code 15853 has been established to report suture *or* staple removal not requiring anesthesia. Code 15854 has been established to report suture *and* staple removal not requiring anesthesia. Codes 15853 and 15854 are add-on codes to be reported with E/M services codes to account for the practice expense involved in the suture and/or staple removal that is not inherent in the E/M codes. Inclusionary parenthetical notes have been added following codes 15853 and 15854 indicating the E/M codes with which they may be reported. An exclusionary parenthetical note has been added restricting the reporting of codes 15853 and 15854 together.

Clinical Example (15851)

A 3-year-old male, who is status post-repair of multiple lacerations, now undergoes suture removal while under general anesthesia.

Description of Procedure (15851)

Cleanse area surrounding the wound(s) with normal saline or soak if crusting inhibits access to sutures. Remove sutures. Observe the wound line(s) for separation during the procedure. Obtain hemostasis with pressure as needed. Apply adhesive strips as needed.

Surgery / Integumentary System 10004-19499

Clinical Example (15853)

A 60-year-old male, who is status post-hernia repair of a 3- to 10-cm defect, undergoes removal of sutures during a separately reportable office or other outpatient evaluation and management service. [**Note:** This is an add-on code. Consider only the work associated with removal of the sutures.]

Description of Procedure (15853)

Clean the area surrounding the wound(s) with normal saline or soak if crusting inhibits access to sutures/staples. Remove the sutures or staples. Observe the wound line(s) for separation during the procedure. Obtain hemostasis with pressure as needed. Apply adhesive strips and sterile dressings as needed.

Clinical Example (15854)

A 60-year-old male, who is status post-hernia repair of a 3- to 10-cm defect, undergoes removal of sutures and staples during a separately reportable office or other outpatient evaluation and management service. [**Note:** This is an add-on code. Consider only the work associated with removal of the sutures and staples.]

Description of Procedure (15854)

Clean the area surrounding the wound(s) with normal saline or soak if crusting inhibits access to sutures/staples. Remove the sutures and staples. Observe the wound line(s) for separation during the procedure. Obtain hemostasis with pressure as needed. Apply adhesive strips and sterile dressings as needed.

Musculoskeletal System

General

Introduction or Removal

▶Manual preparation involves the mixing and preparation of antibiotics or other therapeutic agent(s) with a carrier substance by the physician or other qualified health care professional during the surgical procedure and then shaping the mixture into a drug-delivery device(s) (eg, beads, nails, spacers) for placement in the deep (eg, subfascial), intramedullary, or intra-articular space(s). Codes 20700, 20702, 20704 are add-on codes for the manual preparation and insertion of the drug-delivery device(s). They may be used with any open procedure code except those that include the placement of a "spacer" (eg, 27091, 27488). The add-on codes may be used when infection is present, suspected, or anticipated during the surgery. The location of the primary service determines which of the insertion codes may be selected. If the primary surgery is in the deep (subfascial) region, add-on code 20700 may be reported. If the primary surgery is within the bone or "intramedullary," add-on code 20702 may be reported. If the primary surgery is within the joint, add-on code 20704 may be reported.

Codes 20701, 20703, 20705 are add-on codes used to report removal of drug-delivery device(s). These codes may be typically associated with specific surgeries if the infection has been eradicated. For removal of a drug-delivery device from a deep (subfascial) space performed in conjunction with a primary procedure (ie, complex wound closure [13100-13160], adjacent tissue transfer [14000-14350], or a flap closure [15570-15758]), add-on code 20701 may be reported. For infection that has not been eradicated, see the tissue debridement codes (eg, 11011, 11012, 11042, 11043, 11044, 11045, 11046, 11047) for the primary procedure. If a subsequent new drug-delivery device is placed, 20700 may be additionally reported.

Similarly, for add-on code 20703, removal of drug delivery device from the bone may be associated with different procedures. If the infection has been eradicated and the drug delivery device removal is the only procedure being performed, report 20680 (removal of deep hardware). Bony reconstruction performed in conjunction with eradication of infection may be reported using the reconstruction as the primary procedure. Persistent infection that is treated using an additional bony debridement procedure (eg, 11012, 23180, 23182, 23184, 24140, 24145, 25150, 25151, 26230, 26235, 26236, 27070, 27071, 27360, 27640, 27641, 28122, 28124) may be reported using the debridement as the primary procedure. Amputation (eg, 27290, 27590, 27598) performed in conjunction with delivery of a new, manually prepared drug delivery device may be reported with add-on code 20702.

When joint infection is present, suspected, or anticipated, add-on code 20704 (for manual preparation of an intra-articular drug delivery device) may be reported. Code 20704 may not be reported when the placement of a spacer is included in the code (eg, 27091, 27488) or when antibiotic cement is used for implant fixation.

Add-on code 20705 (for removal of a manually prepared intra-articular drug delivery device) may be typically used in conjunction with a joint stabilization procedure such as arthrodesis (eg, 22532, 22533, 22534, 22548, 22551, 22552, 22554, 22556, 22558, 22585, 22586, 22590, 22595, 22600, 22610, 22614, 22634, 22800, 22802, 22804, 22808, 22810, 22812, 22830, 22853, 22854, 22899, 24800, 24802, 25800, 25805, 25810, 25825,

25830, 26841, 26842, 26843, 26844, 26850, 26852, 26860, 26861, 26862, 26863, 27279, 27280, 27282, 27284, 27286, 27580, 27870, 27871, 28295, 28296, 28298, 28299, 28705, 28715, 28725, 28730, 28735, 28737, 28740, 28750, 28755, 28760, 29907) and revision joint arthroplasties (eg, 23473, 23474 [shoulder], 24370, 24371 [elbow], 25449 [wrist], 27134 [hip], 27487 [knee], and 27703 [ankle]). In the rare circumstance in which only part of the joint is destroyed by infection, a partial arthroplasty may be reported (eg, 23470, 24360, 24361, 24362, 24365, 24366, 25441, 25442, 25443, 25444, 25445, 27125, 27236, 27438, 27440, 27441, 27442, 27443, and 27446).

If no primary service is associated with add-on code 20705 and the joint is left without remaining cartilage or stabilization (ie, flail joint), only 20680 may be reported.◄

Insertion of a prefabricated drug device(s) may not be reported with 20700, 20702, 20704. Report 20680, if removal of drug-delivery device(s) is performed alone. Report 20700, 20701, 20702, 20703, 20704, 20705 once per anatomic location.

+ 20700   Manual preparation and insertion of drug-delivery device(s), deep (eg, subfascial) (List separately in addition to code for primary procedure)

(Use 20700 in conjunction with 11010, 11011, 11012, 11043, 11044, 11046, 11047, 20240, 20245, 20250, 20251, 21010, 21025, 21026, 21501, 21502, 21510, 21627, 21630, 22010, 22015, 23030, 23031, 23035, 23040, 23044, 23170, 23172, 23174, 23180, 23182, 23184, 23334, 23335, 23930, 23931, 23935, 24000, 24134, 24136, 24138, 24140, 24147, 24160, 25031, 25035, 25040, 25145, 25150, 25151, 26070, 26230, 26235, 26236, 26990, 26991, 26992, 27030, 27070, 27071, 27090, 27301, 27303, 27310, 27360, 27603, 27604, 27610, 27640, 27641, 28001, 28002, 28003, 28020, 28120, 28122)

►(Do not report 20700 in conjunction with any services that include placement of a spacer [eg, 11981, 27091, 27488])◄

+ 20701   Removal of drug-delivery device(s), deep (eg, subfascial) (List separately in addition to code for primary procedure)

►(Use 20701 in conjunction with 11010, 11011, 11012, 11043, 11044, 11046, 11047, 13100-13160, 14000-14350, 15570, 15572, 15574, 15576, 15736, 15738, 15740, 15750, 15756, 15757, 15758)◄

(Do not report 20701 in conjunction with 11982)

►(For removal of a deep drug-delivery device only, use 20680)◄

+ 20702   Manual preparation and insertion of drug-delivery device(s), intramedullary (List separately in addition to code for primary procedure)

(Use 20702 in conjunction with 20680, 20690, 20692, 20694, 20802, 20805, 20838, 21510, 23035, 23170, 23180, 23184, 23515, 23615, 23935, 24134, 24138, 24140, 24147, 24430, 24516, 25035, 25145, 25150, 25151, 25400, 25515, 25525, 25526, 25545, 25574, 25575, 27245, 27259, 27360, 27470, 27506, 27640, 27720)

►(Do not report 20702 in conjunction with 11981, 27091, 27488)◄

+ 20703   Removal of drug-delivery device(s), intramedullary (List separately in addition to code for primary procedure)

►(Use 20703 in conjunction with 23485, 24430, 24435, 25400, 25405, 25415, 25420, 25425, 27470, 27472, 27720, 27722, 27724, 27725)◄

(Do not report 20703 in conjunction with 11982)

►(For removal of an intramedullary drug-delivery device as a stand-alone procedure, use 20680)◄

+ 20704   Manual preparation and insertion of drug-delivery device(s), intra-articular (List separately in addition to code for primary procedure)

►(Use 20704 in conjunction with 22864, 22865, 23040, 23044, 23334, 23335, 23473, 23474, 24000, 24160, 24370, 24371, 25040, 25250, 25251, 25449, 26070, 26990, 27030, 27090, 27132, 27134, 27137, 27138, 27301, 27310, 27487, 27603, 27610, 27703, 28020)◄

(Do not report 20704 in conjunction with 11981, 27091, 27488)

+ 20705   Removal of drug-delivery device(s), intra-articular (List separately in addition to code for primary procedure)

►(Use 20705 in conjunction with 22864, 22865, 23040, 23044, 23334, 23473, 23474, 24000, 24160, 24370, 24371, 25040, 25250, 25251, 25449, 26070, 26075, 26080, 26990, 27030, 27090, 27132, 27134, 27137, 27138, 27301, 27310, 27487, 27603, 27610, 27703, 28020)◄

►(Do not report 20705 in conjunction with 11982, 27130, 27447, 27486)◄

►(For arthrodesis after eradicated infection, see 22532, 22533, 22534, 22548, 22551, 22552, 22554, 22556, 22558, 22585, 22586, 22590, 22595, 22600, 22610, 22614, 22634, 22800, 22802, 22804, 22808, 22810, 22812, 22830, 22853, 22854, 22899, 24800, 24802, 25800, 25805, 25810, 25825, 25830, 26841, 26842, 26843, 26844, 26850, 26852, 26860, 26861, 26862, 26863, 27279, 27280, 27282, 27284, 27286, 27580, 27870, 27871, 28295, 28296, 28298, 28299, 28705, 28715, 28725, 28730, 28735, 28737, 28740, 28750, 28755, 28760, 29907)◄

►(For implant removal after failed drug delivery device placement, see 22862, 22864, 23334, 23335, 24160, 25250, 25251, 27090, 27091, 27488, 27704)◄

Surgery / Musculoskeletal System   20100-29999

▶(For partial replacement after successful eradication of infection with removal of drug delivery implant, see 23470, 24360, 24361, 24362, 24365, 24366, 25441, 25442, 25443, 25444, 25445, 27125, 27236, 27438, 27440, 27441, 27442, 27443, 27446)◀

Rationale

Guidelines and parenthetical notes associated with codes 20700-20705 have been added or revised to provide better instructions regarding intent for reporting these services when performed in conjunction with other surgical procedures.

The introductory guidelines and instructional parenthetical notes for these add-on codes have been updated to clarify when these procedures may be additionally reported. Additional instructions have been added to reflect correct reporting that may vary according to whether the infection being addressed by the drug-delivery device has been eradicated or not. If the infection has been eradicated, no additional consideration is necessary to report the service. However, if the device is removed but the infection is still present, the physician may deem it necessary to perform other procedures to address the infection at the same operative session. This can include services such as debridement of the infected area. In these circumstances, it is appropriate to report the appropriate debridement code in conjunction with the device removal code.

The circumstance may also vary according to whether a drug-delivery device is being removed from a site where an infection has been eradicated but requires significant work to close the wound or separate work to address injury(ies) that has not healed. In these circumstances, reporting a code(s) according to the specific repair(s) performed may be appropriate.

The guidelines and parenthetical notes that have been updated for this subsection provide specific information that explains how these codes are intended to be reported. This includes guidance such as how to report deep removal of a drug-delivery device when the infection has been eradicated and the drug-delivery device removal is the only procedure being performed (20680). This also includes instruction for how to report insertion of a drug-delivery device into deep tissue when a spacer is also inserted, how to report implant removal after a failed drug-delivery device placement, and how to report partial replacement after successful eradication of infection with removal of drug-delivery implant. The parenthetical notes have also been updated to reflect more specific listings of codes that may or may not be reported according to the type of instruction being provided.

Replantation

▶(For repair of incomplete amputation of the arm, forearm, hand, digit, thumb, thigh, leg, foot, or toe, report the specific code[s] for repair of bone[s], ligament[s], tendon[s], nerve[s], and/or blood vessel[s] and append modifier 51 or 59 as appropriate)◀

▶(For replantation of complete amputation of the lower extremity, except foot, report the specific code[s] for repair of bone[s], ligament[s], tendon[s], nerve[s], and/or blood vessel[s] and append modifier 51 or 59 as appropriate)◀

20802 Replantation, arm (includes surgical neck of humerus through elbow joint), complete amputation

20805 Replantation, forearm (includes radius and ulna to radial carpal joint), complete amputation

20808 Replantation, hand (includes hand through metacarpophalangeal joints), complete amputation

20816 Replantation, digit, excluding thumb (includes metacarpophalangeal joint to insertion of flexor sublimis tendon), complete amputation

20822 Replantation, digit, excluding thumb (includes distal tip to sublimis tendon insertion), complete amputation

20824 Replantation, thumb (includes carpometacarpal joint to MP joint), complete amputation

20827 Replantation, thumb (includes distal tip to MP joint), complete amputation

20838 Replantation, foot, complete amputation

Rationale

Parenthetical notes previously associated with replantation codes (20802, 20805, 20808, 20816, 20822, 20824, 20827, 20838) implied that use of modifier 52 (reduced services) was appropriate for reporting incomplete replantation procedures. These parenthetical notes have been deleted and two new introductory parenthetical notes have been established to clarify correct reporting. The first new introductory parenthetical note instructs that repair of incomplete amputation at specific anatomical locations is reported with code(s) for repair of bone(s), ligament(s), tendon(s), nerve(s), and/or blood vessel(s) as appropriate, and to append modifier 51 or 59 as appropriate. The additional introductory parenthetical note that follows provides instruction regarding reporting replantation of a complete amputation of the lower extremity, except foot, with code(s) for repair of bone(s), ligament(s), tendon(s), nerve(s), and/or blood vessel(s), and appending modifier 51 or 59 as appropriate.

★=Telemedicine ◀=Audio-only ✚=Add-on code 𝒩=FDA approval pending #=Resequenced code ⊘=Modifier 51 exempt

Spine (Vertebral Column)

Spinal Instrumentation

▲ **22857**   Total disc arthroplasty (artificial disc), anterior approach, including discectomy to prepare interspace (other than for decompression); single interspace, lumbar

(Do not report 22857 in conjunction with 22558, 22845, 22853, 22854, 22859, 49010 when performed at the same level)

22858   Code is out of numerical sequence. See 22853-22861

22859   Code is out of numerical sequence. See 22853-22861

+● **22860**   second interspace, lumbar (List separately in addition to code for primary procedure)

►(Use 22860 in conjunction with 22857)◄

►(For total disc arthroplasty, anterior approach, lumbar, more than two interspaces, use 22899)◄

Rationale

Code 0163T, *Total disc arthroplasty (artificial disc), anterior approach, including discectomy to prepare interspace (other than for decompression), each additional interspace, lumbar (List separately in addition to code for primary procedure),* has been deleted from the Category III codes section and new Category I code 22860 has been added to report total disc arthroplasty of a second interspace performed via anterior approach. In addition, numerous parenthetical notes have been added, deleted, or revised, and code 22857 has been revised to become a parent code to accommodate the addition of new code 22860.

Previously, code 0163T was reported for **each** additional interspace of arthroplasty provided for the procedure described in code 22857. However, it was determined that total disc arthroplasty of more than two interspaces was rare. Therefore, new code 22860 is reported only for the second interspace in conjunction with code 22857. If more than two interspaces are treated, then the unlisted code 22899 is reported for the entire procedure. This is additionally supported by the deletion of the parenthetical note that previously directed users to report code 0163T for additional levels of arthroplasty. In accordance with the deletion of code 0163T, parenthetical notes have been added, deleted, and revised throughout the code set to reflect this change.

Code 22857 has been revised by replacing the comma with a semicolon to allow the use of this code as a parent code for the new child code 22860.

Clinical Example (22857)

A 41-year-old male has progressive low-back pain for several years that is unresponsive to multiple modalities of conservative treatment. Plain X rays and magnetic resonance imaging (MRI) scan show degenerative disc disease at the L5-S1 level. Discograms reproduce concordant pain at the affected level. A total disc arthroplasty is performed using an anterior approach. Postoperative hospital care and office visits are conducted as necessary through the 90-day global.

Description of Procedure (22857)

[Co-Surgeon A: Exposure] Make a left paramedian incision to expose the abdominal muscles of the anterior abdominal wall. Identify and mobilize the deeper rectus muscle within the rectus sheath. Perform anterior retroperitoneal approach to the spine after incision of the posterior sheath, and gradually mobilize and sweep the abdominal contents, including rectum medially. Identify and protect the left ureter; keep it to the left as the peritoneal contents are swept to the right. Place hand-held or self-retaining retractors to maintain the retroperitoneal exposure. Identify the iliac arteries and veins and palpate the sacral promontory. Place a marker for intraoperative fluoroscopic confirmation of the lumbosacral junction. Identify, coagulate or tie, and divide the median sacral vein. Similarly, identify, tie, and divide the iliolumbar vein, as required, to improve mobilization of the iliac vein. Perform dissection around the iliac veins to mobilize these veins laterally for sufficient anterior exposure. As needed, perform mobilization of the vena cava and/or aorta to allow sufficient mobility of the iliac vessels to achieve the necessary exposure. Carefully place manual retraction on the iliac vessels to maintain sufficient midline exposure of the interspace. Examine the bifurcation for degree of stretch and perform additional mobilization as required to prevent venous laceration. Mark the midline and use intraoperative fluoroscopy to confirm midline localization. In addition, perform any subsequent mobilization during the spine component of the procedure, as necessary.

[Co-Surgeon B: Arthroplasty] Incise the annulus using a combination of elevators, rongeurs, and curettes to perform a near-total discectomy. Remove the cartilaginous end plates. Pay particular attention to the posterolateral aspects of the disc space to ensure an adequate cavity for the arthroplasty device. Shape the superior and inferior cortical endplates to obtain the necessary surface for placement of the arthroplasty device. Choose the appropriate prosthesis size based on the internal anatomy and preoperative imaging. Insert the arthroplasty device after templating to confirm appropriate height and width. Prevent laceration by paying attention to the retraction of the iliac vessels during arthroplasty placement. Perform intraoperative fluoroscopy in multiple projections to confirm appropriate alignment and depth. As needed, make adjustments to the arthroplasty device.

[**Co-Surgeon A: Closure**] Relax the retraction on the iliac veins and examine the vessel integrity, and repair if needed. Irrigate and inspect the retroperitoneal exposure for bleeding sites. Examine and inspect the ureter for integrity. Remove the abdominal retractors and examine the integrity of the peritoneum, and repair if needed. As necessary, place and bring out retroperitoneal drains through a separate incision. Close the posterior rectus sheath and close the abdominal musculature in layers using sutures and staples, as indicated.

Clinical Example (22860)

A 43-year-old male, who has just had an anterior approach L4-L5 lumbar total disc arthroplasty, also requires an L5-S1 lumbar total disc arthroplasty, undergoes an anterior approach L5-S1 lumbar total disc arthroplasty. [**Note:** This is an add-on service. Consider only the work associated with the L5-S1 anterior approach lumbar total disc arthroplasty.]

Description of Procedure (22860)

[**Second-level arthroplasty, additional approach work by Co-Surgeon A**] Identify the additional vertebral level using fluoroscopy, mobilize and retract the left iliac artery and vein from left to right to provide sufficient anterior exposure of the additional disc space. Use careful table-mounted or manual retraction on the vessels to maintain sufficient midline exposure of the interspace. Mark the midline and use intraoperative fluoroscopy to confirm midline localization.

[**Second-level arthroplasty work by Co-Surgeon B**] Incise the annulus and use a combination of elevators, rongeurs, and curettes to perform a near total discectomy. Remove the cartilaginous end plates. Pay particular attention to the posterolateral aspects of the disc space to ensure an adequate cavity for the arthroplasty device. Shape the superior and inferior cortical endplates to obtain the necessary surface for placement of the arthroplasty device. Choose the appropriate prosthesis size based on the internal anatomy and preoperative imaging. Confirm the appropriate height and width after templating and insert the arthroplasty device. Prevent laceration by paying attention to the retraction of the iliac vessels during arthroplasty placement. Perform intraoperative fluoroscopy in multiple projections to confirm appropriate alignment and depth. As needed, make adjustments to the arthroplasty device.

[**Second-level arthroplasty, additional closure work by Co-Surgeon A**] Relax the additional retraction on the iliac veins and examine the vessel integrity, and repair if needed. Irrigate the additional retroperitoneal exposure and inspect for bleeding sites.

Pelvis and Hip Joint

Arthrodesis

▶Code 27279 describes percutaneous arthrodesis of the sacroiliac joint using a minimally invasive technique to place an internal fixation device(s) that passes through the ilium, across the sacroiliac joint and into the sacrum, thus transfixing the sacroiliac joint. Report 0775T for the percutaneous placement of an intra-articular stabilization device into the sacroiliac joint using a minimally invasive technique that does not transfix the sacroiliac joint. For percutaneous arthrodesis of the sacroiliac joint utilizing both a transfixation device and intra-articular implant(s), use 27299.◀

27279 Arthrodesis, sacroiliac joint, percutaneous or minimally invasive (indirect visualization), with image guidance, includes obtaining bone graft when performed, and placement of transfixing device

▶(Do not report 27279 in conjunction with 0775T)◀

▶(For percutaneous arthrodesis of the sacroiliac joint utilizing both a transfixation device and intra-articular implant[s], use 27299)◀

▶(For percutaneous arthrodesis of the sacroiliac joint by intra-articular implant[s], use 0775T)◀

(For bilateral procedure, report 27279 with modifier 50)

▲ **27280** Arthrodesis, sacroiliac joint, open, includes obtaining bone graft, including instrumentation, when performed

▶(Do not report 27280 in conjunction with 0775T)◀

▶(For percutaneous/minimally invasive arthrodesis of the sacroiliac joint without fracture and/or dislocation, utilizing a transfixation device, use 27279)◀

(To report bilateral procedure, report 27280 with modifier 50)

★ = Telemedicine   ◀ = Audio-only   ✚ = Add-on code   ✗ = FDA approval pending   # = Resequenced code   ⊘ = Modifier 51 exempt

Surgery / Musculoskeletal System 20100-29999

Rationale

New introductory guidelines and parenthetical notes have been included within the code set to accommodate the editorial revision of code 27280 and the addition of code 0775T. The new guidelines clarify the differences in devices and techniques between code 27279 (internal fixation device transfixes the sacroiliac joint) and 0775T (placement of intra-articular stabilization implant). A parenthetical note has also been added that instructs reporting unlisted code 27299 for instances when both a transfixing device and intra-articular implant are placed.

Refer to the codebook and the Rationale for code 0775T for a full discussion of these changes.

Femur (Thigh Region) and Knee Joint

Repair, Revision, and/or Reconstruction

27415 Osteochondral allograft, knee, open

(For arthroscopic implant of osteochondral allograft, use 29867)

(Do not report 27415 in conjunction with 27416)

▶(For osteochondral xenograft scaffold, use 0737T)◀

27416 Osteochondral autograft(s), knee, open (eg, mosaicplasty) (includes harvesting of autograft[s])

(Do not report 27416 in conjunction with 27415, 29870, 29871, 29875, 29884 when performed at the same session and/or 29874, 29877, 29879, 29885-29887 when performed in the same compartment)

(For arthroscopic osteochondral autograft of knee, use 29866)

▶(For osteochondral xenograft scaffold, use 0737T)◀

Rationale

In accordance with the establishment of code 0737T, instructional parenthetical notes following codes 27415 and 27416 have been added to direct users to code 0737T for xenograft implantation into the articular surface.

Refer to the codebook and the Rationale for code 0737T for a full discussion of these changes.

Respiratory System

Nose

Repair

30465 Repair of nasal vestibular stenosis (eg, spreader grafting, lateral nasal wall reconstruction)

▶(Do not report 30465 in conjunction with 30468, 30469, when performed on the ipsilateral side)◀

(30465 excludes obtaining graft. For graft procedure, see 15769, 20900, 20902, 20910, 20912, 20920, 20922, 20924, 21210, 21235)

▶(For repair of nasal valve collapse with low energy, temperature-controlled [ie, radiofrequency] subcutaneous/submucosal remodeling, use 30469)◀

(30465 is used to report a bilateral procedure. For unilateral procedure, use modifier 52)

30468 Repair of nasal valve collapse with subcutaneous/submucosal lateral wall implant(s)

▶(Do not report 30468 in conjunction with 30465, 30469, when performed on the ipsilateral side)◀

(For repair of nasal vestibular stenosis [eg, spreader grafting, lateral nasal wall reconstruction], use 30465)

▶(For repair of nasal vestibular stenosis or collapse without cartilage graft, lateral wall reconstruction, or subcutaneous/submucosal implant [eg, lateral wall suspension, or stenting without graft or subcutaneous/submucosal implant], use 30999)◀

(30468 is used to report a bilateral procedure. For unilateral procedure, use modifier 52)

● **30469** Repair of nasal valve collapse with low energy, temperature-controlled (ie, radiofrequency) subcutaneous/submucosal remodeling

▶(Do not report 30469 in conjunction with 30465, 30468, when performed on the ipsilateral side)◀

▶(For repair of nasal vestibular stenosis [eg, spreader grafting, lateral nasal wall reconstruction], use 30465)◀

▶(For repair of nasal vestibular lateral wall collapse with subcutaneous/submucosal lateral wall implant[s], use 30468)◀

▶(For repair of nasal vestibular stenosis or collapse without cartilage graft, lateral wall reconstruction, or subcutaneous/submucosal implant [eg, lateral wall suspension or stenting without graft or subcutaneous/submucosal implant], use 30999)◀

▶(30469 is used to report a bilateral procedure. For unilateral procedure, use modifier 52)◀

Surgery / Cardiovascular System 33016-39599

Rationale

Nasal valve collapse repair with low-energy temperature-controlled subcutaneous/submucosal remodeling has always been reported with unlisted code 30999. This procedure allows for remodeling of nasal valve cartilage by opening and improving the airway and nasal airflow.

For CPT 2023, code 30469 has been established to report the repair of nasal valve collapse with low-energy temperature-controlled (ie, radiofrequency) subcutaneous/submucosal remodeling.

Five new parenthetical notes have been added following code 30469 to guide users in the appropriate reporting for these services.

In addition, a parenthetical note has been established following code 30465 to instruct users to use new code 30469 for repair of nasal valve collapse. Existing parenthetical notes following codes 30465 and 30468 have been revised to include new code 30469. An existing parenthetical note following 30468 has been revised by deleting the term "radiofrequency remodeling."

Clinical Example (30469)

A 50-year-old male presents with chronic bilateral nasal airway obstruction that affects breathing and disturbs sleep. The patient is unresponsive to medical therapy and has nasal valve collapse upon examination. The patient is referred for nasal valve collapse repair with low-energy and temperature-controlled subcutaneous remodeling with a radiofrequency device.

Description of Procedure (30469)

Introduce the radiofrequency handpiece into the caudal border of the upper lateral cartilage and apply radiofrequency treatment in three adjacent non-overlapping areas. Perform the treatments in both an active period and a cool-down period. Take meticulous care to perform this in a non-overlapping fashion. Carefully monitor and maintain hemostasis during the procedure. Then repeat the same procedure on the opposite side.

Trachea and Bronchi

Bronchial Thermoplasty

31660 Bronchoscopy, rigid or flexible, including fluoroscopic guidance, when performed; with bronchial thermoplasty, 1 lobe

31661 with bronchial thermoplasty, 2 or more lobes

▶(For radiofrequency destruction of pulmonary nerves of the bronchi, see 0781T, 0782T)◀

Rationale

In accordance with the establishment of codes 0781T and 0782T, an instructional parenthetical note following code 31661 has been added to direct users to codes 0781T and 0782T for radiofrequency destruction of pulmonary nerves of the bronchi.

Refer to the codebook and the Rationale for codes 0781T, 0782T for a full discussion of these changes.

Cardiovascular System

Selective vascular catheterizations should be coded to include introduction and all lesser order selective catheterizations used in the approach (eg, the description for a selective right middle cerebral artery catheterization includes the introduction and placement catheterization of the right common and internal carotid arteries).

Additional second and/or third order arterial catheterizations within the same family of arteries supplied by a single first order artery should be expressed by 36218 or 36248. Additional first order or higher catheterizations in vascular families supplied by a first order vessel different from a previously selected and coded family should be separately coded using the conventions described above.

▶(For monitoring, operation of pump and other nonsurgical services, see 99190-99192, 99291, 99292, 99358, 99359, 99360)◀

(For other medical or laboratory related services, see appropriate section)

(For radiological supervision and interpretation, see 75600-75970)

(For anatomic guidance of arterial and venous anatomy, see Appendix L)

Rationale

In accordance with the deletion of code 99354, the cross-reference parenthetical note for monitoring and operation of pump and other nonsurgical services has been revised to reflect this change.

Refer to the codebook and the Rationale for code 99354 for a full discussion of this change.

Heart and Pericardium

Implantable Hemodynamic Monitors

Transcatheter implantation of a wireless pulmonary artery pressure sensor (33289) establishes an intravascular device used for long-term remote monitoring of pulmonary artery pressures (93264). The hemodynamic data derived from this device is used to guide management of patients with heart failure. Code 33289 includes deployment and calibration of the sensor, right heart catheterization, selective pulmonary artery catheterization, radiological supervision and interpretation, and pulmonary artery angiography, when performed.

33289 Transcatheter implantation of wireless pulmonary artery pressure sensor for long-term hemodynamic monitoring, including deployment and calibration of the sensor, right heart catheterization, selective pulmonary catheterization, radiological supervision and interpretation, and pulmonary artery angiography, when performed

▶(Do not report 33289 in conjunction with 36013, 36014, 36015, 75741, 75743, 75746, 76000, 93451, 93453, 93456, 93457, 93460, 93461, 93568, 93569, 93573, 93593, 93594, 93596, 93597, 93598)◀

(For remote monitoring of an implantable wireless pulmonary artery pressure sensor, use 93264)

Rationale

In accordance with the establishment of codes 93569 and 93573, the exclusionary parenthetical note following code 33289 has been revised with the addition of these new codes to restrict reporting them with code 33289.

Refer to the codebook and the Rationale for codes 93569 and 93573 for a full discussion of these changes.

Cardiac Valves

Pulmonary Valve

Code 33477 is used to report transcatheter pulmonary valve implantation (TPVI). Code 33477 should only be reported once per session.

Code 33477 includes the work, when performed, of percutaneous access, placing the access sheath, advancing the repair device delivery system into position, repositioning the device as needed, and deploying the device(s). Angiography, radiological supervision, and interpretation performed to guide TPVI (eg, guiding device placement and documenting completion of the intervention) are included in the code.

▶Code 33477 includes all cardiac catheterization(s), intraprocedural contrast injection(s), fluoroscopic radiological supervision and interpretation, and imaging guidance performed to complete the pulmonary valve procedure. Do not report 33477 in conjunction with 76000, 93451, 93453, 93454, 93455, 93456, 93457, 93458, 93459, 93460, 93461, 93563, 93566, 93567, 93568, 93569, 93573, 93593, 93594, 93596, 93597, 93598, for angiography intrinsic to the procedure.◀

Code 33477 includes percutaneous balloon angioplasty of the conduit/treatment zone, valvuloplasty of the pulmonary valve conduit, and stent deployment within the pulmonary conduit or an existing bioprosthetic pulmonary valve, when performed. Do not report 33477 in conjunction with 37236, 37237, 92997, 92998 for pulmonary artery angioplasty/valvuloplasty or stenting within the prosthetic valve delivery site.

Codes 92997, 92998 may be reported separately when pulmonary artery angioplasty is performed at a site separate from the prosthetic valve delivery site. Codes 37236, 37237 may be reported separately when pulmonary artery stenting is performed at a site separate from the prosthetic valve delivery site.

▶Diagnostic right heart catheterization and diagnostic angiography codes (93451, 93453, 93454, 93455, 93456, 93457, 93458, 93459, 93460, 93461,93563, 93566, 93567, 93568, 93569, 93573, 93593, 93594, 93596, 93597, 93598) should **not** be used with 33477 to report:

1. Contrast injections, angiography, roadmapping, and/or fluoroscopic guidance for the TPVI,

2. Pulmonary conduit angiography for guidance of TPVI, or

3. Right heart catheterization for hemodynamic measurements before, during, and after TPVI for guidance of TPVI.

Diagnostic right and left heart catheterization codes (93451, 93452, 93453, 93456, 93457, 93458, 93459, 93460, 93461, 93593, 93594, 93595, 93596, 93597, 93598), diagnostic coronary angiography codes (93454, 93455, 93456, 93457, 93458, 93459, 93460, 93461, 93563, 93564), and diagnostic pulmonary angiography codes (93568, 93569, 93573, 93574, 93575) may be reported with 33477, representing separate and distinct services from TPVI, if:

1. No prior study is available and a full diagnostic study is performed, or

2. A prior study is available, but as documented in the medical record:

   a. There is inadequate visualization of the anatomy and/or pathology, or

   b. The patient's condition with respect to the clinical indication has changed since the prior study, or

   c. There is a clinical change during the procedure that requires new evaluation.◀

Other cardiac catheterization services may be reported separately when performed for diagnostic purposes not intrinsic to TPVI.

For same session/same day diagnostic cardiac catheterization services, report the appropriate diagnostic cardiac catheterization code(s) appended with modifier 59 to indicate separate and distinct procedural services from TPVI.

Rationale

In accordance with the establishment of codes 93569-93575, the pulmonary valve guidelines have been revised to include codes 93569-93575, where appropriate, to provide accurate instruction on the reporting of these new codes.

Refer to the codebook and the Rationale for codes 93569-93575 for a full discussion of these changes.

Shunting Procedures

▶Codes 33741, 33745 are typically used to report creation of effective intracardiac blood flow in the setting of congenital heart defects. Code 33741 (transcatheter atrial septostomy) involves the percutaneous creation of improved atrial blood flow (eg, balloon/blade method), typically in infants ≤4 kg with congenital heart disease. Code 33745 is typically used for intracardiac shunt creation by stent placement to establish improved intracardiac blood flow (eg, atrial septum, Fontan fenestration, right ventricular outflow tract, Mustard/Senning/Warden baffles). Code 33746 is used to describe each additional intracardiac shunt creation by stent placement at a separate location during the same session as the primary intervention (33745).◀

Code 33741 includes percutaneous access, placing the access sheath(s), advancement of the transcatheter delivery system, and creation of effective intracardiac atrial blood flow. Codes 33741, 33745 include, when performed, ultrasound guidance for vascular access and fluoroscopic guidance for the intervention. Code 33745 additionally includes intracardiac stent placement, target zone angioplasty preceding or after stent implantation, and complete diagnostic right and left heart catheterization, when performed.

Diagnostic cardiac catheterization is not typically performed at the same session as transcatheter atrial septostomy (33741) and, when performed, may be separately reported. Diagnostic cardiac catheterization is typically performed at the same session with 33745 and the code descriptor includes this work, when performed.

▶Cardiovascular injection procedures for diagnostic angiography reported using 93563, 93565, 93566,

93567, 93568, 93569, 93573, 93574, 93575 are not typically performed at the same session as 33741. Although diagnostic angiography is typically performed during 33745, target vessels and chambers are highly variable and, when performed for an evaluation separate and distinct from the shunt creation, may be reported separately.

Codes 33745, 33746 are used to describe intracardiac stent placement. Multiple stents placed in a single location may only be reported with a single code. When additional, different intracardiac locations are treated in the same session, 33746 may be reported. Codes 33745, 33746 include all balloon angioplasty(ies) performed in the target lesion, including any pre-dilation (whether performed as a primary or secondary dilation), post-dilation following stent placement, or use of larger/smaller balloon, to achieve therapeutic result. Angioplasty in a separate and distinct intracardiac lesion may be reported separately. Use 33746 in conjunction with 33745.

Diagnostic right and left heart catheterization codes (93451, 93452, 93453, 93456, 93457, 93458, 93459, 93460, 93461, 93593, 93594, 93595, 93596, 93597) should not be used in conjunction with 33741, 33745 to report:

1. Fluoroscopic guidance for the intervention, or
2. Limited hemodynamic and angiographic data used solely for purposes of accomplishing the intervention (eg, measurement of atrial pressures before and after septostomy, atrial injections to determine appropriate catheter position).

Diagnostic right and left heart catheterization (93451, 93452, 93453, 93456, 93457, 93458, 93459, 93460, 93461, 93593, 93594, 93595, 93596, 93597) performed at the same session as 33741 may be separately reported, if:

1. No prior study is available, and a full diagnostic study is performed, or
2. A prior study is available, but as documented in the medical record:
   a. There is inadequate visualization of the anatomy and/or pathology, or
   b. The patient's condition with respect to the clinical indication has changed since the prior study, or
   c. There is a clinical change during the procedure that requires a more thorough evaluation.

For same-session diagnostic cardiac angiography for an evaluation separate and distinct from 33741 or 33745, the appropriate contrast injection(s) performed (93563, 93565, 93566, 93567, 93568, 93569, 93573, 93574, 93575) may be reported.◀

33735 Atrial septectomy or septostomy; closed heart (Blalock-Hanlon type operation)

Rationale

The Shunting Procedures subsection guidelines have been revised to clarify when it is appropriate to report new codes 93569-93575 and existing codes 93451-93461 with code 33741 or 33745. The subsection guidelines have also been updated to clarify the intent and correct reporting of codes 33741, 33745, and 33746.

Refer to the codebook and the Rationale for codes 93569-93575 for a full discussion of these changes.

Endovascular Repair of Congenital Heart and Vascular Defects

33897 Percutaneous transluminal angioplasty of native or recurrent coarctation of the aorta

(Do not report 33897 in conjunction with 33210, 34701, 34702, 34703, 34704, 34705, 34706, 36200, 37236, 37246, 75600, 75605, 75625, 93567, 93595, 93596, 93597)

(Do not report 33897 in conjunction with 33894, 33895 for balloon angioplasty of the aorta within the coarctation stent treatment zone)

(For additional congenital right heart diagnostic catheterization performed in same setting as 33897, see 93593, 93594)

(For angioplasty and other transcatheter revascularization interventions of additional upper or lower extremity vessels in same setting, use the appropriate code from the Surgery/Cardiovascular System section)

►Codes 33900, 33901, 33902, 33903, 33904 describe endovascular repair of pulmonary artery stenosis by stent placement. Codes 33900, 33901 describe stent placement within the pulmonary arteries via normal native connections, defined as superior vena cava/inferior vena cava to right atrium, then right ventricle, then pulmonary arteries. Codes 33902, 33903 describe stent placement within the pulmonary arteries, ductus arteriosus, or within a surgical shunt, via abnormal connections or through post-surgical shunts (eg, Blalock-Taussig shunt, Sano shunt, or post Glenn or Fontan procedures). Code 33904 is an add-on code that describes placement of stent(s) in additional vessels or lesions beyond the primary vessel or lesion treated whether access is via normal or abnormal connection.

Codes 33900, 33901, 33902, 33903, 33904 include vascular access and all catheter and guidewire manipulation, fluoroscopy to guide the intervention, any post-diagnostic angiography for roadmapping purposes and post-implant evaluation, stent positioning and balloon inflation for stent delivery, and radiologic supervision and interpretation of the intervention.

Angiography at the same session, as part of a diagnostic cardiac catheterization, may be reported with the appropriate angiographic codes from the Radiology or Medicine/Cardiovascular/Cardiac Catheterization/Injection Procedures sections.

Diagnostic cardiac catheterization and diagnostic angiography codes (93451, 93452, 93453, 93454, 93455, 93456, 93457, 93458, 93459, 93460, 93461, 93563, 93566, 93567, 93568, 93593, 93594, 93596, 93597, 93598) should **not** be used with 33900, 33901, 33902, 33903, 33904 to report:

1. Contrast injections, angiography, roadmapping, and/or fluoroscopic guidance for the TPVI,

2. Pulmonary conduit angiography for guidance of TPVI, or

3. Right heart catheterization for hemodynamic measurements before, during, and after TPVI for guidance of TPVI.

Diagnostic right and left heart catheterization codes (93451, 93452, 93453, 93456, 93457, 93458, 93459, 93460, 93461, 93593, 93594, 93595, 93596, 93597, 93598), diagnostic coronary angiography codes (93454, 93455, 93456, 93457, 93458, 93459, 93460, 93461, 93563, 93564), and diagnostic angiography codes 93565, 93566, 93567, 93568 may be separately reported in conjunction with 33900, 33901, 33902, 33903, 33904, representing separate and distinct services from pulmonary artery revascularization, if:

1. No prior study is available and a full diagnostic study is performed, or

2. A prior study is available, but as documented in the medical record:

   a. There is inadequate visualization of the anatomy and/or pathology, or

   b. The patient's condition with respect to the clinical indication has changed since the prior study, or

   c. There is a clinical change during the procedure that requires new evaluation.

Do not report 33900, 33901, 33902, 33903, 33904 in conjunction with 76000, 93451, 93452, 93453, 93454, 93455, 93456, 93457, 93458, 93459, 93460, 93461, 93563, 93564, 93565, 93566, 93567, 93568, 93593, 93594, 93596, 93597, 93598 for catheterization and angiography services intrinsic to the procedure.

Balloon angioplasty (92997, 92998) within the same target lesion as stent implant, either before or after stent deployment, is not separately reported.

For balloon angioplasty at the same session as 33900, 33901, 33902, 33903, 33904, but for a distinct lesion or in a different artery, see 92997, 92998.

To report percutaneous pulmonary artery revascularization by stent placement in conjunction with

Surgery / Cardiovascular System 33016-39599

diagnostic congenital cardiac catheterization, see 33900, 33901, 33902, 33903, 33904.

For transcatheter intracardiac shunt (TIS) creation by stent placement for congenital cardiac anomalies to establish effective intracardiac flow, see 33745, 33746. ◀

- ● **33900** Percutaneous pulmonary artery revascularization by stent placement, initial; normal native connections, unilateral

- ● **33901** normal native connections, bilateral

- ● **33902** abnormal connections, unilateral

- ● **33903** abnormal connections, bilateral

+● **33904** Percutaneous pulmonary artery revascularization by stent placement, each additional vessel or separate lesion, normal or abnormal connections (List separately in addition to code for primary procedure)

▶(Use 33904 in conjunction with 33900, 33901, 33902, 33903)◀

Rationale

Five new Category I codes (33900-33904) have been added for reporting percutaneous pulmonary artery revascularization procedures performed using both normal native and abnormal connections. A new parenthetical note, new guidelines, and revisions to existing guidelines have also been included to provide instructions to users regarding appropriate reporting for these codes.

Codes 33900-33904 identify percutaneous revascularization procedures used to open the left and right pulmonary arteries. The codes are listed according to catheterization procedures that require initial, "normal/native" (ie, ordinary) connections/pathways (33900, 33901), initial "abnormal" connections (33902, 33903) to access the pulmonary arteries, and any additional vessels addressed during these procedures (33904). In other words, the differences in the code language identify the differences in catheterization efforts that may be needed to eventually access the obstructed pulmonary vessels at issue in the procedure. The descriptors for codes 33900-33903 also take into account laterality (ie, unilateral or bilateral) involved in accessing and treating the pulmonary arterial vessel(s). Code 33904 is used to identify any additional, percutaneously accessed pulmonary vessels and/or lesions that may be revascularized and stented for patency. It is important to note that the language included regarding the use of this code specifies that it may be used for **each additional pulmonary vessel or each separate lesion** that may be accessed and should be used for either additional "normal" or "abnormal" catheterization connections (ie, used in conjunction with codes 33900-33903). Instruction regarding codes for which code 33904 may be reported is also included within the add-on parenthetical note following code 33904.

Guidelines included for the new codes provide information regarding: (1) what the codes are used for; (2) all of the services included as part of the procedures (such as vascular access/catheterization/guidewire manipulation, imaging to guide intervention, post-diagnostic road-mapping, post-implant evaluations, stenting, balloon inflation, and radiologic supervision and interpretation needed for the intervention, and when separate, additional imaging and catheterization procedures may be additionally reported); (3) services that are excluded from reporting in conjunction with codes 33900-33904, as well as when certain services may be separately reported; (4) how to report balloon angioplasty within the same target lesion as the stent placement; (5) how to report balloon angioplasty performed at the same session for a distinct lesion or a different artery; (6) how to report diagnostic congenital cardiac catheterization performed in conjunction with percutaneous pulmonary artery revascularization by stent placement; and (7) how to report transcatheter intracardiac shunt (TIS) creation by stent placement performed for congenital cardiac anomalies to establish effective intracardiac flow.

Clinical Example (33900)

A 2-year-old female with prior surgical repair of tetralogy of fallot in infancy is suspected of having left pulmonary artery stenosis by echocardiography and physical examination. Congenital diagnostic cardiac catheterization demonstrates severe left pulmonary artery stenosis.

Description of Procedure (33900)

With patient under general anesthesia, perform the procedure using fluoroscopic guidance throughout. Inject lidocaine into the access sites as an adjunct to general anesthesia. Obtain vascular access percutaneously, typically in a large vein. The site of venous access may vary due to patient anatomy and vascular access limitations. Obtain arterial access for hemodynamics and pressure monitoring during intervention. Initially place introducer sheaths over a wire in the vein and artery to establish secure access. Remove the wires and dilators and flush the sheaths with heparinized saline. Administer intravenous heparin to achieve therapeutic anticoagulation. Monitor the activated clotting time throughout the procedure and administer additional heparin as needed. Diagnostic cardiac catheterization (separately reportable, 93593-93597), including hemodynamic and angiographic evaluation, is initially performed and demonstrates an indication for further intervention. Use angiograms to measure the lesion, as well as neighboring healthy vessel, which is used for selection of the appropriate balloon and stent sizes. Remove the angiographic catheter and

★ = Telemedicine ◀ = Audio-only ✛ = Add-on code ✚ = FDA approval pending # = Resequenced code ⊘ = Modifier 51 exempt

advance an end-hole catheter with soft guidewire into and beyond the stenotic pulmonary artery. Replace the soft guidewire with a stiff interventional guidewire to secure a stable position in the distal branch to support the remainder of the intervention. Prepare, mount, and hand-crimp the selected stent on the appropriate delivery balloon, which has been de-aired to ensure the lowest possible profile. Remove the diagnostic introducer sheath in the vein and exchange for a larger and longer sheath to accommodate delivery of the balloon-mounted stent. Advance the delivery sheath over the wire to the target location, just distal to the lesion in the pulmonary artery. Remove the dilator and allow the sheath to bleed back to ensure evacuation of any air, then flush with heparinized saline. Load the balloon with mounted stent onto the wire and advance through the long sheath to the tip of the sheath. Adjust the entire system to position the stent, still within the sheath, across the lesion. Once in the appropriate location, partially withdraw the sheath carefully. Perform an angiogram through the side port of the sheath to evaluate the position. Make adjustments as needed and repeat angiography until the position is appropriate. Then withdraw the sheath further, fully exposing the delivery balloon. Inflate the balloon to deliver the stent within the pulmonary artery. Deflate and remove the balloon, maintaining wire position. A larger or higher-pressure balloon catheter may be used to post-dilate the stent to the desired diameter (not additionally reportable). Exchange the balloon for a diagnostic catheter to perform hemodynamic assessment of the result. Perform angiography to assess the positioning of the delivered stent and potential need for additional intervention. Remove all catheters and sheaths and use manual compression or a vascular closure device to achieve hemostasis prior to transferring the patient to the recovery area.

Clinical Example (33901)

A 4-year-old male with history of extreme prematurity, chronic lung disease, and tracheostomy is found to have right ventricular hypertension by echocardiography and bilateral pulmonary artery stenosis on MRI. Congenital diagnostic cardiac catheterization demonstrates severe bilateral pulmonary artery stenosis.

Description of Procedure (33901)

With the patient under general anesthesia, conduct the procedure using fluoroscopic guidance throughout. Inject lidocaine into the access sites as an adjunct to general anesthesia. Obtain vascular access percutaneously, typically in a large vein. The site of venous access may vary due to patient anatomy and any vascular access limitations. Obtain arterial access for hemodynamics and pressure monitoring during intervention. Initially place introducer sheaths over a wire in the vein and artery to establish secure access.

Remove the wires and dilators and flush the sheaths with heparinized saline. Administer intravenous heparin to achieve therapeutic anticoagulation. Monitor the activated clotting time throughout the case, and administer additional heparin as needed. Diagnostic cardiac catheterization (separately reportable, 93593-93597), including hemodynamic and angiographic evaluation, is initially performed and demonstrates an indication for further intervention. After identification of bilateral right and left main pulmonary artery stenosis, use angiograms to measure the lesions, as well as neighboring healthy vessels, which are used for selection of the appropriate balloon and stent sizes. Remove the angiographic catheter and advance an end-hole catheter with soft guidewire into and beyond the stenotic pulmonary artery and extend into the distal right lower lobe branch. Replace the soft guidewire with a stiff interventional guidewire to secure a stable position in the distal branch to support the remainder of the intervention. Prepare, mount, and hand-crimp the selected stent on the appropriate delivery balloon, which has been de-aired to ensure the lowest possible profile. Remove the diagnostic introducer sheath in the vein and exchange for a larger and longer sheath to accommodate delivery of the balloon-mounted stent. Advance the delivery sheath over the wire to the target location, just distal to the lesion in the right pulmonary artery. Remove the dilator and allow the sheath to bleed back to ensure evacuation of any air, then flush with heparinized saline. Load the balloon-mounted stent onto the wire and advance through the long sheath to the tip of the sheath. Adjust the entire system to position the stent, still within the sheath, across the lesion. Once in the appropriate location, partially withdraw the sheath carefully. Perform an angiogram through the side port of the sheath to evaluate the position. Make adjustments as needed and repeat angiography until the position is appropriate. Then withdraw the sheath further, fully exposing the delivery balloon. Inflate the balloon to deliver the stent within the pulmonary artery. Deflate and remove the balloon, maintaining wire position. A larger or higher-pressure balloon catheter may be used to post-dilate the stent to the desired diameter (not additionally reportable). Exchange the balloon for a diagnostic catheter to perform hemodynamic assessment of the result. Angiography is also performed to assess the positioning of the delivered stent and potential need for additional intervention. Then insert the diagnostic catheter and use to retrieve the stiff interventional wire and remove it from the body. Re-insert the soft-tipped guidewire through the catheter and advance into and beyond the stenotic left pulmonary artery and extend into the distal left lower lobe branch. Once again, remove the guidewire and re-insert the stiff interventional wire to secure left-sided wire position for the subsequent intervention. The entire process described above for the right-sided stent is now repeated to address the left pulmonary artery stenosis. Once the left-sided lesion is successfully stented, repeat a final main pulmonary artery angiogram to assess the final results of the bilateral stent implants. Remove all catheters and sheaths and use manual compression or a vascular closure device to achieve hemostasis prior to transferring the patient to the recovery area.

Clinical Example (33902)

A 3-month-old female with pulmonary atresia and intact ventricular septum who underwent surgical Blalock-Thomas-Taussig (BTT) shunt in the neonatal period presents with worsening systemic hypoperfusion, shock, and evidence of acute shunt stenosis. She is brought to the cardiac catheterization laboratory emergently for stenting of the BTT shunt.

Description of Procedure (33902)

With the patient under general anesthesia, perform the procedure using fluoroscopic guidance throughout. Inject lidocaine into the access sites to help minimize hypotension caused by excessive general anesthetic. Obtain vascular access percutaneously, typically in a large vein and an artery. The site of venous access is variable and depends on patient anatomy and any vascular access limitations. Obtain arterial access via a femoral artery but may require carotid artery access. Initially place introducer sheaths over a wire in the vein and artery to establish secure access. Remove the wires and dilators and flush the sheaths with heparinized saline. Administer intravenous heparin to achieve therapeutic anticoagulation. The activated clotting time is monitored throughout the case, and additional heparin is administered, as needed. Diagnostic catheterization varies due to inconsistent venous or arterial access to the pulmonary arteries. Diagnostic cardiac catheterization (separately reportable, 93593-93597), including hemodynamic and angiographic evaluation, is initially performed and demonstrates an indication for further intervention. If the pulmonary arteries originate from the aorta, the diagnostic evaluation would include an aortogram to evaluate the shunt or ductal pathway to the pulmonary arteries for stenosis. Use angiograms to measure the lesion, as well as neighboring healthy vessels, which are used for selection of the appropriate balloon and stent sizes. Remove the angiographic catheter and advance an end-hole catheter with soft guidewire into and beyond the stenotic lesion. Replace the soft guidewire with a stiff interventional guidewire to secure a stable position in the distal branch to support the remainder of the intervention. Prepare, mount, and hand-crimp the selected stent on the appropriate delivery balloon, which has been de-aired to ensure the lowest possible profile. Remove the diagnostic introducer sheath and exchange for a larger and longer sheath to accommodate delivery of the balloon-mounted stent.

Advance the delivery sheath over the wire to the target location, just distal to the lesion. Remove the dilator and allow the sheath to bleed back to ensure evacuation of any air, then flush with heparinized saline. Load the balloon with mounted stent onto the wire and advance through the long sheath to the tip of the sheath. Adjust the entire system to position the stent, still within the sheath, across the lesion. Once in the appropriate location, partially withdraw the sheath carefully. Perform an angiogram through the side port of the sheath to evaluate the position. Make adjustments as needed and repeat the angiography until the position is appropriate. Then withdraw the sheath further, fully exposing the delivery balloon. Inflate the balloon to deliver the stent within the target lesion. Deflate and remove the balloon, maintaining wire position. A larger or higher-pressure balloon catheter may be used to post-dilate the stent to the desired diameter (not additionally reportable). Exchange the balloon for a diagnostic catheter to perform hemodynamic assessment of the result. Also perform angiography to assess the positioning of the delivered stent and potential need for additional intervention. Remove all catheters and sheaths and use manual compression or a vascular closure device to achieve hemostasis prior to transferring the patient to the recovery area.

Clinical Example (33903)

A 5-year-old male with hypoplastic left heart syndrome, status post-Fontan operation, is identified by physical examination and subsequent MRI to have possible bilateral pulmonary artery stenoses. He is brought to the cardiac catheterization laboratory for further evaluation and possible bilateral stent implantation of the right and left main pulmonary arteries.

Description of Procedure (33903)

With the patient under general anesthesia, perform the procedure using fluoroscopic guidance throughout. Inject lidocaine into the access sites to help minimize hypotension caused by excessive general anesthetic. Obtain vascular access percutaneously, typically in a large vein and an artery. The site of venous access is variable and depends on patient anatomy and any vascular access limitations. Obtain arterial access typically in a femoral artery but may require carotid artery access. Initially place introducer sheaths over a wire in the vein and artery to establish secure access. Remove the wires and dilators and flush the sheaths with heparinized saline. Administer intravenous heparin to achieve therapeutic anticoagulation. Monitor the activated clotting time throughout the case, and administer additional heparin as needed. Diagnostic catheterization varies due to inconsistent venous or arterial access to the pulmonary arteries. Diagnostic cardiac catheterization (separately reportable,

93593-93597), including hemodynamic and angiographic evaluation, is initially performed and demonstrates an indication for further intervention. Use angiograms to measure the lesion, as well as neighboring healthy vessels, which is used for selection of the appropriate balloon and stent sizes. Remove the angiographic catheter and advance an end-hole catheter with soft guidewire into and beyond the stenotic left pulmonary artery lesion. Replace the soft guidewire with a stiff interventional guidewire to secure a stable position in the distal branch to support the remainder of the intervention. Prepare, mount, and hand-crimp the selected stent on the appropriate delivery balloon, which has been de-aired to ensure the lowest possible profile. Remove the diagnostic introducer sheath and exchange for a larger and longer sheath to accommodate delivery of the balloon-mounted stent. Advance the delivery sheath over the wire to the target location, just distal to the lesion. Remove the dilator and allow the sheath to bleed back to ensure evacuation of any air, then flush with heparinized saline. Load the balloon with mounted stent onto the wire and advance through the long sheath to the tip of the sheath. Adjust the entire system to position the stent, still within the sheath, across the lesion. Once in the appropriate location, partially withdraw the sheath carefully. Perform an angiogram through the side port of the sheath to evaluate the position. Make adjustments as needed and repeat angiography until the position is appropriate. Then withdraw the sheath further, fully exposing the delivery balloon. Inflate the balloon to deliver the stent within the target lesion. Deflate and remove the balloon, maintaining wire position. A larger or higher-pressure balloon catheter may be used to post-dilate the stent to the desired diameter (not additionally reportable). Exchange the balloon for a diagnostic catheter to perform hemodynamic assessment of the result. Also perform angiography to assess the positioning of the delivered stent and potential need for additional intervention. Then re-insert the soft-tipped guidewire through the catheter and advance into and beyond the stenotic right pulmonary artery and extend into the distal right lower lobe branch. Once again, remove the guidewire and re-insert the stiff interventional wire to secure the right-sided wire position for the subsequent intervention. The entire process described above for the left-sided stent is now repeated to address the right pulmonary artery stenosis. Once the right-sided lesion is successfully stented, repeat a final main pulmonary artery angiogram to assess the final result of the bilateral stent implants. Remove all catheters and sheaths and use manual compression or a vascular closure device to achieve hemostasis prior to transferring the patient to the recovery area.

Clinical Example (33904)

A 4-year-old female, who has just undergone bilateral stent implant via abnormal connections, requires additional stent implants for additional lesions not previously identified during congenital cardiac catheterization for suspected pulmonary artery stenosis. She undergoes additional segmental pulmonary arterial stent implant in the right and left upper branches. [**Note:** This is an add-on code for the additional work related to stent placement of each additional vessel or separate lesion {normal or abnormal} of percutaneous pulmonary artery revascularization. The work related to the first percutaneous pulmonary artery revascularization by stent placement is reported separately as the primary procedure and not included in the work of this add-on code.]

Description of Procedure (33904)

[**Note:** The work for code 33904 begins following completion of primary stent implantation in the left and/or right main pulmonary arteries.] Hemodynamic and angiographic evaluation identifies multiple segmental branch pulmonary artery stenoses. After selective angiography (separately reported) is performed in the right lower lobe segmental branch, advance an end-hole catheter with soft guidewire into and beyond the stenotic right lower lobe lesion. Replace the soft guidewire with a stiff interventional guidewire to secure a stable position in the distal branch to support the remainder of the intervention. Prepare, mount, and hand-crimp the selected stent on the appropriate delivery balloon, which has been de-aired to ensure the lowest possible profile. Advance the delivery sheath over the wire to the target location, just distal to the lesion. Remove the dilator and allow the sheath to bleed back to ensure evacuation of any air, then flush with heparinized saline. Load the balloon with mounted stent onto the wire and advance through the long sheath to the tip of the sheath. Adjust the entire system to position the stent, still within the sheath, across the lesion. Once in the appropriate location, partially withdraw the sheath carefully. Perform an angiogram through the side port of the sheath to evaluate the position. Make adjustments as needed and repeat angiography until the position is appropriate. Then withdraw the sheath further, fully exposing the delivery balloon. Inflate the balloon to deliver the stent within the target lesion. Deflate and remove the balloon, maintaining wire position. A larger or higher-pressure balloon catheter may be used to post-dilate the stent to the desired diameter and is not additionally reportable. Repeat hemodynamic and angiographic evaluation to assess the result. The entire process described above for the right lower lobe stent is now repeated in the right upper lobe, left lower lobe, and left upper lobe to address these additional bilateral segmental stenoses. Remove all catheters and sheaths and use manual compression or a vascular closure device to achieve hemostasis prior to transferring the patient to the recovery area.

Extracorporeal Membrane Oxygenation or Extracorporeal Life Support Services

Prolonged extracorporeal membrane oxygenation (ECMO) or extracorporeal life support (ECLS) is a procedure that provides cardiac and/or respiratory support to the heart and/or lungs, which allows them to rest and recover when sick or injured. ECMO/ECLS supports the function of the heart and/or lungs by continuously pumping some of the patient's blood out of the body to an oxygenator (membrane lung) where oxygen is added to the blood, carbon dioxide (CO_2) is removed, and the blood is warmed before it is returned to the patient. There are two methods that can be used to accomplish ECMO/ECLS. One method is veno-arterial extracorporeal life support, which will support both the heart and lungs. Veno-arterial ECMO/ECLS requires that two cannula(e) are placed—one in a large vein and one in a large artery. The other method is veno-venous extracorporeal life support. Veno-venous ECMO/ECLS is used for lung support only and requires one or two cannula(e), which are placed in a vein.

▶Services directly related to the cannulation, initiation, management, and discontinuation of the ECMO/ECLS circuit and parameters (33946, 33947, 33948, 33949) are distinct from the daily overall management of the patient. The daily overall management of the patient is a factor that will vary greatly depending on the patient's age, disease process, and condition. Daily overall management of the patient may be separately reported using the relevant hospital inpatient or observation care services (99221, 99222, 99223, 99231, 99232, 99233, 99234, 99235, 99236) or critical care or intensive care evaluation and management codes (99291, 99292, 99468, 99469, 99471, 99472, 99475, 99476, 99477, 99478, 99479, 99480).◀

Services directly related to the ECMO/ECLS involve the initial cannulation and repositioning, removing, or adding cannula(e) while the patient is being supported by the ECMO/ECLS. Initiation of the ECMO/ECLS circuit and setting parameters (33946, 33947) is performed by the physician and involves determining the necessary ECMO/ECLS device components, blood flow, gas exchange, and other necessary parameters to manage the circuit. The daily management of the ECMO/ECLS circuit and monitoring parameters (33948, 33949) requires physician oversight to ensure that specific features of the interaction of the circuit with the patient are met. Daily management of the circuit and parameters includes management of blood flow, oxygenation, CO_2 clearance by the membrane lung, systemic response, anticoagulation and treatment of bleeding, and cannula(e) positioning, alarms and safety. Once the patient's heart and/or lung function has sufficiently recovered, the physician will wean the patient from the ECMO/ECLS circuit and finally decannulate the patient. The basic management of the ECMO/ECLS circuit and parameters are similar, regardless of the patient's condition.

ECMO/ECLS commonly involves multiple physicians and supporting nonphysician personnel to manage each patient. Different physicians may insert the cannula(e) and initiate ECMO/ECLS, manage the ECMO/ECLS circuit, and decannulate the patient. In addition, it would be common for one physician to manage the ECMO/ECLS circuit and patient-related issues (eg, anticoagulation, complications related to the ECMO/ECLS devices), while another physician manages the overall patient medical condition and underlying disorders, all on a daily basis. The physicians involved in the patient's care are commonly of different specialties, and significant physician team interaction may be required. Depending on the type of circuit and the patient's condition, there is substantial nonphysician work by ECMO/ECLS specialists, cardiac perfusionists, respiratory therapists, and specially trained nurses who provide long periods of constant attention.

▶If the same physician provides any or all of the services for placing a patient on an ECMO/ECLS circuit, they may report the appropriate codes for the services they performed, which may include codes for the cannula(e) insertion (33951, 33952, 33953, 33954, 33955, 33956), ECMO/ECLS initiation (33946 or 33947), and overall patient management (99221, 99222, 99223, 99231, 99232, 99233, 99234, 99235, 99236, 99291, 99292, 99468, 99469, 99471, 99472, 99475, 99476, 99477, 99478, 99479, 99480).◀

ECMO/ECLS daily management (33948, 33949) and repositioning services (33957, 33958, 33959, 33962, 33963, 33964) may not be reported on the same day as initiation services (33946, 33947) by the same or different individuals.

If different physicians provide parts of the service, each physician may report the correct code(s) for the service(s) they provided, except as noted.

Repositioning of the ECMO/ECLS cannula(e) (33957, 33958, 33959, 33962, 33963, 33964) at the same session as insertion (33951, 33952, 33953, 33954, 33955, 33956) is not separately reportable. Replacement of ECMO/ECLS cannula(e) in the same vessel should only be reported using the insertion code (33951, 33952, 33953, 33954, 33955, 33956). If cannula(e) are removed from one vessel and new cannula(e) are placed in a different vessel, report the appropriate cannula(e) removal (33965, 33966, 33969, 33984, 33985, 33986) and insertion (33951, 33952, 33953, 33954, 33955, 33956) codes. Extensive repair or replacement of an artery may be additionally reported (eg, 35266, 35286, 35371, and 35665). Fluoroscopic guidance used for cannula(e) repositioning (33957, 33958, 33959, 33962, 33963, 33964) is included in the procedure when performed and should not be separately reported.

Daily management codes (33948 and 33949) should not be reported on the same day as initiation of ECMO (33946 or 33947).

Initiation codes (33946 or 33947) should not be reported on the same day as repositioning codes (33957, 33958, 33959, 33962, 33963, 33964). See the CPT codes for ECMO/ECLS Procedure Chart.

Rationale

In accordance with the deletion of codes 99218-99220, the Extracorporeal Membrane Oxygenation or Extracorporeal Life Support Services subsection guidelines have been revised to reflect these changes.

Refer to the codebook and the Rationale for codes 99218-99220 for a full discussion of these changes.

Arteries and Veins

Venous Reconstruction

34501   Valvuloplasty, femoral vein

▶(For insertion of bioprosthetic valve into femoral vein, use 0744T)◀

34502   Reconstruction of vena cava, any method

34510   Venous valve transposition, any vein donor

▶(For insertion of bioprosthetic valve into femoral vein, use 0744T)◀

Rationale

In accordance with the establishment of Category III code 0744T, cross-reference parenthetical notes have been added following codes 34501 and 34510 to reflect this change.

Refer to the codebook and the Rationale for code 0744T for a full discussion of this change.

Excision, Exploration, Repair, Revision

▲ **35883**   Revision, femoral anastomosis of synthetic arterial bypass graft in groin, open; with nonautogenous patch graft (eg, polyester, ePTFE, bovine pericardium)

(For bilateral procedure, use modifier 50)

(Do not report 35883 in conjunction with 35700, 35875, 35876, 35884)

Rationale

Code 35883 has been editorially revised. Prior to 2023, the term "Dacron" was included in the list of patch graft examples in the code descriptor. For 2023, this term has been replaced with "polyester" to conform with the CPT language convention.

Vascular Injection Procedures

Listed services for injection procedures include necessary local anesthesia, introduction of needles or catheter, injection of contrast media with or without automatic power injection, and/or necessary pre- and postinjection care specifically related to the injection procedure.

Selective vascular catheterization should be coded to include introduction and all lesser order selective catheterization used in the approach (eg, the description for a selective right middle cerebral artery catheterization includes the introduction and placement catheterization of the right common and internal carotid arteries).

Additional second and/or third order arterial catheterization within the same family of arteries or veins supplied by a single first order vessel should be expressed by 36012, 36218, or 36248.

Additional first order or higher catheterization in vascular families supplied by a first order vessel different from a previously selected and coded family should be separately coded using the conventions described above.

(For radiological supervision and interpretation, see **Radiology**)

▶(For injection procedures in conjunction with cardiac catheterization, see 93452, 93453, 93454, 93455, 93456, 93457, 93458, 93459, 93460, 93461, 93563, 93564, 93565, 93566, 93567, 93568, 93569, 93573, 93574, 93575)◀

(For chemotherapy of malignant disease, see 96401-96549)

Rationale

In accordance with the establishment of codes 93569-93575, the cross-reference parenthetical note in the Vascular Injection Procedures subsection guidelines that directs users to injection procedures performed in conjunction with cardiac catheterization has been revised with the inclusion of these new codes.

Refer to the codebook and the Rationale for codes 93569-93575 for a full discussion of these changes.

Surgery / Cardiovascular System 33016-39599

Intravenous

36005 Injection procedure for extremity venography (including introduction of needle or intracatheter)

▶(Do not report 36005 in conjunction with 36836, 36837)◀

(For radiological supervision and interpretation, see 75820, 75822)

Intra-Arterial—Intra-Aortic

36140 Introduction of needle or intracatheter, upper or lower extremity artery

▶(Do not report 36140 in conjunction with 36836, 36837)◀

(For insertion of arteriovenous cannula, see 36810-36821)

Rationale

In accordance with the establishment of codes 36836 and 36837, exclusionary parenthetical notes have been added following codes 36005 and 36140 to restrict reporting these codes with codes 36836 and 36837.

Refer to the codebook and the Rationale for codes 36836 and 36837 for a full discussion of these changes.

36215 Selective catheter placement, arterial system; each first order thoracic or brachiocephalic branch, within a vascular family

(For catheter placement for coronary angiography, see 93454-93461)

36216 initial second order thoracic or brachiocephalic branch, within a vascular family

36217 initial third order or more selective thoracic or brachiocephalic branch, within a vascular family

+ 36218 additional second order, third order, and beyond, thoracic or brachiocephalic branch, within a vascular family (List in addition to code for initial second or third order vessel as appropriate)

(Use 36218 in conjunction with 36216, 36217, 36225, 36226)

▶(Do not report 36215, 36216, 36217, 36218 in conjunction with 36836, 36837)◀

(For angiography, see 36222-36228, 75600-75774)

(For transluminal balloon angioplasty [except lower extremity artery[ies] for occlusive disease, intracranial, coronary, pulmonary, or dialysis circuit], see 37246, 37247)

(For transcatheter therapies, see 37200, 37211, 37213, 37214, 37236, 37237, 37238, 37239, 37241, 37242, 37243, 37244, 61624, 61626)

(When arterial [eg, internal mammary, inferior epigastric or free radial artery] or venous bypass graft angiography is performed in conjunction with cardiac catheterization, see the appropriate cardiac catheterization, injection procedure, and imaging supervision code[s] [93454, 93455, 93456, 93457, 93458, 93459, 93460, 93461, 93564, 93593, 93594, 93595, 93596, 93597] in the **Medicine** section. When internal mammary artery angiography only is performed without a concomitant cardiac catheterization, use 36216 or 36217 as appropriate)

Rationale

In accordance with the establishment of codes 36836 and 36837, an exclusionary parenthetical note has been added following code 36218 to restrict reporting codes 36215-36218 with codes 36836 and 36837.

Refer to the codebook and the Rationale for codes 36836 and 36837 for a full discussion of these changes.

36245 Selective catheter placement, arterial system; each first order abdominal, pelvic, or lower extremity artery branch, within a vascular family

36246 initial second order abdominal, pelvic, or lower extremity artery branch, within a vascular family

36247 initial third order or more selective abdominal, pelvic, or lower extremity artery branch, within a vascular family

+ 36248 additional second order, third order, and beyond, abdominal, pelvic, or lower extremity artery branch, within a vascular family (List in addition to code for initial second or third order vessel as appropriate)

(Use 36248 in conjunction with 36246, 36247)

▶(Do not report 36245, 36246, 36247, 36248 in conjunction with 36836, 36837)◀

Rationale

In accordance with the establishment of codes 36836 and 36837, an exclusionary parenthetical note has been added following code 36248 to restrict reporting codes 36245-36248 with codes 36836 and 36837.

Refer to the codebook and the Rationale for codes 36836 and 36837 for a full discussion of these changes.

★=Telemedicine ◀=Audio-only ✚=Add-on code ✗=FDA approval pending #=Resequenced code ⊘=Modifier 51 exempt

Hemodialysis Access, Intervascular Cannulation for Extracorporeal Circulation, or Shunt Insertion

36832 Revision, open, arteriovenous fistula; without thrombectomy, autogenous or nonautogenous dialysis graft (separate procedure)

36833 with thrombectomy, autogenous or nonautogenous dialysis graft (separate procedure)

(For percutaneous thrombectomy within the dialysis circuit, see 36904, 36905, 36906)

(For central dialysis segment angioplasty in conjunction with 36818-36833, use 36907)

(For central dialysis segment stent placement in conjunction with 36818-36833, use 36908)

(Do not report 36832, 36833 in conjunction with 36901, 36902, 36903, 36904, 36905, 36906 for revision of the dialysis circuit)

►Codes 36836, 36837 describe percutaneous arteriovenous fistula creation in the upper extremity for hemodialysis access, including image-guided percutaneous access into a peripheral artery and peripheral vein via single access (36836) or two separate access sites (36837). The artery and vein are approximated and then energy (eg, thermal) is applied to establish the fistulous communication between the two vessels. Fistula maturation procedures promote blood flow through the newly created fistula by augmentation (eg, angioplasty) or redirection (eg, coil embolization of collateral pathways) of blood flow. Codes 36836, 36837 include all vascular access, angiography, imaging guidance, and blood flow redirection or maturation techniques (eg, transluminal balloon angioplasty, coil embolization) performed for fistula creation. These procedures may not be reported separately with 36836, 36837, when performed at the same operative session.◄

#● 36836 Percutaneous arteriovenous fistula creation, upper extremity, single access of both the peripheral artery and peripheral vein, including fistula maturation procedures (eg, transluminal balloon angioplasty, coil embolization) when performed, including all vascular access, imaging guidance and radiologic supervision and interpretation

►(Do not report 36836 in conjunction with 36005, 36140, 36215, 36216, 36217, 36218, 36245, 36246, 36247, 36837, 36901, 36902, 36903, 36904, 36905, 36906, 36907, 36908, 36909, 37236, 37238, 37241, 37242, 37246, 37248, 37252, 75710, 75716, 75820, 75822, 75894, 75898, 76937, 77001)◄

►(For arteriovenous fistula creation via an open approach, see 36800, 36810, 36815, 36818, 36819, 36820, 36821)◄

►(For percutaneous arteriovenous fistula creation in any location other than the upper extremity, use 37799)◄

#● 36837 Percutaneous arteriovenous fistula creation, upper extremity, separate access sites of the peripheral artery and peripheral vein, including fistula maturation procedures (eg, transluminal balloon angioplasty, coil embolization) when performed, including all vascular access, imaging guidance and radiologic supervision and interpretation

►(Do not report 36837 in conjunction with 36005, 36140, 36215, 36216, 36217, 36218, 36245, 36246, 36247, 36836, 36901, 36902, 36903, 36904, 36905, 36906, 36907, 36908, 36909, 37236, 37238, 37241, 37242, 37246, 37248, 37252, 75710, 75716, 75820, 75822, 75894, 75898, 76937, 77001)◄

►(For arteriovenous fistula creation via an open approach, see 36800, 36810, 36815, 36818, 36819, 36820, 36821)◄

►(For percutaneous arteriovenous fistula creation in any location other than the upper extremity, use 37799)◄

Rationale

Two new codes (36836 and 36837), new introductory guidelines, and new and revised parenthetical notes have been added within the Surgery/Cardiovascular System and Radiology subsections to identify the appropriate reporting for percutaneous arteriovenous fistula creation via a single access of both the peripheral artery and peripheral vein (36836) and via separate access sites of the peripheral artery and peripheral vein (36837). Previously, there were only codes for arteriovenous fistula creation via an open approach.

To provide further instruction regarding the intended use of these new series of codes, several parenthetical notes have been added following codes 36836 and 36837. The first exclusionary parenthetical note following codes 36836 and 36837 excludes reporting of those services in conjunction with a number of procedures throughout the code set.

The second and third instructional parenthetical notes following these codes have been added to direct users to the appropriate reporting for arteriovenous fistula creation via an open approach (36800, 36810, 36815, 36818-36821), and reporting unlisted code 37799 for percutaneous arteriovenous fistula creation in any location other than the upper extremity.

In addition, numerous parenthetical notes in the Surgery and Radiology subsections have been added or revised to further clarify the appropriate reporting of these codes.

Clinical Example (36836)

A 65-year-old male with advanced chronic kidney disease will require hemodialysis. Preoperative vascular imaging shows appropriate size and patency of the radial artery and perforating vein with a distance between the respective vessels of <1.5 mm, suitable for percutaneous arteriovenous fistula creation in the upper extremity.

Description of Procedure (36836)

Using ultrasound guidance, access the target vein with a micropuncture needle. Next, using continuous ultrasound guidance, carefully navigate the same needle within the perforator vein and advance to the level of the adjacent artery. After confirming location of the needle on orthogonal views by ultrasound, puncture the artery using the needle. Advance a guidewire through the artery. Exchange the needle over the wire for a sheath until the distal end just enters the artery. Advance a catheter into the artery. Then carefully retract the catheter to grasp the arterial wall, allowing approximation of the artery and vein, which must be confirmed with ultrasound. Apply energy to create the anastomosis. Then remove the catheter and dilate the anastomosis and perforating vein with a balloon to ensure adequate flow under imaging guidance. Remove the balloon, guidewire, and sheath. Obtain hemostasis at the percutaneous venous access site using manual pressure.

Clinical Example (36837)

A 65-year-old male with advanced chronic kidney disease will require hemodialysis. Preoperative vascular imaging shows appropriate size and patency of the radial and ulnar artery, presence of a perforating vein, and radial and ulnar vein within <1 mm of the respective corresponding arteries, suitable for percutaneous arteriovenous fistula creation in the upper extremity.

Description of Procedure (36837)

Obtain ultrasound-guided access in a vein in the extremity and insert a guidewire. Next, introduce a dilator and vascular sheath and perform a venogram of the central veins. Under ultrasound guidance, access the target artery separately. Perform an arteriogram of the entire extremity. Advance a guidewire to the target creation site. Using the arterial guidewire as a roadmap, advance the venous guidewire into the vein and navigate under fluoroscopy to the intended fistula site. Then perform a venogram at the intended fistula site to confirm superficial communication via the presence of a perforator vein. Under fluoroscopic guidance, carefully advance the arterial catheter over the guidewire to the target fistula creation site making sure proper orientation to the venous guide catheter is maintained. Then insert the venous catheter into the sheath and advance over the guidewire to the target fistula creation. Optimally position the catheters and magnetic components and bring into alignment. Confirm correct orientation and

alignment via fluoroscopy in multiple orthogonal projections. Deliver radiofrequency energy to the electrode for 0.7 seconds, creating the arteriovenous fistula. After the arteriovenous fistula has been created, remove the catheters. Obtain an angiogram of the newly created fistula through the arterial sheath or an arterial catheter that has been advanced central to the percutaneous arteriovenous fistula to verify successful arteriovenous fistula creation with outflow in cephalic and/or basilic veins. From the venous access site, navigate a catheter to the brachial vein. Then occlude the brachial vein in the mid-upper extremity by coil embolization to direct more flow to the cephalic and/or basilic veins, which is confirmed by repeat arteriography to evaluate the percutaneous arteriovenous fistula and outflow veins. Then remove the venous and arterial sheaths. Obtain hemostasis at the arterial and venous access sites using manual compression for a minimum of 20 minutes.

36835   Insertion of Thomas shunt (separate procedure)

36836   Code is out of numerical sequence. See 36832-36838

36837   Code is out of numerical sequence. See 36832-36838

Dialysis Circuit

36901   Introduction of needle(s) and/or catheter(s), dialysis circuit, with diagnostic angiography of the dialysis circuit, including all direct puncture(s) and catheter placement(s), injection(s) of contrast, all necessary imaging from the arterial anastomosis and adjacent artery through entire venous outflow including the inferior or superior vena cava, fluoroscopic guidance, radiological supervision and interpretation and image documentation and report;

▶(Do not report 36901 in conjunction with 36833, 36836, 36837, 36902, 36903, 36904, 36905, 36906)◀

36902   with transluminal balloon angioplasty, peripheral dialysis segment, including all imaging and radiological supervision and interpretation necessary to perform the angioplasty

▶(Do not report 36902 in conjunction with 36836, 36837, 36903)◀

36903   with transcatheter placement of intravascular stent(s), peripheral dialysis segment, including all imaging and radiological supervision and interpretation necessary to perform the stenting, and all angioplasty within the peripheral dialysis segment

▶(Do not report 36902, 36903 in conjunction with 36833, 36836, 36837, 36904, 36905, 36906)◀

(Do not report 36901, 36902, 36903 more than once per operative session)

(For transluminal balloon angioplasty within central vein(s) when performed through dialysis circuit, use 36907)

★ = Telemedicine   ◀ = Audio-only   ✚ = Add-on code   ✗ = FDA approval pending   # = Resequenced code   ⊘ = Modifier 51 exempt

(For transcatheter placement of intravascular stent(s) within central vein(s) when performed through dialysis circuit, use 36908)

36904 Percutaneous transluminal mechanical thrombectomy and/or infusion for thrombolysis, dialysis circuit, any method, including all imaging and radiological supervision and interpretation, diagnostic angiography, fluoroscopic guidance, catheter placement(s), and intraprocedural pharmacological thrombolytic injection(s);

▶(Do not report 36904 in conjunction with 36836, 36837)◀

(For open thrombectomy within the dialysis circuit, see 36831, 36833)

36905   with transluminal balloon angioplasty, peripheral dialysis segment, including all imaging and radiological supervision and interpretation necessary to perform the angioplasty

▶(Do not report 36905 in conjunction with 36836, 36837, 36904)◀

36906   with transcatheter placement of intravascular stent(s), peripheral dialysis segment, including all imaging and radiological supervision and interpretation necessary to perform the stenting, and all angioplasty within the peripheral dialysis circuit

▶(Do not report 36906 in conjunction with 36836, 36837, 36901, 36902, 36903, 36904, 36905)◀

(Do not report 36904, 36905, 36906 more than once per operative session)

(For transluminal balloon angioplasty within central vein(s) when performed through dialysis circuit, use 36907)

(For transcatheter placement of intravascular stent(s) within central vein(s) when performed through dialysis circuit, use 36908)

+ 36907 Transluminal balloon angioplasty, central dialysis segment, performed through dialysis circuit, including all imaging and radiological supervision and interpretation required to perform the angioplasty (List separately in addition to code for primary procedure)

(Use 36907 in conjunction with 36818-36833, 36901, 36902, 36903, 36904, 36905, 36906)

▶(Do not report 36907 in conjunction with 36836, 36837, 36908)◀

(Report 36907 once for all angioplasty performed within the central dialysis segment)

+ 36908 Transcatheter placement of intravascular stent(s), central dialysis segment, performed through dialysis circuit, including all imaging and radiological supervision and interpretation required to perform the stenting, and all angioplasty in the central dialysis segment (List separately in addition to code for primary procedure)

(Use 36908 in conjunction with 36818-36833, 36901, 36902, 36903, 36904, 36905, 36906)

▶(Do not report 36908 in conjunction with 36836, 36837, 36907)◀

(Report 36908 once for all stenting performed within the central dialysis segment)

+ 36909 Dialysis circuit permanent vascular embolization or occlusion (including main circuit or any accessory veins), endovascular, including all imaging and radiological supervision and interpretation necessary to complete the intervention (List separately in addition to code for primary procedure)

(Use 36909 in conjunction with 36901, 36902, 36903, 36904, 36905, 36906)

▶(Do not report 36909 in conjunction with 36836, 36837)◀

(For open ligation/occlusion in dialysis access, use 37607)

(36909 includes all permanent vascular occlusions within the dialysis circuit and may only be reported once per encounter per day)

Rationale

In accordance with the establishment of codes 36836 and 36837, exclusionary parenthetical notes have been added or revised following codes 36901-36909 to restrict reporting these codes with codes 36836 and 36837.

Refer to the codebook and the Rationale for codes 36836 and 36837 for a full discussion of these changes.

Endovascular Revascularization (Open or Percutaneous, Transcatheter)

 # 37246 Transluminal balloon angioplasty (except lower extremity artery(ies) for occlusive disease, intracranial, coronary, pulmonary, or dialysis circuit), open or percutaneous, including all imaging and radiological supervision and interpretation necessary to perform the angioplasty within the same artery; initial artery

#+ 37247   each additional artery (List separately in addition to code for primary procedure)

(Use 37247 in conjunction with 37246)

▶(Do not report 37246, 37247 in conjunction with 36836, 36837)◀

(Do not report 37246, 37247 in conjunction with 37215, 37216, 37217, 37218, 37220-37237 when performed in the same artery during the same operative session)

Surgery / Cardiovascular System 33016-39599

(Do not report 37246, 37247 in conjunction with 34841, 34842, 34843, 34844, 34845, 34846, 34847, 34848 for angioplasty[ies] performed, when placing bare metal or covered stents into the visceral branches within the endoprosthesis target zone)

 # 37248 Transluminal balloon angioplasty (except dialysis circuit), open or percutaneous, including all imaging and radiological supervision and interpretation necessary to perform the angioplasty within the same vein; initial vein

#+ 37249 each additional vein (List separately in addition to code for primary procedure)

(Use 37249 in conjunction with 37248)

▶(Do not report 37248, 37249 in conjunction with 36836, 36837)◀

(Do not report 37248, 37249 in conjunction with 37238, 37239 when performed in the same vein during the same operative session)

(Do not report 37248, 37249 in conjunction with 0505T, within the femoral-popliteal segment)

(Do not report 37248, 37249 in conjunction with 0620T within the tibial-peroneal segment)

(For transluminal balloon angioplasty in aorta/visceral artery[ies] in conjunction with fenestrated endovascular repair, see 34841, 34842, 34843, 34844, 34845, 34846, 34847, 34848)

(For transluminal balloon angioplasty in iliac, femoral, popliteal, or tibial/peroneal artery[ies] for occlusive disease, see 37220-37235)

(For transluminal balloon angioplasty in a dialysis circuit performed through the circuit, see 36902, 36903, 36904, 36905, 36906, 36907, 36908)

(For transluminal balloon angioplasty in an intracranial artery, see 61630, 61635)

(For transluminal balloon angioplasty in a coronary artery, see 92920-92944)

(For transluminal balloon angioplasty in a pulmonary artery, see 92997, 92998)

37236 Transcatheter placement of an intravascular stent(s) (except lower extremity artery(s) for occlusive disease, cervical carotid, extracranial vertebral or intrathoracic carotid, intracranial, or coronary), open or percutaneous, including radiological supervision and interpretation and including all angioplasty within the same vessel, when performed; initial artery

+ 37237 each additional artery (List separately in addition to code for primary procedure)

(Use 37237 in conjunction with 37236)

▶(Do not report 37236, 37237 in conjunction with 36836, 36837)◀

(Do not report 37236, 37237 in conjunction with 34841-34848 for bare metal or covered stents placed into the visceral branches within the endoprosthesis target zone)

(For stent placement(s) in iliac, femoral, popliteal, or tibial/peroneal artery(s) for occlusive disease, see 37221, 37223, 37226, 37227, 37230, 37231, 37234, 37235)

(For transcatheter placement of intravascular cervical carotid artery stent(s), see 37215, 37216)

(For transcatheter placement of intracranial stent(s), use 61635)

(For transcatheter placement of intracoronary stent(s), see 92928, 92929, 92933, 92934, 92937, 92938, 92941, 92943, 92944)

(For stenting of visceral arteries in conjunction with fenestrated endovascular repair, see 34841-34848)

(For open or percutaneous antegrade transcatheter placement of intrathoracic carotid/innominate artery stent(s), use 37218)

(For open or percutaneous transcatheter placement of extracranial vertebral artery stent(s), see Category III codes 0075T, 0076T)

(For open retrograde transcatheter placement of intrathoracic common carotid/innominate artery stent(s), use 37217)

(For placement of a stent at the arterial anastomosis of a dialysis circuit with or without transluminal mechanical thrombectomy and/or infusion for thrombolysis, see 36903, 36906)

37238 Transcatheter placement of an intravascular stent(s), open or percutaneous, including radiological supervision and interpretation and including angioplasty within the same vessel, when performed; initial vein

+ 37239 each additional vein (List separately in addition to code for primary procedure)

(Use 37239 in conjunction with 37238)

▶(Do not report 37238, 37239 in conjunction with 36836, 36837)◀

(Do not report 37238, 37239 in conjunction with 0505T, within the femoral-popliteal segment)

(Do not report 37238, 37239 in conjunction with 0620T within the tibial-peroneal segment)

(For placement of a stent[s] within the peripheral segment of the dialysis circuit, see 36903, 36906)

(For transcatheter placement of an intravascular stent[s] within central dialysis segment when performed through the dialysis circuit, use 36908)

Rationale

In accordance with the establishment of codes 36836 and 36837, exclusionary parenthetical notes have been added following codes 37237, 37239, 37247, and 37249 to restrict reporting these codes with codes 36836 and 36837.

Refer to the codebook and the Rationale for codes 36836 and 36837 for a full discussion of these changes.

Vascular Embolization and Occlusion

37241   Vascular embolization or occlusion, inclusive of all radiological supervision and interpretation, intraprocedural roadmapping, and imaging guidance necessary to complete the intervention; venous, other than hemorrhage (eg, congenital or acquired venous malformations, venous and capillary hemangiomas, varices, varicoceles)

(Do not report 37241 in conjunction with 36468, 36470, 36471, 36473, 36474, 36475-36479, 75894, 75898 in the same surgical field)

(For sclerosis of veins or endovenous ablation of incompetent extremity veins, see 36468-36479)

(For dialysis circuit permanent endovascular embolization or occlusion, use 36909)

37242   arterial, other than hemorrhage or tumor (eg, congenital or acquired arterial malformations, arteriovenous malformations, arteriovenous fistulas, aneurysms, pseudoaneurysms)

▶(Do not report 37241, 37242 in conjunction with 36836, 36837)◀

(For percutaneous treatment of extremity pseudoaneurysm, use 36002)

Rationale

In accordance with the establishment of codes 36836 and 36837, an exclusionary parenthetical note has been added following code 37242 to restrict reporting codes 37241 and 37242 with codes 36836 and 36837.

Refer to the codebook and the Rationale for codes 36836 and 36837 for a full discussion of these changes.

Intravascular Ultrasound Services

+ 37252   Intravascular ultrasound (noncoronary vessel) during diagnostic evaluation and/or therapeutic intervention, including radiological supervision and interpretation; initial noncoronary vessel (List separately in addition to code for primary procedure)

+ 37253   each additional noncoronary vessel (List separately in addition to code for primary procedure)

(Use 37253 in conjunction with 37252)

(Use 37252, 37253 in conjunction with 33361, 33362, 33363, 33364, 33365, 33366, 33367, 33368, 33369, 33477, 33880, 33881, 33883, 33884, 33886, 34701, 34702, 34703, 34704, 34705, 34706, 34707, 34708, 34709, 34710, 34711, 34712, 34718, 34841, 34842, 34843, 34844, 34845, 34846, 34847, 34848, 36010, 36011, 36012, 36013, 36014, 36015, 36100, 36140, 36160, 36200, 36215, 36216, 36217, 36218, 36221, 36222, 36223, 36224, 36225, 36226, 36227, 36228, 36245, 36246, 36247, 36248, 36251, 36252, 36253, 36254, 36481, 36555-36571, 36578, 36580, 36581, 36582, 36583, 36584, 36585, 36595, 36901, 36902, 36903, 36904, 36905, 36906, 36907, 36908, 36909, 37184, 37185, 37186, 37187, 37188, 37200, 37211, 37212, 37213, 37214, 37215, 37216, 37218, 37220, 37221, 37222, 37223, 37224, 37225, 37226, 37227, 37228, 37229, 37230, 37231, 37232, 37233, 37234, 37235, 37236, 37237, 37238, 37239, 37241, 37242, 37243, 37244, 37246, 37247, 37248, 37249, 61623, 75600, 75605, 75625, 75630, 75635, 75705, 75710, 75716, 75726, 75731, 75733, 75736, 75741, 75743, 75746, 75756, 75774, 75805, 75807, 75810, 75820, 75822, 75825, 75827, 75831, 75833, 75860, 75870, 75872, 75885, 75887, 75889, 75891, 75893, 75894, 75898, 75901, 75902, 75956, 75957, 75958, 75959, 75970, 76000, 77001, 0075T, 0076T, 0234T, 0235T, 0236T, 0237T, 0238T, 0338T)

▶(Do not report 37252, 37253 in conjunction with 36836, 36837, 37191, 37192, 37193, 37197)◀

Rationale

In accordance with the establishment of codes 36836 and 36837, the exclusionary parenthetical note following code 37253 has been revised with the addition of the new codes.

Refer to the codebook and the Rationale for codes 36836 and 36837 for a full discussion of these changes.

Hemic and Lymphatic Systems

Transplantation and Post-Transplantation Cellular Infusions

Hematopoietic cell transplantation (HCT) refers to the infusion of hematopoietic progenitor cells (HPC) obtained from bone marrow, peripheral blood apheresis, and/or umbilical cord blood. These procedure codes (38240-38243) include physician monitoring of multiple

Surgery / Cardiovascular System 33016-39599

physiologic parameters, physician verification of cell processing, evaluation of the patient during as well as immediately before and after the HPC/lymphocyte infusion, physician presence during the HPC/lymphocyte infusion with associated direct physician supervision of clinical staff, and management of uncomplicated adverse events (eg, nausea, urticaria) during the infusion, which is not separately reportable.

HCT may be autologous (when the HPC donor and recipient are the same person) or allogeneic (when the HPC donor and recipient are not the same person). Code 38241 is used to report any autologous transplant while 38240 is used to report an allogeneic transplant. In some cases allogeneic transplants involve more than one donor and cells from each donor are infused sequentially whereby one unit of 38240 is reported for each donor infused. Code 38242 is used to report a donor lymphocyte infusion. Code 38243 is used to report a HPC boost from the original allogeneic HPC donor. A lymphocyte infusion or HPC boost can occur days, months or even years after the initial hematopoietic cell transplant. HPC boost represents an infusion of hematopoietic progenitor cells from the original donor that is being used to treat post-transplant cytopenia(s). Codes 38240, 38242, and 38243 should not be reported together on the same date of service.

▶If a separately identifiable evaluation and management service is performed on the same date of service, the appropriate E/M service code, including office or other outpatient services, established (99211-99215), hospital inpatient or observation care services (99221-99223, 99231-99239), and inpatient neonatal and pediatric critical care (99471, 99472, 99475, 99476), may be reported using modifier 25 in addition to 38240, 38242 or 38243. Post-transplant infusion management of adverse reactions is reported separately using the appropriate E/M, prolonged service or critical care code(s). In accordance with place of service and facility reporting guidelines, the fluid used to administer the cells and other infusions for incidental hydration (eg, 96360, 96361) are not separately reportable. Similarly, infusion(s) of any medication(s) concurrently with the transplant infusion are not separately reportable. However, hydration or administration of medications (eg, antibiotics, narcotics) unrelated to the transplant are separately reportable using modifier 59.◀

38240   Hematopoietic progenitor cell (HPC); allogeneic transplantation per donor

Rationale

In accordance with the deletion of codes 99217-99220 and 99224-99226, the transplantation and post-transplantation cellular infusions guidelines have been revised.

Refer to the codebook and the Rationale for codes 99217-99220 and 99224-99226 for a full discussion of these changes.

Digestive System

Esophagus

Endoscopy

Esophagoscopy

43197   Esophagoscopy, flexible, transnasal; diagnostic, including collection of specimen(s) by brushing or washing, when performed (separate procedure)

▶(Do not report 43197 in conjunction with 31575, 43191, 43192, 43193, 43194, 43195, 43196, 43198, 43200-43232, 43235-43259, 43266, 43270, 43290, 43291, 43497, 92511, 0652T, 0653T, 0654T)◀

(Do not report 43197 in conjunction with 31231 unless separate type of endoscope [eg, rigid endoscope] is used)

(For transoral esophagoscopy, see 43191, 43200)

43198   with biopsy, single or multiple

▶(Do not report 43198 in conjunction with 31575, 43191, 43192, 43193, 43194, 43195, 43196, 43197, 43200-43232, 43235-43259, 43266, 43270, 43290, 43291, 92511, 0652T, 0653T, 0654T)◀

(Do not report 43198 in conjunction with 31231 unless separate type of endoscope [eg, rigid endoscope] is used)

(For transoral esophagoscopy with biopsy, see 43193, 43202)

Rationale

In accordance with the establishment of codes 43290 and 43291, the exclusionary parenthetical notes following codes 43197 and 43198 have been revised with the addition of the new codes.

Refer to the codebook and the Rationale for codes 43290 and 43291 for a full description of these changes.

Esophagogastroduodenoscopy

43235   Esophagogastroduodenoscopy, flexible, transoral; diagnostic, including collection of specimen(s) by brushing or washing, when performed (separate procedure)

★ = Telemedicine   ◀ = Audio-only   ✛ = Add-on code   ⁄ = FDA approval pending   # = Resequenced code   ⊘ = Modifier 51 exempt

►(Do not report 43235 in conjunction with 43197, 43198, 43210, 43236-43259, 43266, 43270, 43290, 43291, 43497, 44360, 44361, 44363, 44364, 44365, 44366, 44369, 44370, 44372, 44373, 44376, 44377, 44378, 44379)◄

43241   with insertion of intraluminal tube or catheter

►(Do not report 43241 in conjunction with 43197, 43198, 43212, 43235, 43266, 43290, 44360, 44361, 44363, 44364, 44365, 44366, 44369, 44370, 44372, 44373, 44376, 44377, 44378, 44379)◄

(For naso- or oro-gastric tube placement requiring physician's or other qualified health care professional's skill and fluoroscopic guidance, use 43752)

(For nonendoscopic enteric tube placement, see 44500, 74340)

43247   with removal of foreign body(s)

►(Do not report 43247 in conjunction with 43197, 43198, 43235, 43290, 43291, 44360, 44361, 44363, 44364, 44365, 44366, 44369, 44370, 44372, 44373, 44376, 44377, 44378, 44379)◄

(If fluoroscopic guidance is performed, use 76000)

#● 43290   with deployment of intragastric bariatric balloon

►(Do not report 43290 in conjunction with 43197, 43198, 43235, 43241, 43247)◄

#● 43291   with removal of intragastric bariatric balloon(s)

►(Do not report 43291 in conjunction with 43197, 43198, 43235, 43247)◄

43248   with insertion of guide wire followed by passage of dilator(s) through esophagus over guide wire

(Do not report 43248 in conjunction with 43197, 43198, 43235, 43266, 43270, 44360, 44361, 44363, 44364, 44365, 44366, 44369, 44370, 44372, 44373, 44376, 44377, 44378, 44379)

(If fluoroscopic guidance is performed, use 74360)

Rationale

Two codes (43290, 43291) have been established to report esophagogastroduodenoscopy with deployment and removal of an intragastric bariatric balloon device(s).

To support the addition of these new codes, two parenthetical notes have been added to guide users in the appropriate reporting for these services. Several existing parenthetical notes have been revised with the addition of codes 43290 and 43291.

Prior to 2023, there were no CPT codes that described the deployment and/or removal of an intragastric bariatric balloon. This new procedure may be used to assist in the treatment of conditions such as weight loss for the morbid obesity population.

Code 43290 describes the procedure with deployment of intragastric bariatric balloon, and code 43291 describes the removal of intragastric bariatric balloon(s).

To provide further instruction regarding the intent and use of these new codes, two exclusionary parenthetical notes have been added following codes 43290 and 43291. The first exclusionary parenthetical note has been added following code 43290 to restrict reporting code 43290 with codes 43197, 43198, 43235, 43241, and 43247. The second exclusionary parenthetical note has been added following code 43291 to restrict reporting code 43291 with codes 43197, 43198, 43235, and 43247. Additional parenthetical notes following codes 43197, 43198, 43235, 43241, and 43247 have been revised to include codes 43290 and 43291.

Clinical Example (43290)

A 45-year-old female with a body mass index (BMI) of 33, who has not responded to dietary and pharmacologic interventions for weight loss, undergoes endoscopically guided insertion of a gastric balloon.

Description of Procedure (43290)

Assess level of sedation prior to inserting the endoscope. Insert a standard flexible upper endoscope through the mouth into the oropharynx and advance through the esophagus into the proximal stomach. Insufflate the stomach with air after suctioning liquid contents. Perform an examination of the entire stomach in the forward and retroflexed positions. Advance the endoscope through the pylorus into the duodenal bulb. Inspect the duodenum circumferentially after air insufflation. Slowly withdraw the endoscope and re-inspect the stomach and duodenum. After suctioning air to deflate the stomach, withdraw the endoscope into the esophagus, allowing measurement of the squamocolumnar (SC) and gastroesophageal (GE) junctions from the incisors. Assess for presence of a hiatal hernia and examine the esophageal mucosa. When indicated, obtain brushings or washings of suspicious abnormalities. Obtain photodocumentation of appropriate normal landmarks and abnormalities. Withdraw the endoscope. Then advance the intragastric balloon catheter into the stomach based on the markings on the catheter and the prior noted location of the SC junction. Re-insert the scope to confirm and adjust the position of the collapsed intragastric balloon into the body of the stomach. Then withdraw the endoscope to the level of GE junction at which point the stiffening wire is removed from the delivery catheter. Slowly inflate the balloon using saline with or without methylene blue dye. After the intragastric balloon is inflated to the desired volume, disengage the catheter from the intragastric balloon. Inspect the balloon and stomach to make sure there is no evidence of fluid leakage. Then complete removal of the catheter. Obtain photodocumentation confirming intragastric balloon placement in the stomach. Then remove the endoscope and the procedure is complete.

Clinical Example (43291)

A 45-year-old female who is 6 months post-placement of an intragastric balloon presents for removal of the balloon.

Description of Procedure (43291)

Assess level of sedation prior to inserting the endoscope. Insert a standard flexible upper endoscope through the mouth into the oropharynx and advance through the esophagus into the proximal stomach. Insufflate the stomach with air after suctioning liquid contents. Perform an examination of the entire stomach in the forward and retroflexed positions. Inspect the duodenum circumferentially after air insufflation. Slowly withdraw the endoscope and re-inspect the stomach and duodenum. Visualize the previously placed balloon. Insert a needle instrument through the working channel of the endoscope. Use the needle instrument to puncture the balloon. Attach the external portion of the needle catheter to suction and remove the fluid from the balloon. The volume of the fluid is measured to ensure it approximates the same amount that was used to fill the balloon. After careful inspection to ensure the balloon is fully deflated, remove the needle catheter. Use the device-specific retrieval instrument to grasp the deflated balloon. Bring the balloon in apposition to the endoscope. Remove the endoscope and balloon perorally using direct endoscopic guidance. Then re-insert the endoscope to make sure there is no mucosal trauma in the upper gastrointestinal tract. Advance the endoscope through the pylorus into the duodenal bulb. Re-insufflate the stomach. Remove the remaining fluid. Carefully evaluate the stomach and esophagus, allowing measurement of the SC and GE junctions from the incisors. Assess for presence of a hiatal hernia and examine the esophageal mucosa. When indicated, obtain brushings or washings of suspicious abnormalities. Obtain photodocumentation of appropriate normal landmarks and abnormalities. Then remove the endoscope and the procedure is complete.

Laparoscopy

43289   Unlisted laparoscopy procedure, esophagus

43290   Code is out of numerical sequence. See 43246-43249

43291   Code is out of numerical sequence. See 43246-43249

Intestines (Except Rectum)

Other Procedures

44705   Preparation of fecal microbiota for instillation, including assessment of donor specimen

▶(Do not report 44705 in conjunction with 74283, 0780T)◀

(For fecal instillation by oro-nasogastric tube or enema, use 44799)

▶(For instillation of fecal microbiota suspension via rectal enema, use 0780T)◀

Rationale

In support of the establishment of code 0780T, the inclusionary parenthetical note following code 44705 has been revised, and a new cross-reference parenthetical note has been added, to provide guidance for reporting the new code.

Refer to the codebook and the Rationale for code 0780T for a full discussion of these changes.

Biliary Tract

Introduction

47537   Removal of biliary drainage catheter, percutaneous, requiring fluoroscopic guidance (eg, with concurrent indwelling biliary stents), including diagnostic cholangiography when performed, imaging guidance (eg, fluoroscopy), and all associated radiological supervision and interpretation

(Do not report 47537 in conjunction with 47538 for the same access)

▶(For removal of biliary drainage catheter not requiring fluoroscopic guidance, see E/M services and report the appropriate level of service provided [eg, 99202-99215, 99221, 99222, 99223, 99231, 99232, 99233])◀

Rationale

In accordance with the deletion of codes 99217-99220 and 99224-99226, the cross-reference parenthetical note following code 47537 has been revised to reflect these changes.

Refer to the codebook and the Rationale for codes 99217-99220 and 99224-99226 for a full discussion of these changes.

★ = Telemedicine   ◀ = Audio-only   ✚ = Add-on code   ✱ = FDA approval pending   # = Resequenced code   ⊘ = Modifier 51 exempt

Abdomen, Peritoneum, and Omentum

Repair

Hernioplasty, Herniorrhaphy, Herniotomy

►The hernia repair codes in this section are categorized primarily by the type of hernia (inguinal, femoral, lumbar, omphalocele, anterior abdominal, parastomal).◄

Some types of hernias are further categorized as "initial" or "recurrent" based on whether or not the hernia has required previous repair(s).

Additional variables accounted for by some of the codes include patient age and clinical presentation (reducible vs. incarcerated or strangulated).

The excision/repair of strangulated organs or structures such as testicle(s), intestine, ovaries are reported by using the appropriate code for the excision/repair (eg, 44120, 54520, and 58940) in addition to the appropriate code for the repair of the strangulated hernia.

(For debridement of abdominal wall, see 11042, 11043)

(For reduction and repair of intra-abdominal hernia, use 44050)

►(49491-49557, 49600, 49605, 49606, 49610, 49611, 49650, 49651 are unilateral procedures. For bilateral procedure, use modifier 50)◄

►(Do not report modifier 50 in conjunction with 49591-49622)◄

49491 Repair, initial inguinal hernia, preterm infant (younger than 37 weeks gestation at birth), performed from birth up to 50 weeks postconception age, with or without hydrocelectomy; reducible

49555 Repair recurrent femoral hernia; reducible

49557 incarcerated or strangulated

►(49560, 49561 have been deleted. For repair of initial incisional or ventral hernia, see 49591, 49592, 49593, 49594, 49595, 49596)◄

►(49565, 49566 have been deleted. For repair of recurrent incisional or ventral hernia, see 49613, 49614, 49615, 49616, 49617, 49618)◄

►(49568 has been deleted. For implantation of mesh or other prosthesis for anterior abdominal hernia repair, see 49591-49618)◄

►(49570, 49572 have been deleted. For epigastric hernia repair, see 49591-49618)◄

►(49580, 49582 have been deleted. For umbilical hernia repair, younger than age 5 years, see 49591-49618)◄

►(49585, 49587 have been deleted. For umbilical hernia repair, age 5 years and older, see 49591-49618)◄

►(49590 has been deleted. For spigelian hernia repair, see 49591-49618)◄

►Codes 49591-49618 describe repair of an anterior abdominal hernia(s) (ie, epigastric, incisional, ventral, umbilical, spigelian) by any approach (ie, open, laparoscopic, robotic). Codes 49591-49618 are reported only once, based on the total defect size for one or more anterior abdominal hernia(s), measured as the maximal craniocaudal or transverse distance between the outer margins of all defects repaired. For example, "Swiss cheese" defects (ie, multiple separate defects) would be measured from the superior most aspect of the upper defect to the inferior most aspect of the lowest defect. In addition, the hernia defect size should be measured prior to opening the hernia defect(s) (ie, during repair the fascia will typically retract creating a falsely elevated measurement).

When both reducible and incarcerated or strangulated anterior abdominal hernias are repaired at the same operative session, all hernias are reported as incarcerated or strangulated. For example, one 2-cm reducible initial incisional hernia and one 4-cm incarcerated initial incisional hernia separated by 2 cm would be reported as an initial incarcerated hernia repair with a maximum craniocaudal distance of 8 cm (49594).

Inguinal, femoral, lumbar, omphalocele, and/or parastomal hernia repair may be separately reported when performed at the same operative session as anterior abdominal hernia repair by appending modifier 59, as appropriate.

Codes 49621, 49622 describe repair of a parastomal hernia (initial or recurrent) by any approach (ie, open, laparoscopic, robotic). Code 49621 is reported for repair of a reducible parastomal hernia, and code 49622 is reported for an incarcerated or strangulated parastomal hernia.

Implantation of mesh or other prosthesis, when performed, is included in 49591-49622 and may not be separately reported. For total or near total removal of non-infected mesh when performed, use 49623 in conjunction with 49591-49622. For removal of infected mesh, use 11008.◄

● **49591** Repair of anterior abdominal hernia(s) (ie, epigastric, incisional, ventral, umbilical, spigelian), any approach (ie, open, laparoscopic, robotic), initial, including implantation of mesh or other prosthesis when performed, total length of defect(s); less than 3 cm, reducible

● **49592** less than 3 cm, incarcerated or strangulated

● **49593** 3 cm to 10 cm, reducible

● **49594** 3 cm to 10 cm, incarcerated or strangulated

● **49595** greater than 10 cm, reducible

● **49596** greater than 10 cm, incarcerated or strangulated

Measuring Total Length of Anterior Abdominal Hernia Defect(s)
49591-49618

Hernia measurements are performed either in the transverse or craniocaudal dimension. The total length of the defect(s) corresponds to the maximum width or height of an oval drawn to encircle the outer perimeter of all repaired defects. If the defects are not contiguous and are separated by greater than or equal to 10 cm of intact fascia, total defect size is the sum of each defect measured individually.

Codes 49591-49618 are reported only once, based on the total defect size for one or more anterior abdominal hernia(s), measured as the maximal craniocaudal or transverse distance between the outer margins of all defects repaired.

A. Single anterior abdominal hernia defect

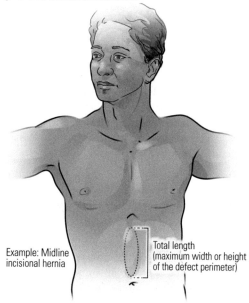

Example: Midline incisional hernia

Total length (maximum width or height of the defect perimeter)

B. Multiple anterior abdominal hernia defects

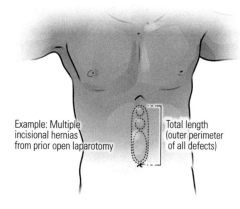

Example: Multiple incisional hernias from prior open laparotomy

Total length (outer perimeter of all defects)

C. Remote anterior abdominal hernia defects

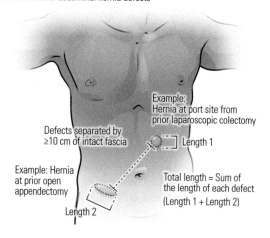

Example: Hernia at port site from prior laparoscopic colectomy

Length 1

Defects separated by ≥10 cm of intact fascia

Example: Hernia at prior open appendectomy

Length 2

Total length = Sum of the length of each defect (Length 1 + Length 2)

#● 49613 Repair of anterior abdominal hernia(s) (ie, epigastric, incisional, ventral, umbilical, spigelian), any approach (ie, open, laparoscopic, robotic), recurrent, including implantation of mesh or other prosthesis when performed, total length of defect(s); less than 3 cm, reducible

#● 49614 less than 3 cm, incarcerated or strangulated

#● 49615 3 cm to 10 cm, reducible

#● 49616 3 cm to 10 cm, incarcerated or strangulated

#● 49617 greater than 10 cm, reducible

#● 49618 greater than 10 cm, incarcerated or strangulated

#● 49621 Repair of parastomal hernia, any approach (ie, open, laparoscopic, robotic), initial or recurrent, including implantation of mesh or other prosthesis, when performed; reducible

#● 49622 incarcerated or strangulated

#+● 49623 Removal of total or near total non-infected mesh or other prosthesis at the time of initial or recurrent anterior abdominal hernia repair or parastomal hernia repair, any approach (ie, open, laparoscopic, robotic) (List separately in addition to code for primary procedure)

▶(Use 49623 in conjunction with 49591-49622)◀

▶(For removal of infected mesh, use 11008)◀

49600 Repair of small omphalocele, with primary closure

(Do not report modifier 63 in conjunction with 49600)

49610 Repair of omphalocele (Gross type operation); first stage

49611 second stage

(Do not report modifier 63 in conjunction with 49610, 49611)

(For diaphragmatic or hiatal hernia repair, see 39503, 43332)

(For surgical repair of omentum, use 49999)

★ = Telemedicine ◀ = Audio-only + = Add-on code 𝙽 = FDA approval pending # = Resequenced code ⊘ = Modifier 51 exempt

49613	Code is out of numerical sequence. See 49595-49605
49614	Code is out of numerical sequence. See 49595-49605
49615	Code is out of numerical sequence. See 49595-49605
49616	Code is out of numerical sequence. See 49595-49605
49617	Code is out of numerical sequence. See 49595-49605
49618	Code is out of numerical sequence. See 49595-49605
49621	Code is out of numerical sequence. See 49595-49605
49622	Code is out of numerical sequence. See 49595-49605
49623	Code is out of numerical sequence. See 49595-49605

Rationale

Repair of a recurrent incisional or ventral hernia; reducible (49565), was identified by the AMA/Specialty Society Relative Value Scale (RVS) Update Committee (RUC) Relativity Assessment Workgroup (RAW) as a service performed less than 50% of the time in the inpatient setting, which included inpatient hospital E/M service codes in the Centers for Medicare & Medicaid Services (CMS) time/visit database and had Medicare utilization over 5,000.

In response to this analysis, along with several coding issues and a need to update these services to reflect current clinical practice, the abdominal hernia repair procedures, guidelines, and instructional, inclusionary, exclusionary, and cross-reference parenthetical notes have been updated.

In accordance with the deletion of hernia repair codes 49560-4959 and 49652-49657 and the establishment of new hernia repair codes 49591-49622 and add-on code 49623, the Hernioplasty, Herniorrhaphy, Herniotomy subsection guidelines have been revised, deleted, and new guidelines have been established to clarify correct reporting of the new codes.

Parenthetical notes that followed the guidelines have been deleted and new parenthetical notes established to reflect the new and deleted codes.

Codes 49560, 49561, 49565, and 49566, which describe the repair of initial or recurrent incisional or ventral hernia, reducible, incarcerated or strangulated, have been deleted and two parenthetical notes have been established. One parenthetical note to instruct users which codes to use for repair of initial incisional or ventral hernia and one parenthetical note to instruct users which codes to use for repair of recurrent incisional or ventral hernia have been added.

Add-on code 49568, which describes implantation of mesh or other prosthesis for open incisional or ventral hernia repair, and its corresponding parenthetical note and coding

tip have been deleted. However, because the new hernia repair codes 49591-49622 include the implantation of mesh or other prosthesis when performed, a separate code is not needed. In addition, because deleted code 49568 also described the implantation of mesh for closure of debridement for a necrotizing soft tissue infection, code 15778 has been established to report the implantation of absorbable mesh or other prosthesis for delayed closure of defect(s) due to soft tissue infection or trauma. Codes 49570-49590, which describe repair of epigastric, umbilical, spigelian, incarcerated, or strangulated hernia, have been deleted as these are all anterior abdominal hernias that will be reported with the new codes in 2023. Multiple instructional parenthetical notes have been added to instruct users on the deleted codes and the correct use of the new codes 49591-49618.

Six new codes (49591-49596) have been established to report initial anterior abdominal hernia repair and six new codes (49613-49618) have been established to report recurrent anterior abdominal hernia repair. Two new codes (49621, 49622) have been established to report parastomal hernia repair and one add-on code (49623) has been established to report the removal of noninfected mesh or other prosthesis. In addition, new parenthetical notes have been added to guide users in the appropriate reporting for these services.

Three new illustrations have been created to instruct users on measuring total length of anterior abdominal hernia defect(s) repair.

Clinical Example (49591)

A 55-year-old male presents with a painful mass through the umbilicus that disappears in supine position. He undergoes hernia repair of a defect that is less than 3 cm with placement of mesh.

Description of Procedure (49591)

Make an infraumbilical incision. Dissect the subcutaneous tissues surrounding the hernia sac. Detach the overlying umbilical dermis from the hernia sac. Circumferentially dissect the fascia surrounding the periphery of the hernia sac. Open the hernia sac and divide adhesions to the hernia sac. Then excise the hernia sac. Measure the hernia defect at less than 3 cm in diameter. Select a mesh to provide adequate overlap of the hernia defect. Insert the mesh preperitoneal or intraperitoneal and suture to the abdominal wall. Close the hernia defect with interrupted sutures over the top the mesh. Excise redundant umbilical skin. Suture the umbilical dermis to the abdominal fascia. Perform a layered closure.

Clinical Example (49592)

A 55-year-old male presents with a history of painful swelling in the umbilical region. Physical examination reveals an umbilical hernia that is tender and nonreducible by manual manipulation. He undergoes hernia repair of a defect that is less than 3 cm with placement of mesh.

Description of Procedure (49592)

Make an infraumbilical skin incision. Dissect the subcutaneous tissues surrounding the hernia sac. Detach the overlying umbilical dermis from the hernia sac. This is exacerbated by the location of the incarcerated hernia contents occupying the central space of the operative field making the dissection more challenging. Separation is performed without damaging the intra-abdominal contents incarcerated in the hernia sac. Open the hernia sac and inspect the contents. Perform adhesiolysis to free omentum and intestines incarcerated within the hernia sac. Inspect the reduced hernia contents for viability. Excise the hernia sac. The hernia defect is measured and found to span less than 3 cm. Suture a mesh with adequate overlap of the abdominal wall to the abdominal wall circumferentially. Close the hernia defect over the mesh. Excise redundant skin as appropriate. Suture the umbilical dermis to the abdominal fascia.

Clinical Example (49593)

A 60-year-old obese male with a prior laparotomy has developed a bulge in the midline incision. The defect has been increasing in size during follow-up. He has symptoms of pain and local tenderness. He has had no history of incarceration or bowel obstruction. Physical examination reveals a reducible incisional hernia. He undergoes hernia repair of a defect that is 3 to 10 cm with placement of mesh.

Description of Procedure (49593)

Obtain abdominal access and create a pneumoperitoneum with placement of a needle/trocar in the left upper quadrant. Insert the camera and verify safe entry. Place additional trocars in the lateral abdomen under direct vision. A large field of adhesions occupies approximately half of the anterior abdominal wall correlating with the extent of the prior laparotomy. Divide adhesions to the abdominal wall sharply to free the anterior abdominal wall adequately for subsequent mesh landing. Visualize the hernia defect. Take great care to avoid injury to the intestine or other intra-abdominal contents. Each separate defect within the overall hernia defect contains a separate component of adipose and intestine that requires safe reduction. Clear the falciform ligament and preperitoneal fat from the abdominal wall fascia to expose the posterior fascia. Measure and sum all of the

defects with a minimum length of 3 cm and maximum length of 10 cm. Create peritoneal flaps for placement of mesh. When appropriate, approximate the fascial defect with sutures. Select a mesh to provide adequate overlap of the hernia defect. Introduce the mesh into the peritoneal cavity through a trocar and orient. Reduce insufflation to facilitate mesh conformity to the anterior abdominal wall. Secure the mesh to the abdominal wall utilizing multiple sutures and tacks. Perform complete camera survey of the abdomen and contents to inspect for bleeding and visceral injury. Irrigate as necessary. Close fascial incisions from laparoscopic ports larger than 1 cm in diameter with a suture passer. Close skin incisions according to surgeon preference.

Clinical Example (49594)

A 60-year-old obese male with a prior laparotomy has developed an incisional hernia in the midline incision. Over the past few months, the defect has become chronically protuberant. He reports increasing pain and discomfort. Physical examination reveals a hernia that is tender and nonreducible by manual manipulation. He undergoes hernia repair of a defect that is 3 to 10 cm with placement of mesh.

Description of Procedure (49594)

Obtain abdominal access and create a safe pneumoperitoneum with placement of a needle/trocar in the left upper quadrant. Insert the camera and verify safe entry. Place additional trocars in the lateral abdomen under direct vision. A large field of adhesions occupies approximately half of the abdominal wall correlating with the extent of the prior laparotomy. Sharply divide adhesions to the abdominal wall to free the anterior abdominal wall adequately for subsequent mesh landing. Carefully reduce the incarcerated/strangulated bowel, mesentery and omentum with dissection of the adhesions and sac to clear the defects for repair. Take care to avoid injury to the incarcerated intestine and omentum. Each separate defect within the overall hernia defect contains a separate component of adipose and intestine that requires safe reduction. This requires manipulation both intra-abdominally with minimally invasive instrumentation and extra-abdominally with palpation and pressure applied to the abdominal wall to reduce the incarcerated contents. Examine the reduced tissue for viability and any inadvertent injury. Reduce the hernia sac and resect as needed to expose the fascial edges of the defect(s). Visualize the hernia defect. Clear the falciform ligament and preperitoneal fat from the abdominal wall fascia to expose the posterior fascia. Measure and sum all of the defects with a minimum of 3 cm and maximum of 10 cm. Create peritoneal flaps for placement of mesh. When appropriate, approximate the fascial defect with sutures. Select a mesh to provide

★=Telemedicine   ◀=Audio-only   ✚=Add-on code   ✐=FDA approval pending   #=Resequenced code   ⊘=Modifier 51 exempt

adequate overlap of the hernia defect. Introduce the mesh into the peritoneal cavity through a trocar and orient. Reduce insufflation to facilitate mesh conformity to the anterior abdominal wall. Secure the mesh to the abdominal wall utilizing multiple sutures and tacks. Perform a complete camera survey of the abdomen and contents to inspect for bleeding and visceral injury and perform a final viability assessment of the material once incarcerated in the hernia sac. Irrigate as necessary. Close fascial incisions from laparoscopic ports larger than 1 cm with a suture passer. Close skin incisions according to surgeon preference.

Clinical Example (49595)

A 64-year-old obese male with a prior laparotomy has developed incisional hernias with defects of varying sizes at multiple points. He has symptoms of pain and tenderness at the sites. Physical examination reveals multiple reducible incisional hernias. He undergoes hernia repair of a defect that totals more than 10 cm with placement of mesh.

Description of Procedure (49595)

Obtain abdominal access and create a safe pneumoperitoneum with placement of a needle/trocar. Because the hernia extends across the majority of the anterior abdominal wall, select the location for insertion of the needle/trocar based on prior surgical history and the safest location to avoid intra-abdominal injury. Insert the camera and verify safe entry. Place additional trocars in the lateral abdomen, and in additional areas as needed, all under direct vision. A field of adhesions occupies the entire anterior abdominal wall correlating with the extent of the prior laparotomy. Sharply divide the adhesions to free the anterior abdominal wall completely taking great care to avoid injury to the intestine. Each separate defect within the entire hernia defect contains adipose and intestinal components and requires a safe and effective clearance of tissue. Visualize the hernia defect. Clear the falciform ligament and preperitoneal fat from the abdominal wall fascia to expose the posterior fascia to include wide lateral clearance for adequate later mesh coverage. Create peritoneal flaps for placement of mesh. Approximate the fascial defect with sutures placed along the entire length of the defect. Calculate the appropriate size mesh after total defect length is documented. Adequate overlap of at least 5 cm in all directions is included in the calculation. Remove a trocar from the abdominal wall and dilate the track to allow insertion of the large mesh into the peritoneal cavity. Orient the mesh intra-abdominally. Reduce insufflation to facilitate mesh conformity to the anterior abdominal wall. Secure the mesh to the abdominal wall utilizing multiple sutures and numerous tacks. The suture the peritoneal flaps over the mesh to protect it from the abdominal viscera. Perform a

complete camera survey of the abdomen and contents to inspect for bleeding and visceral injury. Irrigate as necessary. Close fascial incisions from laparoscopic ports larger than 1 cm with a suture passer. Close skin incisions according to surgeon preference.

Clinical Example (49596)

A 64-year-old obese male with a prior laparotomy has developed incisional hernias with defects of varying sizes at multiple points. The defects have been increasing in size during follow-up with increasing symptoms. Physical examination reveals multiple tender and nonreducible incisional hernias. He undergoes hernia repair of a defect that totals more than 10 cm with placement of mesh.

Description of Procedure (49596)

Obtain abdominal access and create a safe pneumoperitoneum with placement of a needle/trocar. As the hernia extends across the majority of the anterior abdominal wall, select a location for insertion of the needle/trocar based on the prior surgical history and the safest location to avoid intra-abdominal injury. Insert the camera and verify safe entry. Place additional trocars in the lateral abdomen under direct vision. A large field of adhesions occupies the entire anterior abdominal wall correlating with the extent of the prior laparotomy. Sharply divide adhesions to free the anterior abdominal wall completely taking great care to avoid injury to the intestine. Each separate defect within the entire hernia defect contains adipose and intestinal components and requires a safe and effective clearance of tissue. Carefully reduce the incarcerated/strangulated bowel, mesentery, and omentum with dissection of the adhesions and sac to clear all the defects for repair. Take care to avoid injury to the incarcerated tissue. This requires manipulation both intra-abdominally with minimally invasive instrumentation and extra-abdominally with palpation and pressure applied to the abdominal wall to reduce the incarcerated contents. Examine the reduced tissue for viability and any inadvertent injury. Clear the falciform ligament and preperitoneal fat from the abdominal wall fascia to expose all defects and enough surface for mesh overlap. Reduce and resect the hernia sac as needed to expose the fascial edges of the defect(s). Visualize the hernia defect. Measure the defects with a minimum craniocaudal length greater than 10 cm. Create peritoneal flaps for placement of mesh. Approximate the fascial defect with sutures placed along the entirety of the defect. Calculate the appropriate size mesh after total defect length is documented. Adequate overlap of at least 5 cm in all directions is included in the calculation. Remove a trocar from the abdominal wall and dilate the track to allow insertion of the large mesh into the peritoneal cavity. Orient the mesh intra-abdominally. Reduce insufflation to facilitate mesh conformity to the anterior abdominal wall. Secure the mesh to the abdominal wall utilizing sutures and tacks. Then suture the peritoneal flaps over the mesh to protect it from the abdominal viscera. Perform a complete camera survey of the abdomen and contents to inspect for bleeding and visceral injury and perform a final viability assessment of the material once incarcerated in the hernia sac. Irrigate as necessary. Close fascial incisions for laparoscopic ports larger than 1 cm with a suture passer. Close skin incisions according to surgeon preference.

Clinical Example (49613)

A 60-year-old obese male has a surgical history of a prior laparotomy with a resultant hernia in the incision. The prior hernia was repaired 5 years ago. He now has a bulge in the midepigastric area for 2 months that disappears when he lies down. Physical examination reveals a small recurrent reducible incisional hernia. He undergoes hernia repair of a defect that is less than 3 cm with placement of mesh.

Description of Procedure (49613)

Obtain abdominal access and create a safe pneumoperitoneum with placement of a needle/trocar in the left upper quadrant. Insert the camera and verify safe entry. Place additional trocars in the lateral abdomen under direct vision. Perform adhesiolysis to clear adhesions between omentum, small intestines, and colon from the abdominal wall and prior mesh. Visualize the hernia defect. Sharply divide the adhesions to the abdominal wall to free the anterior abdominal wall completely. Clear the falciform ligament and preperitoneal fat from the abdominal wall fascia to expose the posterior fascia. Create peritoneal flaps for placement of mesh. Approximate the fascial defect with sutures. Measure the hernia defect at less than 3 cm in diameter. Select a mesh to provide adequate overlap of the hernia defect. Introduce a mesh into the peritoneal cavity through a trocar and orient. Reduce insufflation to facilitate mesh conformity to the anterior abdominal wall. Secure the mesh to the abdominal wall utilizing sutures and/or tacks. Then suture the peritoneal flaps over the mesh to protect it from the abdominal viscera. Perform a complete camera survey of the abdomen and contents to inspect for bleeding and visceral injury. Irrigate as necessary. Close fascial incisions for laparoscopic ports larger than 1 cm with a suture passer. Close skin incisions according to surgeon preference.

Clinical Example (49614)

A 60-year-old obese male has a surgical history of a prior laparotomy with a resultant hernia in the incision. The prior hernia was repaired 5 years ago. He now has a small bulge in the midepigastric area for 2 months that previously disappeared when supine. The bulge is now

irreducible and tender. Physical examination reveals a small recurrent incarcerated incisional hernia. He undergoes hernia repair of a defect that is less than 3 cm with placement of mesh.

Description of Procedure (49614)

Obtain abdominal access and create a safe pneumoperitoneum with placement of a needle/trocar in the left upper quadrant. Insert the camera and verify a safe entry. Place additional trocars in the lateral abdomen under direct vision. Carefully reduce the incarcerated/strangulated bowel, mesentery, and omentum with dissection of the adhesions from any previous mesh to expose and to clear the defect for repair. This requires manipulation both intra-abdominally with minimally invasive instrumentation and extra-abdominally with palpation and pressure applied to the abdominal wall to reduce the incarcerated contents. Examine the reduced tissue for viability and any inadvertent injury. Reduce the hernia sac and resect as needed to expose the fascial edges of the defect(s). Visualize the hernia defect. Clear the falciform ligament and preperitoneal fat from the abdominal wall fascia to expose the posterior fascia. Create peritoneal flaps for placement of mesh. Suture the fascial defect. Introduce a mesh into the peritoneal cavity through a trocar and orient. Reduce insufflation to facilitate mesh conformity to the anterior abdominal wall. Secure the mesh to the abdominal wall utilizing sutures and/or tacks. Then suture the peritoneal flaps over the mesh to protect it from the abdominal viscera. Perform a complete camera survey of the abdomen and contents to inspect for bleeding and visceral injury and perform a final viability assessment of the material once incarcerated in the hernia sac. Irrigate as necessary. Close fascial incisions from laparoscopic ports larger than 1 cm with a suture passer. Close skin incisions according to surgeon preference.

Clinical Example (49615)

A 60-year-old obese male presents with a large bulge in midepigastric area that disappears when he lies down. His surgical history includes a prior laparotomy with resultant hernia that was repaired 5 years ago. Physical examination reveals a large recurrent reducible incisional hernia. He undergoes hernia repair of a defect that is 3 to 10 cm with placement of mesh.

Description of Procedure (49615)

Obtain abdominal access and create a safe pneumoperitoneum with placement of a needle/trocar in the left upper quadrant. Insert the camera and verify safe entry. Place additional trocars in the lateral abdomen under direct vision. A large field of adhesions occupies approximately half of the anterior abdominal wall correlating with the extent of the prior laparotomy and hernia repair. Sharply divide adhesions to the abdominal wall to free the anterior abdominal wall completely. Perform the careful process of adhesiolysis to clear adhesions from between omentum, small intestines and colon, and the abdominal wall and prior mesh. Each separate defect within the entire hernia defect contains adipose and intestinal components and requires a safe and effective clearance of tissue. Visualize the hernia defect. Clear the falciform ligament and preperitoneal fat from the abdominal wall fascia to expose the posterior fascia. Create peritoneal flaps for placement of mesh. Suture the fascial defect the entire length. Select a mesh to provide adequate overlap of the hernia defect. Introduce a mesh into the peritoneal cavity through a trocar and orient. Reduce insufflation to facilitate mesh conformity to the anterior abdominal wall. Secure the mesh to the abdominal wall utilizing sutures and/or tacks. Then suture the peritoneal flaps over the mesh to protect it from the abdominal viscera. Perform a complete camera survey of the abdomen and contents to inspect for bleeding and visceral injury. Irrigate as necessary. Close fascial incisions for laparoscopic ports larger than 1 cm with a suture passer. Close skin incisions according to surgeon preference.

Clinical Example (49616)

A 60-year-old obese male presents with an irreducible mass in the midline of the abdomen. He has a history of a previous laparotomy with an incisional hernia from that operation that was repaired 5 years ago. Over the course of the last few months, he has developed a recurrence that has been slowly increasing in size. Suddenly, the hernia is not reducible, and the mass is tender with severe, unremitting pain. He undergoes hernia repair of a defect that is 3 to 10 cm with placement of mesh.

Description of Procedure (49616)

Obtain abdominal access and create a safe pneumoperitoneum with placement of a needle/trocar in the left upper quadrant. Insert the camera and verify safe entry. Place additional trocars in the lateral abdomen under direct vision. A large field of adhesions occupies approximately half of the anterior abdominal wall correlating with the extent of the prior laparotomy and hernia repair. Carefully reduce the incarcerated/strangulated bowel, mesentery, and omentum with dissection of the adhesions from prior mesh to expose and to clear the defects for repair. This requires manipulation both intra-abdominally with minimally invasive instrumentation and extra-abdominally with palpation and pressure applied to the abdominal wall to reduce the incarcerated contents. Examine the reduced tissue for viability and any inadvertent injury. Reduce the hernia sac and resect as needed to expose the fascial edges of the defect(s). Visualize the hernia defect(s).

Create peritoneal flaps for placement of mesh. Clear the falciform ligament and preperitoneal fat from the abdominal wall fascia to expose the posterior fascia. Measure all of the defects. Approximate the fascial defect with suture. Select a mesh to provide adequate overlap of the hernia defect. Introduce a mesh into the peritoneal cavity through a trocar and orient. Reduce insufflation to facilitate mesh conformity to the anterior abdominal wall. Secure the mesh to the abdominal wall utilizing numerous sutures and/or tacks. Then suture the peritoneal flaps over the mesh to protect it from the abdominal viscera. Perform a complete camera survey of the abdomen and contents to inspect for bleeding and visceral injury and perform a final viability assessment of the material once incarcerated in the hernia sac. Irrigate as necessary. Close fascial incisions for laparoscopic ports larger than 1 cm with a suture passer. Close skin incisions according to surgeon preference.

Clinical Example (49617)

A 60-year-old obese male presents with an irreducible mass in the midline of the abdomen. He has a history of a previous laparotomy with an incisional hernia from that operation that was repaired 5 years ago. Over the course of the last few months, he has developed a recurrence that has been slowly increasing in size but is reducible. He undergoes hernia repair of a defect that totals more than 10 cm with placement of mesh.

Description of Procedure (49617)

Obtain abdominal access and create a safe pneumoperitoneum with placement of a needle/trocar. Because the hernia extends across the majority of the anterior abdominal wall, select the location for insertion of the needle/trocar based on the prior surgical history and the safest location to avoid intra-abdominal injury. Insert the camera and verify safe entry. Place additional trocars in the lateral abdomen, and in additional areas as needed, all under direct vision. A field of adhesions occupies the entire anterior abdominal wall correlating with the extent of the prior laparotomy and hernia repair. Perform the careful process of adhesiolysis to clear adhesions from between omentum, small intestines and colon, and the abdominal wall and prior mesh. Each separate defect within the entire hernia defect contains adipose and intestinal components and requires a safe and effective clearance of tissue. Visualize the hernia defect. Clear the falciform ligament and preperitoneal fat from the abdominal wall fascia to expose the posterior fascia to include wide lateral clearance for adequate later mesh coverage. Create peritoneal flaps for placement of mesh. Approximate the fascial defect with sutures placed along the entire length of the defect. Calculate the appropriate size mesh after total defect length is documented. Adequate overlap of at least 5 cm in all directions is included in the calculation. Remove a trocar from the abdominal wall and dilate the track to allow insertion of the large mesh into the peritoneal cavity. Orient the mesh intra-abdominally. Reduce insufflation to facilitate mesh conformity to the anterior abdominal wall. Secure the mesh to the abdominal wall utilizing multiple sutures and numerous tacks. Then suture the peritoneal flaps over the mesh to protect it from the abdominal viscera. Perform a complete camera survey of the abdomen and contents to inspect for bleeding and visceral injury. Irrigate as necessary. Close fascial incisions from laparoscopic ports larger than 1 cm with a suture passer. Close skin incisions according to surgeon preference.

Clinical Example (49618)

A 60-year-old obese male presents with an irreducible mass in the midline of the abdomen. He has a history of a previous laparotomy with an incisional hernia from that operation that was repaired 5 years ago. Over the course of the last few months, he has developed a recurrence that has been slowly increasing in size and is now tender and irreducible. He undergoes hernia repair of a defect that totals more than 10 cm with placement of mesh.

Description of Procedure (49618)

Obtain abdominal access and create a safe pneumoperitoneum with placement of a needle/trocar. Because the hernia extends across the majority of the anterior abdominal wall, select the location for insertion of the needle/trocar based on the prior surgical history and the safest location to avoid intra-abdominal injury. Insert the camera and verify safe entry. Place additional trocars in the lateral abdomen under direct vision. A large field of adhesions occupies the entire anterior abdominal wall correlating with the extent of the prior laparotomy. Perform the careful process of adhesiolysis to clear adhesions from between omentum, small intestines and colon, and the abdominal wall and prior mesh. Each separate defect within the entire hernia defect contains adipose and intestinal components and requires a safe and effective clearance of tissue. Carefully reduce the incarcerated/strangulated bowel, mesentery, and omentum with dissection of the adhesions and sac to clear all the defects for repair. Take care to avoid injury to the incarcerated tissue. This requires manipulation both intra-abdominally with minimally invasive instrumentation and extra-abdominally with palpation and pressure applied to the abdominal wall to reduce the incarcerated contents. Examine the reduced tissue for viability and any inadvertent injury. Clear the falciform ligament and preperitoneal fat from the abdominal wall fascia to expose all defects and enough surface for mesh overlap. Reduce the hernia sac and resect as needed to expose the fascial edges of the defect(s). Visualize the hernia defect. Measure the defects with a minimum

craniocaudal length greater than 10 cm. Create peritoneal flaps for placement of mesh. Approximate the fascial defect with sutures placed along the entirety of the defect. Calculate the appropriate size mesh after total defect length is documented. Adequate overlap of at least 5 cm in all directions is included in the calculation. Remove a trocar from the abdominal wall and dilate the track to allow insertion of the large mesh into the peritoneal cavity. Orient the mesh intra-abdominally. Reduce insufflation to facilitate mesh conformity to the anterior abdominal wall. Secure the mesh to the abdominal wall utilizing sutures and tacks. Then suture the peritoneal flaps over the mesh to protect it from the abdominal viscera. Perform a complete camera survey of the abdomen and contents to inspect for bleeding and visceral injury and perform a final viability assessment of the material once incarcerated in the hernia sac. Irrigate as necessary. Close fascial incisions for laparoscopic ports larger than 1 cm with a suture passer. Close skin incisions according to surgeon preference.

Clinical Example (49621)

A 70-year-old male with history of rectal cancer with subsequent abdominoperineal resection and end colostomy presents with a worsening bulge around his stoma when coughing, pain and discomfort around the stoma, and difficulty keeping the stoma appliance in place due to leakage. CT scan revealed small bowel in the hernia sac. He undergoes parastomal hernia repair with placement of mesh.

Description of Procedure (49621)

Obtain abdominal access and create a safe pneumoperitoneum with placement of a needle/trocar. Insert the camera and verify safe entry. Place additional trocars in the lateral abdomen under direct vision. A large field of adhesions occupies the anterior abdominal wall surrounding the stoma site. Take down adhesions around the stoma sharply, avoiding injury to the stoma intestinal component traversing the abdominal wall. Perform the careful process of adhesiolysis to clear adhesions from between omentum, small intestines and colon, and the abdominal wall and prior mesh when present. Identify the hernia sac and take down adhesions within the sac. Excise the hernia sac. Narrow the hernia defect with suture, taking care to leave the appropriate size fascial defect for the colostomy yet avoiding an opportunity for intestinal contents to traverse the abdominal wall beside it allowing a recurrence. Mobilize the colon proximal to the colostomy to ensure that there is no tension on the colostomy. Insert the appropriate size mesh into the peritoneal cavity and fashion around the colostomy to cover the hernia defect also avoiding narrowing of the colostomy or offering space for material to traverse the abdominal wall beside it allowing a recurrence. Use sutures and tacks to anchor the mesh to

★ =Telemedicine ◀ =Audio-only ✚ =Add-on code ⇗ =FDA approval pending # =Resequenced code ⊘ =Modifier 51 exempt

the anterior abdominal wall. Perform a complete laparoscopic survey to inspect for bleeding and visceral injury. Irrigate as necessary. Obtain hemostasis. Close fascial incisions for laparoscopic ports larger than 1 cm with a suture passer. Close skin incisions according to surgeon preference. Remove the temporary closure suture from the stoma. Assess patency of the stoma prior to completion of the procedure.

Clinical Example (49622)

A 70-year-old male with history of rectal cancer, colon resection, and sigmoid colostomy presents with a worsening parastomal hernia associated with pain. The hernia cannot be reduced, and a CT scan indicates incarcerated small bowel loops in the parastomal hernia sac. He undergoes parastomal hernia repair with placement of mesh.

Description of Procedure (49622)

Obtain abdominal access and create a safe pneumoperitoneum with placement of a needle/trocar. Insert the camera and verify safe entry. Place additional trocars in the lateral abdomen under direct vision. A large field of adhesions occupies the anterior abdominal wall surrounding the stoma site. Take down adhesions around the stoma sharply, avoiding injury to the stoma intestinal component traversing the abdominal wall. Perform the careful process of adhesiolysis to clear adhesions from between omentum, small intestines and colon, and the abdominal wall and prior mesh when present. Initiate the reduction of the incarcerated material. This requires manipulation both intra-abdominally with minimally invasive instrumentation and extra-abdominally with palpation and pressure applied to the abdominal wall to reduce the incarcerated contents. Examine the reduced tissue for viability and any inadvertent injury. Identify the hernia sac and take down adhesions within the sac and excise the hernia sac. Narrow the hernia defect with suture, taking care to leave the appropriate size fascial defect for the colostomy yet avoiding an opportunity for intestinal contents to traverse the abdominal wall beside it allowing a recurrence. Mobilize the colon proximal to the colostomy to ensure that there is no tension on the colostomy. Insert the appropriate size mesh into the peritoneal cavity and fashion around the colostomy to cover the hernia defect also avoiding narrowing of the colostomy or offering space for material to traverse the abdominal wall beside it allowing a recurrence. Use sutures and tacks to anchor the mesh to the anterior abdominal wall to secure the mesh. Perform a completion laparoscopic survey to inspect for bleeding and visceral injury and perform a final viability assessment of the material once incarcerated in the hernia sac. Irrigate as necessary. Obtain hemostasis. Close fascial incisions for laparoscopic ports larger than

1 cm with a suture passer. Close skin incisions according to surgeon preference. Remove the temporary closure suture from the stoma. Assess patency of the stoma prior to completion of the procedure.

Clinical Example (49623)

At the time of hernia repair, a 64-year-old obese male who had mesh placed with a prior hernia repair now requires removal of the mesh to allow for an adequate repair of a new hernia. [**Note:** This is an add-on code. Only consider the additional work related to mesh removal.]

Description of Procedure (49623)

Utilizing electrocautery and sharp dissection, dissect the previously placed mesh from the abdominal wall fascia. Take care to prevent damage to the abdominal wall and intra-abdominal contents while removing the mesh in its entirety. Identify prior sutures and tacks and dissect from the abdominal wall. Obtain hemostasis in the abdominal wall over the surface area of the excised mesh.

Laparoscopy

49650	Laparoscopy, surgical; repair initial inguinal hernia
49651	repair recurrent inguinal hernia

▶(49652, 49653 have been deleted. To report laparoscopic repair of ventral, umbilical, spigelian, or epigastric hernia, see 49591-49618)◀

▶(49654, 49655 have been deleted. To report laparoscopic repair of incisional hernia, see 49591-49618)◀

▶(49656, 49657 have been deleted. To report laparoscopic repair of recurrent incisional hernia, see 49613, 49614, 49615, 49616, 49617, 49618)◀

Rationale

Codes 49652-49657, which were used to report laparoscopic surgical repair of a ventral, umbilical, spigelian, epigastric, or incisional hernia, have been deleted. Corresponding instructional parenthetical notes also have been deleted. Parenthetical notes have been established to inform users of the deleted codes and to instruct reporting of the new codes.

Refer to the codebook and the Rationale for abdominal hernia repair codes for a full discussion of these changes.

Urinary System

Kidney

Incision

▶Nephrolithotomy is the surgical removal of stones from the kidney, and pyelolithotomy is the surgical removal of stones from the renal pelvis. This section of the guidelines refers to the removal of stones from the kidney or renal pelvis using a percutaneous antegrade approach. Breaking and removing stones is separate from accessing the kidney (ie, 50040, 50432, 50433, 52334), accessing the kidney with dilation of the tract to accommodate an endoscope used in an endourologic procedure (ie, 50437), or dilation of a previously established tract to accommodate an endoscope used in an endourologic procedure (ie, 50436). These procedures include the antegrade removal of stones in the calyces, renal pelvis, and/or ureter with the antegrade placement of catheters, stents, and tubes, but do not include retrograde placement of catheters, stents, and tubes.

Code 50080 describes nephrolithotomy or pyelolithotomy using a percutaneous antegrade approach with endoscopic instruments to break and remove kidney stones of 2 cm or smaller.

Code 50081 includes the elements of 50080, but it is reported for stones larger than 2 cm, branching, stones in multiple locations, ureteral stones, or in patients with complicated anatomy.

Creation of percutaneous access or dilation of the tract to accommodate large endoscopic instruments used in stone removals (50436, 50437) is not included in 50080, 50081, and may be reported separately, if performed. Codes 50080, 50081 include placement of any stents or drainage catheters that remain indwelling after the procedure.

Report one unit of 50080 or 50081 per side (ie, per kidney), regardless of the number of stones broken and/or removed or locations of the stones. For bilateral procedure, report 50080, 50081 with modifier 50. When 50080 is performed on one side and 50081 is performed on the contralateral side, modifier 50 is not applicable. Placement of additional accesses, if needed, into the kidney, and removal of stones through other approaches (eg, open or retrograde) may be reported separately, if performed.◀

▲ **50080** Percutaneous nephrolithotomy or pyelolithotomy, lithotripsy, stone extraction, antegrade ureteroscopy, antegrade stent placement and nephrostomy tube placement, when performed, including imaging guidance; simple (eg, stone[s] up to 2 cm in single location of kidney or renal pelvis, nonbranching stones)

▲ **50081** complex (eg, stone[s] > 2 cm, branching stones, stones in multiple locations, ureter stones, complicated anatomy)

▶(50080, 50081 may only be reported once per side. For bilateral procedure, report 50080, 50081 with modifier 50)◀

▶(Do not report 50080, 50081 in conjunction with 50430, 50431, 50433, 50434, 50435, if performed on the same side)◀

▶(For establishment of nephrostomy without nephrolithotomy, see 50040, 50432, 50433, 52334)◀

▶(For dilation of an existing percutaneous access for an endourologic procedure, use 50436)◀

▶(For dilation of an existing percutaneous access for an endourologic procedure with new access into the collecting system, use 50437; for additional new access into the kidney, use 50437 for each new access that is dilated for an endourologic procedure)◀

▶(For removal of stone without lithotripsy, use 50561)◀

▶(For cystourethroscopy with insertion of ureteral guidewire through kidney to establish a percutaneous nephrostomy, retrograde, use 52334)◀

Rationale

Codes 50080 and 50081 have been revised. New guidelines and parenthetical notes have been added regarding these codes.

Prior to 2023, codes 50080 and 50081 described percutaneous nephrostolithotomy or pyelostolithotomy with or without dilation, endoscopy, lithotripsy, stenting, or basket extraction. The terms "nephrostolithotomy" and "pyelostolithotomy" are no longer used in current clinical practice. In addition, the terminology describing some of the components of the procedure (ie, dilation, endoscopy, stenting, basket extraction) no longer accurately describe how these procedures are performed.

Effective in 2023, codes 50080 and 50081 have been revised with terminology that accurately reflects current clinical practice. The outdated terms "nephrostolithotomy" and "pyelostolithotomy" have been revised to "nephrolithotomy" and "pyelolithotomy." "Endoscopy" has been revised to the more specific term "antegrade ureteroscopy." "Stenting" has been revised to specify antegrade stent placement. Nephrostomy tube placement has been added to the descriptor. "Basket extraction" has been revised to the more general term "stone extraction." All of these procedures are included in the codes when they are performed. As such, the "with or without" language has been revised to "when performed" to match the current CPT language convention. An exclusionary parenthetical note has been added restricting use of

★=Telemedicine ◀=Audio-only ✚=Add-on code ✺=FDA approval pending #=Resequenced code ⦰=Modifier 51 exempt

codes 50430, 50431, 50433, 50434, and 50435 with codes 50080 and 50081, if the procedure is performed on the same side. Dilation has been removed from codes 50080 and 50081. Dilation of an existing percutaneous access is reported with dilation code 50436. Dilation of an existing percutaneous access with new access into the collecting system and additional new access into the kidney is reported with dilation code 50437. Cross-reference parenthetical notes directing users to these dilation codes have been added following codes 50080 and 50081. Codes 50080 and 50081 include imaging guidance.

Code 50080 is reported for stone(s) up to 2 cm in a single location of the kidney or renal pelvis, or for nonbranching stones (ie, stones that do not branch from one location into other locations). Code 50081 is reported for complex procedures (eg, removal of stone[s] greater than 2 cm in size, branching stones, stones in multiple locations, stones in the ureter, or in patients with complicated anatomy). When the procedure described by code 50080 or 50081 is performed bilaterally (ie, on both kidneys), one unit is reported with modifier 50, *Bilateral Procedure,* appended. In the instance when the procedure represented by code 50080 is performed in one kidney and the procedure represented by code 50081 is performed in the contralateral kidney, modifier 50 would not be appended.

Clinical Example (50080)

A 68-year-old male with a 1.8-cm calculus in the lower pole of the kidney undergoes a percutaneous nephrolithotomy. [**Note:** Initial access and dilation are separately reported.]

Description of Procedure (50080)

Insert a rigid nephroscope through the previously placed Amplatz sheath and identify the stone. Insert the handheld lithotripter through the nephroscope and fragment the stone as much as possible. Extract the fragments with grasping forceps and/or suction. Once the limits of rigid nephroscopy have been reached (due to angulation), insert a flexible nephroscope to access calyces inaccessible with the rigid nephroscope. Remove calyceal stones with a stone basket or fragment with a laser and then remove the fragments with a stone basket. Perform antegrade ureteroscopy to ascertain there are no fragments in the ureter. Pass the flexible ureteroscope through the access sheath into the calyx and into the renal pelvis. Identify the ureteropelvic junction and pass the ureteroscope through the junction and into the ureter. Assess the entire length of the ureter for injury from passage of guidewires/catheters. Then withdraw the ureteroscope. At the completion of the nephrolithotomy, remove the nephroscope. During the entire procedure, the operating surgeon tracks the use of fluids and

pressures in real time to ensure no fluid mismatch. Remove the Amplatz sheath. Obtain fluoroscopic images over the ipsilateral lung to ascertain there is no evidence of a pneumothorax or hydrothorax. Place a nephrostomy tube. Perform a nephrostogram to determine proper positioning of the nephrostomy tube.

Clinical Example (50081)

A 66-year-old male with a staghorn (branched) calculus filling the entire renal pelvis and most calyces undergoes a percutaneous nephrolithotomy. [**Note:** Initial access and dilation are separately reported.]

Description of Procedure (50081)

Insert a rigid nephroscope through the previously placed sheath and identify the large stone. Insert the handheld lithotripter through the nephroscope and fragment the stone as much as possible. Extract fragments with grasping forceps and/or suction. Once the limits of rigid nephroscopy have been reached (due to angulation), utilize additional nephrostomy access into the kidney in a similar fashion. Again, carry out rigid nephroscopy of calyceal and remaining renal pelvis stone. Once this is complete, insert a flexible nephroscope to access calyces inaccessible with the rigid nephroscope. Remove calyceal stones with a stone basket or fragment with a laser and then remove the fragments with a stone basket. Perform antegrade ureteroscopy to ascertain there are no fragments in the ureter. Pass the flexible ureteroscope through the access sheath into the calyx and into the renal pelvis. Identify the ureteropelvic junction and pass the ureteroscope through it into the ureter. Assess the entire length of the ureter for injury from passage of guidewires/catheters. Assess the ureter for primary stones or stone fragments. Remove small fragments with a stone basket. For larger stones, pass a laser fiber and fragment the stone(s). Irrigate small fragments down the length of the ureter or remove with a stone basket. Once the ureter is deemed to be free of stone fragments, withdraw the ureteroscope. At the completion of the nephrolithotomy, remove the nephroscope. During the entire procedure the operating surgeon tracks the use of fluids and pressures in real time to ensure no fluid mismatch. Remove the Amplatz sheath. Obtain fluoroscopic images over the ipsilateral lung to ascertain there is no evidence of a pneumothorax or hydrothorax. Place a nephrostomy tube in each access. Perform a nephrostogram to ascertain proper positioning of the nephrostomy tube(s).

Introduction

Other Introduction (Injection/Change/Removal) Procedures

 # 50436   Dilation of existing tract, percutaneous, for an endourologic procedure including imaging guidance (eg, ultrasound and/or fluoroscopy) and all associated radiological supervision and interpretation, with postprocedure tube placement, when performed;

 # 50437   including new access into the renal collecting system

▶(Do not report 50436, 50437 in conjunction with 50382, 50384, 50430, 50431, 50432, 50433, 52334, 74485)◀

▶(For nephrolithotomy, see 50080, 50081)◀

▶(For dilation of an existing percutaneous access for an endourologic procedure with a new access into the collecting system, use 50437; for additional new access into the kidney, use 50437 for each new access that is dilated for an endourologic procedure)◀

(For endoscopic surgery, see 50551-50561)

(For retrograde percutaneous nephrostomy, use 52334)

Rationale

In accordance with the revision of codes 50080 and 50081, the exclusionary parenthetical note and the cross-reference parenthetical note directing users to codes 50080 and 50081 following code 50437 have been revised, and an instructional parenthetical note has been added to reflect these changes.

Refer to the codebook and the Rationale for codes 50080 and 50081 for a full discussion of these changes.

Bladder

Transurethral Surgery

Ureter and Pelvis

52334   Cystourethroscopy with insertion of ureteral guide wire through kidney to establish a percutaneous nephrostomy, retrograde

▶(For percutaneous nephrolithotomy, see 50080, 50081; for establishment of percutaneous nephrostomy, see 50432, 50433)◀

(For cystourethroscopy, with ureteroscopy and/or pyeloscopy, see 52351-52356)

(For cystourethroscopy with incision, fulguration, or resection of congenital posterior urethral valves or obstructive hypertrophic mucosal folds, use 52400)

(Do not report 52334 in conjunction with 50437, 52000, 52351)

Rationale

In accordance with the revision of codes 50080 and 50081, the cross-reference parenthetical note following code 52334 that directs users to codes 50080 and 50081 has been revised.

Refer to the codebook and the Rationale for codes 50080 and 50081 for a full discussion of these changes.

Male Genital System

Prostate

Excision

55821   Prostatectomy (including control of postoperative bleeding, vasectomy, meatotomy, urethral calibration and/or dilation, and internal urethrotomy); suprapubic, subtotal, 1 or 2 stages

55831   retropubic, subtotal

▶(For laparoscopy, surgical prostatectomy, simple subtotal, use 55867)◀

Rationale

A new parenthetical note following code 55831 has been established to instruct users to report code 55867 for laparoscopic simple subtotal prostatectomy.

Refer to the codebook and the Rationale for code 55867 for a full discussion of these changes.

Laparoscopy

55866   Laparoscopy, surgical prostatectomy, retropubic radical, including nerve sparing, includes robotic assistance, when performed

(For open procedure, use 55840)

▶(For laparoscopy, surgical prostatectomy, simple subtotal, use 55867)◀

★=Telemedicine   ◀=Audio-only   ✚=Add-on code   ✔=FDA approval pending   #=Resequenced code   ⊘=Modifier 51 exempt

● **55867**   Laparoscopy, surgical prostatectomy, simple subtotal (including control of postoperative bleeding, vasectomy, meatotomy, urethral calibration and/or dilation, and internal urethrotomy), includes robotic assistance, when performed

▶(For open subtotal prostatectomy, see 55821, 55831)◀

Rationale

There are CPT codes that report simple prostatectomy (55821, 55831), open radical prostatectomy (55840, 55842, 55845), and laparoscopic radical prostatectomy (55866), but not specifically for laparoscopic simple prostatectomy. Previously laparoscopic simple prostatectomy has been reported using only unlisted codes.

Code 55867 has been established to report laparoscopic simple prostatectomy and a corresponding parenthetical note has been established following code 55867 to instruct users to report code 55821 or 55831 for open subtotal prostatectomy.

In addition, a new parenthetical note following code 55866 has been established to instruct users to use code 55867 for laparoscopic simple prostatectomy.

Clinical Example (55867)

A 65-year-old male who is symptomatic due to obstruction from prostatic enlargement chose to undergo laparoscopic simple suprapubic prostatectomy.

Description of Procedure (55867)

Make a suprapubic incision and introduce a needle. Confirm an intraperitoneal position and create a pneumoperitoneum. Place a midline trocar and insert a zero-degree lens camera. Inspect the abdomen and pelvis for visceral injury or abnormal anatomy. Make five additional incisions after appropriate measurements, and place five additional trocars under direct vision. Adjust the table to place the patient in a steep Trendelenburg position and advance the robot. The four robotic arms are individually docked and pressure points are checked. Make appropriate adjustments to the robotic arms at the surgical console. Next, introduce the laparoscope and mobilize the colon so it is away from the bladder. Make an incision in the posterior bladder wall. Place several stay sutures in the bladder wall to expose the base of the bladder. Identify the ureteral orifices and survey the prostate anatomy to assess for median lobe location and relational anatomy to the bladder. Make an incision at the junction of the prostate and the bladder neck. Carry the incision circumferentially along the capsule of the prostate out laterally and distally. Rock the prostate back and forth and continue dissection along the lateral pedicle plane to define the apex of the prostate

posteriorly. Unfasten the final attachments and place the specimen into the endosac and place out of the surgical field. Decrease the pneumoperitoneum and inspect the entire surgical field for evidence of bleeding. Once hemostasis is obtained, advance the bladder neck to the urethral mucosa using fine monofilament suture. Hemostasis is also achieved using cautery and suture. Close the posterior bladder wall with suture. Pass a catheter into the bladder and test the closure by placing 200 ml of saline into the bladder to distend it. Place a drain through one of the abdominal side ports. Inspect all six trocar sites and all surgical sites at 5-mm Hg pressure before the trocars are removed under direct vision. Extract the specimen by enlarging the midline incision and transferring the endosac bag to this area, where it is removed. Close the rectus fascia using suture, inject local anesthetic into all five of the trocar incisions, and close the trocar incisions with interrupted 2-0 nylon sutures. Place sterile dressings over each incision and secure the catheter to the patient's thigh with a catheter strap.

Maternity Care and Delivery

▶The services normally provided in uncomplicated maternity cases include antepartum care, delivery, and postpartum care. Pregnancy confirmation during a problem-oriented or preventive visit is not considered as part of antepartum care and should be reported using the appropriate E/M service codes 99202, 99203, 99204, 99205, 99211, 99212, 99213, 99214, 99215, 99242, 99243, 99244, 99245, 99281, 99282, 99283, 99284, 99285, 99384, 99385, 99386, 99394, 99395, 99396 for that visit.◀

Antepartum care includes the initial prenatal history and physical examination; subsequent prenatal history and physical examinations; recording of weight, blood pressures, fetal heart tones, routine chemical urinalysis, and monthly visits up to 28 weeks gestation; biweekly visits to 36 weeks gestation; and weekly visits until delivery. Any other visits or services within this time period should be coded separately.

▶Delivery services include admission to the hospital, the admission history and physical examination, management of uncomplicated labor, vaginal delivery (with or without episiotomy, with or without forceps), or cesarean delivery. When reporting delivery only services (59409, 59514, 59612, 59620), report inpatient postdelivery management and discharge services using E/M service codes (99238, 99239). Delivery and postpartum services (59410, 59515, 59614, 59622) include delivery services and all inpatient and outpatient postpartum services. Medical complications of pregnancy (eg, cardiac problems, neurological problems, diabetes, hypertension,

Surgery / Nervous System   61000-64999

toxemia, hyperemesis, preterm labor, premature rupture of membranes, trauma) and medical problems complicating labor and delivery management may require additional resources and may be reported separately. ◄

Postpartum care only services (59430) include office or other outpatient visits following vaginal or cesarean section delivery.

For surgical complications of pregnancy (eg, appendectomy, hernia, ovarian cyst, Bartholin cyst), see services in the **Surgery** section.

If all or part of the antepartum and/or postpartum patient care is provided except delivery due to termination of pregnancy by abortion or referral to another physician or other qualified health care professional for delivery, see the antepartum and postpartum care codes 59425, 59426, and 59430.

(For circumcision of newborn, see 54150, 54160)

Rationale

In accordance with the deletion of codes 99217 and 99241, the Maternity Care and Delivery subsection guidelines have been revised to reflect these changes.

Refer to the codebook and the Rationale for codes 99217 and 99241 for a full discussion of these changes.

Nervous System

Extracranial Nerves, Peripheral Nerves, and Autonomic Nervous System

Introduction/Injection of Anesthetic Agent (Nerve Block), Diagnostic or Therapeutic

Somatic Nerves

Codes 64400-64489 describe the introduction/injection of an anesthetic agent and/or steroid into the somatic nervous system for diagnostic or therapeutic purposes. For injection or destruction of genicular nerve branches, see 64454, 64624, respectively.

Codes 64400-64450, 64454 describe the injection of an anesthetic agent(s) and/or steroid into a nerve plexus, nerve, or branch. These codes are reported once per nerve plexus, nerve, or branch as described in the descriptor regardless of the number of injections performed along the nerve plexus, nerve, or branch described by the code.

►Imaging guidance and localization may be reported separately for 64400, 64405, 64408, 64420, 64421, 64425, 64430, 64435, 64449, 64450. Imaging guidance and any injection of contrast are inclusive components of 64415, 64416, 64417, 64445, 64446, 64447, 64448, 64451, 64454. ◄

Codes 64455, 64479, 64480, 64483, 64484 are reported for single or multiple injections on the same site. For 64479, 64480, 64483, 64484, imaging guidance (fluoroscopy or CT) and any injection of contrast are inclusive components and are not reported separately. For 64455, imaging guidance (ultrasound, fluoroscopy, CT) and localization may be reported separately.

Codes 64461, 64462, 64463 describe injection of a paravertebral block (PVB). Codes 64486, 64487, 64488, 64489 describe injection of a transversus abdominis plane (TAP) block. Imaging guidance and any injection of contrast are inclusive components of 64461, 64462, 64463, 64486, 64487, 64488, 64489 and are not reported separately.

64400   Injection(s), anesthetic agent(s) and/or steroid; trigeminal nerve, each branch (ie, ophthalmic, maxillary, mandibular)

▲ 64415   brachial plexus, including imaging guidance, when performed

►(Do not report 64415 in conjunction with 76942, 77002, 77003)◄

▲ 64416   brachial plexus, continuous infusion by catheter (including catheter placement), including imaging guidance, when performed

►(Do not report 64416 in conjunction with 01996, 76942, 77002, 77003)◄

▲ 64417   axillary nerve, including imaging guidance, when performed

►(Do not report 64417 in conjunction with 76942, 77002, 77003)◄

▲ 64445   sciatic nerve, including imaging guidance, when performed

►(Do not report 64445 in conjunction with 76942, 77002, 77003)◄

▲ 64446   sciatic nerve, continuous infusion by catheter (including catheter placement), including imaging guidance, when performed

►(Do not report 64446 in conjunction with 01996, 76942, 77002, 77003)◄

▲ 64447   femoral nerve, including imaging guidance, when performed

►(Do not report 64447 in conjunction with 01996, 76942, 77002, 77003)◄

▲ 64448   femoral nerve, continuous infusion by catheter (including catheter placement), including imaging guidance, when performed

▶(Do not report 64448 in conjunction with 01996, 76942, 77002, 77003)◀

Rationale

Introductory guidelines, code descriptors, and parenthetical notes have been revised to identify when imaging guidance is inclusive in nerve injection procedures and when imaging guidance may be separately reported.

The guidelines in the Surgery/Extracranial Nerves, Peripheral Nerves, and Autonomic Nervous System, Introduction/Injection of Anesthetic Agent (Nerve Block), Diagnostic or Therapeutic, Somatic Nerves subsection have been revised to provide instruction that imaging guidance and localization may be separately reported, when performed with nerve injection represented by codes 64405, 64408, 64420, 64421, 64425, 64430, 64435, and 64449. The guidelines also have been revised to specify that codes 64415-64417 and 64445-64448 include imaging guidance and any injection of contrast as inclusive components.

In addition, the code descriptors have also been revised for those codes (64415-64417, 64445-64448) that inherently include imaging guidance. To reiterate this, parenthetical notes have also been added or revised to restrict reporting of the specific image guidance procedures (eg, 76942, 77002, 77003) for these nerve injection services.

These changes have been incorporated throughout the CPT code set to help users differentiate reporting for nerve injection procedures that include imaging guidance and those codes that do not include imaging guidance.

In addition, exclusionary parenthetical notes following codes 76942, 77002, and 77003 have been revised by addition and/or deletion of codes to direct users regarding the appropriate reporting of injection services in conjunction with image guidance.

Lastly, the headings and code listings in the Extracranial Nerves, Peripheral Nerves, and Autonomic Nervous System, Introduction/Injection of Anesthetic Agent (Nerve Block), Diagnostic or Therapeutic table have been revised to provide guidance and clarity on how to correctly report these revised services.

Clinical Example (64415)

A 66-year-old female will undergo surgery on her shoulder and the surgeon consults the anesthesiologist for opioid-sparing postoperative pain management. A brachial plexus block with ultrasound guidance is performed to relieve her pain and improve her function.

Description of Procedure (64415)

Identify the appropriate skin and bony landmarks bordering the brachial plexus. With ultrasound imaging, visualize the nerve(s) and identify the skin entry point. Create a local anesthetic skin wheal. Under ultrasound guidance, advance a needle toward the brachial plexus and confirm the correct position. Under continuous ultrasound imaging, inject a local anesthetic solution with or without adjuvants into the fascial compartment containing the brachial plexus using intermittent aspiration and injection. Remove the needle. After cleaning the site, place an occlusive dressing.

Clinical Example (64416)

A 54-year-old female will undergo surgery on her shoulder and the surgeon consults the anesthesiologist for opioid-sparing postoperative pain management. A brachial plexus block with a catheter and a continuous infusion of local anesthetic with ultrasound guidance is performed to relieve her pain and improve her function.

Description of Procedure (64416)

Identify the appropriate skin and bony landmarks bordering the brachial plexus. With ultrasound imaging, visualize the nerve(s) and identify the skin entry point. Create a local anesthetic skin wheal. Under ultrasound guidance, advance a needle toward the brachial plexus and confirm the correct position. Under continuous ultrasound imaging, inject a local anesthetic or crystalloid solution into the fascial compartment containing the brachial plexus using intermittent aspiration and injection. Advance a catheter carefully under ultrasound guidance to lie next to the brachial plexus then remove the needle. Inject local anesthetic via the catheter. Secure the catheter and place an occlusive dressing.

Clinical Example (64417)

A 68-year-old male will undergo surgery on his arm and the surgeon consults the anesthesiologist for opioid-sparing postoperative pain management. An axillary nerve block with ultrasound guidance is performed to relieve his pain and improve his function.

Description of Procedure (64417)

Identify the appropriate skin and bony landmarks bordering the axillary nerve. With ultrasound imaging, visualize the nerve(s) and identify the skin entry point. Create a local anesthetic skin wheal. Under ultrasound guidance, advance a needle toward the target nerve(s) and confirm the correct position. Inject a local anesthetic solution with or without adjuvants around the target nerve using intermittent aspiration and injection. Remove the needle. After cleaning the site, place an occlusive dressing.

Clinical Example (64445)

A 25-year-old female will undergo surgery for a right trimalleolar fracture open reduction and fixation and the surgeon consults the anesthesiologist for opioid-sparing postoperative pain management. A sciatic nerve block with ultrasound guidance is performed to relieve her pain and improve her function.

Description of Procedure (64445)

Identify the appropriate skin and bony landmarks bordering the sciatic nerve. With ultrasound imaging, visualize the nerve(s) and identify the skin entry point. Create a local anesthetic skin wheal. Under ultrasound guidance, advance a needle toward the sciatic nerve and confirm the correct position. Under continuous ultrasound imaging, inject a local anesthetic solution with or without adjuvants into the fascial compartment containing the sciatic nerve using intermittent aspiration and injection. Remove the needle. After cleaning the site, place an occlusive dressing.

Clinical Example (64446)

A 30-year-old male will undergo surgery for major reconstruction of his left foot and ankle and the surgeon consults the anesthesiologist for opioid-sparing postoperative pain management. A continuous sciatic nerve block with a catheter and a continuous infusion of local anesthetic with ultrasound guidance is performed to relieve his pain and improve his function.

Description of Procedure (64446)

Identify the appropriate skin and bony landmarks bordering the sciatic nerve. With ultrasound imaging, visualize the nerve(s) and identify the skin entry point. Create a local anesthetic skin wheal. Under ultrasound guidance, advance a needle toward the sciatic nerve and confirm the correct position. Under continuous ultrasound imaging, inject a local anesthetic or crystalloid solution into the fascial compartment containing the sciatic nerve using intermittent aspiration and injection. Advance a catheter carefully under ultrasound guidance to lie next to the sciatic nerve. Then remove the needle. Inject a local anesthetic via the catheter. Secure the catheter and place an occlusive dressing.

Clinical Example (64447)

A 30-year-old male will undergo surgery for a right anterior cruciate ligament repair and the surgeon consults the anesthesiologist for opioid-sparing postoperative pain management. A femoral nerve block with ultrasound guidance is performed to manage postoperative pain and improve his function.

Description of Procedure (64447)

Identify the appropriate skin and bony landmarks bordering the femoral nerve. With ultrasound guidance, visualize the nerve(s) and identify the skin entry point. Create a local anesthetic skin wheal. Under ultrasound guidance, advance a needle toward the femoral nerve and confirm the correct position. Under continuous ultrasound imaging, inject a local anesthetic solution with or without adjuvants into the fascial compartment containing the femoral nerve using intermittent aspiration and injection. Remove the needle. After cleaning the site, place an occlusive dressing.

Clinical Example (64448)

A 65-year-old male will undergo surgery for a right total knee replacement and the surgeon consults the anesthesiologist for opioid-sparing postoperative pain management. A continuous femoral nerve block with a catheter and a continuous infusion of local anesthetic with ultrasound guidance is performed to manage postoperative pain and improve his function.

Description of Procedure (64448)

Identify the appropriate skin and bony landmarks bordering the femoral nerve. With ultrasound imaging, visualize the nerve(s) and identify the skin entry point. Create a local anesthetic skin wheal. Under ultrasound guidance, advance a needle toward the femoral nerve and confirm the correct position. Under continuous ultrasound imaging, inject a local anesthetic or crystalloid solution into the fascial compartment containing the femoral nerve using intermittent aspiration and injection. Advance a catheter carefully under ultrasound guidance to lie next to the femoral nerve. Remove the needle. Inject a local anesthetic via the catheter. Secure the catheter and place an occlusive dressing.

Paraverterbral Spinal Nerves and Branches

▶Codes 64490, 64491, 64492, 64493, 64494, 64495 describe the introduction/injection of a diagnostic or therapeutic agent into the paravertebral facet joint or into the nerves that innervate that joint by level. Facet joints are paired joints with one pair at each vertebral level. Imaging guidance and localization are required for the performance of paravertebral facet joint injections described by 64490, 64491, 64492, 64493, 64494, 64495. If imaging is not used, report 20552, 20553. If ultrasound guidance is used, report 0213T, 0214T, 0215T, 0216T, 0217T, 0218T.

When determining a level, count the number of facet joints injected, not the number of nerves injected. Therefore, if multiple nerves of the same facet joint are injected, it would be considered as a single level. The add-on codes are reported when second, third, or additional levels are injected during the same session.

When the procedure is performed bilaterally at the same level, report one unit of the primary code with modifier 50.

When the procedure is performed on the left side at one level and the right side at a different level in the same region, report one unit of the primary procedure and one unit of the add-on code.

When the procedure is performed bilaterally at one level and unilaterally at a different level(s), report one unit of the primary procedure for each level and append modifier 50 for the bilateral procedure. If the procedure is performed unilaterally at different levels, report one unit of the primary procedure and the appropriate add-on code(s).◄

Extracranial Nerves, Peripheral Nerves, and Autonomic Nervous System			
Introduction/Injection of Anesthetic Agent (Nerve Block), Diagnostic or Therapeutic			
Code(s)	**Unit**	▶**Imaging Guidance Included**◄	▶**Imaging Guidance Separately Reported, When Performed**◄
Somatic Nerve			
▶64400-64408	1 unit per plexus, nerve, or branch injected regardless of the number of injections		X
64415-64417	1 unit per plexus, nerve, or branch injected regardless of the number of injections	X	
64418-64435	1 unit per plexus, nerve, or branch injected regardless of the number of injections		X
64445-64448	1 unit per plexus, nerve, or branch injected regardless of the number of injections	X	
64449	1 unit per plexus, nerve, or branch injected regardless of the number of injections		X
64450	1 unit per plexus, nerve, or branch injected regardless of the number of injections◄		X
64451	1 unit for any number of nerves innervating the sacroiliac joint injected regardless of the number of injections	X	
64454	1 unit for any number of genicular nerve branches, with a required minimum of three nerve branches	X	
64455	1 or more injections per level		X
64479	1 or more injections per level	X	
+64480	1 or more additional injections per level (add-on)	X	
64483	1 or more injections per level	X	
+64484	1 or more additional injections per level (add-on)	X	
64461	1 injection site	X	
+64462	1 or more additional injections per code (add-on)	X	
64463	1 or more injections per code	X	
64486-64489	By injection site	X	
Destruction by Neurolytic Agent (Eg, Chemical, Thermal, Electrical, or Radiofrequency), Chemodenervation			
Code(s)	**Unit**	▶**Imaging Guidance Included**◄	▶**Imaging Guidance Separately Reported, When Performed**◄
Somatic Nerves			
64624	1 unit for any number of genicular nerve branches, with a required minimum of three nerve branches	X	

Surgery / Nervous System 61000-64999

▶Procedure	Cervical/ Thoracic	Lumbar/ Sacral
Multiple nerves injected at the same level	64490 X 1	64493 X 1
1 level injected unilaterally	64490 X 1	64493 X 1
1 level injected bilaterally	64490 50 X 1	64493 50 X 1
1 level injected bilaterally and 1 level injected unilaterally	64490 50 X 1 64491 X 1	64493 50 X 1 64494 X 1
2 levels injected unilaterally	64490 X 1 64491 X 1	64493 X 1 64494 X 1
2 levels injected bilaterally	64490 50 X 1 64491 X 2	64493 50 X 1 64494 X 2
3 or more levels injected unilaterally	64490 X 1 64491 X 1 64492 X 1	64493 X 1 64494 X 1 64495 X 1
3 or more levels injected bilaterally	64490 50 X 1 64491 X 2 64492 X 2	64493 50 X 1 64494 X 2 64495 X 2◀

(For bilateral paravertebral facet injection procedures, report 64490, 64493 with modifier 50. Report add-on codes 64491, 64492, 64494, 64495 twice, when performed bilaterally. Do not report modifier 50 in conjunction with 64491, 64492, 64494, 64495)

(For paravertebral facet injection of the T12-L1 joint, or nerves innervating that joint, use 64490)

▶(For unilateral paravertebral facet injection of the T12-L1 and L1-L2 levels or nerves innervating that joint, use 64490 and 64494 once)◀

▶(For bilateral paravertebral facet injection of the T12-L1 and L1-L2 levels or nerves innervating that joint, use 64490 with modifier 50 once and 64494 twice)◀

64490 Injection(s), diagnostic or therapeutic agent, paravertebral facet (zygapophyseal) joint (or nerves innervating that joint) with image guidance (fluoroscopy or CT), cervical or thoracic; single level

+ 64491 second level (List separately in addition to code for primary procedure)

(Use 64491 in conjunction with 64490)

+ 64492 third and any additional level(s) (List separately in addition to code for primary procedure)

(Use 64492 in conjunction with 64490, 64491)

64493 Injection(s), diagnostic or therapeutic agent, paravertebral facet (zygapophyseal) joint (or nerves innervating that joint) with image guidance (fluoroscopy or CT), lumbar or sacral; single level

(For injection, anesthetic agent, nerves innervating the sacroiliac joint, use 64451)

+ 64494 second level (List separately in addition to code for primary procedure)

▶(Use 64494 in conjunction with 64490, 64493)◀

+ 64495 third and any additional level(s) (List separately in addition to code for primary procedure)

(Use 64495 in conjunction with 64493, 64494)

Rationale

New guidelines and instructional parenthetical notes have been added for paravertebral spinal nerves and branches injection codes 64490-64495.

Prior to 2023, there was confusion about how "level" is defined in codes 64490-64495 and what constitutes a procedure described by these codes as "bilateral" (ie, whether bilateral is only applicable on one level). Effective for 2023, guidelines and parenthetical notes have been added to provide clear definitions of "level" and appropriate reporting of various scenarios in which the procedures described by these codes are performed bilaterally.

Codes 64490-64495 describe injection/introduction of an agent into the paravertebral facet joint or nerves that innervate that joint, by level. The guidelines clarify that facet joints are paired, with one pair at each vertebral level. Multiple nerves of the same facet joint may be injected, and this would constitute injection of a single level. When multiple nerves that innervate a single facet joint are injected (ie, single level), then one unit is reported regardless of the number of nerves injected at that level. Codes 64491 and 64492 are add-on codes for the second and third and any additional cervical or thoracic vertebral levels injected and are reported with cervical or thoracic primary procedure code 64490. Similarly, codes 64494 and 64495 are add-on codes that are reported for the second and third and any additional lumbar or sacral vertebral levels injected and are reported with lumbar or sacral primary procedure code 64493.

Because facet joints are paired at each vertebral level, there is more than one possible bilateral injection procedure scenario. When reviewing a procedure report, it would be most useful to first determine the number of levels at which injections were performed and assign a code (eg, 64490 for the first level, 64491 for the second level). Next, determine if one facet joint or both facet joints at each level were injected. This will help in determining which vertebral levels were injected bilaterally, if any, for which the procedure code will need modifier 50 appended. For example, when injections are performed bilaterally at one vertebral level (ie, in both facet joints at that level), then one unit of the code is reported with modifier 50, *Bilateral Procedure*. In another

★ = Telemedicine ◀ = Audio-only + = Add-on code ⁄ = FDA approval pending # = Resequenced code ⊘ = Modifier 51 exempt

example, injections may be performed bilaterally at one vertebral level, and at the same session, another injection is performed unilaterally at a different vertebral level. In this scenario, a code is reported for each level that is injected, and modifier 50 would be appended to the code for the level at which the procedure was performed bilaterally. The new guidelines include a table that serves as a guide to reporting various scenarios in which multiple levels are injected and in which bilateral injections are performed.

Instructional parenthetical notes have been added that provide reporting instructions for unilateral and bilateral injection procedures performed at the T12-L1 and L1-L2 vertebral levels. The inclusionary parenthetical note following code 64494 has been revised to include code 64490.

Neurostimulators (Peripheral Nerve)

64566 Posterior tibial neurostimulation, percutaneous needle electrode, single treatment, includes programming

(Do not report 64566 in conjunction with 64555, 95970-95972)

▶(For peripheral nerve transcutaneous magnetic stimulation, see 0766T, 0767T, 0768T, 0769T)◀

Rationale

In accordance with the establishment of Category III codes 0766T-0769T, a cross-reference parenthetical note has been added following code 64566 to reflect these changes.

Refer to the codebook and the Rationale for codes 0766T-0769T for a full discussion of these changes.

Eye and Ocular Adnexa

Anterior Segment

Anterior Chamber

Incision

65850 Trabeculotomy ab externo

▶(Do not report 65850 in conjunction with 0730T)◀

▶(For trabeculotomy by laser, including optical coherence tomography [OCT] image guidance, use 0730T)◀

65855 Trabeculoplasty by laser surgery

▶(Do not report 65855 in conjunction with 65860, 65865, 65870, 65875, 65880, 0730T)◀

(For trabeculectomy, use 66170)

▶(For trabeculotomy by laser, including optical coherence tomography [OCT] image guidance, use 0730T)◀

Rationale

In accordance with the establishment of Category III code 0730T, parenthetical notes have been added and revised following codes 65850 and 65855.

Refer to the codebook and the Rationale for code 0730T for a full discussion of these changes.

Anterior Sclera

Excision

▲ **66174** Transluminal dilation of aqueous outflow canal (eg, canaloplasty); without retention of device or stent

(Do not report 66174 in conjunction with 65820)

▲ **66175** with retention of device or stent

Rationale

Codes 66174 and 66175 have been revised to include the example "canaloplasty" in parentheses. The codes have been revised to align with the FDA terminology for approved transluminal dilation of aqueous outflow canal service and provide clarification for coders, billers, payers, and physicians.

Auditory System

External Ear

Removal

69209 Removal impacted cerumen using irrigation/lavage, unilateral

(Do not report 69209 in conjunction with 69210 when performed on the same ear)

(For bilateral procedure, report 69209 with modifier 50)

(For removal of impacted cerumen requiring instrumentation, use 69210)

▶(For cerumen removal that is not impacted, see E/M service code, which may include new or established patient office or other outpatient services [99202-99215], hospital inpatient or observation care [99221-99223, 99231-99233], hospital inpatient or observation discharge day management [99238, 99239], consultations [99242, 99243, 99244, 99245, 99252, 99253, 99254, 99255], emergency department services [99281-99285], nursing facility services [99304-99316], home or residence services [99341-99350])◀

69210   Removal impacted cerumen requiring instrumentation, unilateral

(Do not report 69210 in conjunction with 69209 when performed on the same ear)

(For bilateral procedure, report 69210 with modifier 50)

(For removal of impacted cerumen achieved with irrigation and/or lavage but without instrumentation, use 69209)

▶(For cerumen removal that is not impacted, see E/M service code, which may include new or established patient office or other outpatient services [99202-99215], hospital inpatient or observation care [99221-99223, 99231-99233], hospital inpatient or observation discharge day management [99238, 99239], consultations [99242, 99243, 99244, 99245, 99252, 99253, 99254, 99255], emergency department services [99281-99285], nursing facility services [99304-99316], home or residence services [99341-99350])◀

Rationale

In accordance with the deletion of codes 99217-99220, 99224-99226, 99241, 99318, and 99324-99337, the cross-reference parenthetical notes following codes 69209 and 69210 have been revised to reflect these changes.

Refer to the codebook and the Rationale for codes 99217-99220, 99224-99226, 99241, 99318, and 99324-99337 for a full discussion of these changes.

Middle Ear

Osseointegrated Implants

▶The following codes are for implantation of an osseointegrated implant into the skull. These devices treat hearing loss through surgical placement of an abutment or device into the skull that facilitates transduction of acoustic energy to be received by the better-hearing inner ear or both inner ears when the implant is coupled to a speech processor and vibratory element. This coupling may occur in a percutaneous or a transcutaneous fashion. Other middle ear and mastoid procedures (69501-69676) may be performed for different indications and may be reported separately, when performed.◀

 # 69714   Implantation, osseointegrated implant, skull; with percutaneous attachment to external speech processor

(69715 has been deleted. To report mastoidectomy performed at the same operative session as osseointegrated implant placement, revision, replacement, or removal, see 69501-69676)

#▲ 69716   with magnetic transcutaneous attachment to external speech processor, within the mastoid and/or resulting in removal of less than 100 sq mm surface area of bone deep to the outer cranial cortex

#● 69729   with magnetic transcutaneous attachment to external speech processor, outside of the mastoid and resulting in removal of greater than or equal to 100 sq mm surface area of bone deep to the outer cranial cortex

#▲ 69717   Replacement (including removal of existing device), osseointegrated implant, skull; with percutaneous attachment to external speech processor

(69718 has been deleted. To report mastoidectomy performed at the same operative session as osseointegrated implant placement, revision, replacement, or removal, see 69501-69676)

#▲ 69719   with magnetic transcutaneous attachment to external speech processor, within the mastoid and/or involving a bony defect less than 100 sq mm surface area of bone deep to the outer cranial cortex

#● 69730   with magnetic transcutaneous attachment to external speech processor, outside the mastoid and involving a bony defect greater than or equal to 100 sq mm surface area of bone deep to the outer cranial cortex

#▲ 69726   Removal, entire osseointegrated implant, skull; with percutaneous attachment to external speech processor

▶(To report partial removal of the device [ie, abutment only], use appropriate evaluation and management code)◀

#▲ 69727   with magnetic transcutaneous attachment to external speech processor, within the mastoid and/or involving a bony defect less than 100 sq mm surface area of bone deep to the outer cranial cortex

#● 69728   with magnetic transcutaneous attachment to external speech processor, outside the mastoid and involving a bony defect greater than or equal to 100 sq mm surface area of bone deep to the outer cranial cortex

Rationale

Three codes have been added and five codes have been revised for osseointegrated implant procedures. In addition, the subsection guidelines have been revised and a parenthetical note added regarding these codes.

In CPT 2022, codes 69714-69719, 69726, and 69727 were added and revised for reporting implantation, revision/replacement, and removal of an osseointegrated implant in the skull. For CPT 2023, code 69716 has been revised and code 69729 has been established to clarify the intraservice work involved in osseointegrated implantations, differentiating within and outside the mastoid and between percutaneous (69714) and transcutaneous attachments. Codes that mirror the implantation codes also have been added and revised for replacement (69717, 69719, 69730) and removal (69726-69728) procedures.

In addition, the removal codes 69726-69728 have been revised to specify the removal of the entire osseointegrated implant. An instructional parenthetical note has been added following code 69726 indicating the use of an evaluation and management code when only a partial removal of the device (ie, abutment only) is performed.

Finally, the term "reparative" in reference to middle ear and mastoid procedure codes 69501-69676 has been deleted from the guidelines.

Clinical Example (69716)

A 48-year-old male with congenital left conductive hearing loss seeks intervention for improved quality of life at work and socially. A magnetic transcutaneous bone-anchored hearing device is placed behind the left ear.

Description of Procedure (69716)

Make an incision followed by a meticulous dissection through the pericranium. Perform a subpericranial dissection and create a subpericranial pocket for the implant coil and magnet. Then identify the area for the transducer using the template and mark on the outer table of the skull in the region of the sinodural angle. Then drill surgical guide and fixation holes taking care not to penetrate the sigmoid sinus or the dura overlying the temporal lobe of the brain. Measure this area for appropriate depth to accommodate the fixation screw.

Then drill the skull overlying the sinodural angle, less than 100 sq mm, to create a well in the bone to accommodate the transducer device, again staying just superficial to the dura and sigmoid sinus. Place the entire device, including the coil, magnet, and transducer portions. Fix the device to the skull using the fixation screw to a specific torque setting. Carefully measure the thickness of the flap overlying the magnet and coil portion of the device and precisely trim to a specific thickness to allow for transcutaneous transmission. Irrigate the wound and obtain hemostasis. Close the wound in a layered fashion.

Clinical Example (69717)

A 16-year-old female with chronic otitis media and conductive hearing loss who previously received a percutaneous bone-anchored implant has chronic inflammation at the abutment site, which has been unresponsive to medical therapy. The device is removed, and a new device placed at a different site.

Description of Procedure (69717)

Make an incision followed by a meticulous dissection to the pericranium. Perform a subpericranial dissection and remove the previous implant abutment. Drill the cranial bone surrounding the osseointegrated titanium fixture in the patient's skull around the implant. Remove the fixture. Thoroughly inspect the wound for the cause of the patient's original complication related to the implant. Identify, template, and mark the area for the new placement of the implant on the outer table of the skull. Perform a dissection and incise the pericranium and dissect away from the cranial bone to expose an area for implant placement. Drill a new pilot guide hole through the cranium and instrument the deep portion of the guide hole to ascertain the possible presence of dural contact and lack of sigmoid sinus exposure. Depending on this deep instrumentation, possibly deepen the pilot hole. Then widen the final guide hole with spiral drilling to achieve a larger opening to receive the implant. Install the implanted fixture in the cranial bone to very specific torque settings. Secure this implanted fixture to the transcutaneous abutment. Thin the overlying flap and surrounding soft tissues to a maximal thickness to allow for transcutaneous attachment to the processor. Make a separate incision in the overlying skin of the flap to allow the percutaneous abutment to extend through the soft tissue flap. Irrigate the wound and obtain hemostasis. Close the wound in layered fashion. Create a small bolster immediately surrounding the abutment and fix a locking cap to the abutment to keep the small abutment bolster in place and with appropriate pressure.

Clinical Example (69719)

A 59-year-old female with right conductive hearing loss previously had placement of a right magnetic transcutaneous bone-anchored hearing device that has malfunctioned. She undergoes removal and replacement of the device.

Description of Procedure (69719)

Make an incision followed by a meticulous dissection through the pericranium. Perform a subpericranial dissection and remove the previous implant. Thoroughly inspect the wound for the cause of the patient's original complication related to the implant. Create a subpericranial pocket for the implant coil and magnet. Identify area for the new placement of the transducer using the template and mark on the outer table of the skull. Then drill surgical guide and fixation holes, taking care not to penetrate the dura overlying the temporal lobe of the brain. Measure this area for appropriate depth to accommodate the fixation screw. Then drill the skull, less than 100 sq mm, to create a well in the bone to accommodate the transducer device, again staying just superficial to the dura. Place the entire device, including the coil, magnet, and transducer portions. Fix the device to the skull using the fixation screw to a specific torque setting. Carefully measure the thickness of the flap overlying the magnet and coil portion of the device and precisely trim to a specific thickness to allow for transcutaneous transmission. Irrigate the wound and obtain hemostasis. Close the wound in a layered fashion.

Clinical Example (69726)

A 48-year-old female with left single-sided deafness previously had placement of a percutaneous bone-anchored implant. It worked well but the patient has now developed discomfort at the device site. The device is removed in its entirety.

Description of Procedure (69726)

Make an incision followed by a meticulous dissection through the pericranium. Perform a subpericranial dissection and expose the previous implant. Drill around the cranial bone surrounding the osseointegrated titanium fixture in patient's skull to free the implant. Thoroughly inspect wound for cause of patient's original complication related to the implant. Irrigate the wound and obtain hemostasis. Debride and then close the wound where the external abutment of the implant occurs followed by closure of the linear incision anterior to the implant site in a layered fashion.

Clinical Example (69727)

A 62-year-old male with right mixed-hearing loss previously had a magnetic transcutaneous bone-anchored implant that had worked well but has now become infected. The device is removed.

Description of Procedure (69727)

Make an incision followed by a meticulous dissection through the pericranium. Perform a subpericranial dissection and expose the previous implant. Drill out the cranial bone surrounding the osseointegrated titanium transducer and the respective fixture screws in the patient's skull to free the implant. Thoroughly inspect the wound for the cause of patient's original complication related to the implant. Irrigate the wound and obtain hemostasis. Close the wound in layered fashion.

Clinical Example (69728)

A 52-year-old female with left mixed-hearing loss, whose previously placed magnetic transcutaneous bone-anchored implant in the retrosigmoid cranium that had worked well has become infected, is having the device removed.

Description of Procedure (69728)

Make an incision followed by a meticulous dissection through the pericranium. Perform a subpericranial dissection and expose the previous implant. Drill out the cranial bone surrounding the osseo-integrated titanium transducer and the respective fixture screws in the patient's skull to free the implant. Thoroughly inspect the wound for the cause of the patient's original complication related to the implant. Irrigate the wound and obtain hemostasis. Close the wound in layered fashion.

Clinical Example (69729)

A 59-year-old female with right mixed-hearing loss from chronic ear disease with history of surgical treatment seeks intervention for improved quality of life at work and socially. A magnetic transcutaneous bone-anchored hearing device is placed in the right retrosigmoid location because the right mastoid is contracted and inflamed.

Description of Procedure (69729)

Make an incision followed by meticulous dissection through the pericranium. Perform a subpericranial dissection and create a subpericranial pocket for the implant coil and magnet. Identify the area for the transducer using the template and mark on the outer table of the skull in the region of the sinodural angle. Then drill surgical guide and fixation holes taking care not to penetrate the sigmoid sinus or the dura overlying the temporal lobe of the brain. Measure this area for appropriate depth to accommodate the fixation screw. Then drill the skull overlying the sinodural angle, greater than or equal to 100 sq mm, to create a well in the bone to accommodate the transducer device, again staying just superficial to the dura and sigmoid sinus. Place the entire device, including the coil, magnet, and transducer portions. Fix the device to the skull using the fixation screw to a specific torque setting. Carefully measure the thickness of the flap overlying the magnet and coil portion of the device and precisely trim to a specific thickness to allow for transcutaneous transmission. Irrigate the wound and obtain hemostasis. Close the wound in layered fashion.

Clinical Example (69730)

A 49-year-old female with right mixed-hearing loss and history of right therapeutic mastoidectomy with tympanoplasty, whose previously placed magnetic transcutaneous bone-anchored hearing device in the right retrosigmoid region has malfunctioned, undergoes removal and replacement of the device.

Description of Procedure (69730)

Make an incision followed by a meticulous dissection through the pericranium. Perform a subpericranial dissection and remove the previous implant. Thoroughly inspect the wound for the cause of the patient's original complication related to the implant. Create a subpericranial pocket for the implant coil and magnet. Then identify the area for the new placement of the transducer using the template and mark on the outer table of the skull. Drill surgical guide and fixation holes taking care not to penetrate the dura overlying the temporal lobe of the brain. Measure this area for appropriate depth to accommodate the fixation screw. Then drill the skull, greater than or equal to 100 sq mm, to create a well in the bone to accommodate the transducer device, again staying just superficial to the dura. Place the entire device, including the coil, magnet, and transducer portions. Fix the device to the skull using the fixation screw to a specific torque setting. Carefully measure the thickness of the flap overlying the magnet and coil portion of the device and precisely trim to a specific thickness to allow for transcutaneous transmission. Irrigate the wound and obtain hemostasis. Close the wound in a layered fashion.

Other Procedures

69720   Decompression facial nerve, intratemporal; lateral to geniculate ganglion

69725   including medial to geniculate ganglion

69728   Code is out of numerical sequence. See 69670-69705

69729   Code is out of numerical sequence. See 69670-69705

69730   Code is out of numerical sequence. See 69670-69705

Inner Ear

Introduction

69930   Cochlear device implantation, with or without mastoidectomy

▶(For implantation of vestibular device, use 0725T)◀

Rationale

In accordance with the establishment of Category III code 0725T, a cross-reference parenthetical note directing users to the new code has been added following code 69930.

Refer to the codebook and the Rationale for code 0725T for a full discussion of this change.

Notes

Radiology

Summary of Additions, Deletions, and Revisions

The summary of changes shows the actual changes that have been made to the code descriptors.

New codes appear with a bullet (●) and are indicated as "Code added." Revised codes are preceded with a triangle (▲). Within revised codes, or if a code symbol has been deleted, the deleted language and code symbol appear with a ~~strikethrough~~, while new text appears <u>underlined</u>.

The ✗ symbol is used to identify codes for vaccines that are pending FDA approval. The # symbol is used to identify codes that have been resequenced. CPT add-on codes are annotated by the ✚ symbol. The ⊘ symbol is used to identify codes that are exempt from the use of modifier 51. The ★ symbol is used to identify codes that may be used for reporting telemedicine services. The ✕ symbol is used to identify a proprietary laboratory analyses (PLA) test that has an identical descriptor as another PLA test. A PLA code that satisfies Category I code criteria and has been accepted by the CPT Editorial Panel is annotated with the ↕ symbol. The ◀ symbol is used to identify codes that may be used to report audio-only telemedicine services when appended by modifier 93 **(see Appendix T)**.

Code	Description
▲76882	Ultrasound, limited, joint or <u>focal evaluation of </u>other nonvascular extremity structure(s) (eg, joint space, peri-articular tendon[s], muscle[s], nerve[s], other soft-tissue structure[s], or soft-tissue mass[es]), real-time with image documentation
●76883	Code added
▲78803	tomographic (SPECT), single area (eg, head, neck, chest, pelvis) <u>or acquisition</u>, single day imaging
#▲78830	tomographic (SPECT) with concurrently acquired computed tomography (CT) transmission scan for anatomical review, localization and determination/detection of pathology, single area (eg, head, neck, chest, pelvis) <u>or acquisition</u>, single day imaging
#▲78831	tomographic (SPECT), minimum 2 areas (eg, pelvis and knees, <u>chest and </u>abdomen ~~and pelvis~~) <u>or separate acquisitions (eg, lung ventilation and perfusion)</u>, single day imaging, or single area <u>or acquisition</u>~~imaging~~ over 2 or more days
#▲78832	tomographic (SPECT) with concurrently acquired computed tomography (CT) transmission scan for anatomical review, localization and determination/detection of pathology, minimum 2 areas (eg, pelvis and knees, <u>chest and </u>abdomen ~~and pelvis~~) <u>or separate acquisitions (eg, lung ventilation and perfusion)</u>, single day imaging, or single area <u>or acquisition</u>~~imaging~~ over 2 or more days

Radiology

Diagnostic Radiology (Diagnostic Imaging)

Vascular Procedures

Aorta and Arteries

75705 Angiography, spinal, selective, radiological supervision and interpretation

75710 Angiography, extremity, unilateral, radiological supervision and interpretation

▶(Do not report 75710 in conjunction with 36836, 36837)◀

75716 Angiography, extremity, bilateral, radiological supervision and interpretation

▶(Do not report 75716 in conjunction with 36836, 36837)◀

Rationale

In accordance with the establishment of codes 36836 and 36837, exclusionary parenthetical notes have been added following codes 75710 and 75716 to restrict reporting of these codes with codes 36836 and 36837.

Refer to the codebook and the Rationale for codes 36836 and 36837 for a full discussion of these changes.

75726 Angiography, visceral, selective or supraselective (with or without flush aortogram), radiological supervision and interpretation

(For selective angiography, each additional visceral vessel studied after basic examination, use 75774)

75743 Angiography, pulmonary, bilateral, selective, radiological supervision and interpretation

▶(For selective pulmonary arterial angiography during cardiac catheterization, see 93569, 93573)◀

▶(For selective pulmonary venous angiography during cardiac catheterization, each distinct vein, use 93574)◀

▶(For selective pulmonary angiography of major aortopulmonary collateral arteries [MAPCAs] arising off the aorta or its systemic branches, use 93575)◀

75746 Angiography, pulmonary, by nonselective catheter or venous injection, radiological supervision and interpretation

▶(For nonselective pulmonary arterial angiography by catheter injection performed at the time of cardiac catheterization, use 93568, which includes imaging supervision, interpretation, and report)◀

75756 Angiography, internal mammary, radiological supervision and interpretation

(For internal mammary angiography performed at the time of cardiac catheterization, see 93455, 93457, 93459, 93461, 93564, which include imaging supervision, interpretation, and report)

+ 75774 Angiography, selective, each additional vessel studied after basic examination, radiological supervision and interpretation (List separately in addition to code for primary procedure)

(Use 75774 in addition to code for specific initial vessel studied)

(Do not report 75774 as part of diagnostic angiography of the extracranial and intracranial cervicocerebral vessels. It may be appropriate to report 75774 for diagnostic angiography of upper extremities and other vascular beds performed in the same session)

(For angiography, see 75600-75756)

(For catheterizations, see codes 36215-36248)

▶(For cardiac catheterization procedures, see 93452-93462, 93563, 93564, 93565, 93566, 93567, 93568, 93569, 93573, 93574, 93575, 93593, 93594, 93595, 93596, 93597)◀

(For radiological supervision and interpretation of dialysis circuit angiography performed through existing access[es] or catheter-based arterial access, use 36901 with modifier 52)

Rationale

In accordance with the establishment of codes 93569-93575, parenthetical notes have been added and revised following codes 75743, 75746, and 75774 to reflect these changes.

Refer to the codebook and the Rationale for codes 93569-93575 for a full discussion of these changes.

Veins and Lymphatics

75810 Splenoportography, radiological supervision and interpretation

75820 Venography, extremity, unilateral, radiological supervision and interpretation

▶(Do not report 75820 in conjunction with 36836, 36837)◀

★ = Telemedicine   ◀ = Audio-only   ✚ = Add-on code   ⚕ = FDA approval pending   # = Resequenced code   ⊘ = Modifier 51 exempt

75822 Venography, extremity, bilateral, radiological supervision and interpretation

▶(Do not report 75822 in conjunction with 36836, 36837)◀

Rationale

In accordance with the establishment of codes 36836 and 36837, exclusionary parenthetical notes have been added following codes 75820 and 75822 to restrict reporting of these codes with codes 36836 and 36837.

Refer to the codebook and the Rationale for codes 36836 and 36837 for a full discussion of these changes.

75825 Venography, caval, inferior, with serialography, radiological supervision and interpretation

Transcatheter Procedures

Code 75958 includes the analogous services for placement of each proximal thoracic endovascular extension. Code 75959 includes the analogous services for placement of a distal thoracic endovascular extension(s) placed during a procedure after the primary repair.

75894 Transcatheter therapy, embolization, any method, radiological supervision and interpretation

▶(Do not report 75894 in conjunction with 36475, 36476, 36478, 36479, 36836, 36837, 37241, 37242, 37243, 37244)◀

Rationale

In accordance with the establishment of codes 36836 and 36837, the exclusionary parenthetical note following code 75894 has been revised with the addition of the new codes.

Refer to the codebook and the Rationale for codes 36836 and 36837 for a full discussion of these changes.

75898 Angiography through existing catheter for follow-up study for transcatheter therapy, embolization or infusion, other than for thrombolysis

▶(Do not report 75898 in conjunction with 36836, 36837, 37211, 37212, 37213, 37214, 37241, 37242, 37243, 37244, 61645, 61650, 61651)◀

(For thrombolysis infusion management other than coronary, see 37211-37214, 61645)

(For non-thrombolysis infusion management other than coronary, see 61650, 61651)

Rationale

In accordance with the establishment of codes 36836 and 36837, the exclusionary parenthetical note following code 75898 has been revised with the addition of the new codes.

Refer to the codebook and the Rationale for codes 36836 and 36837 for a full discussion of these changes.

75901 Mechanical removal of pericatheter obstructive material (eg, fibrin sheath) from central venous device via separate venous access, radiologic supervision and interpretation

75984 Change of percutaneous tube or drainage catheter with contrast monitoring (eg, genitourinary system, abscess), radiological supervision and interpretation

(For percutaneous replacement of gastrostomy, duodenostomy, jejunostomy, gastro-jejunostomy, or cecostomy [or other colonic] tube including fluoroscopic imaging guidance, see 49450-49452)

(To report exchange of a percutaneous nephrostomy catheter, use 50435)

(For percutaneous cholecystostomy, use 47490)

(For percutaneous biliary procedures, including radiological supervision and interpretation, see 47531-47544)

▶(For percutaneous nephrolithotomy or pyelolithotomy, see 50080, 50081)◀

(For removal and/or replacement of an internally dwelling ureteral stent via a transurethral approach, see 50385-50386)

Rationale

In accordance with the revision of codes 50080 and 50081, the cross-reference parenthetical note following code 75984 that directs users to codes 50080 and 50081 has been revised.

Refer to the codebook and the Rationale for codes 50080 and 50081 for a full discussion of these changes.

Diagnostic Ultrasound

Extremities

Code 76881 represents a complete evaluation of a specific joint in an extremity. Code 76881 requires ultrasound examination of all of the following joint elements: joint space (eg, effusion), peri-articular soft-tissue structures that surround the joint (ie, muscles, tendons, other soft-tissue structures), and any identifiable abnormality. In some circumstances, additional evaluations such as dynamic imaging or stress maneuvers may be performed as part of the complete evaluation. Code 76881 also requires permanently recorded images and a written report containing a description of each of the required elements or reason that an element(s) could not be visualized (eg, absent secondary to surgery or trauma).

When fewer than all of the required elements for a "complete" exam (76881) are performed, report the "limited" code (76882).

►Code 76882 represents a limited evaluation of a joint or focal evaluation of a structure(s) in an extremity other than a joint (eg, soft-tissue mass, fluid collection, or nerve[s]). Limited evaluation of a joint includes assessment of a specific anatomic structure(s) (eg, joint space only [effusion] or tendon, muscle, and/or other soft-tissue structure[s] that surround the joint) that does not assess all of the required elements included in 76881. Code 76882 also requires permanently recorded images and a written report containing a description of each of the elements evaluated.

Comprehensive evaluation of a nerve is defined as evaluation of the nerve throughout its course in an extremity. Documentation of the entire course of a nerve throughout an extremity includes the acquisition and permanent archive of cine clips and static images to demonstrate the anatomy.◄

For spectral and color Doppler evaluation of the extremities, use 93925, 93926, 93930, 93931, 93970, or 93971 as appropriate.

76881   Ultrasound, complete joint (ie, joint space and peri-articular soft-tissue structures), real-time with image documentation

▲ **76882**   Ultrasound, limited, joint or focal evaluation of other nonvascular extremity structure(s) (eg, joint space, peri-articular tendon[s], muscle[s], nerve[s], other soft-tissue structure[s], or soft-tissue mass[es]), real-time with image documentation

     ►(Do not report 76882 in conjunction with 76883)◄

● **76883**   Ultrasound, nerve(s) and accompanying structures throughout their entire anatomic course in one extremity, comprehensive, including real-time cine imaging with image documentation, per extremity

Rationale

Diagnostic ultrasound code 76882 has been revised. Code 76883 has been established to report ultrasound of nerve(s) and accompanying structures in one extremity. The Diagnostic Ultrasound/Extremities subsection guidelines have been revised and an exclusionary note following code 76882 has been added.

Prior to 2023, code 76882 described limited ultrasound of a joint or other nonvascular extremity structure and was intended to describe a focal evaluation (ie, evaluation of a specific location on or around a specific structure, such as a cyst) of structures in the extremity such as a joint space or nerve. Within the extremities, there are nerves that pass through more than one structure. For example, the median nerve transverses the wrist, elbow, and shoulder joints. In certain circumstances, an ultrasound of a nerve throughout its entire anatomic course in the extremity is necessary (eg, for non-localized neuropathy in the extremity). This is a comprehensive ultrasound evaluation of the nerve in the extremity. Code 76882 is not intended to describe this type of ultrasound evaluation.

Effective in 2023, code 76883 has been established to report comprehensive diagnostic ultrasound of nerves and accompanying structures throughout their entire course in one extremity. To clarify the distinction between limited ultrasound of nerves described in code 76882 and ultrasound of a nerve's entire anatomic course described in code 76883, code 76882 has been revised with the addition of the term "focal evaluation." An exclusionary parenthetical note has been added restricting the use of code 76882 with code 76883. The Diagnostic Ultrasound/Extremities subsection guidelines have been revised to clarify that code 76882 includes a focal evaluation of a structure(s) and to define comprehensive evaluation of a nerve in an extremity.

Clinical Example (76882)

A 36-year-old male presents with an acute injury to his Achilles tendon, sustained while playing soccer. No open wounds are noted. X rays are negative for osseous pathology. Mild erythema and edema are noted at the posterior lower leg. Ultrasound is performed to evaluate the Achilles tendon.

Description of Procedure (76882)

Supervise the sonographer performing the examination, as well as personally scan the patient to perform dynamic maneuvers and/or confirm the sonographer's impression as needed. This includes obtaining images in multiple planes through the specific area of concern (ie, Achilles tendon) and evaluating for abnormalities of a specific structure or any pathology in the area. Document normal anatomic structure and assess any pathologic

★=Telemedicine   ◀=Audio-only   ✛=Add-on code   ⁄=FDA approval pending   #=Resequenced code   ⊘=Modifier 51 exempt

findings including evidence of tendinosis, tendon tear, or paratenonitis. Perform measurements of tendon thinning and tear separation to assist in determining patient management options. Compare to the contralateral side as needed. Dictate a report for the patient's chart.

Clinical Example (76883)

A 45-year-old female presents with progressive atrophy and weakness of the intrinsic muscles on the left hand associated with altered sensation on the medial aspect of the hand. An ultrasound of the left ulnar nerve and accompanying structures is ordered to assess for a disorder involving the ulnar nerve.

Description of Procedure (76883)

Perform a focused H&P, position patient for procedure, and instruct the patient to report any pain or paresthesia felt during the examination from the ultrasound probe, which may reflect nerve entrapment. Use a high-frequency linear transducer and identify the nerve of interest first distally, inspecting the nerve itself and any pertinent surrounding structures, such as a ganglion cyst, anomalous muscle, bone spur, or tenosynovitis. Then follow the nerve proximally, throughout the entire length of the limb, making measurements of cross-sectional area and quantifying vascularity, mobility, and echogenicity of the nerve at potential sites of entrapment, as well as taking long axis views to evaluate for changes in morphology. For the ulnar nerve, this would include Guyon's canal in the wrist, the cubital tunnel distal to the elbow, the retrocondylar groove at the elbow, the upper arm (ligament of Struthers), and the axilla. At areas of enlargement, assess the underlying joint for osteophytes or effusions and examine the affected muscles for signs of denervation (in the case of the ulnar nerve, atrophy and increased echogenicity of the first dorsal interosseous, abductor digiti minimi, flexor digitorum profundus, and flexor carpi ulnaris muscles), with comparison to unaffected muscles as clinically indicated. Compare suspected abnormalities to the contralateral side. Record cine loops of any identified areas of entrapment or pathology. Dictate a report for the patient's chart.

Ultrasonic Guidance Procedures

76936 Ultrasound guided compression repair of arterial pseudoaneurysm or arteriovenous fistulae (includes diagnostic ultrasound evaluation, compression of lesion and imaging)

+ 76937 Ultrasound guidance for vascular access requiring ultrasound evaluation of potential access sites, documentation of selected vessel patency, concurrent realtime ultrasound visualization of vascular needle entry, with permanent recording and reporting (List separately in addition to code for primary procedure)

▶(Do not report 76937 in conjunction with 33274, 33275, 36568, 36569, 36572, 36573, 36584, 36836, 36837, 37191, 37192, 37193, 37760, 37761, 76942)◀

(Do not report 76937 in conjunction with 0505T, 0620T for ultrasound guidance for vascular access)

(If extremity venous non-invasive vascular diagnostic study is performed separate from venous access guidance, see 93970, 93971)

Rationale

In accordance with the establishment of codes 36836 and 36837, the exclusionary parenthetical note following code 76937 has been revised with the addition of the new codes.

Refer to the codebook and the Rationale for codes 36836 and 36837 for a full discussion of these changes.

76940 Ultrasound guidance for, and monitoring of, parenchymal tissue ablation

(Do not report 76940 in conjunction with 20982, 20983, 32994, 32998, 50250, 50542, 76942, 76998, 0582T, 0600T, 0601T)

(For ablation, see 47370-47382, 47383, 50592, 50593)

76942 Ultrasonic guidance for needle placement (eg, biopsy, aspiration, injection, localization device), imaging supervision and interpretation

▶(Do not report 76942 in conjunction with 10004, 10005, 10006, 10021, 10030, 19083, 19285, 20604, 20606, 20611, 27096, 32408, 32554, 32555, 32556, 32557, 37760, 37761, 43232, 43237, 43242, 45341, 45342, 46948, 55874, 64415, 64416, 64417, 64445, 64446, 64447, 64448, 64479, 64480, 64483, 64484, 64490, 64491, 64493, 64494, 64495, 76975, 0213T, 0214T, 0215T, 0216T, 0217T, 0218T, 0232T, 0481T, 0582T)◀

(For harvesting, preparation, and injection[s] of platelet rich plasma, use 0232T)

Rationale

In accordance with the revisions to codes 64415-64418 and 64445-64448, the exclusionary parenthetical note following code 76942 has been revised to preclude its use with codes 64415-64417 and 64445-64448.

Refer to the codebook and the Rationale for codes 64415-64418 and 64445-64448 for a full discussion of these changes.

Radiologic Guidance

Fluoroscopic Guidance

(Do not report guidance codes 77001, 77002, 77003 for services in which fluoroscopic guidance is included in the descriptor)

+ 77001 Fluoroscopic guidance for central venous access device placement, replacement (catheter only or complete), or removal (includes fluoroscopic guidance for vascular access and catheter manipulation, any necessary contrast injections through access site or catheter with related venography radiologic supervision and interpretation, and radiographic documentation of final catheter position) (List separately in addition to code for primary procedure)

▶(Do not report 77001 in conjunction with 33957, 33958, 33959, 33962, 33963, 33964, 36568, 36569, 36572, 36573, 36584, 36836, 36837, 77002)◀

(If formal extremity venography is performed from separate venous access and separately interpreted, use 36005 and 75820, 75822, 75825, or 75827)

Rationale

In accordance with the establishment of codes 36836 and 36837, the exclusionary parenthetical note following code 77001 has been revised with the addition of the new codes.

Refer to the codebook and the Rationale for codes 36836 and 36837 for a full discussion of these changes.

+ 77002 Fluoroscopic guidance for needle placement (eg, biopsy, aspiration, injection, localization device) (List separately in addition to code for primary procedure)

▶(Use 77002 in conjunction with 10160, 20206, 20220, 20225, 20520, 20525, 20526, 20550, 20551, 20552, 20553, 20555, 20600, 20605, 20610, 20612, 20615, 21116, 21550, 23350, 24220, 25246, 27093, 27095, 27369, 27648, 32400, 32553, 36002, 38220, 38221, 38222, 38505, 38794, 41019, 42400, 42405, 47000, 47001, 48102, 49180, 49411, 50200, 50390, 51100, 51101, 51102, 55700, 55876, 60100, 62268, 62269, 64400, 64405, 64408, 64418, 64420, 64421, 64425, 64430, 64435, 64450, 64455, 64505, 64600, 64605)◀

(77002 is included in all arthrography radiological supervision and interpretation codes. See **Administration of Contrast Material[s]** introductory guidelines for reporting of arthrography procedures)

Rationale

In accordance with the revisions to codes 64415-64418 and 64445-64448, the inclusionary parenthetical note following code 77002 has been revised by removing the code range 64400-64448 and specifically indicating its use with codes 64400, 64405, 64408, 64418, 64420, 64421, 64425, 64430, and 64435.

Refer to the codebook and the Rationale for codes 64415-64418 and 64445-64448 for a full discussion of these changes.

+ 77003 Fluoroscopic guidance and localization of needle or catheter tip for spine or paraspinous diagnostic or therapeutic injection procedures (epidural or subarachnoid) (List separately in addition to code for primary procedure)

(Use 77003 in conjunction with 61050, 61055, 62267, 62273, 62280, 62281, 62282, 62284, 64449, 64510, 64517, 64520, 64610, 96450)

▶(Do not report 77003 in conjunction with 62270, 62272, 62320, 62321, 62322, 62323, 62324, 62325, 62326, 62327, 62328, 62329, 64415, 64416, 64417, 64445, 64446, 64447, 64448, 0627T, 0628T)◀

Rationale

In accordance with the revisions to codes 64415-64417 and 64445-64448, an exclusionary parenthetical note following code 77003 has been revised to preclude its use with codes 64415-64417 and 64445-64448.

Refer to the codebook and the Rationale for codes 64415-64417 and 64445-64448 for a full discussion of these changes.

Radiation Oncology

Hyperthermia

Hyperthermia treatments as listed in this section include external (superficial and deep), interstitial, and intracavitary.

Radiation therapy when given concurrently is listed separately.

★ = Telemedicine   ◀ = Audio-only   + = Add-on code   ✚ = FDA approval pending   # = Resequenced code   ⊘ = Modifier 51 exempt

Hyperthermia is used only as an adjunct to radiation therapy or chemotherapy. It may be induced by a variety of sources (eg, microwave, ultrasound, low energy radio-frequency conduction, or by probes).

The listed treatments include management during the course of therapy and follow-up care for three months after completion.

▶Preliminary consultation is not included (see **evaluation and management** services).◀

Physics planning and interstitial insertion of temperature sensors, and use of external or interstitial heat generating sources are included.

Rationale

In accordance with the changes to evaluation and management consultation codes 99241-99255, the instructional parenthetical note regarding preliminary consultation in the Hyperthermia subsection has been revised to reflect these changes.

Refer to the codebook and the Rationale for codes 99241-99255 for a full discussion of these changes.

Nuclear Medicine

Diagnostic

Cardiovascular System

78451   Myocardial perfusion imaging, tomographic (SPECT) (including attenuation correction, qualitative or quantitative wall motion, ejection fraction by first pass or gated technique, additional quantification, when performed); single study, at rest or stress (exercise or pharmacologic)

(Do not report 78451 in conjunction with 78800, 78801, 78802, 78803, 78804, 78830, 78831, 78832, 78835)

▶(For absolute quantification of myocardial blood flow [AQMBF] with single-photon emission computed tomography [SPECT], use 0742T)◀

78452   multiple studies, at rest and/or stress (exercise or pharmacologic) and/or redistribution and/or rest reinjection

(Do not report 78452 in conjunction with 78800, 78801, 78802, 78803, 78804, 78830, 78831, 78832, 78835)

▶(For absolute quantification of myocardial blood flow [AQMBF] with single-photon emission computed tomography [SPECT], use 0742T)◀

#+ 78434   Absolute quantitation of myocardial blood flow (AQMBF), positron emission tomography (PET), rest and pharmacologic stress (List separately in addition to code for primary procedure)

(Use 78434 in conjunction with 78431, 78492)

(For CT coronary calcium scoring, use 75571)

(For myocardial imaging by planar or SPECT, see 78451, 78452, 78453, 78454)

▶(For absolute quantification of myocardial blood flow [AQMBF] with single-photon emission computed tomography [SPECT], use 0742T)◀

Rationale

In accordance with the establishment of Category III code 0742T, cross-reference parenthetical notes directing users to the new code have been added following codes 78451, 78452, and 78434.

Refer to the codebook and the Rationale for code 0742T for a full discussion of this change.

Other Procedures

(For specific organ, see appropriate heading)

78800   Radiopharmaceutical localization of tumor, inflammatory process or distribution of radiopharmaceutical agent(s) (includes vascular flow and blood pool imaging, when performed); planar, single area (eg, head, neck, chest, pelvis), single day imaging

(For specific organ, see appropriate heading)

78801   planar, 2 or more areas (eg, abdomen and pelvis, head and chest), 1 or more days imaging or single area imaging over 2 or more days

78802   planar, whole body, single day imaging

 # 78804   planar, whole body, requiring 2 or more days imaging

▲ 78803   tomographic (SPECT), single area (eg, head, neck, chest, pelvis) or acquisition, single day imaging

78804   Code is out of numerical sequence. See 78801-78811

(For imaging bone infectious or inflammatory disease with a bone imaging radiopharmaceutical, see 78300, 78305, 78306, 78315)

#▲ 78830   tomographic (SPECT) with concurrently acquired computed tomography (CT) transmission scan for anatomical review, localization and determination/detection of pathology, single area (eg, head, neck, chest, pelvis) or acquisition, single day imaging

#▲ **78831**   tomographic (SPECT), minimum 2 areas (eg, pelvis and knees, chest and abdomen) or separate acquisitions (eg, lung ventilation and perfusion), single day imaging, or single area or acquisition over 2 or more days

#▲ **78832**   tomographic (SPECT) with concurrently acquired computed tomography (CT) transmission scan for anatomical review, localization and determination/detection of pathology, minimum 2 areas (eg, pelvis and knees, chest and abdomen) or separate acquisitions (eg, lung ventilation and perfusion), single day imaging, or single area or acquisition over 2 or more days

(For cerebrospinal fluid studies that require injection procedure, see 61055, 61070, 62320, 62321, 62322, 62323)

Rationale

Codes 78803 and 78830-78832 have been editorially revised to further clarify the intended use of these codes to differentiate when a single area or single acquisition is examined vs when two or more separate acquisitions with two radiopharmaceuticals are performed on the same date of service or over two or more days. The intent and use of these codes remain the same.

The codes included for this section have been revised to differentiate: (1) the area(s) and acquisition provided for the procedure(s) and (2) whether or not an acquired computed tomography transmission scan was completed for the anatomical review. The differentiation includes addition of the term "or acquisition" to all four codes and "separate acquisitions" to codes 78831 and 78832. Previously, these codes did not differentiate according to acquisition—only according to the anatomic area observed and/or according to single or multiple days used for the procedures. Adding the term "acquisition" to each of the codes allows for more specific reporting (ie, according to area or acquisitions performed). For example, two different acquisitions performed for the same area on the same day (such as a lung ventilation—the study to identify the flow of air through the lung tubes—vs a lung perfusion imaging—that examines the infiltration of oxygen into the lung tissues) necessitates a mechanism of reporting that allows for differentiation for multiple acquisitions performed on the same anatomical area on the same day at different times using different tracers. By adding the term "separate acquisition" within the descriptors for codes 78831 and 78832, users are provided a way to identify not only studies of different areas or studies of the same area performed on different days but also studies in which the acquisitions are separate and distinct even though they may be provided for the same anatomic location and on the same day.

As a result, codes 78803 and 78830-78832 have been editorially revised by adding the term "or acquisition" to clarify that acquisition may be performed for any of these codes. Addition of this term to codes 78803 and 78830 allows users to report when a single area (eg, pelvis and knees, chest and abdomen) is examined/imaged on a single day or when a single acquisition is performed. (**Note:** A "single area" is inherently understood to be performed using a single acquisition of images). If a "*concurrently acquired computed tomography (CT) transmission scan for anatomical review, localization and determination/detection of pathology*" is also performed, then code 78830 should be reported.

Addition of the term "separate acquisition" to codes 78831 and 78832 clarifies that multiple acquisitions may be reported when separate anatomic areas are examined or when a singular anatomic area is examined twice with a different tracer on the same day. Similar to code 78830, if a "*concurrently acquired computed tomography (CT) transmission scan for anatomical review, localization and determination/detection of pathology*" is also performed, then code 78832 should be reported.

Examples of the anatomic areas have also been included or moved within each of the codes to help users understand the locations for which these procedures may be performed. For codes 78831 and 78832, the phrase "(eg, lung ventilation and perfusion)" has been added within each code descriptor along with the term "or acquisition."

★ = Telemedicine   ◀ = Audio-only   ✛ = Add-on code   ✒ = FDA approval pending   # = Resequenced code   ⊘ = Modifier 51 exempt

Pathology and Laboratory

Summary of Additions, Deletions, and Revisions

The summary of changes shows the actual changes that have been made to the code descriptors.

New codes appear with a bullet (●) and are indicated as "Code added." Revised codes are preceded with a triangle (▲). Within revised codes, or if a code symbol has been deleted, the deleted language and code symbol appear with a ~~strikethrough~~, while new text appears <u>underlined</u>.

The ⚡ symbol is used to identify codes for vaccines that are pending FDA approval. The # symbol is used to identify codes that have been resequenced. CPT add-on codes are annotated by the ✚ symbol. The ⊘ symbol is used to identify codes that are exempt from the use of modifier 51. The ★ symbol is used to identify codes that may be used for reporting telemedicine services. The ✂ symbol is used to identify a proprietary laboratory analyses (PLA) test that has an identical descriptor as another PLA test. A PLA code that satisfies Category I code criteria and has been accepted by the CPT Editorial Panel is annotated with the ↕ symbol. The ◀ symbol is used to identify codes that may be used to report audio-only telemedicine services when appended by modifier 93 **(see Appendix T)**.

Code	Description
#●81418	Code added
#●81441	Code added
▲81445	Targeted genomic sequence analysis panel, solid organ neoplasm~~, DNA analysis, and RNA analysis when performed~~, 5-50 genes (eg, *ALK, BRAF, CDKN2A, EGFR, ERBB2, KIT, KRAS, MET, NRAS, PDGFRA, PDGFRB, PGR, PIK3CA, PTEN, RET*), interrogation for sequence variants and copy number variants or rearrangements, if performed; <u>DNA analysis or combined DNA and RNA analysis</u>
●81449	Code added
▲81450	Targeted genomic sequence analysis panel, hematolymphoid neoplasm or disorder~~, DNA analysis, and RNA analysis when performed~~, 5-50 genes (eg, *BRAF, CEBPA, DNMT3A, EZH2, FLT3, IDH1, IDH2, JAK2, KIT, KRAS, MLL, NOTCH1, NPM1, NRAS*), interrogation for sequence variants, and copy number variants or rearrangements, or isoform expression or mRNA expression levels, if performed; <u>DNA analysis or combined DNA and RNA analysis</u>
●81451	Code added
▲81455	Targeted genomic sequence analysis panel, solid organ or hematolymphoid neoplasm <u>or disorder</u>, ~~DNA analysis, and RNA analysis when performed,~~ 51 or greater genes (eg, *ALK, BRAF, CDKN2A, CEBPA, DNMT3A, EGFR, ERBB2, EZH2, FLT3, IDH1, IDH2, JAK2, KIT, KRAS, MET, MLL, NOTCH1, NPM1, NRAS, PDGFRA, PDGFRB, PGR, PIK3CA, PTEN, RET*), interrogation for sequence variants and copy number variants or rearrangements, <u>or isoform expression or mRNA expression levels,</u> if performed; <u>DNA analysis or combined DNA and RNA analysis</u>
●81456	Code added
#●84433	Code added
●87467	Code added
●87468	Code added
●87469	Code added
●87478	Code added
#●87484	Code added

▲=Revised code ●=New code ▶◀=Contains new or revised text ✂=Duplicate PLA test ↕=Category I PLA

Code	Description
#●87913	Code added
~~0012U~~	~~Germline disorders, gene rearrangement detection by whole genome next-generation sequencing, DNA, whole blood, report of specific gene rearrangement(s)~~
~~0013U~~	~~Oncology (solid organ neoplasia), gene rearrangement detection by whole genome next-generation sequencing, DNA, fresh or frozen tissue or cells, report of specific gene rearrangement(s)~~
~~0014U~~	~~Hematology (hematolymphoid neoplasia), gene rearrangement detection by whole genome next-generation sequencing, DNA, whole blood or bone marrow, report of specific gene rearrangement(s)~~
▲0022U	Targeted genomic sequence analysis panel, <u>cholangiocarcinoma and </u>non-small cell lung neoplasia, DNA and RNA analysis, <u>1-</u>23 genes, interrogation for sequence variants and rearrangements, reported as presence/absence of variants and associated therapy(ies) to consider
~~0056U~~	~~Hematology (acute myelogenous leukemia), DNA, whole genome next-generation sequencing to detect gene rearrangement(s), blood or bone marrow, report of specific gene rearrangement(s)~~
▲0090U	Oncology (cutaneous melanoma), mRNA gene expression profiling by RT-PCR of 23 genes (14 content and 9 housekeeping), utilizing formalin-fixed paraffin-embedded <u>(FFPE)</u> tissue, algorithm reported as a categorical result (ie, benign, <u>intermediate</u>~~indeterminate~~, malignant)
~~0097U~~	~~Gastrointestinal pathogen, multiplex reverse transcription and multiplex amplified probe technique, multiple types or subtypes, 22 targets (Campylobacter [C. jejuni/C. coli/C. upsaliensis], Clostridium difficile [C. difficile] toxin A/B, Plesiomonas shigelloides, Salmonella, Vibrio [V. parahaemolyticus/V. vulnificus/V. cholerae], including specific identification of Vibrio cholerae, Yersinia enterocolitica, Enteroaggregative Escherichia coli [EAEC], Enteropathogenic Escherichia coli [EPEC], Enterotoxigenic Escherichia coli [ETEC] lt/st, Shiga-like toxin-producing Escherichia coli [STEC] stx1/stx2 [including specific identification of the E. coli O157 serogroup within STEC], Shigella/Enteroinvasive Escherichia coli [EIEC], Cryptosporidium, Cyclospora cayetanensis, Entamoeba histolytica, Giardia lamblia [also known as G. intestinalis and G. duodenalis], adenovirus F 40/41, astrovirus, norovirus GI/GII, rotavirus A, sapovirus [Genogroups I, II, IV, and V])~~
~~0151U~~	~~Infectious disease (bacterial or viral respiratory tract infection), pathogen specific nucleic acid (DNA or RNA), 33 targets, real-time semi-quantitative PCR, bronchoalveolar lavage, sputum, or endotracheal aspirate, detection of 33 organismal and antibiotic resistance genes with limited semi-quantitative results~~
~~0208U~~	~~Oncology (medullary thyroid carcinoma), mRNA, gene expression analysis of 108 genes, utilizing fine needle aspirate, algorithm reported as positive or negative for medullary thyroid carcinoma~~
▲0229U	*BCAT1 (Branched chain amino acid transaminase 1)* ~~or~~ <u>and</u> *IKZF1 (IKAROS family zinc finger 1)* (eg, colorectal cancer) promoter methylation analysis
▲0276U	Hematology (inherited thrombocytopenia), genomic sequence analysis of ~~23~~ <u>42</u> genes, blood, buccal swab, or amniotic fluid
●0285U	Code added
●0286U	Code added
●0287U	Code added
●0288U	Code added
●0289U	Code added
●0290U	Code added
●0291U	Code added
●0292U	Code added
●0293U	Code added

★ = Telemedicine　◀ = Audio-only　✚ = Add-on code　✗ = FDA approval pending　# = Resequenced code　⊘ = Modifier 51 exempt

Code	Description
●0294U	Code added
●0295U	Code added
●0296U	Code added
●0297U	Code added
●0298U	Code added
●0299U	Code added
●0300U	Code added
●0301U	Code added
●0302U	Code added
●0303U	Code added
●0304U	Code added
●0305U	Code added
●0306U	Code added
●0307U	Code added
●0308U	Code added
●0309U	Code added
●0310U	Code added
●0311U	Code added
●0312U	Code added
●0313U	Code added
●0314U	Code added
●0315U	Code added
●0316U	Code added
●0317U	Code added
●0318U	Code added
●0319U	Code added
●0320U	Code added
●0321U	Code added
●0322U	Code added
●0323U	Code added
●0324U	Code added
●0325U	Code added
●0326U	Code added

Code	Description
●0327U	Code added
●0328U	Code added
●0329U	Code added
●0330U	Code added
●0331U	Code added
●0332U	Code added
●0333U	Code added
●0334U	Code added
●0335U	Code added
●0336U	Code added
●0337U	Code added
●0338U	Code added
●0339U	Code added
●0340U	Code added
●0341U	Code added
●0342U	Code added
●0343U	Code added
●0344U	Code added
●0345U	Code added
●0346U	Code added
●0347U	Code added
●0348U	Code added
●0349U	Code added
●0350U	Code added
●0351U	Code added
●0352U	Code added
●0353U	Code added
●0354U	Code added

★=Telemedicine ◀=Audio-only ✚=Add-on code ✔=FDA approval pending #=Resequenced code ⊘=Modifier 51 exempt

Pathology and Laboratory

Pathology Clinical Consultations

80503 Pathology clinical consultation; for a clinical problem, with limited review of patient's history and medical records and straightforward medical decision making

When using time for code selection, 5-20 minutes of total time is spent on the date of the consultation.

▶(For consultations involving the examination and evaluation of the patient, see evaluation and management services)◀

80504 for a moderately complex clinical problem, with review of patient's history and medical records and moderate level of medical decision making

When using time for code selection, 21-40 minutes of total time is spent on the date of the consultation.

80505 for a highly complex clinical problem, with comprehensive review of patient's history and medical records and high level of medical decision making

When using time for code selection, 41-60 minutes of total time is spent on the date of the consultation.

+ 80506 prolonged service, each additional 30 minutes (List separately in addition to code for primary procedure)

(Use 80506 in conjunction with 80505)

(Do not report 80503, 80504, 80505, 80506 in conjunction with 88321, 88323, 88325)

(Prolonged pathology clinical consultation service of less than 15 additional minutes is not reported separately)

▶(For consultations involving the examination and evaluation of the patient, see evaluation and management services)◀

Rationale

In accordance with the changes to the evaluation and management consultation codes 99241-99255, the cross-reference parenthetical notes following codes 80503 and 80506 have been revised to reflect these changes.

Refer to the codebook and the Rationale for codes 99241-99255 for a full discussion of these changes.

Genomic Sequencing Procedures and Other Molecular Multianalyte Assays

▶Genomic sequencing procedures (GSPs) and other molecular multianalyte assays GSPs are DNA or RNA sequence analysis methods that simultaneously assay multiple genes or genetic regions relevant to a clinical situation. They may target specific combinations of genes or genetic material, or assay the exome or genome. The technology typically used for genomic sequencing is referred to as next generation sequencing (NGS) or massively parallel sequencing (MPS) although other technologies may be employed. GSPs are performed on nucleic acids from germline or neoplastic samples. Examples of applications include aneuploidy analysis of cell-free circulating fetal DNA, gene panels for somatic alterations in neoplasms, and sequence analysis of the exome or genome to determine the cause of developmental delay. The exome and genome procedures are designed to evaluate the genetic material in totality or near totality. Although commonly used to identify sequence (base) changes, they can also be used to identify copy number, structural changes, and abnormal zygosity patterns which may be performed in combination or may require separately performed methods and analyses. Another unique feature of GSPs is the ability to "re-query" or re-evaluate the sequence data (eg, complex phenotype such as developmental delay is reassessed when new genetic knowledge is attained, or for a separate unrelated clinical indication). The analyses listed below represent groups of genes that are often performed by GSPs; however, the analyses may also be performed by other molecular techniques (eg, polymerase chain reaction [PCR] methods and microarrays). These codes should be used when the components of the descriptor(s) are fulfilled regardless of the technique used to provide the analysis, unless specifically noted in the code descriptor. When a GSP assay includes gene(s) that is listed in more than one code descriptor, the code for the most specific test for the primary disorder sought should be reported, rather than reporting multiple codes for the same gene(s). When all of the components of the descriptor are not performed, use individual Tier 1 codes, Tier 2 codes, or 81479 (Unlisted molecular pathology procedure).

Testing for somatic alterations in neoplasms may be reported differently based on whether combined methods and analyses are used for both DNA and RNA analytes, or if separate methods and analyses are used for each analyte (DNA analysis only, RNA analysis only). For targeted genomic sequence DNA analysis or DNA and RNA analysis using a single combined method, report

81445, 81450, or 81455. For targeted genomic sequence RNA analysis when performed using a separate method, report 81449, 81451, 81456. For targeted genomic sequence DNA analysis and RNA analysis performed separately rather than via a combined method, report 81445, 81450, or 81455 for the DNA analysis and report 81449, 81451, or 81456 for the RNA analysis. ◄

Low-pass sequencing: a method of genome sequencing intended for cytogenomic analysis of chromosomal abnormalities, such as that performed for trait mapping or copy number variation, typically performed to an average depth of sequencing ranging from 0.1 to 5X.

The assays in this section represent discrete genetic values, properties, or characteristics in which the measurement or analysis of each analyte is potentially of independent medical significance or useful in medical management. In contrast to multianalyte assays with algorithmic analyses (MAAAs), the assays in this section do not represent algorithmically combined results to obtain a risk score or other value, which in itself represents a new and distinct medical property that is of independent medical significance relative to the individual, component test results.

81413   Cardiac ion channelopathies (eg, Brugada syndrome, long QT syndrome, short QT syndrome, catecholaminergic polymorphic ventricular tachycardia); genomic sequence analysis panel, must include sequencing of at least 10 genes, including *ANK2, CASQ2, CAV3, KCNE1, KCNE2, KCNH2, KCNJ2, KCNQ1, RYR2,* and *SCN5A*

81414   duplication/deletion gene analysis panel, must include analysis of at least 2 genes, including KCNH2 and KCNQ1

(For genomic sequencing panel testing for cardiomyopathies, use 81439)

(Do not report 81413, 81414 in conjunction with 81439 when performed on the same date of service)

#● 81418   Drug metabolism (eg, pharmacogenomics) genomic sequence analysis panel, must include testing of at least 6 genes, including *CYP2C19, CYP2D6,* and *CYP2D6* duplication/deletion analysis

Rationale

New code 81418 has been added to the Genomic Sequencing Procedures and Other Molecular Multianalyte Assays subsection to report a drug metabolism (eg, pharmacogenomics) genomic sequence analysis panel.

The genomic sequencing procedures (GSP) subsection includes analyses of genes that are relevant to specific clinical conditions (eg, aortic dysfunction or dilation, hereditary breast cancer–related disorders). The GSP codes include, but are not limited to, specific genes or types of genes in the analysis. Code 81418 is distinct from

other GSP codes because this is a drug metabolism (eg, pharmacogenomics) genomic sequence analysis panel.

Prior to the addition of code 81418, there was no specific code to report a drug metabolism (eg, pharmacogenomics) genomic sequence analysis panel. In order to report code 81418, at least 6 genes, including CYP2C19 and CYP2D6, must be sequenced, and CYP2D6 duplication/deletion (copy number variation) analysis must be performed.

Clinical Example (81418)

A 66-year-old male diagnosed with colon cancer presents to his physician with disorientation and confusion after taking a tricyclic antidepressant. A peripheral blood sample is submitted for pharmacogenetic panel testing.

Description of Procedure (81418)

Isolate high-quality genomic DNA from whole blood and subject to hydrolysis probe technique to detect common variants in CYPC19, CYP2D6, CYP2C9, CYP2B6, CYP3A4, and CYP3A5 and duplications and deletions in CYP2D6. The pathologist or other qualified health care professional (QHP) analyzes the data and composes a report.

81418   Code is out of numerical sequence. See 81414-81416

81439   Hereditary cardiomyopathy (eg, hypertrophic cardiomyopathy, dilated cardiomyopathy, arrhythmogenic right ventricular cardiomyopathy), genomic sequence analysis panel, must include sequencing of at least 5 cardiomyopathy-related genes (eg, *DSG2, MYBPC3, MYH7, PKP2, TTN*)

(Do not report 81439 in conjunction with 81413, 81414 when performed on the same date of service)

(For genomic sequencing panel testing for cardiac ion channelopathies, see 81413, 81414)

#● 81441   Inherited bone marrow failure syndromes (IBMFS) (eg, Fanconi anemia, dyskeratosis congenita, Diamond-Blackfan anemia, Shwachman-Diamond syndrome, GATA2 deficiency syndrome, congenital amegakaryocytic thrombocytopenia) sequence analysis panel, must include sequencing of at least 30 genes, including *BRCA2, BRIP1, DKC1, FANCA, FANCB, FANCC, FANCD2, FANCE, FANCF, FANCG, FANCI, FANCL, GATA1, GATA2, MPL, NHP2, NOP10, PALB2, RAD51C, RPL11, RPL35A, RPL5, RPS10, RPS19, RPS24, RPS26, RPS7, SBDS, TERT,* and *TINF2*

Pathology and Laboratory 80047-89398, 0001U-0284U

★ = Telemedicine   ◀ = Audio-only   ✚ = Add-on code   ✚ = FDA approval pending   # = Resequenced code   ⊘ = Modifier 51 exempt

Rationale

Code 81441 has been added to the Genomic Sequencing Procedures and Other Molecular Multianalyte Assays subsection to report inherited bone marrow failure syndromes (IBMFS).

Code 81441 is used to report the specific genomic sequencing procedure for at least the 30 genes identified in IBMFS. The specific genes included for analysis are listed within the code descriptor for this service.

Clinical Example (81441)

A 5-year-old male presents with severe pancytopenia. A comprehensive inherited bone marrow failure syndrome panel is ordered.

Description of Procedure (81441)

Isolate high-quality DNA from the patient's sample. Enrich DNA targets for at least 30 genes, including BRCA2, BRIP1, DKC1, FANCA, FANCB, FANCC, FANCD2, FANCE, FANCF, FANCG, FANCI, FANCL, GATA1, GATA2, MPL, NHP2, NOP10, PALB2, RAD51C, RPL11, RPL35A, RPL5, RPS10, RPS19, RPS24, RPS26, RPS7, SBDS, TERT, and TINF2. Perform massively parallel DNA sequencing of the coding regions and intron/exon boundaries and analyze results. The pathologist or other QHP composes a report that specifies and classifies any genetic variants.

81440   Nuclear encoded mitochondrial genes (eg, neurologic or myopathic phenotypes), genomic sequence panel, must include analysis of at least 100 genes, including *BCS1L, C10orf2, COQ2, COX10, DGUOK, MPV17, OPA1, PDSS2, POLG, POLG2, RRM2B, SCO1, SCO2, SLC25A4, SUCLA2, SUCLG1, TAZ, TK2,* and *TYMP*

81441   Code is out of numerical sequence. See 81437-81442

▲ **81445**   Targeted genomic sequence analysis panel, solid organ neoplasm, 5-50 genes (eg, *ALK, BRAF, CDKN2A, EGFR, ERBB2, KIT, KRAS, MET, NRAS, PDGFRA, PDGFRB, PGR, PIK3CA, PTEN, RET*), interrogation for sequence variants and copy number variants or rearrangements, if performed; DNA analysis or combined DNA and RNA analysis

81448   Code is out of numerical sequence. See 81437-81442

● **81449**   RNA analysis

(For copy number assessment by microarray, use 81406)

▲ **81450**   Targeted genomic sequence analysis panel, hematolymphoid neoplasm or disorder, 5-50 genes (eg, *BRAF, CEBPA, DNMT3A, EZH2, FLT3, IDH1, IDH2, JAK2, KIT, KRAS, MLL, NOTCH1, NPM1, NRAS*), interrogation for sequence variants, and copy number variants or

rearrangements, or isoform expression or mRNA expression levels, if performed; DNA analysis or combined DNA and RNA analysis

● **81451**   RNA analysis

(For copy number assessment by microarray, use 81406)

▲ **81455**   Targeted genomic sequence analysis panel, solid organ or hematolymphoid neoplasm or disorder, 51 or greater genes (eg, *ALK, BRAF, CDKN2A, CEBPA, DNMT3A, EGFR, ERBB2, EZH2, FLT3, IDH1, IDH2, JAK2, KIT, KRAS, MET, MLL, NOTCH1, NPM1, NRAS, PDGFRA, PDGFRB, PGR, PIK3CA, PTEN, RET*), interrogation for sequence variants and copy number variants or rearrangements, or isoform expression or mRNA expression levels, if performed; DNA analysis or combined DNA and RNA analysis

● **81456**   RNA analysis

(For copy number assessment by microarray, use 81406)

▶(For targeted genomic sequence DNA analysis and RNA analysis performed separately rather than via a combined method, report 81445, 81450, 81455 for the DNA analysis and report 81449, 81451, 81456 for the RNA analysis)◀

▶(For targeted genomic sequence RNA analysis using a separate method, see 81449, 81451, 81456)◀

Rationale

Targeted genomic sequence analysis panel codes 81445, 81450, and 81455 have been revised. Codes 81449, 81451, and 81456 have been established. The guidelines for the Genomic Sequencing Procedures and Other Molecular Multianalyte Assays subsection have been revised.

Prior to 2023, codes 81445, 81450, and 81455 described GSPs used for somatic mutation detection in oncology specimens in which DNA analysis was always performed and included RNA analysis when it was performed. However, it was not inclusive of other possibilities. There are at least four scenarios for targeted genomic sequence analysis using DNA- and/or RNA-based analyses: (1) only DNA is analyzed; (2) DNA and RNA are analyzed using a *single combined method*; (3) DNA and RNA are *analyzed separately* rather than via a combined method; and (4) only RNA is analyzed. To reflect current clinical practice, codes 81445, 81450, and 81455 have been revised to describe DNA analysis or *combined* DNA and RNA analysis (ie, using a single combined method). In addition, code 81455 has been revised to include testing for hematolymphoid disorders and to describe isoform expression or mRNA expression levels. Codes 81449, 81451, and 81456 have been established to describe targeted genomic sequence analysis for *RNA only*. When targeted genomic sequence DNA analysis or DNA and

---

Pathology and Laboratory 80047-89398, 0001U-0284U

RNA analysis using a single combined method is performed, code 81445, 81450, or 81455 is reported, as appropriate. When DNA and RNA analysis are *performed separately* rather than via a combined method, code 81445, 81450, or 81455 is reported for the DNA analysis, and code 81449, 81451, or 81456 is reported for the RNA analysis. When only RNA analysis is performed, code 81449, 81451, or 81456 is reported.

The Genomic Sequencing Procedures and Other Molecular Multianalyte Assays subsection guidelines have been revised and parenthetical notes have been added following code 81456 to provide instruction on appropriate reporting of the new and revised codes.

Clinical Example (81445)

A 50-year-old female presents with a thyroid nodule. Fine-needle aspiration is performed and sent for evaluation. Initial pathology review showed a follicular lesion of indeterminate diagnosis. Residual tissue is submitted for targeted genomic DNA sequence analysis of a panel of 12 genes known to be important in thyroid cancer.

Description of Procedure (81445)

Isolate high-quality DNA from the patient's tumor tissue and perform massively parallel sequencing on the tumor DNA, looking for mutations in 12 genes. Send the analytical results to a pathologist or other QHP for identification of mutations, interpretation, and preparation of a written report that specifies the patient's mutation status, which may contain information about diagnosis, prognosis, and patient management, to include information about targeted drug therapy.

Clinical Example (81449)

A 52-year-old female presents with a lung nodule. Needle biopsy is performed and sent for evaluation. Initial pathology shows a non-small cell malignancy. Residual tissue is submitted for a targeted genomic RNA sequence panel of 19 genes with common gene rearrangements and sequence variants known to be important in lung cancer.

Description of Procedure (81449)

Isolate high-quality RNA from the patient's tumor tissue and perform massively parallel sequencing on the tumor RNA, looking for mutations in 19 genes. Send the analytical results to a pathologist or other QHP for identification of mutations, interpretation, and preparation of a written report that specifies the patient's mutation status, which may contain information about diagnosis, prognosis, and patient management, to include information about targeted drug therapy.

Clinical Example (81450)

A 55-year-old male presents with an elevated white blood cell (WBC) count with 80% blasts, anemia, and thrombocytopenia. The pathologic diagnosis was acute myeloid leukemia (AML). Cytogenetic studies were normal, stratifying the patient as intermediate risk for survival. Blood is submitted for targeted genomic sequence analysis of a panel of 25 genes known to be informative in patients with AML.

Description of Procedure (81450)

Isolate high-quality DNA from the patient's blood and perform massively parallel sequencing on the DNA, looking for mutations in 25 genes. Send the analytical results to a pathologist or other QHP for identification of mutations, interpretation, and preparation of a written report that specifies the patient's mutation status, which may contain information about diagnosis, prognosis, and patient management, to include information about targeted drug therapy.

Clinical Example (81451)

A 45-year-old female presents with an elevated WBC count with 85% blasts, anemia, and thrombocytopenia. The pathologic diagnosis was AML. Cytogenetic studies were normal. Blood is submitted for a targeted genomic RNA sequence panel of 32 genes with recurrent gene rearrangements known to be important in patients with AML.

Description of Procedure (81451)

Isolate high-quality RNA from the patient's tumor tissue and perform massively parallel sequencing on the tumor RNA, looking for mutations in 32 genes. Send the analytical results to a pathologist or other QHP for identification of mutations, interpretation, and preparation of a written report that specifies the patient's mutation status, which may contain information about diagnosis, prognosis, and patient management, to include information about targeted drug therapy.

Clinical Example (81455)

A 65-year-old male presents with lung and liver lesions. Pathologic evaluation of biopsies of these lesions reveals a poorly differentiated neoplasm of uncertain primary origin. Tumor tissue is submitted for a targeted genomic sequence analysis of a panel of 250 genes known to be informative in a broad array of cancers.

★ = Telemedicine ◀ = Audio-only ✚ = Add-on code ⅄ = FDA approval pending # = Resequenced code ⊘ = Modifier 51 exempt

Description of Procedure (81455)

Isolate high-quality DNA from the patient's tumor tissue and perform massively parallel sequencing on the tumor DNA, looking for mutations in 250 genes, which may be genomic targets for therapeutic management. Send the analytical results to a pathologist or other QHP for identification of mutations, interpretation, and preparation of a written report that specifies the patient's mutation status, which may contain information about diagnosis, prognosis, and patient management, to include information about targeted drug therapy.

Clinical Example (81456)

A 57-year-old male presents with colon and liver lesions. Pathologic evaluation of biopsies of these lesions reveals a poorly differentiated neoplasm of uncertain primary origin. Tumor tissue is submitted for a targeted genomic RNA sequence analysis of a panel of 70 genes with recurrent sequence variants, and gene rearrangements known to be informative in a broad array of cancers.

Description of Procedure (81456)

Isolate high-quality RNA from the patient's tumor tissue and perform massively parallel sequencing on the tumor RNA, looking for mutations in 70 genes. Send the analytical results to a pathologist or other QHP for identification of mutations, interpretation, and preparation of a written report that specifies the patient's mutation status, which may contain information about diagnosis, prognosis, and patient management, to include information about targeted drug therapy.

Chemistry

	84430	Thiocyanate
#●	84433	Thiopurine S-methyltransferase (TPMT)

Rationale

A new Category I code 84433 has been established in the Chemistry subsection to report testing for thiopurine S-methyltransferase. Prior to CPT 2023, there was no specific CPT code that described enzyme-activity testing for thiopurine S-methyltransferase. The addition of this new code can aid in identifying individuals at greater risk of hepatotoxicity from thiopurine dose increase.

Clinical Example (84433)

A 42-year-old female with rheumatoid arthritis will be starting therapy with azathioprine (AZA). Thiopurine methyltransferase (TPMT) activity testing is ordered to calculate the correct dosage of AZA.

Description of Procedure (84433)

Submit whole blood and perform liquid chromatography/tandem mass spectrometry (LC-MS/MS). Calculate enzyme activity and report results.

84431	Thromboxane metabolite(s), including thromboxane if performed, urine
	(For concurrent urine creatinine determination, use 84431 in conjunction with 82570)
84433	Code is out of numerical sequence. See 84425-84432

Microbiology

87301	Infectious agent antigen detection by immunoassay technique (eg, enzyme immunoassay [EIA], enzyme-linked immunosorbent assay [ELISA], fluorescence immunoassay [FIA], immunochemiluminometric assay [IMCA]), qualitative or semiquantitative; adenovirus enteric types 40/41
87324	Clostridium difficile toxin(s)
87327	Cryptococcus neoformans
	(For Cryptococcus latex agglutination, use 86403)
	▶(For quantitative hepatitis B surface antigen [HBsAg], use 87467)◀

Rationale

In accordance with the establishment of code 87467, an instructional parenthetical note has been added following code 87340 to direct users to the appropriate code to report for this new service.

Refer to the codebook and the Rationale for code 87467 for a full discussion of these changes.

	87340	hepatitis B surface antigen (HBsAg)
		▶(For quantitative hepatitis B surface antigen [HBsAg], use 87467)◀
	87451	polyvalent for multiple organisms, each polyvalent antiserum
●	87467	Hepatitis B surface antigen (HBsAg), quantitative
		▶(For qualitative hepatitis B surface antigen [HBsAg], use 87340)◀

Pathology and Laboratory 80047-89398, 0001U-0284U

Rationale

Code 87467 has been established in the Microbiology subsection to report quantitative hepatitis B surface antigen (HBsAg). In addition, two cross-reference parenthetical notes have been added to direct users to report the appropriate codes when performing this service.

Code 87467 describes specific analyte testing for HBsAg. The current CPT codes do not indicate what analyte is being tested, only how the analyte is tested.

Of the two parenthetical notes that have been added, the first cross-reference parenthetical note following code 87340 directs users to the specific code for reporting quantitative HBsAg. The second cross-reference parenthetical note following code 87467 instructs the use of code 87340 when reporting for qualitative HBsAg.

Clinical Example (87467)

A 35-year-old female is found to have chronic hepatitis B (CHB) with positive hepatitis B surface antigen (HBsAg), negative hepatitis B e antigen (HBeAg), and low hepatitis B virus (HBV) DNA level. A quantitative hepatitis B surface antigen (HBsAg) level in serum is ordered to monitor the progression of CHB.

Description of Procedure (87467)

Perform quantitative measurement of hepatitis B surface antigen (HBsAg) in serum by immunoassay and report the result.

● 87468	Infectious agent detection by nucleic acid (DNA or RNA); Anaplasma phagocytophilum, amplified probe technique	
● 87469	Babesia microti, amplified probe technique	
87471	Bartonella henselae and Bartonella quintana, amplified probe technique	
87472	Bartonella henselae and Bartonella quintana, quantification	
87475	Borrelia burgdorferi, direct probe technique	
87476	Borrelia burgdorferi, amplified probe technique	
● 87478	Borrelia miyamotoi, amplified probe technique	
87480	Candida species, direct probe technique	
87481	Candida species, amplified probe technique	
87482	Candida species, quantification	

87483	central nervous system pathogen (eg, Neisseria meningitidis, Streptococcus pneumoniae, Listeria, Haemophilus influenzae, E. coli, Streptococcus agalactiae, enterovirus, human parechovirus, herpes simplex virus type 1 and 2, human herpesvirus 6, cytomegalovirus, varicella zoster virus, Cryptococcus), includes multiplex reverse transcription, when performed, and multiplex amplified probe technique, multiple types or subtypes, 12-25 targets
87484	Code is out of numerical sequence. See 87496-87500
87485	Chlamydia pneumoniae, direct probe technique
87497	cytomegalovirus, quantification
#● 87484	Ehrlichia chaffeensis, amplified probe technique

Rationale

Four new infectious agent detection codes (87468, 87469, 87478, 87484) have been added to the Microbiology subsection to identify new procedures for infectious agent detection by nucleic acid using an amplified probe technique of four different tick-borne bacterial illnesses.

Four infectious agent detection codes that are specific to detection of *Anaplasma phagocytophilum*, *Babesia microti*, *Borrelia miyamotoi*, and *Ehrlichia chaffeensis* have been established for early detection of diseases that are transferred/spread via ticks. As is noted within each descriptor, the codes utilize an amplified probe technique to identify strands of DNA/RNA associated with each bacterium. Because these codes are listed in alphabetical order, the former parent code (87471) has been changed to a child code to accommodate alphabetical listing of each new code, including listing of *Anaplasma phagocytophilum* at the beginning of the code as the newly assigned parent code.

Clinical Example (87468)

A 42-year-old male presents with fever, headache, muscle aches, and chills and reports exposure to ticks. The physician orders tick-borne testing by polymerase chain reaction (PCR) that includes detection of Anaplasma phagocytophilum.

Description of Procedure (87468)

Submit the patient's blood for nucleic acid extraction and purification, followed by PCR to detect Anaplasma phagocytophilum. Report the result.

★ = Telemedicine   ◀ = Audio-only   ✚ = Add-on code   ✔ = FDA approval pending   # = Resequenced code   ⊘ = Modifier 51 exempt

Clinical Example (87469)

A 42-year-old male presents with fever, headache, muscle aches, and chills and reports exposure to ticks. The physician orders tick-borne testing by PCR that includes detection of Babesia microti.

Description of Procedure (87469)

Submit the patient's blood for nucleic acid extraction and purification, followed by PCR to detect Babesia microti. Report the result.

Clinical Example (87478)

A 42-year-old male presents with fever, headache, muscle aches, and chills and reports exposure to ticks. The physician orders tick-borne testing by PCR that includes detection of Borrelia miyamotoi.

Description of Procedure (87478)

Submit the patient's blood for nucleic acid extraction and purification, followed by PCR to detect Borrelia miyamotoi. Report the result.

Clinical Example (87484)

A 42-year-old male presents with fever, headache, muscle aches, and chills and reports exposure to ticks. The physician orders tick-borne testing by PCR that includes detection of Ehrlichia chaffeensis.

Description of Procedure (87484)

Submit the patient's blood for nucleic acid extraction and purification, followed by PCR to detect Ehrlichia chaffeensis. Report the result.

87498	enterovirus, amplified probe technique, includes reverse transcription when performed
87635	severe acute respiratory syndrome coronavirus 2 (SARS-CoV-2) (coronavirus disease [COVID-19]), amplified probe technique
87636	severe acute respiratory syndrome coronavirus 2 (SARS-CoV-2) (coronavirus disease [COVID-19]) and influenza virus types A and B, multiplex amplified probe technique
87637	severe acute respiratory syndrome coronavirus 2 (SARS-CoV-2) (coronavirus disease [COVID-19]), influenza virus types A and B, and respiratory syncytial virus, multiplex amplified probe technique

(For nucleic acid detection of multiple respiratory infectious agents, not including severe acute respiratory syndrome coronavirus 2 [SARS-CoV-2] [coronavirus disease {COVID-19}], see 87631, 87632, 87633)

(For nucleic acid detection of multiple respiratory infectious agents, including severe acute respiratory syndrome coronavirus 2 [SARS-CoV-2] [coronavirus disease {COVID-19}] in conjunction with additional target[s] beyond influenza virus types A and B and respiratory syncytial virus, see 87631, 87632, 87633)

▶(For infectious agent genotype analysis by nucleic acid [DNA or RNA] for severe acute respiratory syndrome coronavirus 2 [SARS-CoV-2] [coronavirus disease {COVID-19}], mutation identification in targeted region[s], use 87913)◀

▶(For SARS-CoV-2 variant analysis, use 87913)◀

# 87910		Infectious agent genotype analysis by nucleic acid (DNA or RNA); cytomegalovirus

(For infectious agent drug susceptibility phenotype prediction for HIV-1, use 87900)

(For Human Papillomavirus [HPV] for high-risk types [ie, genotyping], of five or greater separately reported HPV types, use 0500T)

87901		HIV-1, reverse transcriptase and protease regions
# 87906		HIV-1, other region (eg, integrase, fusion)

(For infectious agent drug susceptibility phenotype prediction for HIV-1, use 87900)

# 87912		Hepatitis B virus
87902		Hepatitis C virus
#● 87913		severe acute respiratory syndrome coronavirus 2 (SARS-CoV-2) (coronavirus disease [COVID-19]), mutation identification in targeted region(s)

▶(For infectious agent detection by nucleic acid [DNA or RNA] for severe acute respiratory syndrome coronavirus 2 [SARS-CoV-2] [coronavirus disease {COVID-19}], see 87635, 87636, 87637)◀

▶(For SARS-CoV-2 variant analysis, use 87913)◀

Rationale

Code 87913 has been established to report severe acute respiratory syndrome coronavirus 2 (SARS-CoV-2) (coronavirus disease [COVID-19]) mutation identification in targeted region(s) using infectious agent genotype analysis by nucleic acid (DNA or RNA). This genotype analysis is performed to identify the presence of SARS-CoV-2 variants with mutations in one or more genes that may be responsible for resistance to SARS-CoV-2 vaccine. This test may be performed on patients who have developed SARS-CoV-2 after having been fully vaccinated.

A cross-reference parenthetical note has been added following code 87913 directing users to codes 87635, 87636, and 87637 for infectious agent detection by nucleic acid (DNA or RNA) for SARS-CoV-2 (COVID-19). An

Pathology and Laboratory 80047-89398, 0001U-0284U

Pathology and Laboratory 80047-89398, 0001U-0284U

instructional parenthetical note has also been added instructing users to report 87913 for SARS-CoV-2 variant analysis. In accordance with the establishment of code 87913, two parenthetical notes have been added following code 87637 directing users to code 87913.

Clinical Example (87913)

A 71-year-old male is admitted with fever and new onset cough. A nasopharyngeal swab specimen is positive for SARS-CoV-2 RNA. The same specimen is submitted for SARS-CoV-2 variant genotype analysis.

Description of Procedure (87913)

Subject the SARS-CoV-2 RNA-positive clinical specimen to viral nucleic acid extraction and purification, followed by reverse transcription-polymerase chain reaction (RT-PCR) of the viral genomic targets. The amplified cDNA products undergo probe hybridization to detect specific nucleotide base substitutions, and presumptive viral lineage is determined by specific pattern of these substitutions. Report results.

87913   Code is out of numerical sequence. See 87899-87904

Surgical Pathology

88302   **Level II** - Surgical pathology, gross and microscopic examination

Appendix, incidental

Fallopian tube, sterilization

Fingers/toes, amputation, traumatic

Foreskin, newborn

Hernia sac, any location

Hydrocele sac

Nerve

Skin, plastic repair

Sympathetic ganglion

Testis, castration

Vaginal mucosa, incidental

Vas deferens, sterilization

▶(Use 0751T in conjunction with 88302 when the digitization of glass microscope slides is performed)◀

Rationale

In support of the establishment of code 0751T, a parenthetical note has been established following code 88302 to refer users to code 0751T when the digitization of glass microscope slides is performed.

Refer to the codebook and the Rationale for code 0751T for a full discussion of these changes.

88304   **Level III** - Surgical pathology, gross and microscopic examination

Abortion, induced

Abscess

Aneurysm - arterial/ventricular

Anus, tag

Appendix, other than incidental

Artery, atheromatous plaque

Bartholin's gland cyst

Bone fragment(s), other than pathologic fracture

Bursa/synovial cyst

Carpal tunnel tissue

Cartilage, shavings

Cholesteatoma

Colon, colostomy stoma

Conjunctiva - biopsy/pterygium

Cornea

Diverticulum - esophagus/small intestine

Dupuytren's contracture tissue

Femoral head, other than fracture

Fissure/fistula

Foreskin, other than newborn

Gallbladder

Ganglion cyst

Hematoma

Hemorrhoids

Hydatid of Morgagni

Intervertebral disc

Joint, loose body

Meniscus

Mucocele, salivary

Neuroma - Morton's/traumatic

Pilonidal cyst/sinus

★ = Telemedicine   ◀ = Audio-only   ✦ = Add-on code   ✎ = FDA approval pending   # = Resequenced code   ⊘ = Modifier 51 exempt

Polyps, inflammatory - nasal/sinusoidal

Skin - cyst/tag/debridement

Soft tissue, debridement

Soft tissue, lipoma

Spermatocele

Tendon/tendon sheath

Testicular appendage

Thrombus or embolus

Tonsil and/or adenoids

Varicocele

Vas deferens, other than sterilization

Vein, varicosity

▶(Use 0752T in conjunction with 88304 when the digitization of glass microscope slides is performed)◀

Rationale

In support of the establishment of code 0752T, a parenthetical note has been established following code 88304 to refer users to code 0752T when the digitization of glass microscope slides is performed.

Refer to the codebook and the Rationale for code 0752T for a full discussion of these changes.

88305 **Level IV** - Surgical pathology, gross and microscopic examination

Abortion - spontaneous/missed

Artery, biopsy

Bone marrow, biopsy

Bone exostosis

Brain/meninges, other than for tumor resection

Breast, biopsy, not requiring microscopic evaluation of surgical margins

Breast, reduction mammoplasty

Bronchus, biopsy

Cell block, any source

Cervix, biopsy

Colon, biopsy

Duodenum, biopsy

Endocervix, curettings/biopsy

Endometrium, curettings/biopsy

Esophagus, biopsy

Extremity, amputation, traumatic

Fallopian tube, biopsy

Fallopian tube, ectopic pregnancy

Femoral head, fracture

Fingers/toes, amputation, non-traumatic

Gingiva/oral mucosa, biopsy

Heart valve

Joint, resection

Kidney, biopsy

Larynx, biopsy

Leiomyoma(s), uterine myomectomy - without uterus

Lip, biopsy/wedge resection

Lung, transbronchial biopsy

Lymph node, biopsy

Muscle, biopsy

Nasal mucosa, biopsy

Nasopharynx/oropharynx, biopsy

Nerve, biopsy

Odontogenic/dental cyst

Omentum, biopsy

Ovary with or without tube, non-neoplastic

Ovary, biopsy/wedge resection

Parathyroid gland

Peritoneum, biopsy

Pituitary tumor

Placenta, other than third trimester

Pleura/pericardium - biopsy/tissue

Polyp, cervical/endometrial

Polyp, colorectal

Polyp, stomach/small intestine

Prostate, needle biopsy

Prostate, TUR

Salivary gland, biopsy

Sinus, paranasal biopsy

Skin, other than cyst/tag/debridement/plastic repair

Small intestine, biopsy

Soft tissue, other than tumor/mass/lipoma/debridement

Spleen

Stomach, biopsy

Synovium

Testis, other than tumor/biopsy/castration

Thyroglossal duct/brachial cleft cyst

Tongue, biopsy

Tonsil, biopsy

Trachea, biopsy

Ureter, biopsy

Urethra, biopsy

Urinary bladder, biopsy

Uterus, with or without tubes and ovaries, for prolapse

Vagina, biopsy

Vulva/labia, biopsy

▶(Use 0753T in conjunction with 88305 when the digitization of glass microscope slides is performed)◀

Rationale

In support of the establishment of code 0753T, a parenthetical note has been established following code 88305 to refer users to code 0753T when the digitization of glass microscope slides is performed.

Refer to the codebook and the Rationale for code 0753T for a full discussion of these changes.

88307 **Level V** - Surgical pathology, gross and microscopic examination

Adrenal, resection

Bone - biopsy/curettings

Bone fragment(s), pathologic fracture

Brain, biopsy

Brain/meninges, tumor resection

Breast, excision of lesion, requiring microscopic evaluation of surgical margins

Breast, mastectomy - partial/simple

Cervix, conization

Colon, segmental resection, other than for tumor

Extremity, amputation, non-traumatic

Eye, enucleation

Kidney, partial/total nephrectomy

Larynx, partial/total resection

Liver, biopsy - needle/wedge

Liver, partial resection

Lung, wedge biopsy

Lymph nodes, regional resection

Mediastinum, mass

Myocardium, biopsy

Odontogenic tumor

Ovary with or without tube, neoplastic

Pancreas, biopsy

Placenta, third trimester

Prostate, except radical resection

Salivary gland

Sentinel lymph node

Small intestine, resection, other than for tumor

Soft tissue mass (except lipoma) - biopsy/simple excision

Stomach - subtotal/total resection, other than for tumor

Testis, biopsy

Thymus, tumor

Thyroid, total/lobe

Ureter, resection

Urinary bladder, TUR

Uterus, with or without tubes and ovaries, other than neoplastic/prolapse

▶(Use 0754T in conjunction with 88307 when the digitization of glass microscope slides is performed)◀

Rationale

In support of the establishment of code 0754T, a parenthetical note has been established following code 88307 to refer users to code 0754T when the digitization of glass microscope slides is performed.

Refer to the codebook and the Rationale for code 0754T for a full discussion of these changes.

88309 **Level VI** - Surgical pathology, gross and microscopic examination

Bone resection

Breast, mastectomy - with regional lymph nodes

Colon, segmental resection for tumor

Colon, total resection

Esophagus, partial/total resection

★=Telemedicine ◀=Audio-only ✛=Add-on code ✎=FDA approval pending #=Resequenced code ⊘=Modifier 51 exempt

Extremity, disarticulation

Fetus, with dissection

Larynx, partial/total resection - with regional lymph nodes

Lung - total/lobe/segment resection

Pancreas, total/subtotal resection

Prostate, radical resection

Small intestine, resection for tumor

Soft tissue tumor, extensive resection

Stomach - subtotal/total resection for tumor

Testis, tumor

Tongue/tonsil -resection for tumor

Urinary bladder, partial/total resection

Uterus, with or without tubes and ovaries, neoplastic

Vulva, total/subtotal resection

►(Use 0755T in conjunction with 88309 when the digitization of glass microscope slides is performed)◄

(Do not report 88302-88309 on the same specimen as part of Mohs surgery)

(For fine needle aspiration biopsy, see 10004, 10005, 10006, 10007, 10008, 10009, 10010, 10011, 10012, 10021)

(For evaluation of fine needle aspirate, see 88172-88173)

Rationale

In support of the establishment of code 0755T, a parenthetical note has been established following code 88309 to refer users to code 0755T when the digitization of glass microscope slides is performed.

Refer to the codebook and the Rationale for code 0755T for a full discussion of these changes.

+ **88311** Decalcification procedure (List separately in addition to code for surgical pathology examination)

88312 Special stain including interpretation and report; Group I for microorganisms (eg, acid fast, methenamine silver)

►(Use 0756T in conjunction with 88312 when the digitization of glass microscope slides is performed)◄

(Report one unit of 88312 for each special stain, on each surgical pathology block, cytologic specimen, or hematologic smear)

Rationale

In support of the establishment of code 0756T, a parenthetical note has been established following code 88312 to refer users to code 0756T when the digitization of glass microscope slides is performed.

Refer to the codebook and the Rationale for code 0756T for a full discussion of these changes.

88313 Group II, all other (eg, iron, trichrome), except stain for microorganisms, stains for enzyme constituents, or immunocytochemistry and immunohistochemistry

►(Use 0757T in conjunction with 88313 when the digitization of glass microscope slides is performed)◄

(Report one unit of 88313 for each special stain, on each surgical pathology block, cytologic specimen, or hematologic smear)

(For immunocytochemistry and immunohistochemistry, use 88342)

Rationale

In support of the establishment of code 0757T, a parenthetical note has been established following code 88313 to refer users to code 0757T when the digitization of glass microscope slides is performed.

Refer to the codebook and the Rationale for code 0757T for a full discussion of these changes.

+ **88314** histochemical stain on frozen tissue block (List separately in addition to code for primary procedure)

(Use 88314 in conjunction with 17311-17315, 88302-88309, 88331, 88332)

►(Use 0758T in conjunction with 88314 when the digitization of glass microscope slides is performed)◄

(Do not report 88314 with 17311-17315 for routine frozen section stain [eg, hematoxylin and eosin, toluidine blue], performed during Mohs surgery. When a nonroutine histochemical stain on frozen tissue during Mohs surgery is utilized, report 88314 with modifier 59)

(Report one unit of 88314 for each special stain on each frozen surgical pathology block)

(For a special stain performed on frozen tissue section material to identify enzyme constituents, use 88319)

(For determinative histochemistry to identify chemical components, use 88313)

Pathology and Laboratory 80047-89398, 0001U-0284U

Pathology and Laboratory 80047-89398, 0001U-0284U

Rationale

In support of the establishment of code 0758T, a parenthetical note has been established following code 88314 to refer users to code 0758T when the digitization of glass microscope slides is performed.

Refer to the codebook and the Rationale for code 0758T for a full discussion of these changes.

88319   Group III, for enzyme constituents

▶(Use 0759T in conjunction with 88319 when the digitization of glass microscope slides is performed)◀

(For each stain on each surgical pathology block, cytologic specimen, or hematologic smear, use one unit of 88319)

(For detection of enzyme constituents by immunohistochemical or immunocytochemical technique, use 88342)

Rationale

In support of the establishment of code 0759T, a parenthetical note has been established following code 88319 to refer users to code 0759T when the digitization of glass microscope slides is performed.

Refer to the codebook and the Rationale for code 0759T for a full discussion of these changes.

88342   Immunohistochemistry or immunocytochemistry, per specimen; initial single antibody stain procedure

▶(Use 0760T in conjunction with 88342 when the digitization of glass microscope slides is performed)◀

(For quantitative or semiquantitative immunohistochemistry, see 88360, 88361)

Rationale

In support of the establishment of code 0760T, a parenthetical note has been established following code 88342 to refer users to code 0760T when the digitization of glass microscope slides is performed.

Refer to the codebook and the Rationale for code 0760T for a full discussion of these changes.

#✚ 88341   each additional single antibody stain procedure (List separately in addition to code for primary procedure)

(Use 88341 in conjunction with 88342)

▶(Use 0761T in conjunction with 88341 when the digitization of glass microscope slides is performed)◀

(For multiplex antibody stain procedure, use 88344)

Rationale

In support of the establishment of code 0761T, a parenthetical note has been established following code 88341 to refer users to code 0761T when the digitization of glass microscope slides is performed.

Refer to the codebook and the Rationale for code 0761T for a full discussion of these changes.

88344   each multiplex antibody stain procedure

▶(Use 0762T in conjunction with 88344 when the digitization of glass microscope slides is performed)◀

(Do not use more than one unit of 88341, 88342, or 88344 for the same separately identifiable antibody per specimen)

(Do not report 88341, 88342, 88344 in conjunction with 88360, 88361 unless each procedure is for a different antibody)

(When multiple separately identifiable antibodies are applied to the same specimen [ie, multiplex antibody stain procedure], use one unit of 88344)

(When multiple antibodies are applied to the same slide that are not separately identifiable, [eg, antibody cocktails], use 88342, unless an additional separately identifiable antibody is also used, then use 88344)

Rationale

In support of the establishment of code 0762T, a parenthetical note has been established following code 88344 to refer users to code 0762T when the digitization of glass microscope slides is performed.

Refer to the codebook and the Rationale for code 0762T for a full discussion of these changes.

88360   Morphometric analysis, tumor immunohistochemistry (eg, Her-2/neu, estrogen receptor/progesterone receptor), quantitative or semiquantitative, per specimen, each single antibody stain procedure; manual

▶(Use 0763T in conjunction with 88360 when the digitization of glass microscope slides is performed)◀

★ = Telemedicine   ◀ = Audio-only   ✚ = Add-on code   � = FDA approval pending   # = Resequenced code   ⊘ = Modifier 51 exempt

Rationale

In support of the establishment of code 0763T, a parenthetical note has been established following code 88360 to refer users to code 0763T when the digitization of glass microscope slides is performed.

Refer to the codebook and the Rationale for code 0763T for a full discussion of these changes.

Proprietary Laboratory Analyses

►(0012U has been deleted)◄

►(0013U has been deleted)◄

►(0014U has been deleted)◄

▲ **0022U** Targeted genomic sequence analysis panel, cholangiocarcinoma and non-small cell lung neoplasia, DNA and RNA analysis, 1-23 genes, interrogation for sequence variants and rearrangements, reported as presence/absence of variants and associated therapy(ies) to consider

►(0056U has been deleted)◄

▲ **0090U** Oncology (cutaneous melanoma), mRNA gene expression profiling by RT-PCR of 23 genes (14 content and 9 housekeeping), utilizing formalin-fixed paraffin-embedded (FFPE) tissue, algorithm reported as a categorical result (ie, benign, intermediate, malignant)

►(0097U has been deleted)◄

►(0151U has been deleted)◄

►(0208U has been deleted)◄

▲ **0229U** *BCAT1 (Branched chain amino acid transaminase 1)* and *IKZF1 (IKAROS family zinc finger 1)* (eg, colorectal cancer) promoter methylation analysis

▲ **0276U** Hematology (inherited thrombocytopenia), genomic sequence analysis of 42 genes, blood, buccal swab, or amniotic fluid

● **0285U** Oncology, response to radiation, cell-free DNA, quantitative branched chain DNA amplification, plasma, reported as a radiation toxicity score

● **0286U** *CEP72 (centrosomal protein, 72-KDa), NUDT15 (nudix hydrolase 15)* and *TPMT (thiopurine S-methyltransferase)* (eg, drug metabolism) gene analysis, common variants

● **0287U** Oncology (thyroid), DNA and mRNA, next-generation sequencing analysis of 112 genes, fine needle aspirate or formalin-fixed paraffin-embedded (FFPE) tissue, algorithmic prediction of cancer recurrence, reported as a categorical risk result (low, intermediate, high)

● **0288U** Oncology (lung), mRNA, quantitative PCR analysis of 11 genes (*BAG1, BRCA1, CDC6, CDK2AP1, ERBB3, FUT3, IL11, LCK, RND3, SH3BGR, WNT3A*) and 3 reference genes (*ESD, TBP, YAP1*), formalin-fixed paraffin-embedded (FFPE) tumor tissue, algorithmic interpretation reported as a recurrence risk score

● **0289U** Neurology (Alzheimer disease), mRNA, gene expression profiling by RNA sequencing of 24 genes, whole blood, algorithm reported as predictive risk score

● **0290U** Pain management, mRNA, gene expression profiling by RNA sequencing of 36 genes, whole blood, algorithm reported as predictive risk score

● **0291U** Psychiatry (mood disorders), mRNA, gene expression profiling by RNA sequencing of 144 genes, whole blood, algorithm reported as predictive risk score

● **0292U** Psychiatry (stress disorders), mRNA, gene expression profiling by RNA sequencing of 72 genes, whole blood, algorithm reported as predictive risk score

● **0293U** Psychiatry (suicidal ideation), mRNA, gene expression profiling by RNA sequencing of 54 genes, whole blood, algorithm reported as predictive risk score

● **0294U** Longevity and mortality risk, mRNA, gene expression profiling by RNA sequencing of 18 genes, whole blood, algorithm reported as predictive risk score

● **0295U** Oncology (breast ductal carcinoma in situ), protein expression profiling by immunohistochemistry of 7 proteins (COX2, FOXA1, HER2, Ki-67, p16, PR, SIAH2), with 4 clinicopathologic factors (size, age, margin status, palpability), utilizing formalin-fixed paraffin-embedded (FFPE) tissue, algorithm reported as a recurrence risk score

● **0296U** Oncology (oral and/or oropharyngeal cancer), gene expression profiling by RNA sequencing of at least 20 molecular features (eg, human and/or microbial mRNA), saliva, algorithm reported as positive or negative for signature associated with malignancy

● **0297U** Oncology (pan tumor), whole genome sequencing of paired malignant and normal DNA specimens, fresh or formalin-fixed paraffin-embedded (FFPE) tissue, blood or bone marrow, comparative sequence analyses and variant identification

● **0298U** Oncology (pan tumor), whole transcriptome sequencing of paired malignant and normal RNA specimens, fresh or formalin-fixed paraffin-embedded (FFPE) tissue, blood or bone marrow, comparative sequence analyses and expression level and chimeric transcript identification

● **0299U** Oncology (pan tumor), whole genome optical genome mapping of paired malignant and normal DNA specimens, fresh frozen tissue, blood, or bone marrow, comparative structural variant identification

Pathology and Laboratory 80047-89398, 0001U-0284U

● **0300U** Oncology (pan tumor), whole genome sequencing and optical genome mapping of paired malignant and normal DNA specimens, fresh tissue, blood, or bone marrow, comparative sequence analyses and variant identification

● **0301U** Infectious agent detection by nucleic acid (DNA or RNA), Bartonella henselae and Bartonella quintana, droplet digital PCR (ddPCR);

● **0302U** following liquid enrichment

● **0303U** Hematology, red blood cell (RBC) adhesion to endothelial/subendothelial adhesion molecules, functional assessment, whole blood, with algorithmic analysis and result reported as an RBC adhesion index; hypoxic

● **0304U** normoxic

● **0305U** Hematology, red blood cell (RBC) functionality and deformity as a function of shear stress, whole blood, reported as a maximum elongation index

● **0306U** Oncology (minimal residual disease [MRD]), next-generation targeted sequencing analysis, cell-free DNA, initial (baseline) assessment to determine a patient-specific panel for future comparisons to evaluate for MRD

▶(Do not report 0306U in conjunction with 0307U)◀

● **0307U** Oncology (minimal residual disease [MRD]), next-generation targeted sequencing analysis of a patient-specific panel, cell-free DNA, subsequent assessment with comparison to previously analyzed patient specimens to evaluate for MRD

▶(Do not report 0307U in conjunction with 0306U)◀

● **0308U** Cardiology (coronary artery disease [CAD]), analysis of 3 proteins (high sensitivity [hs] troponin, adiponectin, and kidney injury molecule-1 [KIM-1]), plasma, algorithm reported as a risk score for obstructive CAD

● **0309U** Cardiology (cardiovascular disease), analysis of 4 proteins (NT-proBNP, osteopontin, tissue inhibitor of metalloproteinase-1 [TIMP-1], and kidney injury molecule-1 [KIM-1]), plasma, algorithm reported as a risk score for major adverse cardiac event

● **0310U** Pediatrics (vasculitis, Kawasaki disease [KD]), analysis of 3 biomarkers (NT-proBNP, C-reactive protein, and T-uptake), plasma, algorithm reported as a risk score for KD

● **0311U** Infectious disease (bacterial), quantitative antimicrobial susceptibility reported as phenotypic minimum inhibitory concentration (MIC)–based antimicrobial susceptibility for each organism identified

▶(Do not report 0311U in conjunction with 87076, 87077, 0086U)◀

● **0312U** Autoimmune diseases (eg, systemic lupus erythematosus [SLE]), analysis of 8 IgG autoantibodies and 2 cell-bound complement activation products using enzyme-linked immunosorbent immunoassay (ELISA), flow cytometry and indirect immunofluorescence, serum, or plasma and whole blood, individual components reported along with an algorithmic SLE-likelihood assessment

● **0313U** Oncology (pancreas), DNA and mRNA next-generation sequencing analysis of 74 genes and analysis of CEA (CEACAM5) gene expression, pancreatic cyst fluid, algorithm reported as a categorical result (ie, negative, low probability of neoplasia or positive, high probability of neoplasia)

● **0314U** Oncology (cutaneous melanoma), mRNA gene expression profiling by RT-PCR of 35 genes (32 content and 3 housekeeping), utilizing formalin-fixed paraffin-embedded (FFPE) tissue, algorithm reported as a categorical result (ie, benign, intermediate, malignant)

● **0315U** Oncology (cutaneous squamous cell carcinoma), mRNA gene expression profiling by RT-PCR of 40 genes (34 content and 6 housekeeping), utilizing formalin-fixed paraffin-embedded (FFPE) tissue, algorithm reported as a categorical risk result (ie, Class 1, Class 2A, Class 2B)

● **0316U** Borrelia burgdorferi (Lyme disease), OspA protein evaluation, urine

● **0317U** Oncology (lung cancer), four-probe FISH (3q29, 3p22.1, 10q22.3, 10cen) assay, whole blood, predictive algorithm-generated evaluation reported as decreased or increased risk for lung cancer

● **0318U** Pediatrics (congenital epigenetic disorders), whole genome methylation analysis by microarray for 50 or more genes, blood

● **0319U** Nephrology (renal transplant), RNA expression by select transcriptome sequencing, using pretransplant peripheral blood, algorithm reported as a risk score for early acute rejection

● **0320U** Nephrology (renal transplant), RNA expression by select transcriptome sequencing, using posttransplant peripheral blood, algorithm reported as a risk score for acute cellular rejection

● **0321U** Infectious agent detection by nucleic acid (DNA or RNA), genitourinary pathogens, identification of 20 bacterial and fungal organisms and identification of 16 associated antibiotic-resistance genes, multiplex amplified probe technique

● **0322U** Neurology (autism spectrum disorder [ASD]), quantitative measurements of 14 acyl carnitines and microbiome-derived metabolites, liquid chromatography with tandem mass spectrometry (LC-MS/MS), plasma, results reported as negative or positive for risk of metabolic subtypes associated with ASD

● **0323U** Infectious agent detection by nucleic acid (DNA and RNA), central nervous system pathogen, metagenomic next-generation sequencing, cerebrospinal fluid (CSF), identification of pathogenic bacteria, viruses, parasites, or fungi

● **0324U** Oncology (ovarian), spheroid cell culture, 4-drug panel (carboplatin, doxorubicin, gemcitabine, paclitaxel), tumor chemotherapy response prediction for each drug

● **0325U** Oncology (ovarian), spheroid cell culture, poly (ADP-ribose) polymerase (PARP) inhibitors (niraparib, olaparib, rucaparib, velparib), tumor response prediction for each drug

● **0326U** Targeted genomic sequence analysis panel, solid organ neoplasm, cell-free circulating DNA analysis of 83 or more genes, interrogation for sequence variants, gene copy number amplifications, gene rearrangements, microsatellite instability and tumor mutational burden

● **0327U** Fetal aneuploidy (trisomy 13, 18, and 21), DNA sequence analysis of selected regions using maternal plasma, algorithm reported as a risk score for each trisomy, includes sex reporting, if performed

● **0328U** Drug assay, definitive, 120 or more drugs and metabolites, urine, quantitative liquid chromatography with tandem mass spectrometry (LC-MS/MS), includes specimen validity and algorithmic analysis describing drug or metabolite and presence or absence of risks for a significant patient-adverse event, per date of service

● **0329U** Oncology (neoplasia), exome and transcriptome sequence analysis for sequence variants, gene copy number amplifications and deletions, gene rearrangements, microsatellite instability and tumor mutational burden utilizing DNA and RNA from tumor with DNA from normal blood or saliva for subtraction, report of clinically significant mutation(s) with therapy associations

● **0330U** Infectious agent detection by nucleic acid (DNA or RNA), vaginal pathogen panel, identification of 27 organisms, amplified probe technique, vaginal swab

● **0331U** Oncology (hematolymphoid neoplasia), optical genome mapping for copy number alterations and gene rearrangements utilizing DNA from blood or bone marrow, report of clinically significant alterations

● **0332U** Oncology (pan-tumor), genetic profiling of 8 DNA-regulatory (epigenetic) markers by quantitative polymerase chain reaction (qPCR), whole blood, reported as a high or low probability of responding to immune checkpoint–inhibitor therapy

● **0333U** Oncology (liver), surveillance for hepatocellular carcinoma (HCC) in high-risk patients, analysis of methylation patterns on circulating cell-free DNA (cfDNA) plus measurement of serum of AFP/AFP-L3 and oncoprotein des-gamma-carboxy-prothrombin (DCP), algorithm reported as normal or abnormal result

● **0334U** Oncology (solid organ), targeted genomic sequence analysis, formalin-fixed paraffin-embedded (FFPE) tumor tissue, DNA analysis, 84 or more genes, interrogation for sequence variants, gene copy number amplifications, gene rearrangements, microsatellite instability and tumor mutational burden

● **0335U** Rare diseases (constitutional/heritable disorders), whole genome sequence analysis, including small sequence changes, copy number variants, deletions, duplications, mobile element insertions, uniparental disomy (UPD), inversions, aneuploidy, mitochondrial genome sequence analysis with heteroplasmy and large deletions, short tandem repeat (STR) gene expansions, fetal sample, identification and categorization of genetic variants

▶(Do not report 0335U in conjunction with 81425, 0212U)◀

● **0336U** Rare diseases (constitutional/heritable disorders), whole genome sequence analysis, including small sequence changes, copy number variants, deletions, duplications, mobile element insertions, uniparental disomy (UPD), inversions, aneuploidy, mitochondrial genome sequence analysis with heteroplasmy and large deletions, short tandem repeat (STR) gene expansions, blood or saliva, identification and categorization of genetic variants, each comparator genome (eg, parent)

▶(Do not report 0336U in conjunction with 81426, 0213U)◀

● **0337U** Oncology (plasma cell disorders and myeloma), circulating plasma cell immunologic selection, identification, morphological characterization, and enumeration of plasma cells based on differential CD138, CD38, CD19, and CD45 protein biomarker expression, peripheral blood

● **0338U** Oncology (solid tumor), circulating tumor cell selection, identification, morphological characterization, detection and enumeration based on differential EpCAM, cytokeratins 8, 18, and 19, and CD45 protein biomarkers, and quantification of HER2 protein biomarker–expressing cells, peripheral blood

● **0339U** Oncology (prostate), mRNA expression profiling of *HOXC6* and *DLX1*, reverse transcription polymerase chain reaction (RT-PCR), first-void urine following digital rectal examination, algorithm reported as probability of high-grade cancer

● **0340U** Oncology (pan-cancer), analysis of minimal residual disease (MRD) from plasma, with assays personalized to each patient based on prior next-generation sequencing of the patient's tumor and germline DNA, reported as absence or presence of MRD, with disease-burden correlation, if appropriate

● **0341U** Fetal aneuploidy DNA sequencing comparative analysis, fetal DNA from products of conception, reported as normal (euploidy), monosomy, trisomy, or partial deletion/duplication, mosaicism, and segmental aneuploid

● **0342U**   Oncology (pancreatic cancer), multiplex immunoassay of C5, C4, cystatin C, factor B, osteoprotegerin (OPG), gelsolin, IGFBP3, CA125 and multiplex electrochemiluminescent immunoassay (ECLIA) for CA19-9, serum, diagnostic algorithm reported qualitatively as positive, negative, or borderline

● **0343U**   Oncology (prostate), exosome-based analysis of 442 small noncoding RNAs (sncRNAs) by quantitative reverse transcription polymerase chain reaction (RT-qPCR), urine, reported as molecular evidence of no-, low-, intermediate- or high-risk of prostate cancer

● **0344U**   Hepatology (nonalcoholic fatty liver disease [NAFLD]), semiquantitative evaluation of 28 lipid markers by liquid chromatography with tandem mass spectrometry (LC-MS/MS), serum, reported as at-risk for nonalcoholic steatohepatitis (NASH) or not NASH

● **0345U**   Psychiatry (eg, depression, anxiety, attention deficit hyperactivity disorder [ADHD]), genomic analysis panel, variant analysis of 15 genes, including deletion/duplication analysis of *CYP2D6*

● **0346U**   Beta amyloid, Aß40 and Aß42 by liquid chromatography with tandem mass spectrometry (LC-MS/MS), ratio, plasma

● **0347U**   Drug metabolism or processing (multiple conditions), whole blood or buccal specimen, DNA analysis, 16 gene report, with variant analysis and reported phenotypes

● **0348U**   Drug metabolism or processing (multiple conditions), whole blood or buccal specimen, DNA analysis, 25 gene report, with variant analysis and reported phenotypes

● **0349U**   Drug metabolism or processing (multiple conditions), whole blood or buccal specimen, DNA analysis, 27 gene report, with variant analysis, including reported phenotypes and impacted gene-drug interactions

● **0350U**   Drug metabolism or processing (multiple conditions), whole blood or buccal specimen, DNA analysis, 27 gene report, with variant analysis and reported phenotypes

● **0351U**   Infectious disease (bacterial or viral), biochemical assays, tumor necrosis factor-related apoptosis-inducing ligand (TRAIL), interferon gamma-induced protein-10 (IP-10), and C-reactive protein, serum, algorithm reported as likelihood of bacterial infection

● **0352U**   Infectious disease (bacterial vaginosis and vaginitis), multiplex amplified probe technique, for detection of bacterial vaginosis–associated bacteria (BVAB-2, Atopobium vaginae, and Megasphera type 1), algorithm reported as detected or not detected and separate detection of Candida species (C. albicans, C. tropicalis, C. parapsilosis, C. dubliniensis), Candida glabrata/Candida krusei, and trichomonas vaginalis, vaginal-fluid specimen, each result reported as detected or not detected

● **0353U**   Infectious agent detection by nucleic acid (DNA), Chlamydia trachomatis and Neisseria gonorrhoeae, multiplex amplified probe technique, urine, vaginal, pharyngeal, or rectal, each pathogen reported as detected or not detected

● **0354U**   Human papilloma virus (HPV), high-risk types (ie, 16, 18, 31, 33, 45, 52 and 58) qualitative mRNA expression of E6/E7 by quantitative polymerase chain reaction (qPCR)

Rationale

A total of 70 new proprietary laboratory analyses (PLA) codes have been established for the CPT 2023 code set. PLA test codes are released and posted online at https://www.ama-assn.org/practice-management/cpt/cpt-pla codes on a quarterly basis (Fall, Winter, Spring, and Summer). New codes are effective the quarter following their publication online. Other changes include the deletion of seven codes (0012U-0014U, 0056U, 0097U, 0151U, 0208U), the revision of four codes (0022U, 0090U, 0229U, 0276U), the revision of test names only (0240U, 0241U), and the deletion of a laboratory name (0166U).

Clinical Example (0022U)

A 61-year-old female was recently diagnosed with stage IV intrahepatic cholangiocarcinoma, based on core needle biopsy taken from tumor mass. Physician requests molecular profiling to inform therapy options, including FDA-approved therapies.

Description of Procedure (0022U)

Isolate and subject high-quality genomic DNA and RNA from the patient's formalin-fixed paraffin-embedded (FFPE) tumor sample to massively parallel sequencing of 23 genes (EGFR, BRAF, ROS1, KRAS, MET, PIK3CA, AKT1, ALK, CDK4, DDR2, ERBB2, ERBB3, FGFR2, FGFR3, HRAS, KIT, MAP2K1, MAP2K2, MTOR, NRAS, PDGFRA, RAF1, RET) to identify the specific mutations related to targeted therapies. The pathologist or other QHP analyzes the data and composes a report specifying the patient's mutation status. Edit and sign the report and communicate the results to the appropriate caregivers.

Clinical Example (0090U)

A 72-year-old female undergoes biopsy of a suspicious mole on her upper arm. The pathologist examining the biopsy specimen microscopically cannot determine whether it is a benign nevus (mole) or a malignant melanoma. A gene expression profiling test is ordered to establish the correct diagnosis. If the diagnosis is a

★ = Telemedicine   ◀ = Audio-only   ✦ = Add-on code   ✗ = FDA approval pending   # = Resequenced code   ⊘ = Modifier 51 exempt

benign nevus, no further treatment is necessary. If the diagnosis is malignant melanoma, complete surgical excision (and possibly a sentinel lymph node biopsy) is indicated.

Description of Procedure (0090U)

Obtain the existing biopsy specimen from the referring pathology laboratory. Extract RNA from the neoplasm and use a clinically validated qRT-PCR method to determine the expression levels of 14 genes known to be overexpressed in malignant melanomas and 9 reference genes. Compare the expression levels of the 14 melanoma-specific genes to the baseline expression of the 9 reference genes using a proprietary algorithm to produce a clinically reportable numeric score.

Clinical Example (0285U)

An 80-year-old male presents with high-grade prostate cancer. Blood is obtained before and after pelvic radiation treatment to evaluate risk for radiation toxicity.

Description of Procedure (0285U)

Prepare plasma cell-free DNA (cfDNA) from a blood specimen and quantify using branched chain DNA technology. A qualified laboratory professional compiles the report with the cfDNA level and risk of radiation toxicity, which is communicated to the ordering provider.

Clinical Example (0286U)

An 11-year-old female with relapsed acute lymphocytic leukemia is treated with continuing chemotherapy, including thiopurines in combination with methotrexate, vincristine, and oral prednisolone. A blood sample is submitted for CEP72, NUDT15, and TPMT pharmacogenetic testing to assess to patient's ability to clear toxic thiopurine metabolites and to assess her risk for vincristine-induced peripheral neuropathy (VIPN).

Description of Procedure (0286U)

Isolate high-quality genomic DNA from whole blood or saliva and subject to hydrolysis probe RT-PCR of the TPMT, NUDT15 genes for the common variants (ie, TPMT*2, *3, *4, *8, *24; NUDT15*2, *3, *4, *5, *6, *7, *8, *9, g.48045719 + g.48045720, g.48037847 + g.48037849; CEP72 rs924607). The pathologist or other QHP analyzes the data and composes a report.

Clinical Example (0287U)

A 41-year-old female presents with a 2.5-cm thyroid nodule with no suspicious lymph nodes on ultrasound. Fine-needle aspiration (FNA) cytology was malignant. The FNA sample was submitted to assess risk and plan the appropriate surgery.

Description of Procedure (0287U)

Analyze DNA and mRNA isolated from a thyroid fine-needle aspirate or from FFPE tissue by targeted next-generation sequencing to test for genomic alterations in 112 genes. Subject the findings to algorithmic analysis and report the risk category to the ordering provider.

Clinical Example (0288U)

A 50-year-old male with NSCLC follow up with his surgeon. Tumor tissue is submitted to determine patient recurrence risk and to plan appropriate chemotherapy.

Description of Procedure (0288U)

Perform quantitative PCR using RNA from FFPE lung tumor tissue. Combine algorithmic interpretation of RNA expression from 14 genes to generate a risk score (low, intermediate, high). A qualified laboratory professional reviews the findings and results are communicated to the ordering physician.

Clinical Example (0289U)

A 55-year-old female presents with forgetfulness, depression, stress, and a family history of dementia. Blood is obtained to objectively assess biomarkers for her memory functioning, predict short-term risk and long-term risk for clinical worsening and developing Alzheimer disease, as well as to inform treatment.

Description of Procedure (0289U)

Isolate RNA from blood and sequence 24 genes associated with Alzheimer disease to determine biomarker gene expression levels. Apply a proprietary algorithm. A qualified laboratory professional compiles the report that is communicated to the ordering provider detailing risk and medication suggestions.

Clinical Example (0290U)

A 35-year-old male presents with limiting back pain, depression, and substance abuse history. Blood is obtained to assess biomarkers for his pain intensity, predict short- and long-term risk of increasing pain, and treatment planning.

Description of Procedure (0290U)

Isolate RNA from blood and sequence 36 genes associated with pain to determine biomarker gene expression levels. Apply a proprietary algorithm. A qualified laboratory professional compiles the report that is communicated to the ordering provider detailing risk and medication suggestions.

Clinical Example (0291U)

A 25-year-old female presents with a history of depression, a poor response to antidepressants, and occasional suicidal ideation. Blood is obtained to assess biomarkers for her mood state, predict short- and long-term risk of worsening mood, and treatment planning.

Description of Procedure (0291U)

Isolate RNA from blood and sequence 144 genes associated with mood disorders to determine biomarker gene expression levels. Apply a proprietary algorithm. A qualified laboratory professional compiles the report that is communicated to the ordering provider detailing risk and medication suggestions.

Clinical Example (0292U)

A 23-year-old male presents with suicidal thoughts, depression, post-traumatic stress disorder (PTSD), and chronic pain. Blood is obtained to assess biomarkers for his stress levels, predict short- and long-term risk of increasing stress, and treatment planning.

Description of Procedure (0292U)

Isolate RNA from blood and sequence 72 genes associated with stress disorders to determine biomarker gene expression levels. Apply a proprietary algorithm. A qualified laboratory professional compiles the report that is communicated to the ordering provider detailing risk and medication suggestions.

Clinical Example (0293U)

A 23-year-old male veteran presents with suicidal thoughts and a history of depression, PTSD, and chronic pain. Blood is obtained to assess biomarkers for his current suicidality state, predict short- and long-term risk of suicide, and treatment planning.

Description of Procedure (0293U)

Isolate RNA from blood and sequence 54 genes associated with suicide risk to determine biomarker gene expression levels. Apply a proprietary algorithm. A qualified laboratory professional compiles the report that is communicated to the ordering provider detailing risk and medication suggestions.

Clinical Example (0294U)

A 53-year-old male presents with past depression, stress, decreased physical energy, and concentration ability. Blood is obtained to assess biomarkers to predict longevity, short- and long-term risk of death, and treatment planning.

Description of Procedure (0294U)

Isolate RNA from blood and sequence 18 genes associated with longevity to determine biomarker gene expression levels. Apply a proprietary algorithm. A qualified laboratory professional compiles the report that is communicated to the ordering provider detailing mortality risk and medication suggestions.

Clinical Example (0295U)

A 65-year-old female with ductal carcinoma in situ has tissue submitted for immunohistochemistry and algorithmic analysis with four clinicopathologic factors.

Description of Procedure (0295U)

Perform immunochemistry for 7 biomarkers on tissue sections to determine protein expression of 7 markers. Combine expression results with four clinicopathologic factors and apply an algorithm to produce a risk of recurrence and benefit from radiation therapy. A qualified laboratory professional generates a report that is reviewed by a pathologist and communicated to the ordering physician.

Clinical Example (0296U)

A 65-year-old asymptomatic male presents with a 30 pack-per-year smoking history. Given his smoking history and age, a saliva sample is submitted to assess the patient's oral cancer risk.

Description of Procedure (0296U)

Extract mRNA from saliva and analyze by high-throughput sequencing. Analyze the molecular features using a proprietary algorithm to determine the presence or absence of an oral malignancy. A qualified laboratory professional compiles results, reviews, and reports to the ordering provider.

Clinical Example (0297U)

A 20-year-old male presents with a mediastinal hepatosplenic gamma delta T-cell lymphoma. His oncologist submits whole blood and biopsy of the mediastinal mass for whole genome sequencing comparative analysis to identify specific drug therapies or entry into a clinical trial.

★ = Telemedicine   ◀ = Audio-only   ✚ = Add-on code   ⁄ = FDA approval pending   # = Resequenced code   ⊘ = Modifier 51 exempt

Description of Procedure (0297U)

Isolate high-quality DNA from normal tissue and malignant tissue and perform whole genome sequencing to identify variants present only in the malignant tissue. A qualified laboratory professional prepares a report suggesting treatment options. Review the report and send to the ordering physician.

Clinical Example (0298U)

A 20-year-old male presents with a mediastinal hepatosplenic gamma delta T-cell lymphoma. His oncologist submits whole blood and biopsy of the mediastinal mass for whole transcriptome comparative analysis to identify specific drug therapies or entry into a clinical trial.

Description of Procedure (0298U)

RNA isolated from normal tissue and malignant tissue undergoes whole transcriptome sequencing to identify expression level changes and chimeric transcripts present only in the malignant tissue. A qualified laboratory professional prepares a report suggesting treatment options. Review the report and send to the ordering physician.

Clinical Example (0299U)

A 20-year-old male presents with a mediastinal hepatosplenic gamma delta T-cell lymphoma. His oncologist submits whole blood and biopsy of the mediastinal mass for whole genome optical mapping comparative analysis to identify specific drug therapies or entry into a clinical trial.

Description of Procedure (0299U)

Isolate ultra-high molecular weight DNA and normal and malignant tissue undergoes whole genome optical genome mapping to identify structural variants present only in the malignant tissue. A qualified laboratory professional prepares a report suggesting treatment options. Review the report and send to the ordering physician.

Clinical Example (0300U)

A 20-year-old male presents with a mediastinal hepatosplenic gamma delta T-cell lymphoma. His oncologist submits whole blood and biopsy of the mediastinal mass for whole genome sequencing and optical genome mapping comparative analysis to identify specific drug therapies or entry into a clinical trial.

Description of Procedure (0300U)

Isolate ultra-high molecular weight DNA and perform normal and malignant tissue and whole genome sequencing and optical genome mapping to identify variants present only in the malignant tissue. A qualified laboratory professional prepares a report suggesting treatment options. Review the report and send to the ordering physician.

Clinical Example (0301U)

A 22-year-old male presents with poor appetite, fatigue, fever, joint pain, and adenopathy following a recent cat scratch on his left arm. Blood is submitted for evaluation of cat scratch disease (Bartonellosis).

Description of Procedure (0301U)

Extract high-quality DNA from blood or body fluid, and detected Bartonella DNA is counted using droplet digital PCR. A qualified laboratory professional evaluates a graphic representation of the droplet distribution, composes a report, and sends it to the ordering provider.

Clinical Example (0302U)

A 22-year-old male presents with poor appetite, fatigue, fever, joint pain, and adenopathy following a recent cat scratch on his left arm. Blood is submitted for evaluation of cat scratch disease (Bartonellosis).

Description of Procedure (0302U)

Inoculate blood or body fluid into Bartonella alpha proteobacteria growth medium liquid enrichment and incubate for 7 days. Extract high-quality DNA, and detected Bartonella DNA is counted by droplet digital PCR. A qualified laboratory professional evaluates a graphic representation of the droplet distribution, composes a report, and sends it to the ordering provider.

Clinical Example (0303U)

A 32-year-old female with increasing sickle cell crises is treated and compliant with her hydroxyurea and folic acid treatment. She has done well on hydroxyurea but her physician suspects possible nocturnal hypoxia leading to pain crises. Whole blood is submitted to assess her likelihood of adverse events from nocturnal hypoxia.

Pathology and Laboratory 80047-89398, 0001U-0284U

Description of Procedure (0303U)

Inject whole blood into protein-functionalized microfluidic channels at physiologically relevant shear stress. Remove non-adherent cells using a buffer wash. Scan the middle of the microchannel using light microscopy and count the number of adherent cells. Determine red blood cell (RBC)-adhesion index and report to the ordering physician.

Clinical Example (0304U)

A 28-year-old male with recurrent sickle cell crises and one episode of acute chest pain is advised to begin hydroxyurea therapy. Whole blood is submitted before hydroxyurea treatment to correlate medication use, after 3 to 6 months, with clinical improvement and decreased RBC-adhesion under normoxic conditions.

Description of Procedure (0304U)

Inject whole blood into protein-functionalized microfluidic channels at a single physiologically relevant shear stress. Remove non-adherent cells using a buffer wash. Scan the middle of the microchannel using light microscopy and count the number of adherent cells. Determine RBC-adhesion index and report to the ordering provider.

Clinical Example (0305U)

A 22-year-old male with recurrent sickle cell pain crises is not responsive to hydroxyurea, despite compliance with treatment. Treatment modification is planned. Whole blood is submitted to determine RBC deformity before treatment to correlate hydroxyurea treatment use after 6 months.

Description of Procedure (0305U)

Shear whole blood between two concentric cylinders and apply shear stress. A QHP reviews the results and reports the finding to the ordering provider.

Clinical Example (0306U)

A 64-year-old male with stage II NSCLC has a blood sample submitted to create a patient-specific profile to be used for subsequent monitoring for minimal residual disease (MRD).

Description of Procedure (0306U)

Isolate cell-free DNA from plasma. Perform targeted sequencing analysis and create a patient-specific profile. Generate a qualitative report and send to the ordering provider. Save profile results for future comparisons.

Clinical Example (0307U)

A 65-year-old male with stage II NSCLC has completed surgery and adjuvant chemotherapy. His oncologist submits a blood sample for comparison to a previously collected patient-specific profile to evaluate for minimal residual disease.

Description of Procedure (0307U)

Isolate cell-free DNA from plasma. Use targeted sequencing analysis with a patient-specific panel using a previously analyzed specimen to determine the presence or absence of tumor-specific DNA. Generate and send a qualitative report to the ordering physician.

Clinical Example (0308U)

A 60-year-old male presents with a history of type 2 diabetes, hypertension, and a family history of heart disease. He recently experienced shortness of breath with exertion. Plasma is submitted to assess his risk for obstructive coronary artery disease.

Description of Procedure (0308U)

Combine plasma immunoassay results for high sensitivity (HS) troponin, adiponectin, and kidney injury molecule-1 (KIM-1) using a proprietary algorithm to generate a risk score for obstructive coronary artery disease. A qualified laboratory professional reviews the results and issues a report to the ordering provider.

Clinical Example (0309U)

A 57-year-old female presents with diabetes, peripheral artery disease, and hypertension with recent dyspnea on exertion. Plasma is submitted to determine the risk of a major adverse cardiac event.

Description of Procedure (0309U)

Perform plasma immunoassay and combine results for NT-proBNP, osteopontin, tissue inhibitor of metalloproteinase-1 (TIMP-1), and KIM-1 using a proprietary algorithm to generate a risk score for cardiovascular disease. A qualified laboratory professional reviews the results and issues a report to the ordering provider.

Clinical Example (0310U)

A 2-year-old male presents with fever, rash, diarrhea, and strawberry tongue. Plasma is submitted to determine the likelihood of Kawasaki disease.

★ = Telemedicine   ◀ = Audio-only   ✚ = Add-on code   ✐ = FDA approval pending   # = Resequenced code   ⊘ = Modifier 51 exempt

Description of Procedure (0310U)

Perform plasma immunoassay and combine results for NT-proBNP, C-reactive protein, and T-uptake using a proprietary algorithm to generate a risk score for Kawasaki disease. A qualified laboratory professional reviews the results and issues a report to the ordering provider.

Clinical Example (0311U)

A 68-year-old female with diabetes mellitus presents to the emergency department with dysuria and increased urinary frequency. Blood cultures detect E. coli, and an aliquot of the positive culture is submitted to determine which antibiotic is best to treat the infection.

Description of Procedure (0311U)

Subject a positive blood culture to phenotypic minimum inhibitory concentration (MIC)–based antimicrobial susceptibility testing. The laboratory provides the MIC value with interpretation of susceptibility or resistance to various antimicrobials. A qualified laboratory professional reviews the findings and prepares a report for the ordering provider.

Clinical Example (0312U)

A 28-year-old female presents with a 5-year history of arthralgia, myalgia, and fatigue, not responsive to non-steroidal anti-inflammatory drugs (NSAIDs) along with other findings suggestive of autoimmune disease. Serum and whole blood are submitted to better characterize her presentation.

Description of Procedure (0312U)

Test plasma or serum for 8 biomarkers (ie, anti-dsDNA, anti-CCP, ANA, anti-Sm, anti-SS-B/La, anti-CENP, anti-Scl-70, anti-Jo-1) by enzyme-linked immunosorbent assay (ELISA) and indirect immunofluorescence (IIF) and test whole blood by flow cytometry for 2 CB-CAPs (ie, EC4d and BC4d). A proprietary algorithm yields a negative, tier-2 positive, or tier-1 positive result corresponding to an increasing likelihood of systemic lupus erythematosus (SLE) when placed in the appropriate clinical context.

Clinical Example (0313U)

A 51-year-old male is referred with abdominal pain and a 2.8-cm pancreatic cyst. Pancreatic cyst fluid obtained at the time of FNA biopsy is sent to establish the cyst type and potential risk of progression.

Description of Procedure (0313U)

Analyze DNA and mRNA isolated from a pancreatic cyst fluid sample by targeted next-generation sequencing to test for genomic alterations in 74 genes and by qRT-PCR for expression of the CEA (CEACAM5) gene. Subject the findings to algorithmic analysis to categorize as negative or positive for specific alterations associated with different cyst types and risk of progression. Issue a report to the ordering provider.

Clinical Example (0314U)

A 55-year-old female undergoes biopsy of a suspicious "mole" on her left cheek. The biopsy is indeterminate by standard microscopy. A gene expression profiling test is ordered to establish the diagnosis.

Description of Procedure (0314U)

Extract RNA from a FFPE specimen. Compare the expression levels of 32 content genes to the expression of 3 reference genes using RT-PCR and evaluate using a proprietary algorithm to produce a categorical result. A qualified laboratory professional evaluates the findings and provides results to the ordering provider.

Clinical Example (0315U)

A 74-year-old male undergoes biopsy of a suspicious lesion on his scalp that is determined to be an invasive cutaneous squamous cell carcinoma. A gene expression profiling test is ordered to assess the patient's risk for regional or distant metastasis.

Description of Procedure (0315U)

Extract RNA from a FFPE specimen. Compare the expression levels of 34 content genes to the expression of 6 reference genes using RT-PCR and evaluate using a proprietary algorithm to produce a categorical risk result (ie, class 1, class 2A, class 2B). A qualified laboratory professional evaluates the findings and provides the results to the ordering provider.

Clinical Example (0316U)

A 38-year-old male presents with a history of tick exposure after a hunting trip one month ago with a bullseye rash at the bite site and flu-like symptoms. Urine is submitted for detection of possible OspA protein.

Description of Procedure (0316U)

Inoculate urine with nanoparticles to capture OspA protein and then centrifuge to concentrate the protein target. Wash concentrate and test to detect OspA protein. A qualified laboratory professional evaluates results and sends a report to the ordering provider.

Clinical Example (0317U)

A 49-year-old nonsmoking male presents with a 1-cm solid nodule as an incidental finding on CT scan. To evaluate next steps, blood is submitted to determine the risk for lung cancer.

Description of Procedure (0317U)

Whole blood undergoes immunomagnetic separation and cells are fixed to glass slides. Perform fluorescence in situ hybridization (FISH) for 3q29, 3p22.1, 10q22.3, and 10cen and scan using an automated microscope. A qualified laboratory professional analyzes images using an algorithm. A pathologist or other QHP reviews the assessment and issues a report to the ordering provider.

Clinical Example (0318U)

A 6-year-old female presents to a geneticist with delays and hypotonia. The patient also has a history of feeding difficulties, obesity, and behavior problems. Blood is submitted for evaluation of congenital epigenetic disorders.

Description of Procedure (0318U)

Extract DNA from peripheral blood to undergo bisulfite conversion and PCR amplification. Hybridize DNA to a methylation microarray chip with over 850,000 CpG sites across the genome used to assess genome-wide methylation. Analyze the results using a proprietary algorithm to identify validated epigenetic signatures and methylation abnormalities. A qualified laboratory professional generates and issues a clinical report to the ordering provider.

Clinical Example (0319U)

A 26-year-old female with sickle cell nephropathy presents with progression and requires a kidney transplant. A compatible live donor was identified. Pretransplant blood was submitted to determine the risk of early (6 months) acute rejection to assist in immunosuppression management.

Description of Procedure (0319U)

Isolate high-quality genomic RNA from whole blood and subject to targeted transcriptome next-generation sequencing. Profile a select transcriptomic signature using an empirically derived algorithm. Report results as a risk score for early acute kidney transplant rejection. The pathologist or other QHP analyzes the data and composes a report.

Clinical Example (0320U)

A 60-year-old male post-kidney transplant presents with a low-grade fever and mild weight gain but a normal estimated glomerular filtration rate (eGFR). Blood was submitted to determine the risk for clinical or subclinical acute cellular rejection.

Description of Procedure (0320U)

Isolate high-quality genomic RNA from whole blood and subject to targeted transcriptome next-generation sequencing. Profile a select transcriptomic signature using an empirically derived algorithm. Report results as a risk score for kidney transplant rejection. The pathologist or other QHP analyzes the data and composes a report.

Clinical Example (0321U)

A 72-year-old female with recurrent urinary tract infection (UTI) is hospitalized with urosepsis. A urine specimen is submitted for organism identification and antibiotic resistance.

Description of Procedure (0321U)

Submit urine for analysis by PCR for Acinetobacter baumannii, Candida albicans, Candida glabrata, Citrobacter freundii, Coagulase Negative Staph, Enterobacter aerogenes, Enterobacter cloacae, Enterococcus faecalis, Enterococcus faecium, Escherichia coli, Klebsiella oxytoca, Klebsiella pneumoniae, Morganella morganii, Pantoea agglomerans, Proteus mirabilis, Proteus vulgaris, Pseudomonas aeruginosa, Serratia marcescens, Staphylococcus aureus, and Streptococcus agalactiae. Determine antimicrobial resistance (ABR) by PCR using a culture-based antimicrobial susceptibility test (CTX-M group 1, 2, 9, 8/25, TEM, mecA, QnrA, QnrS, Qnr B, vanA1, vanA2, vanB, dfrA5, dfrA1, Sul1, Sul2, nfsA, SHV, KPC) for specific pathogen isolates. A laboratory professional reviews the results and issues a report to the ordering provider.

★ = Telemedicine   ◀ = Audio-only   ✛ = Add-on code   ✗ = FDA approval pending   # = Resequenced code   ⊘ = Modifier 51 exempt

Clinical Example (0322U)

An 18-month-old scores well below expected developmental milestones using the modified checklist for autism in toddlers (MCHAT). Based on this and other clinical information, autism is suspected. Fasting plasma is submitted to evaluate the patient further for autism spectrum disorder (ASD).

Description of Procedure (0322U)

Subject plasma to LC-MS/MS analysis to measure levels of 3-indoxyl sulfate, 4-ethylphenyl sulfate, CMPF, cortisone, decanoylcarnitine, dodecanedioic acid, glutarylcarnitine, hexanoylcarnitine, hydroxybutyryl-carnitine, indoleacetic acid, indolelactic acid, octanoylcarnitine, palmitoylcarnitine, and p-cresol sulfate. Perform analysis to compare the levels to the metabolic subtypes associated with ASD. Determine the quantitative measurement of the metabolites and identify the presence of any metabolic imbalance. A qualified laboratory professional reviews and reports results to the ordering provider.

Clinical Example (0323U)

A 50-year-old female presents following multiple hospitalizations for symptoms related to SLE and anti-cardiolipin antibody syndrome. Cerebrospinal fluid (CSF) studies revealed a progressive, worsening lymphocytic pleocytosis with low glucose and high protein. CSF was submitted for metagenomic next-generation sequencing.

Description of Procedure (0323U)

Extract nucleic acid from a CSF specimen and prepare separate sequencing libraries for DNA and RNA. Following sequencing, bioinformatic data analysis identifies and classifies the microbial reads based on comparison to a curated, validated database and compared to background control samples. A qualified laboratory professional interprets the findings and issues a report to the ordering physician.

Clinical Example (0324U)

A 65-year-old female with epithelial ovarian cancer has fresh tumor tissue submitted to assess the tumor's response to carboplatin, doxorubicin, gemcitabine, and paclitaxel.

Description of Procedure (0324U)

Grow cells isolated from tumor specimens in culture as spheroids, expose to poly (ADP-ribose) polymerase (PARP) inhibitors (carboplatin, doxorubicin, gemcitabine, paclitaxel), and assess for cell viability via luminescence. A qualified laboratory professional reviews the data and issues a report indicating tumor-specific drug responses.

Clinical Example (0325U)

A 65-year-old female with epithelial ovarian cancer has fresh tissue from the tumor submitted to assess the tumor's response to PARP inhibitors.

Description of Procedure (0325U)

Grow cells isolated from tumor specimens in culture as spheroids, expose to PARP inhibitors (niraparib, olaparib, rucaparib, velparib), and assess for cell viability via luminescence. A qualified laboratory professional reviews the data and issues a report indicating tumor-specific drug responses.

Clinical Example (0326U)

A 65-year-old female with stage IV lung adenocarcinoma had a blood sample submitted to examine the patient's tumor genomic composition, including tumor-mutation burden and microsatellite instability.

Description of Procedure (0326U)

Isolate cell-free circulating DNA from whole blood and subject to targeted next-generation sequencing of 83 genes for nucleotide substitutions, insertion-deletion mutations (indels), copy number amplifications, genomic fusions/rearrangements, tumor mutational burden, and microsatellite instability. The pathologist or other QHP analyzes the data and composes a report.

Clinical Example (0327U)

A 30-year-old female presents in her first trimester of pregnancy. Blood is submitted for single nucleotide polymorphism analysis from cell-free DNA to assess risk for abnormalities in chromosomes 13, 18, and 21.

Description of Procedure (0327U)

Extract cell-free DNA and perform targeted amplification and sequencing of single nucleotide polymorphisms. Analyze maternal and fetal genotype information to determine risk for aneuploidy. A qualified laboratory professional composes a report specifying the risk of trisomy 13, 18, and 21, (and fetal sex, if requested). Results are communicated to the ordering physician.

Clinical Example (0328U)

A 70-year-old male presents for spinal fusion. The provider submits urine for drug testing to identify the presence of drugs contraindicated at the time of surgery.

Description of Procedure (0328U)

Analyze urine by LC-MS/MS to identify and quantitate total drugs and metabolites present. Perform specimen validity. A qualified laboratory professional reviews results using an algorithm to determine adverse event risk and reports the findings to the ordering provider.

Clinical Example (0329U)

A 65-year-old male was recently diagnosed with metastatic lung cancer. An FFPE tissue specimen is submitted for comprehensive tumor profiling to assess the patient's suitability for treatment with targeted therapies.

Description of Procedure (0329U)

Extract DNA from tumor and normal samples. Isolate RNA from the tumor sample. Subject each separately to next-generation sequencing. DNA analysis identifies nucleotide substitutions, indels, copy number amplifications and deletions, and RNA analysis identifies genomic fusions/rearrangements and transcript variants. Calculate tumor-mutation burden and microsatellite instability from DNA mutational results. Query cancer-specific mutations against a proprietary gene-drug database to identify therapeutic associations. The pathologist or other QHP analyzes the data and composes a report.

Clinical Example (0330U)

A 32-year-old female presents with vulvovaginal itching, burning, irritation, and pelvic pain. A vaginal swab is submitted to determine possible infectious cause(s) of the patient's symptoms.

Description of Procedure (0330U)

Evaluate a vaginal swab and/or dirty catch urine using high-throughput molecular PCR to identify 27 possible organisms, including Atopobium vaginae, BVAB2, Chlamydia trachomatis, Enterococcus faecalis, Escherichia coli, Gardnerella vaginalis, Haemophilus ducreyi, Lactobacillus crispatus, Lactobacillus jensenii, Megasphaera species (type 1), Mobiluncus curtisii, Mobiluncus mulieris, Mycoplasma genitalium, Mycoplasma hominis, Ureaplasma urealyticum, Neisseria gonorrhoeae, Staphylococcus aureus, Streptococcus agalactiae (GBS), Treponema pallidum (syphilis), Candida albicans, Candida glabrata, Candida

krusei, Candida parapsilosis, Candida tropicalis, Trichomonas vaginalis, herpes simplex virus type 1 (HSV-1), and herpes simplex virus type 2 (HSV-2). A qualified laboratory professional reviews results and reports the findings to the ordering provider.

Clinical Example (0331U)

A 40-year-old female presents with fatigue, shortness of breath, and a white blood cell (WBC) count with 80% blasts. A bone marrow aspirate sample is submitted for optical genome mapping for cancer cytogenomic analysis.

Description of Procedure (0331U)

Isolate DNA from whole blood or bone marrow and subject to optical genome mapping for copy number variants and fusions/rearrangements. The pathologist or other QHP analyzes the data and composes a report.

Clinical Example (0332U)

A 48-year-old male with metastatic urothelial cancer visits his oncologist to discuss treatment options. His physician submits a blood sample to assess the patient's response to anti-PD-L1 therapy.

Description of Procedure (0332U)

Whole blood undergoes chemical fixation, enzyme digestion, ligation, and purification to isolate DNA fragments. Amplifies DNA using specific primers and probes using qPCR. An algorithm assigns a probability score, defining the patient's response profile to immune checkpoint inhibitor (ICI) therapies as "low probability" or "high probability." Issue a report to the ordering physician.

Clinical Example (0333U)

A 65-year-old male presents to a hepatologist with liver cirrhosis. The patient is monitored with ultrasound every 6 months to detect early-stage liver cancer. The hepatologist orders blood test, instead of an ultrasound.

Description of Procedure (0333U)

Draw blood to perform next-generation sequencing of 77 CpG sites (28 genes) using cfDNA from plasma. Use an immunoanalyzer to determine the concentrations of 3 serum proteins: alpha-fetoprotein (AFP), AFP-L3%, and des-gamma-carboxyprothrombin (DCP). Generate an algorithm report.

★ = Telemedicine　◀ = Audio-only　✛ = Add-on code　✔ = FDA approval pending　# = Resequenced code　⊘ = Modifier 51 exempt

Clinical Example (0334U)

A 65-year-old female with stage IV lung adenocarcinoma has a tissue sample submitted to examine her tumor genomic composition, including tumor-mutation burden and microsatellite instability.

Description of Procedure (0334U)

Isolate tumor DNA from FFPE tumor tissue and subject to targeted next-generation sequencing of 84 genes for nucleotide substitutions, indels, copy number amplifications, genomic fusions/rearrangements, tumor mutational burden, and microsatellite instability. The pathologist or other QHP analyzes the data and composes a report.

Clinical Example (0335U)

A 35-year-old pregnant female presents for her 12-week fetal ultrasound, which shows abnormal nuchal translucency. Amniotic fluid is submitted to assess the fetus for constitutional/heritable genomic changes.

Description of Procedure (0335U)

Isolate and sequence amniotic genomic DNA. A clinical variant scientist examines variants and correlates them with clinical findings, using American College of Medical Genetics and Genomics (ACMG) guidelines. The analyst or other QHP composes and reviews the report and sends to the ordering provider.

Clinical Example (0336U)

A 35-year-old pregnant female presents for her 12-week fetal ultrasound, which shows abnormal nuchal translucency. A sample from the parent is submitted for comparison with the proband sample.

Description of Procedure (0336U)

Isolate genomic DNA from blood and sequence. A clinical variant scientist examines variants and correlates them with a proband sample. The analyst or other QHP composes and reviews the report and sends to the ordering provider.

Clinical Example (0337U)

A 60-year-old male with multiple myeloma presents to his hematologist for his quarterly follow-up. Bone marrow biopsy 6 months ago indicated complete response (CR). Examination and laboratory test results 3 months ago suggested CR, but assay showed elevated plasma cells. A repeat specimen is submitted to further evaluate for recurrence.

Description of Procedure (0337U)

Subject blood to fixation, immunomagnetic selection, and immunofluorescence staining for protein biomarkers associated with malignant and normal plasma cells. Stained cells are detected, identified, morphologically characterized, and enumerated relative to control standards via proprietary imaging software. A qualified laboratory professional reviews and reports results to the ordering provider.

Clinical Example (0338U)

A 38-year-old female with a history of metastatic triple negative breast cancer and bone metastasis treated with standard chemotherapy now has multiple lung lesions inaccessible to biopsy. The oncologist submits a blood sample to evaluate CTC-HER2 status to evaluate the potential need for HER2 targeted therapy.

Description of Procedure (0338U)

Subject blood to fixation, immunomagnetic selection, and immunofluorescence staining for protein biomarkers associated with tumor cells. Stained cells are identified, morphologically characterized, enumerated, and scored for HER2 protein biomarker positivity relative to controls via proprietary imaging software. A qualified laboratory professional reviews images and generates a report with absolute and HER2-positive cell count. Send reviewed report to the ordering physician.

Clinical Example (0339U)

A 45-year-old male presents with an abnormal prostate-specific antigen (PSA) test. Urine is submitted to evaluate risk for prostate cancer.

Description of Procedure (0339U)

Subject urine collected following digital rectal examination to RT-PCR to quantify the levels of HOXC6 and DLX1 mRNA levels relative to KLK3 mRNA. Combine mRNA measurements using an algorithm that includes the patient's age, serum PSA, and DRE findings. Determine the likelihood that biopsy will detect grade group 2 or higher prostate cancer. A qualified laboratory professional reviews and reports results to the ordering provider.

Clinical Example (0340U)

A 65-year-old male presents following curative intent surgery for stage IIb colorectal cancer. Blood is submitted to assess the patient for minimal residual disease.

Description of Procedure (0340U)

Start the test workflow with tumor tissue collection for whole exome sequencing (WES) to detect tumor-associated mutations that are specific to each patient. Extract circulating tumor DNA from blood plasma collected in tubes using proprietary methods. Run customized PCR assays to detect presence or absence of tumor-derived clonal variants within circulating plasma. When at least two tumor-derived variants are detected, issue a report with a positive result and ctDNA quantity. When fewer than two tumor-derived variants are observed, issue a negative result.

Clinical Example (0341U)

A 31-year-old female presents to her physician with a positive noninvasive prenatal screening for DiGeorge syndrome. Maternal blood is submitted to identify risk for presence of the DiGeorge deletion and determine the need for amniocentesis.

Description of Procedure (0341U)

Isolate fetal trophoblasts from maternal blood. Process up to five cells for whole genome amplification and next-generation sequencing. Analyze each cell for aneuploidy and pathogenic deletions or duplications. A qualified laboratory professional interprets the findings (eg, any copy number abnormality) and reports the findings to the ordering physician.

Clinical Example (0342U)

A 64-year-old asymptomatic female presents to her gastrointestinal specialist for annual surveillance for pancreatic cancer, given a strong family history.

Description of Procedure (0342U)

Analyze serum using a multiplex immunoassay for C5, C4, cystatin C, factor B, OPG, gelsolin, IGFBP3, and CA125 and combine with a separately measured CA19-9. Analyze results using a proprietary algorithm predicting risk of pancreatic cancer. A qualified laboratory professional reviews and reports findings to the ordering physician.

Clinical Example (0343U)

A 50-year-old male presents with clinical suspicion of prostate cancer. A urine sample is submitted to determine presence or absence of molecular evidence of prostate cancer.

Description of Procedure (0343U)

Isolate exosomal RNA from urine and assay by high-density real-time qPCR. Summarize and analyze fluorescent signal outputs for 442 small noncoding RNA sequences by a biostatistical algorithm to determine molecular evidence of no-risk, low-risk, intermediate-risk, or high-risk prostate cancer. A qualified laboratory professional reviews the findings and reports the results to the ordering provider.

Clinical Example (0344U)

A 52-year-old male presents with type 2 diabetes, elevated transaminases, and a body mass index of 32. Serum is submitted to determine if the patient is at higher risk of progressive non-alcoholic steatohepatitis (NASH).

Description of Procedure (0344U)

Perform high-pressure liquid chromatography coupled to high resolution mass spectrometry on serum lipid extracts. Combine results using two proprietary algorithms to generate a risk score for non-alcoholic NASH and at-risk NASH. A qualified laboratory professional reviews the results and issues a report to the ordering provider.

Clinical Example (0345U)

A 45-year-old female presents with anxiety and major depressive disorder history. She has been prescribed antidepressants but complains her depressive symptoms have not improved. A cheek swab is submitted for a 15-gene pharmacogenomic panel.

Description of Procedure (0345U)

Isolate DNA from a buccal swab specimen. Perform genotyping and capillary electrophoresis to determine genotypes and to detect specific mutations. Analyze data using a proprietary algorithm, and gene-drug interactions are reported as use-as-directed, moderate gene-drug interaction, or significant gene-drug interaction.

Clinical Example (0346U)

A 60-year-old female with a family history of Alzheimer disease presents to her physician following several episodes of recent confusion. She is back to her cognitive baseline at the visit. Plasma is submitted for amyloid beta 42/40 ratio.

★ = Telemedicine ◀ = Audio-only ✚ = Add-on code ✒ = FDA approval pending # = Resequenced code ⊘ = Modifier 51 exempt

Description of Procedure (0346U)

Immunoprecipitate Aß40 and Aß42 peptides from plasma and then enzymatically digest, desalt, and concentrate by solid-phase extraction, and subject to LC-MS/MS analysis. A qualified laboratory professional quantifies concentrations of both Aß40 and Aß42, and calculates the ratio of Aß42 to Aß40 and report results to the ordering physician.

Clinical Example (0347U)

A 46-year-old male has been unsuccessfully treated with several antidepressant medications. A buccal swab is submitted for a pharmacogenomic panel to evaluate drug metabolism.

Description of Procedure (0347U)

A whole blood or buccal sample undergoes DNA extraction and PCR amplification. Analyze genetic results and assign phenotypes. A qualified laboratory professional approves and reports results to the ordering provider.

Clinical Example (0348U)

A 46-year-old male has been unsuccessfully treated with several antidepressant medications. A buccal swab is submitted for a pharmacogenomic panel to evaluate drug metabolism.

Description of Procedure (0348U)

A whole blood or buccal sample undergoes DNA extraction and PCR amplification. Generate a comprehensive gene and drug report based on the findings. A qualified laboratory professional approves and reports results to the ordering provider.

Clinical Example (0349U)

A 46-year-old male has been unsuccessfully treated with several antidepressant medications. A buccal swab is submitted for a pharmacogenomic panel to evaluate drug metabolism response.

Description of Procedure (0349U)

A blood or buccal sample undergoes DNA extraction and PCR amplification. Generate a comprehensive gene and drug report based on the findings. A qualified laboratory professional approves and reports results to the ordering provider.

Clinical Example (0350U)

A 46-year-old male has been unsuccessfully treated with several antidepressant medications. A buccal swab is submitted for a pharmacogenomic panel to evaluate drug metabolism.

Description of Procedure (0350U)

A blood or buccal sample undergoes DNA extraction and PCR amplification. Analyze genetic results and assign phenotypes. A qualified laboratory professional approves and reports results to the ordering provider.

Clinical Example (0351U)

A 64-year-old male presents with a five-day history of dry cough, fever, weakness, and wheezing. Serum is submitted to evaluate the likelihood of a bacterial or viral infection.

Description of Procedure (0351U)

Evaluate serum biochemically for tumor necrosis factor-related apoptosis-inducing ligand (TRAIL), interferon gamma-induced protein-10 (IP-10), and C-reactive protein. A proprietary algorithm yields a score conveying risk for bacterial vs viral infection. A qualified laboratory professional reviews and reports results to the ordering provider.

Clinical Example (0352U)

A 26-year-old female presents with increased vaginal discharge, foul-smelling odor, and itching for 5 days. Examination is consistent with bacterial vaginosis and vaginitis. A vaginal swab is collected to determine the cause of the symptoms.

Description of Procedure (0352U)

Pipette a sample of the vaginal swab transport media into cartridge and analyze using RT-PCR amplification for detection of target DNA. Positive/negative results for bacterial vaginosis algorithm (BVAB-2, atopobium vaginae, and megasphera type 1), Candida species (C. albicans, C. tropicalis, C. parapsilosis, C. dubliniensis), Candida glabrata/Candida krusei, and Trichomonas vaginalis are reported. The qualified laboratory professional communicates results to the ordering provider.

Clinical Example (0353U)

A 19-year-old male presents with dysuria following recent unprotected oral and vaginal intercourse. A whitish discharge was seen after applying pressure along the penile shaft. Urine is collected for a nucleic acid amplification test (NAAT) to test for Chlamydia trachomatis and Neisseria gonorrhoeae DNA.

Description of Procedure (0353U)

Pipette a sample of the transport media from a collected specimen into a cartridge and analyze using RT-PCR amplification for detection of target DNA. Results for Chlamydia trachomatis and Neisseria gonorrhoeae are reported as postive or negative. A qualified laboratory professional reviews and reports to the ordering provider.

Clinical Example (0354U)

A 37-year-old female presents to her gynecologist. A specimen is submitted to evaluate for the presence of high-risk HPV mRNA E6/E7 expression.

Description of Procedure (0354U)

Isolate nucleic acids from a cervical specimen. Amplify mRNA of E6/E7 high-risk HPV genotypes and analyze to determine presence or absence of each genotype. A qualified laboratory professional prepares a genotype report and sends it to the ordering physician.

★ = Telemedicine   ◀ = Audio-only   ✚ = Add-on code   ✘ = FDA approval pending   # = Resequenced code   ⊘ = Modifier 51 exempt

Medicine

Summary of Additions, Deletions, and Revisions

The summary of changes shows the actual changes that have been made to the code descriptors.

New codes appear with a bullet (●) and are indicated as "Code added." Revised codes are preceded with a triangle (▲). Within revised codes, or if a code symbol has been deleted, the deleted language and code symbol appear with a ~~strikethrough~~, while new text appears <u>underlined</u>.

The ✔ symbol is used to identify codes for vaccines that are pending FDA approval. The # symbol is used to identify codes that have been resequenced. CPT add-on codes are annotated by the ✚ symbol. The ⊘ symbol is used to identify codes that are exempt from the use of modifier 51. The ★ symbol is used to identify codes that may be used for reporting telemedicine services. The ✕ symbol is used to identify a proprietary laboratory analyses (PLA) test that has an identical descriptor as another PLA test. A PLA code that satisfies Category I code criteria and has been accepted by the CPT Editorial Panel is annotated with the ↑↓ symbol. The ◀ symbol is used to identify codes that may be used to report audio-only telemedicine services when appended by modifier 93 (**see Appendix T**).

Code	Description
●0003A	Code added
●0004A	Code added
#●0051A	Code added
#●0052A	Code added
#●0053A	Code added
#●0054A	Code added
#●0071A	Code added
#●0072A	Code added
#●0073A	Code added
#●0074A	Code added
#●0081A	Code added
#●0082A	Code added
#●0083A	Code added
●0013A	Code added
#●0064A	Code added
#●0094A	Code added
▲0031A	Immunization administration by intramuscular injection of severe acute respiratory syndrome coronavirus 2 (SARS-CoV-2) (coronavirus disease [COVID-19]) vaccine, DNA, spike protein, adenovirus type 26 (Ad26) vector, preservative free, 5x10^{10} viral particles/0.5 mL dosage~~;~~; single dose

Code	Description
●0034A	Code added
●0104A	Code added
●0111A	Code added
●0112A	Code added
#●91305	Code added
#●91307	Code added
#●91308	Code added
#●91306	Code added
#●91311	Code added
#●91309	Code added
#✔●91310	Code added
#✔●90584	Code added
✔●90678	Code added
▲90739	Hepatitis B vaccine (HepB), CpG-adjuvanted, adult dosage, 2 dose or 4 dose schedule, for intramuscular use
▲92065	Orthoptic training; performed by a physician or other qualified health care professional
●92066	Code added
▲92229	point-of-care autonomousautomated analysis and report, unilateral or bilateral
▲92284	Diagnostic Ddark adaptation examination with interpretation and report
+▲93568	for nonselective pulmonary arterial angiography (List separately in addition to code for primary procedure)
+●93569	Code added
#+●93573	Code added
#+●93574	Code added
#+●93575	Code added
●95919	Code added
●96202	Code added
+●96203	Code added
▲98975	Remote therapeutic monitoring (eg, respiratory system status, musculoskeletal system status, therapy adherence, therapy response); initial set-up and patient education on use of equipment
▲98976	device(s) supply with scheduled (eg, daily) recording(s) and/or programmed alert(s) transmission to monitor respiratory system, each 30 days
▲98977	device(s) supply with scheduled (eg, daily) recording(s) and/or programmed alert(s) transmission to monitor musculoskeletal system, each 30 days
●98978	Code added

★=Telemedicine ◀=Audio-only +=Add-on code ✔=FDA approval pending #=Resequenced code ⊘=Modifier 51 exempt

Medicine 90281-99607

Medicine

Immunization Administration for Vaccines/Toxoids

▶Report vaccine immunization administration codes (90460, 90461, 90471-90474, 0001A, 0002A, 0003A, 0004A, 0011A, 0012A, 0013A, 0021A, 0022A, 0031A, 0034A, 0041A, 0042A, 0051A, 0052A, 0053A, 0054A, 0064A, 0071A, 0072A, 0073A, 0074A, 0081A, 0082A, 0083A, 0094A, 0104A, 0111A, 0112A) in addition to the vaccine and toxoid code(s) (90476-90759, 91300-91311).◀

Report codes 90460 and 90461 only when the physician or other qualified health care professional provides face-to-face counseling of the patient/family during the administration of a vaccine other than when performed for severe acute respiratory syndrome coronavirus 2 (SARS-CoV-2) (coronavirus disease [COVID-19]) vaccines. For immunization administration of any vaccine, other than SARS-CoV-2 (coronavirus disease [COVID-19]) vaccines, that is not accompanied by face-to-face physician or other qualified health care professional counseling to the patient/family/guardian or for administration of vaccines to patients over 18 years of age, report codes 90471-90474. (See also **Instructions for Use of the CPT Codebook** for definition of reporting qualifications.)

▶Report 0001A, 0002A, 0003A, 0004A, 0011A, 0012A, 0013A, 0021A, 0022A, 0031A, 0034A, 0041A, 0042A, 0051A, 0052A, 0053A, 0054A, 0064A, 0071A, 0072A, 0073A, 0074A, 0081A, 0082A, 0083A, 0094A, 0104A, 0111A, 0112A for immunization administration of SARS-CoV-2 (coronavirus disease [COVID-19]) vaccines only. Each administration code is specific to each individual vaccine product (eg, 91300-91311), the dosage schedule (eg, first dose, second dose), and counseling, when performed. The appropriate administration code is chosen based on the type of vaccine and the specific dose number the patient receives in the schedule. For example, 0012A is reported for the second dose of vaccine 91301. Do not report 90460-90474 for the administration of SARS-CoV-2 (coronavirus disease [COVID-19]) vaccines. Codes related to SARS-CoV-2 (coronavirus disease [COVID-19]) vaccine administration are listed in Appendix Q, with their associated vaccine code descriptors, vaccine administration codes, patient age, vaccine manufacturer, vaccine name(s), National Drug Code (NDC) Labeler Product ID, and interval between doses. In order to report these codes, the vaccine must fulfill the code descriptor and must be the vaccine represented by the manufacturer and vaccine name listed in Appendix Q.

If a significant separately identifiable evaluation and management service (eg, new or established patient office or other outpatient services [99202-99215], office or other outpatient consultations [99242, 99243, 99244, 99245], emergency department services [99281-99285], preventive medicine services [99381-99429]) is performed, the appropriate E/M service code should be reported in addition to the vaccine and toxoid administration codes.◀

Rationale

In accordance with the deletion of code 99241, the Immunization Administration for Vaccines/Toxoids guidelines have been revised to reflect this change.

Refer to the codebook and the Rationale for code 99241 for a full discussion of this change.

90460 Immunization administration through 18 years of age via any route of administration, with counseling by physician or other qualified health care professional; first or only component of each vaccine or toxoid administered

+ 90461 each additional vaccine or toxoid component administered (List separately in addition to code for primary procedure)

(Use 90460 for each vaccine administered. For vaccines with multiple components [combination vaccines], report 90460 in conjunction with 90461 for each additional component in a given vaccine)

▶(Do not report 90460, 90461 in conjunction with 91300-91311, unless both a severe acute respiratory syndrome coronavirus 2 [SARS-CoV-2] [coronavirus disease {COVID-19}] vaccine/toxoid product and at least one vaccine/toxoid product from 90476-90759 are administered at the same encounter)◀

90471 Immunization administration (includes percutaneous, intradermal, subcutaneous, or intramuscular injections); 1 vaccine (single or combination vaccine/toxoid)

(Do not report 90471 in conjunction with 90473)

+ 90472 each additional vaccine (single or combination vaccine/toxoid) (List separately in addition to code for primary procedure)

(Use 90472 in conjunction with 90460, 90471, 90473)

▶(Do not report 90471, 90472 in conjunction with 91300-91311, unless both a severe acute respiratory syndrome coronavirus 2 [SARS-CoV-2] [coronavirus disease {COVID-19}] vaccine/toxoid product and at least one vaccine/toxoid product from 90476-90759 are administered at the same encounter)◀

(For immune globulins, see 90281-90399. For administration of immune globulins, see 96365, 96366, 96367, 96368, 96369, 96370, 96371, 96374)

(For intravesical administration of BCG vaccine, see 51720, 90586)

90473 Immunization administration by intranasal or oral route; 1 vaccine (single or combination vaccine/toxoid)

(Do not report 90473 in conjunction with 90471)

✚ 90474 each additional vaccine (single or combination vaccine/toxoid) (List separately in addition to code for primary procedure)

(Use 90474 in conjunction with 90460, 90471, 90473)

▶(Do not report 90473, 90474 in conjunction with 91300-91311, unless both a severe acute respiratory syndrome coronavirus 2 [SARS-CoV-2] [coronavirus disease {COVID-19}] vaccine/toxoid product and at least one vaccine/toxoid product from 90476-90759 are administered at the same encounter)◀

0001A Immunization administration by intramuscular injection of severe acute respiratory syndrome coronavirus 2 (SARS-CoV-2) (coronavirus disease [COVID-19]) vaccine, mRNA-LNP, spike protein, preservative free, 30 mcg/0.3 mL dosage, diluent reconstituted; first dose

0002A second dose

● 0003A third dose

● 0004A booster dose

▶(Report 0001A, 0002A, 0003A, 0004A for the administration of vaccine 91300)◀

▶(Do not report 0001A, 0002A, 0003A, 0004A in conjunction with 91305, 91307, 91308)◀

#● 0051A Immunization administration by intramuscular injection of severe acute respiratory syndrome coronavirus 2 (SARS-CoV-2) (coronavirus disease [COVID-19]) vaccine, mRNA-LNP, spike protein, preservative free, 30 mcg/0.3 mL dosage, tris-sucrose formulation; first dose

#● 0052A second dose

#● 0053A third dose

#● 0054A booster dose

▶(Report 0051A, 0052A, 0053A, 0054A for the administration of vaccine 91305)◀

▶(Do not report 0051A, 0052A, 0053A, 0054A in conjunction with 91300, 91307, 91308)◀

#● 0071A Immunization administration by intramuscular injection of severe acute respiratory syndrome coronavirus 2 (SARS-CoV-2) (coronavirus disease [COVID-19]) vaccine, mRNA-LNP, spike protein, preservative free, 10 mcg/0.2 mL dosage, diluent reconstituted, tris-sucrose formulation; first dose

#● 0072A second dose

#● 0073A third dose

#● 0074A booster dose

▶(Report 0071A, 0072A, 0073A, 0074A for the administration of vaccine 91307)◀

▶(Do not report 0071A, 0072A, 0073A, 0074A in conjunction with 91300, 91305, 91308)◀

#● 0081A Immunization administration by intramuscular injection of severe acute respiratory syndrome coronavirus 2 (SARS-CoV-2) (coronavirus disease [COVID-19]) vaccine, mRNA-LNP, spike protein, preservative free, 3 mcg/0.2 mL dosage, diluent reconstituted, tris-sucrose formulation; first dose

#● 0082A second dose

#● 0083A third dose

▶(Report 0081A, 0082A, 0083A for the administration of vaccine 91308)◀

▶(Do not report 0081A, 0082A, 0083A in conjunction with 91300, 91305, 91307)◀

0012A second dose

● 0013A third dose

▶(Report 0011A, 0012A, 0013A for the administration of vaccine 91301)◀

▶(Do not report 0011A, 0012A, 0013A in conjunction with 91306, 91309, 91311)◀

#● 0064A Immunization administration by intramuscular injection of severe acute respiratory syndrome coronavirus 2 (SARS-CoV-2) (coronavirus disease [COVID-19]) vaccine, mRNA-LNP, spike protein, preservative free, 50 mcg/0.25 mL dosage, booster dose

▶(Report 0064A for the administration of vaccine 91306)◀

▶(Do not report 0064A in conjunction with 91301, 91309, 91311)◀

#● 0094A Immunization administration by intramuscular injection of severe acute respiratory syndrome coronavirus 2 (SARS-CoV-2) (coronavirus disease [COVID-19]) vaccine, mRNA-LNP, spike protein, preservative free, 50 mcg/0.5 mL dosage, booster dose

▶(Report 0094A for the administration of vaccine 91309)◀

▶(Do not report 0094A in conjunction with 91301, 91306, 91311)◀

0021A Immunization administration by intramuscular injection of severe acute respiratory syndrome coronavirus 2 (SARS-CoV-2) (coronavirus disease [COVID-19]) vaccine, DNA, spike protein, chimpanzee adenovirus Oxford 1 (ChAdOx1) vector, preservative free, 5x10^10 viral particles/0.5 mL dosage; first dose

0022A second dose

Medicine 90281-99607

★=Telemedicine   ◀=Audio-only   ✚=Add-on code   𝒩=FDA approval pending   #=Resequenced code   ⊘=Modifier 51 exempt

▲ **0031A**　Immunization administration by intramuscular injection of severe acute respiratory syndrome coronavirus 2 (SARS-CoV-2) (coronavirus disease [COVID-19]) vaccine, DNA, spike protein, adenovirus type 26 (Ad26) vector, preservative free, 5×10^{10} viral particles/0.5 mL dosage; single dose

● **0034A**　　　booster dose

▶(Report 0031A, 0034A for the administration of vaccine 91303)◀

0041A　Immunization administration by intramuscular injection of severe acute respiratory syndrome coronavirus 2 (SARS-CoV-2) (coronavirus disease [COVID-19]) vaccine, recombinant spike protein nanoparticle, saponin-based adjuvant, preservative free, 5 mcg/0.5 mL dosage; first dose

0042A　　　second dose

(Report 0041A, 0042A for the administration of vaccine 91304)

0051A　Code is out of numerical sequence. See 0003A-0022A

0052A　Code is out of numerical sequence. See 0003A-0022A

0053A　Code is out of numerical sequence. See 0003A-0022A

0054A　Code is out of numerical sequence. See 0003A-0022A

0064A　Code is out of numerical sequence. See 0003A-0022A

0071A　Code is out of numerical sequence. See 0003A-0022A

0072A　Code is out of numerical sequence. See 0003A-0022A

0073A　Code is out of numerical sequence. See 0003A-0022A

0074A　Code is out of numerical sequence. See 0003A-0022A

0081A　Code is out of numerical sequence. See 0003A-0022A

0082A　Code is out of numerical sequence. See 0003A-0022A

0083A　Code is out of numerical sequence. See 0003A-0022A

0094A　Code is out of numerical sequence. See 0003A-0022A

● **0104A**　Immunization administration by intramuscular injection of severe acute respiratory syndrome coronavirus 2 (SARS-CoV-2) (coronavirus disease [COVID-19]) vaccine, monovalent, preservative free, 5 mcg/0.5 mL dosage, adjuvant AS03 emulsion, booster dose

▶(Report 0104A for the administration of vaccine 91310)◀

● **0111A**　Immunization administration by intramuscular injection of severe acute respiratory syndrome coronavirus 2 (SARS-CoV-2) (coronavirus disease [COVID-19]) vaccine, mRNA-LNP, spike protein, preservative free, 25 mcg/0.25 mL dosage; first dose

● **0112A**　　　second dose

▶(Report 0111A, 0112A for the administration of vaccine 91311)◀

▶(Do not report 0111A, 0112A in conjunction with 91301, 91306, 91309)◀

Rationale

New vaccine product (91305-91311) and administration codes (0003A, 0004A, 0013A, 0034A, 0051A-0054A, 0064A, 0071A-0074A, 0081A-0083A, 0094A, 0104A, 0111A, 0112A) have been established for reporting new severe acute respiratory syndrome coronavirus 2 (SARS-CoV-2) (coronavirus disease [COVID-19]) vaccine products and administrations. In addition, new parenthetical notes have been added and changes have been made to the Appendix Q listing, to code 0031A, and to existing guidelines and parenthetical notes throughout the CPT code set to accommodate the new code additions.

To address the urgent health care need and facilitate the curtailing of the rapid pandemic spread of the COVID-19 virus throughout the United States, Emergency Use Authorization (EUA) continues to be provided by the Food and Drug Administration (FDA) for the development of new vaccine products and their administrations. This has been enacted to continue to allow more rapid development of vaccine codes from multiple manufacturers and make COVID vaccine products available earlier for code development.

As a result, new codes have been included within the Vaccine, Toxoids subsection to allow: (1) reporting of separate COVID-19 vaccine product codes according to the manufacturer providing the vaccine product and (2) reporting of specific administration codes that are unique to the various COVID-19 vaccine products. This is exemplified by the inclusion of seven new codes for COVID vaccine products (91305-91311), as well as 20 COVID-19 vaccine administration codes (0003A, 0004A, 0013A, 0034A, 0051A-0054A, 0064A, 0071A-0074A, 0081A-0083A, 0094A, 0104A, 0111A, 0112A), that are only reported according to the COVID-19 vaccine product administered.

CPT code convention typically uses common language within a code descriptor to accurately identify the procedure or vaccine and removes focus from proprietary language that may be specific to a particular manufacturer. However, due to the unique needs of making these products available to address the pandemic and to allow specific, accurate tracking for each manufacturer's product (and the administration needed for that product), separate codes have been assigned for COVID-19 vaccine products that would ordinarily be assigned a single code. Differentiation is exemplified within the code descriptor according to elements that would not ordinarily be used in a CPT vaccine code descriptor. Use of components such as notation of use of spike protein in the compilation and indication of the type of vector used (eg, chimpanzee adenovirus Oxford 1 [ChAdOx1]) provide differentiation that is not ordinarily included within a vaccine product code. As a result, each COVID-19 vaccine product code

Medicine　90281-99607

includes language within its descriptor that is different from other COVID vaccines. This applies similarly to the administration codes needed to administer the vaccine product and includes specificity down to the number of the dose (eg, first dose, second dose) or the type of dose (eg, booster dose). **Note:** Currently, it has been determined that specific booster-dose administrations will not be separately identified with a different code beyond noting that it is a booster dose (eg, a second booster dose is identified by the same administration code as the first booster dose).

Use of separate codes for the administration of COVID-19 vaccine products is unique to COVID-19 vaccine reporting. To eliminate confusion, instructions have been included and updated throughout the code set wherever vaccine administrations are discussed. This includes instruction within the Evaluation and Management (E/M) and Medicine sections that direct the use of the special COVID-19 administration codes only for the specific COVID-19 product for which it was created. These instructions also restrict the use of non-COVID-19 administration codes (90460-90474) in conjunction with COVID-19 vaccine product codes, unless both a COVID vaccine/toxoid product and at least one vaccine/toxoid product from codes 90476-90759 are administered at the same encounter. It also includes instructions for differentiating reporting for different administration types for COVID-19 products manufactured by the same manufacturer.

To further assist users in the appropriate reporting of COVID-19 vaccine services, guidelines and parenthetical notes throughout the code set have been updated or added to accommodate the addition of the new codes, provide instructions regarding codes that may or may not be reported together, direct users to appropriate codes for non-COVID vaccine administrations, and provide instructions regarding the appropriate codes to use for COVID-19 vaccine products and administrations. In addition, Appendix Q has been included and updated to further assist users in differentiating and selecting the appropriate vaccine product codes and the associated administration code(s).

The table in Appendix Q consists of the individual COVID-19 vaccine product codes (91300-91311) and their associated immunization administration codes (0001A-0004A, 0011A-0013A, 0021A, 0022A, 0031A, 0034A, 0041A, 0042A, 0051A-0054A, 0064A, 0071A-0074A, 0081A-0083A, 0094A, 0104A, 0111A, 0112A), manufacturer name, vaccine name(s), 10- and 11-digit National Drug Code (NDC) Labeler Product ID, and interval between doses. New within the Appendix Q table is the addition of a column that provides the age of the patient for the product. This table allows easy visualization of all information related to a particular

COVID vaccine product and administration code. Each of the elements noted within the table provides users with information that helps to differentiate the various COVID-19 vaccine products and administration codes.

Finally, on the AMA's COVID-19 CPT® Coding and Guidance webpage (https://www.ama-assn.org/find-covid-19-vaccine-codes), a built-in tool has also been included to assist vaccine product code and administration code selection. The AMA COVID-19 webpage should be consulted for frequent updates to CPT codes for COVID-19 vaccines and services.

Clinical Example (0003A)

A 33-year-old individual seeks immunization against SARS-CoV-2 to decrease the risk of contracting this disease, consistent with evidence-supported guidelines. The individual is offered and accepts an intramuscular injection of SARS-CoV-2 vaccine for this purpose.

Description of Procedure (0003A)

The physician or other qualified health care professional (QHP) reviews the patient's chart to confirm that vaccination to decrease the risk of COVID-19 is indicated. Counsel the patient on the benefits and risks of vaccination to decrease the risk of COVID-19 and obtain consent. Administer the third dose of the COVID-19 vaccine by intramuscular injection in the upper arm. Monitor the patient for any adverse reaction. Update the patient's immunization record (and registry when applicable) to reflect the vaccine administered.

Clinical Example (0004A)

A 33-year-old individual who was previously immunized with a primary series seeks booster immunization against SARS-CoV-2 to decrease the risk of contracting this disease, consistent with evidence-supported guidelines. The individual is offered and accepts an intramuscular injection of SARS-CoV-2 vaccine for this purpose.

Description of Procedure (0004A)

The physician or other QHP reviews the patient's chart to confirm that vaccination to decrease the risk of COVID-19 is indicated. Counsel the patient on the benefits and risks of vaccination to decrease the risk of COVID-19 and obtain consent. Administer the booster dose of the COVID-19 vaccine by intramuscular injection in the upper arm. Monitor the patient for any adverse reaction. Update the patient's immunization record (and registry when applicable) to reflect the vaccine administered.

Clinical Example (0013A)

A 33-year-old individual seeks immunization against SARS-CoV-2 to decrease the risk of contracting this disease, consistent with evidence-supported guidelines. The individual is offered and accepts an intramuscular injection of SARS-CoV-2 vaccine for this purpose.

Description of Procedure (0013A)

The physician or other QHP reviews the patient's chart to confirm that vaccination to decrease the risk of COVID-19 is indicated. Counsel the patient on the benefits and risks of vaccination to decrease the risk of COVID-19 and obtain consent. Administer the third dose of the COVID-19 vaccine by intramuscular injection in the upper arm. Monitor the patient for any adverse reaction. Update the patient's immunization record (and registry when applicable) to reflect the vaccine administered.

Clinical Example (0034A)

A 33-year-old individual, who was previously immunized with a primary series, seeks booster immunization against SARS-CoV-2 to decrease the risk of contracting this disease, consistent with evidence-supported guidelines. The individual is offered and accepts an intramuscular injection of SARS-CoV-2 vaccine for this purpose.

Description of Procedure (0034A)

The physician or other QHP reviews the patient's chart to confirm that vaccination to decrease the risk of COVID-19 is indicated. Counsel the patient on the benefits and risks of vaccination to decrease the risk of COVID-19 and obtain consent. Administer the booster dose of the COVID-19 vaccine by intramuscular injection in the upper arm. Monitor the patient for any adverse reaction. Update the patient's immunization record (and registry when applicable) to reflect the vaccine administered.

Clinical Example (0051A)

A 33-year-old individual seeks immunization against SARS-CoV-2 to decrease the risk of contracting this disease, consistent with evidence-supported guidelines. The individual is offered and accepts an intramuscular injection of SARS-CoV-2 vaccine for this purpose.

Description of Procedure (0051A)

The physician or other QHP reviews the patient's chart to confirm that vaccination to decrease the risk of COVID-19 is indicated. Counsel the patient on the benefits and risks of vaccination to decrease the risk of COVID-19 and obtain consent. Administer the first dose of the COVID-19 vaccine by intramuscular injection in the upper arm. Monitor the patient for any adverse reaction. Update the patient's immunization record (and registry when applicable) to reflect the vaccine administered.

Clinical Example (0052A)

A 33-year-old individual seeks immunization against SARS-CoV-2 to decrease the risk of contracting this disease, consistent with evidence-supported guidelines. The individual is offered and accepts an intramuscular injection of SARS-CoV-2 vaccine for this purpose.

Description of Procedure (0052A)

The physician or other QHP reviews the patient's chart to confirm that vaccination to decrease the risk of COVID-19 is indicated. Counsel the patient on the benefits and risks of vaccination to decrease the risk of COVID-19 and obtain consent. Administer the second dose of the COVID-19 vaccine by intramuscular injection in the upper arm. Monitor the patient for any adverse reaction. Update the patient's immunization record (and registry when applicable) to reflect the vaccine administered.

Clinical Example (0053A)

A 33-year-old individual seeks immunization against SARS-CoV-2 to decrease the risk of contracting this disease, consistent with evidence-supported guidelines. The individual is offered and accepts an intramuscular injection of SARS-CoV-2 vaccine for this purpose.

Description of Procedure (0053A)

The physician or other QHP reviews the patient's chart to confirm that vaccination to decrease the risk of COVID-19 is indicated. Counsel the patient on the benefits and risks of vaccination to decrease the risk of COVID-19 and obtain consent. Administer the third dose of the COVID-19 vaccine by intramuscular injection in the upper arm. Monitor the patient for any adverse reaction. Update the patient's immunization record (and registry when applicable) to reflect the vaccine administered.

Medicine 90281-99607

Clinical Example (0054A)

A 33-year-old individual who was previously immunized with a primary series seeks booster immunization against SARS-CoV-2 to decrease the risk of contracting this disease, consistent with evidence-supported guidelines. The individual is offered and accepts an intramuscular injection of SARS-CoV-2 vaccine for this purpose.

Description of Procedure (0054A)

The physician or other QHP reviews the patient's chart to confirm that vaccination to decrease the risk of COVID-19 is indicated. Counsel the patient on the benefits and risks of vaccination to decrease the risk of COVID-19 and obtain consent. Administer the booster dose of the COVID-19 vaccine by intramuscular injection in the upper arm. Monitor the patient for any adverse reaction. Update the patient's immunization record (and registry when applicable) to reflect the vaccine administered.

Clinical Example (0064A)

A 33-year-old individual who was previously immunized with a primary series seeks booster immunization against SARS-CoV-2 to decrease the risk of contracting this disease, consistent with evidence-supported guidelines. The individual is offered and accepts an intramuscular injection of SARS-CoV-2 vaccine for this purpose.

Description of Procedure (0064A)

The physician or other QHP reviews the patient's chart to confirm that vaccination to decrease the risk of COVID-19 is indicated. Counsel the patient on the benefits and risks of vaccination to decrease the risk of COVID-19 and obtain consent. Administer the booster dose of the COVID-19 vaccine by intramuscular injection in the upper arm. Monitor the patient for any adverse reaction. Update the patient's immunization record (and registry when applicable) to reflect the vaccine administered.

Clinical Example (0071A)

A parent or guardian of an 8-year-old child seeks immunization against SARS-CoV-2 to decrease the risk of contracting this disease, consistent with evidence-supported guidelines. The parent or guardian is offered and agreed to an intramuscular injection of SARS-CoV-2 vaccine for the child for this purpose.

Description of Procedure (0071A)

The physician or other QHP reviews the patient's chart to confirm that vaccination to decrease the risk of COVID-19 is indicated. Counsel the parent or guardian on the benefits and risks of vaccination to decrease the

risk of COVID-19 and obtain consent. Administer the first dose of the COVID-19 vaccine by intramuscular injection in the upper arm. Monitor the patient for any adverse reaction. Update the patient's immunization record (and registry when applicable) to reflect the vaccine administered.

Clinical Example (0072A)

A parent or guardian of an 8-year-old child seeks immunization against SARS-CoV-2 to decrease the risk of contracting this disease, consistent with evidence-supported guidelines. The parent or guardian is offered and agreed to an intramuscular injection of SARS-CoV-2 vaccine for the child for this purpose.

Description of Procedure (0072A)

The physician or other QHP reviews the patient's chart to confirm that vaccination to decrease the risk of COVID-19 is indicated. Counsel the parent or guardian on the benefits and risks of vaccination to decrease the risk of COVID-19 and obtain consent. Administer the first dose of the COVID-19 vaccine by intramuscular injection in the upper arm. Monitor the patient for any adverse reaction. Update the patient's immunization record (and registry when applicable) to reflect the vaccine administered.

Clinical Example (0073A)

A parent or guardian of an 8-year-old child seeks immunization against SARS-CoV-2 to decrease the risk of contracting this disease, consistent with evidence-supported guidelines. The parent or guardian is offered and agrees to an intramuscular injection of SARS-CoV-2 vaccine for the child for this purpose.

Description of Procedure (0073A)

The physician or other QHP reviews the patient's chart to confirm that vaccination to decrease the risk of COVID-19 is indicated. Counsel the parent or guardian on the benefits and risks of vaccination to decrease the risk of COVID-19 and obtain consent. Administer the third dose of the COVID-19 vaccine by intramuscular injection in the upper arm. Monitor the patient for any adverse reaction. Update the patient's immunization record (and registry when applicable) to reflect the vaccine administered.

Clinical Example (0074A)

A parent/guardian seeks booster immunization for their 5-year-old child who was previously immunized with a primary series against SARS-CoV-2 to decrease the risk of contracting this disease, consistent with evidence-supported guidelines. The parent/guardian is offered and accepts, on the child's behalf, an intramuscular injection of SARS-CoV-2 vaccine for this purpose.

Description of Procedure (0074A)

The physician or other QHP reviews the patient's chart to confirm that vaccination to decrease the risk of COVID-19 is indicated. The parent/guardian is counseled on the benefits and risks of vaccination to decrease the risk of COVID-19 and obtain consent. Administer the booster dose of the COVID-19 vaccine by intramuscular injection in the upper arm. Monitor the patient for any adverse reaction. Update the patient's immunization record (and registry when applicable) to reflect the vaccine administered.

Clinical Example (0081A)

A parent or guardian of a 1-year-old child seeks immunization against SARS-CoV-2 to decrease the risk of contracting this disease, consistent with evidence-supported guidelines. The parent or guardian is offered and agrees to an intramuscular injection of SARS-CoV-2 vaccine for the child for this purpose.

Description of Procedure (0081A)

The physician or other QHP reviews the patient's chart to confirm that vaccination to decrease the risk of COVID-19 is indicated. Counsel the parent or guardian on the benefits and risks of vaccination to decrease the risk of COVID-19 and obtain consent. Administer the first dose of the COVID-19 vaccine by intramuscular injection. Monitor the patient for any adverse reaction. Update the patient's immunization record (and registry when applicable) to reflect the vaccine administered.

Clinical Example (0082A)

A parent or guardian of a 1-year-old child seeks immunization against SARS-CoV-2 to decrease the risk of contracting this disease, consistent with evidence-supported guidelines. The parent or guardian is offered and agrees to an intramuscular injection of SARS-CoV-2 vaccine for the child for this purpose.

Description of Procedure (0082A)

The physician or other QHP reviews the patient's chart to confirm that vaccination to decrease the risk of COVID-19 is indicated. Counsel the parent or guardian on the benefits and risks of vaccination to decrease the risk of COVID-19 and obtain consent. Administer the second dose of the COVID-19 vaccine by intramuscular injection. Monitor the patient for any adverse reaction. Update the patient's immunization record (and registry when applicable) to reflect the vaccine administered.

Clinical Example (0083A)

A parent or guardian of a 1-year-old child seeks immunization against SARS-CoV-2 to decrease the risk of contracting this disease, consistent with evidence-supported guidelines. The parent or guardian is offered and agrees to an intramuscular injection of SARS-CoV-2 vaccine for the child for this purpose.

Description of Procedure (0083A)

The physician or other QHP reviews the patient's chart to confirm that vaccination to decrease the risk of COVID-19 is indicated. Counsel the parent or guardian on the benefits and risks of vaccination to decrease the risk of COVID-19 and obtain consent. Administer the third dose of the COVID-19 vaccine by intramuscular injection. Monitor the patient for any adverse reaction. Update the patient's immunization record (and registry when applicable) to reflect the vaccine administered.

Clinical Example (0094A)

A 33-year-old individual who was previously immunized with a primary series seeks booster immunization against SARS-CoV-2 to decrease the risk of contracting this disease, consistent with evidence-supported guidelines. The individual is offered and accepts an intramuscular injection of SARS-CoV-2 vaccine for this purpose.

Description of Procedure (0094A)

The physician or other QHP reviews the patient's chart to confirm that vaccination to decrease the risk of COVID-19 is indicated. Counsel the patient on the benefits and risks of vaccination to decrease the risk of COVID-19 and obtain consent. Administer the booster dose of the COVID-19 vaccine by intramuscular injection in the upper arm. Monitor the patient for any adverse reaction. Update the patient's immunization record (and registry when applicable) to reflect the vaccine administered.

Clinical Example (0104A)

A 33-year-old individual who was previously immunized with a primary series seeks booster immunization against SARS-CoV-2 to decrease the risk of contracting this disease, consistent with evidence-supported guidelines. The individual is offered and accepts an intramuscular injection of SARS-CoV-2 vaccine for this purpose.

Description of Procedure (0104A)

The physician or other QHP reviews the patient's chart to confirm that vaccination to decrease the risk of COVID-19 is indicated. Counsel the patient on the benefits and risks of vaccination to decrease the risk of COVID-19 and obtain consent. Administer the booster

Medicine 90281-99607

dose of the COVID-19 vaccine by intramuscular injection in the upper arm. Monitor the patient for any adverse reaction. Update the patient's immunization record (and registry when applicable) to reflect the vaccine administered.

Clinical Example (0111A)

A parent or guardian of a 1-year-old child seeks immunization against SARS-CoV-2 to decrease the risk of contracting this disease, consistent with evidence-supported guidelines. The parent or guardian is offered and agrees to an intramuscular injection of SARS-CoV-2 vaccine for the child for this purpose.

Description of Procedure (0111A)

The physician or other QHP reviews the patient's chart to confirm that vaccination to decrease the risk of COVID-19 is indicated. Counsel the parent or guardian on the benefits and risks of vaccination to decrease the risk of COVID-19 and obtain consent. Administer the first dose of the COVID-19 vaccine by intramuscular injection. Monitor the patient for any adverse reaction. Update the patient's immunization record (and registry when applicable) to reflect the vaccine administered.

Clinical Example (0112A)

A parent or guardian of a 1-year-old child seeks immunization against SARS-CoV-2 to decrease the risk of contracting this disease, consistent with evidence-supported guidelines. The parent or guardian is offered and agrees to an intramuscular injection of SARS-CoV-2 vaccine for the child for this purpose.

Description of Procedure (0112A)

The physician or other QHP reviews the patient's chart to confirm that vaccination to decrease the risk of COVID-19 is indicated. Counsel the parent or guardian on the benefits and risks of vaccination to decrease the risk of COVID-19 and obtain consent. Administer the second dose of the COVID-19 vaccine by intramuscular injection. Monitor the patient for any adverse reaction. Update the patient's immunization record (and registry when applicable) to reflect the vaccine administered.

Vaccines, Toxoids

To assist users to report the most recent new or revised vaccine product codes, the American Medical Association (AMA) currently uses the CPT website (ama-assn.org/cpt-cat-i-vaccine-codes), which features updates of CPT Editorial Panel actions regarding these products. See the Introduction section of the CPT code set for a complete list of the dates of release and implementation.

The CPT Editorial Panel, in recognition of the public health interest in vaccine products, has chosen to publish new vaccine product codes prior to approval by the US Food and Drug Administration (FDA). These codes are indicated with the ⁄ symbol and will be tracked by the AMA to monitor FDA approval status. Once the FDA status changes to approval, the ⁄ symbol will be removed. CPT users should refer to the AMA CPT website (ama-assn.org/cpt-cat-i-vaccine-codes) for the most up-to-date information on codes with the ⁄ symbol.

▶Codes 90476-90759, 91300-91311 identify the vaccine product **only**. To report the administration of a vaccine/toxoid other than SARS-CoV-2 (coronavirus disease [COVID-19]), the vaccine/toxoid product codes (90476-90759) must be used in addition to an immunization administration code(s) (90460, 90461, 90471, 90472, 90473, 90474). To report the administration of a SARS-CoV-2 (coronavirus disease [COVID-19]) vaccine, the vaccine/toxoid product codes (91300-91311) should be reported with the corresponding immunization administration codes (0001A, 0002A, 0003A, 0004A, 0011A, 0012A, 0013A, 0021A, 0022A, 0031A, 0034A, 0041A, 0042A, 0051A, 0052A, 0053A, 0054A, 0064A, 0071A, 0072A, 0073A, 0074A, 0081A, 0082A, 0083A, 0094A, 0104A, 0111A, 0112A). All SARS-CoV-2 (coronavirus disease [COVID-19]) vaccine codes in this section are listed in Appendix Q with their associated vaccine code descriptors, vaccine administration codes, patient age, vaccine manufacturer, vaccine name(s), NDC Labeler Product ID, and interval between doses. In order to report these codes, the vaccine must fulfill the code descriptor and must be the vaccine represented by the manufacturer and vaccine name listed in Appendix Q.

Do not report 90476-90759 in conjunction with the SARS-CoV-2 (coronavirus disease [COVID-19]) immunization administration codes 0001A, 0002A, 0003A, 0004A, 0011A, 0012A, 0013A, 0021A, 0022A, 0031A, 0034A, 0041A, 0042A 0051A, 0052A, 0053A, 0054A, 0064A, 0071A, 0072A, 0073A, 0074A, 0081A, 0082A, 0083A, 0094A, 0104A, 0111A, 0112A, unless both a SARS-CoV-2 (coronavirus disease [COVID-19]) vaccine/toxoid product and at least one vaccine/toxoid product from 90476-90759 are administered at the same encounter.

★ = Telemedicine   ◀ = Audio-only   ✚ = Add-on code   ⁄ = FDA approval pending   # = Resequenced code   ⊘ = Modifier 51 exempt

Modifier 51 should not be reported with vaccine/toxoid codes 90476-90759, 91300-91311, when reported in conjunction with administration codes 90460, 90461, 90471, 90472, 90473, 90474, 0001A, 0002A, 0003A, 0004A, 0011A, 0012A, 0013A, 0021A, 0022A, 0031A, 0034A, 0041A, 0042A, 0051A, 0052A, 0053A, 0054A, 0064A, 0071A, 0072A, 0073A, 0074A, 0081A, 0082A, 0083A, 0094A, 0104A, 0111A, 0112A.◀

If a significantly separately identifiable Evaluation and Management (E/M) service (eg, office or other outpatient services, preventive medicine services) is performed, the appropriate E/M service code should be reported in addition to the vaccine and toxoid administration codes.

To meet the reporting requirements of immunization registries, vaccine distribution programs, and reporting systems (eg, Vaccine Adverse Event Reporting System) the exact vaccine product administered needs to be reported. Multiple codes for a particular vaccine are provided in the CPT codebook when the schedule (number of doses or timing) differs for two or more products of the same vaccine type (eg, hepatitis A, Hib) or the vaccine product is available in more than one chemical formulation, dosage, or route of administration.

The "when administered to" age descriptions included in CPT vaccine codes are not intended to identify a product's licensed age indication. The term "preservative free" includes use for vaccines that contain no preservative and vaccines that contain trace amounts of preservative agents that are not present in a sufficient concentration for the purpose of preserving the final vaccine formulation. The absence of a designation regarding a preservative does not necessarily indicate the presence or absence of preservative in the vaccine. Refer to the product's prescribing information (PI) for the licensed age indication before administering vaccine to a patient.

Separate codes are available for combination vaccines (eg, Hib-HepB, DTap-IPV/Hib). It is inappropriate to code each component of a combination vaccine separately. If a specific vaccine code is not available, the unlisted procedure code should be reported, until a new code becomes available.

▶The vaccine/toxoid abbreviations listed in codes 90476-90759, 91300-91311 reflect the most recent US vaccine abbreviation references used in the Advisory Committee on Immunization Practices (ACIP) recommendations at the time of CPT code set publication. Interim updates to vaccine code descriptors will be made following abbreviation approval by the ACIP on a timely basis via the AMA CPT website (ama-assn.org/cpt-cat-i-vaccine-codes). The accuracy of the ACIP vaccine abbreviation designations in the CPT code set does not affect the validity of the vaccine code and its reporting function.

For the purposes of severe acute respiratory syndrome coronavirus 2 (SARS-CoV-2) (coronavirus disease [COVID-19]) vaccinations, codes 0003A, 0013A,

0053A, 0073A, and 0083A represent the administration of a third dose when the initial immune response following a two-dose primary vaccine series is likely to be insufficient (eg, immunocompromised patient). In contrast, the booster dose codes 0004A, 0034A, 0054A, 0064A, 0074A, 0094A, and 0104A represent the administration of a dose of vaccine when the initial immune response to a primary vaccine series was sufficient, but has likely waned over time.◀

(For immune globulins, see 90281-90399. For administration of immune globulins, see 96365-96375)

 # 91300 Severe acute respiratory syndrome coronavirus 2 (SARS-CoV-2) (coronavirus disease [COVID-19]) vaccine, mRNA-LNP, spike protein, preservative free, 30 mcg/0.3 mL dosage, diluent reconstituted, for intramuscular use

▶(Report 91300 with administration codes 0001A, 0002A, 0003A, 0004A)◀

▶Do not report 91300 in conjunction with administration codes 0051A, 0052A, 0053A, 0054A, 0071A, 0072A, 0073A, 0074A, 0081A, 0082A, 0083A)◀

#● 91305 Severe acute respiratory syndrome coronavirus 2 (SARS-CoV-2) (coronavirus disease [COVID-19]) vaccine, mRNA-LNP, spike protein, preservative free, 30 mcg/0.3 mL dosage, tris-sucrose formulation, for intramuscular use

▶(Report 91305 with administration codes 0051A, 0052A, 0053A, 0054A)◀

▶Do not report 91305 in conjunction with administration codes 0001A, 0002A, 0003A, 0004A, 0071A, 0072A, 0073A, 0074A, 0081A, 0082A, 0083A)◀

#● 91307 Severe acute respiratory syndrome coronavirus 2 (SARS-CoV-2) (coronavirus disease [COVID-19]) vaccine, mRNA-LNP, spike protein, preservative free, 10 mcg/0.2 mL dosage, diluent reconstituted, tris-sucrose formulation, for intramuscular use

▶(Report 91307 with administration codes 0071A, 0072A, 0073A, 0074A)◀

▶(Do not report 91307 in conjunction with administration codes 0001A, 0002A, 0003A, 0004A, 0051A, 0052A, 0053A, 0054A, 0081A, 0082A, 0083A)◀

#● 91308 Severe acute respiratory syndrome coronavirus 2 (SARS-CoV-2) (coronavirus disease [COVID-19]) vaccine, mRNA-LNP, spike protein, preservative free, 3 mcg/0.2 mL dosage, diluent reconstituted, tris-sucrose formulation, for intramuscular use

▶(Report 91308 with administration codes 0081A, 0082A, 0083A)◀

▶(Do not report 91308 in conjunction with administration codes 0001A, 0002A, 0003A, 0004A, 0051A, 0052A, 0053A, 0054A, 0071A, 0072A, 0073A, 0074A)◀

 # 91301 Severe acute respiratory syndrome coronavirus 2 (SARS-CoV-2) (coronavirus disease [COVID-19]) vaccine, mRNA-LNP, spike protein, preservative free, 100 mcg/0.5 mL dosage, for intramuscular use

▶(Report 91301 with administration codes 0011A, 0012A, 0013A)◀

▶(Do not report 91301 in conjunction with administration codes 0064A, 0094A, 0111A, 0112A)◀

#● 91306 Severe acute respiratory syndrome coronavirus 2 (SARS-CoV-2) (coronavirus disease [COVID-19]) vaccine, mRNA-LNP, spike protein, preservative free, 50 mcg/0.25 mL dosage, for intramuscular use

▶(Report 91306 with administration code 0064A)◀

▶(Do not report 91306 in conjunction with administration codes 0011A, 0012A, 0013A, 0094A, 0111A, 0112A)◀

#● 91311 Severe acute respiratory syndrome coronavirus 2 (SARS-CoV-2) (coronavirus disease [COVID-19]) vaccine, mRNA-LNP, spike protein, preservative free, 25 mcg/0.25 mL dosage, for intramuscular use

▶(Report 91311 with administration codes 0111A, 0112A)◀

▶(Do not report 91311 in conjunction with administration codes 0011A, 0012A, 0013A, 0064A, 0094A)◀

#● 91309 Severe acute respiratory syndrome coronavirus 2 (SARS-CoV-2) (coronavirus disease [COVID-19]) vaccine, mRNA-LNP, spike protein, preservative free, 50 mcg/0.5 mL dosage, for intramuscular use

▶(Report 91309 with administration code 0094A)◀

▶(Do not report 91309 in conjunction with administration codes 0011A, 0012A, 0013A, 0064A, 0111A, 0112A)◀

#✔ 91302 Severe acute respiratory syndrome coronavirus 2 (SARS-CoV-2) (coronavirus disease [COVID-19]) vaccine, DNA, spike protein, chimpanzee adenovirus Oxford 1 (ChAdOx1) vector, preservative free, 5x10^{10} viral particles/0.5 mL dosage, for intramuscular use

(Report 91302 with administration codes 0021A, 0022A)

 # 91303 Severe acute respiratory syndrome coronavirus 2 (SARS-CoV-2) (coronavirus disease [COVID-19]) vaccine, DNA, spike protein, adenovirus type 26 (Ad26) vector, preservative free, 5x10^{10} viral particles/0.5 mL dosage, for intramuscular use

▶(Report 91303 with administration codes 0031A, 0034A)◀

 # 91304 Severe acute respiratory syndrome coronavirus 2 (SARS-CoV-2) (coronavirus disease [COVID-19]) vaccine, recombinant spike protein nanoparticle, saponin-based adjuvant, preservative free, 5 mcg/0.5 mL dosage, for intramuscular use

(Report 91304 with administration codes 0041A, 0042A)

#✔● 91310 Severe acute respiratory syndrome coronavirus 2 (SARS-CoV-2) (coronavirus disease [COVID-19]) vaccine, monovalent, preservative free, 5 mcg/0.5 mL dosage, adjuvant AS03 emulsion, for intramuscular use

▶(Report 91310 with administration code 0104A)◀

90476 Adenovirus vaccine, type 4, live, for oral use

Rationale

To accommodate the addition of new codes for reporting COVID-19 vaccine products, codes 91305-91311 and associated parenthetical notes have been added and the existing Vaccines, Toxoids subsection guidelines and related parenthetical notes have been revised.

Refer to the codebook and the Rationale for codes 0003A-0112A for a full discussion of these changes.

Clinical Example (91305)

A 33-year-old individual seeks immunization against SARS-CoV-2 to decrease the risk of contracting this disease, consistent with evidence-supported guidelines. The individual is offered and accepts an intramuscular injection of SARS-CoV-2 vaccine for this purpose.

Description of Procedure (91305)

The physician or other QHP determines that the SARS-CoV-2 vaccine is appropriate for this patient and dispenses the vaccine according to the dose scheduled in the administration code for the SARS-CoV-2 vaccine.

Clinical Example (91306)

A 33-year-old individual seeks immunization against SARS-CoV-2 to decrease the risk of contracting this disease, consistent with evidence-supported guidelines. The individual is offered and accepts an intramuscular injection of SARS-CoV-2 vaccine for this purpose.

Description of Procedure (91306)

The physician or other QHP determines that the SARS-CoV-2 vaccine is appropriate for this patient and dispenses the vaccine according to the dose scheduled in the administration code for the SARS-CoV-2 vaccine.

Clinical Example (91307)

A parent or guardian of an 8-year-old child seeks immunization against SARS-CoV-2 to decrease the risk of contracting this disease, consistent with evidence-supported guidelines. The parent or guardian is offered and agreed to an intramuscular injection of SARS-CoV-2 vaccine for the child for this purpose.

★ = Telemedicine   ◀ = Audio-only   ✚ = Add-on code   ✔ = FDA approval pending   # = Resequenced code   ⊘ = Modifier 51 exempt

Medicine 90281-99607

Description of Procedure (91307)

The physician or other QHP determines that the SARS-CoV-2 vaccine is appropriate for this patient and dispenses the vaccine according to the dose scheduled in the administration code for the SARS-CoV-2 vaccine.

Clinical Example (91308)

A parent or guardian of a 1-year-old child seeks immunization against SARS-CoV-2 to decrease the risk of contracting this disease, consistent with evidence-supported guidelines. The parent or guardian is offered and agrees to an intramuscular injection of SARS-CoV-2 vaccine for the child for this purpose.

Description of Procedure (91308)

The physician or other QHP determines that the SARS-CoV-2 vaccine is appropriate for this patient and dispenses the vaccine according to the dose scheduled in the administration code for the SARS-CoV-2 vaccine.

Clinical Example (91309)

A 33-year-old individual who was previously immunized with a primary series seeks booster immunization against SARS-CoV-2 to decrease the risk of contracting this disease, consistent with evidence-supported guidelines. The individual is offered and accepts an intramuscular injection of SARS-CoV-2 vaccine for this purpose.

Description of Procedure (91309)

The physician or other QHP determines that the SARS-CoV-2 vaccine is appropriate for this patient and dispenses the booster vaccine according to the dose scheduled in the administration code for the SARS-CoV-2 vaccine.

Clinical Example (91310)

A 33-year-old individual who was previously immunized with a primary series seeks booster immunization against SARS-CoV-2 to decrease the risk of contracting this disease, consistent with evidence-supported guidelines. The individual is offered and accepts an intramuscular injection of SARS-CoV-2 vaccine for this purpose.

Description of Procedure (91310)

The physician or other QHP determines that the SARS-CoV-2 vaccine is appropriate for this patient and dispenses the booster vaccine according to the dose scheduled in the administration code for the SARS-CoV-2 vaccine.

Clinical Example (91311)

A parent or guardian of a 1-year-old child seeks immunization against SARS-CoV-2 to decrease the risk of contracting this disease, consistent with evidence-supported guidelines. The parent or guardian is offered and agrees to an intramuscular injection of SARS-CoV-2 vaccine for the child for this purpose.

Description of Procedure (91311)

The physician or other QHP determines that the SARS-CoV-2 vaccine is appropriate for this patient and dispenses the vaccine according to the dose scheduled in the administration code for the SARS-CoV-2 vaccine.

90584	Code is out of numerical sequence. See 90585-90632
90586	Bacillus Calmette-Guerin vaccine (BCG) for bladder cancer, live, for intravesical use
#✚● 90584	Dengue vaccine, quadrivalent, live, 2 dose schedule, for subcutaneous use

Rationale

New vaccine product code 90584 has been established in the Vaccines, Toxoids subsection to report quadrivalent dengue vaccine. Code 90584 describes a live dengue vaccine that requires a two-dose schedule. Administration of the vaccine is reported separately using codes 90460-90474 (immunization administration for vaccines/toxoids). Code 90584 carries the US FDA approval-pending symbol (✚); therefore, interim updates on the FDA status of this code will be reflected on the AMA CPT website (https://www.ama-assn.org/system/files/vaccine-long-descriptors.pdf) on a semiannual basis (July 1 and January 1).

The Centers for Disease Control and Prevention Advisory Committee on Immunization Practices (ACIP) has not assigned a US vaccine abbreviation for this vaccine. Visit the AMA CPT website for updates on the US vaccine abbreviation status for this vaccine.

Clinical Example (90584)

A 30-year-old female seeks immunization against dengue fever to decrease the risk of contracting dengue fever consistent with evidence-supported guidelines. She is offered and accepts an intramuscular injection of dengue vaccine for this purpose.

Medicine 90281-99607

Medicine 90281-99607

Description of Procedure (90584)

The physician or other QHP selects the appropriate dosage of the vaccine for injection. Report the administration of the vaccine separately from the vaccine.

90676   Rabies vaccine, for intradermal use

90677   Code is out of numerical sequence. See 90670-90676

✖● **90678**   Respiratory syncytial virus vaccine, preF, subunit, bivalent, for intramuscular use

Rationale

New vaccine product code 90678 has been established in the Vaccines, Toxoids subsection to report respiratory syncytial virus (RSV) vaccine. The vaccine is bivalent and includes subunit preF as an important component of the vaccine. Administration of the vaccine is reported separately using codes 90460-90474 (immunization administration for vaccines/toxoids). Code 90584 carries the US FDA approval-pending symbol (✖); therefore, interim updates on the FDA status of this code will be reflected on the AMA CPT website (https://www.ama-assn.org/system/files/vaccine-long-descriptors.pdf) on a semiannual basis (July 1 and January 1).

The Centers for Disease Control and Prevention Advisory Committee on Immunization Practices (ACIP) has not assigned a US vaccine abbreviation for this vaccine. Visit the AMA CPT website for updates on the US vaccine abbreviation status for this vaccine.

Clinical Example (90678)

A 30-year-old pregnant female presents for a routine prenatal visit at 26 weeks gestation. The physician reviews the patient's immunization record and determines that the patient should receive the respiratory syncytial virus, subunit, preF, bivalent vaccine and orders its administration.

Description of Procedure (90678)

A registered nurse administers the respiratory syncytial virus vaccine by intramuscular injection.

90738   Japanese encephalitis virus vaccine, inactivated, for intramuscular use

▲ **90739**   Hepatitis B vaccine (HepB), CpG-adjuvanted, adult dosage, 2 dose or 4 dose schedule, for intramuscular use

Rationale

Vaccine product code 90739 has been revised to note that it may be used to report a two- or four-dose schedule for hepatitis B vaccination. In addition, the term "CpG-adjuvanted" has also been added to the descriptor to note that an enhancer that improves protection has been added to the vaccine.

Psychiatry

▶Psychiatry services include diagnostic services, psychotherapy, and other services to an individual, family, or group. Patient condition, characteristics, or situational factors may require services described as being with interactive complexity. Services may be provided to a patient in crisis. Services are provided in all settings of care and psychiatry services codes are reported without regard to setting. Services may be provided by a physician or other qualified health care professional. Some psychiatry services may be reported with **evaluation and management services** (99202-99255, 99281-99285, 99304-99316, 99341-99350) or other services when performed. **Evaluation and management services** (99202-99285, 99304-99316, 99341-99350) may be reported for treatment of psychiatric conditions, rather than using **psychiatry services** codes, when appropriate.

Hospital inpatient or observation care in treating a psychiatric inpatient or partial hospitalization may be initial or subsequent in nature (see 99221-99233).

Some patients receive hospital evaluation and management services only and others receive hospital evaluation and management services and other procedures. If other procedures such as electroconvulsive therapy or psychotherapy are rendered in addition to hospital evaluation and management services, these may be listed separately (eg, hospital inpatient or observation care services [99221-99223, 99231-99233] plus electroconvulsive therapy [90870]), or when psychotherapy is done, with appropriate code(s) defining psychotherapy services.◀

Consultation for psychiatric evaluation of a patient includes examination of a patient and exchange of information with the primary physician and other informants such as nurses or family members, and preparation of a report. These services may be reported using consultation codes (see **Consultations**).

(Do not report 90785-90899 in conjunction with 90839, 90840, 97151, 97152, 97153, 97154, 97155, 97156, 97157, 97158, 0362T, 0373T)

Rationale

In accordance with the deletion of codes 99318, 99324-99328, and 99334-99337 and the revision of codes 99221-99223 and 99231-99233, the Psychiatry subsection guidelines have been revised to reflect these changes.

Refer to the codebook and the Rationale for codes 99318, 99324-99328, 99334-99337, 99221-99223, and 99231-99233 for a full discussion of these changes.

Psychiatric Diagnostic Procedures

★◄ **90791**   Psychiatric diagnostic evaluation

★◄ **90792**   Psychiatric diagnostic evaluation with medical services

►(Do not report 90791 or 90792 in conjunction with 99202-99316, 99341-99350, 99366-99368, 99401-99443, 97151, 97152, 97153, 97154, 97155, 97156, 97157, 97158, 0362T, 0373T)◄

(Use 90785 in conjunction with 90791, 90792 when the diagnostic evaluation includes interactive complexity services)

Rationale

In accordance with the deletion of codes 99318, 99324-99328, and 99334-99337, the exclusionary parenthetical note following code 90792 has been revised to reflect these changes.

Refer to the codebook and the Rationale for codes 99318, 99324-99328, and 99334-99337 for a full discussion of these changes.

Psychotherapy

Psychotherapy is the treatment of mental illness and behavioral disturbances in which the physician or other qualified health care professional, through definitive therapeutic communication, attempts to alleviate the emotional disturbances, reverse or change maladaptive patterns of behavior, and encourage personality growth and development.

The psychotherapy service codes 90832-90838 include ongoing assessment and adjustment of psychotherapeutic interventions, and may include involvement of informants in the treatment process.

Codes 90832, 90833, 90834, 90836, 90837, 90838 describe psychotherapy for the individual patient, although times are for face-to-face services with patient and may include informant(s). The patient must be present for all or a majority of the service.

See codes 90846, 90847 when utilizing family psychotherapy techniques, such as focusing on family dynamics. Do not report 90846, 90847 for family psychotherapy services less than 26 minutes. Codes 90832, 90833, 90834, 90836, 90837, 90838 may be reported on the same day as codes 90846, 90847, when the services are separate and distinct.

In reporting, choose the code closest to the actual time (ie, 16-37 minutes for 90832 and 90833, 38-52 minutes for 90834 and 90836, and 53 or more minutes for 90837 and 90838). Do not report psychotherapy of less than 16 minutes duration. (See instructions for the usage of time in the Introduction of the CPT code set.)

Psychotherapy provided to a patient in a crisis state is reported with codes 90839 and 90840 and cannot be reported in addition to the psychotherapy codes 90832-90838. For psychotherapy for crisis, see "Other Psychotherapy."

Code 90785 is an add-on code to report interactive complexity services when provided in conjunction with the psychotherapy codes 90832-90838. For family psychotherapy, see 90846, 90847. The amount of time spent by a physician or other qualified health care professional providing interactive complexity services should be reflected in the timed service code for psychotherapy (90832, 90834, 90837) or the psychotherapy add-on code performed with an evaluation and management service (90833, 90836, 90838).

Some psychiatric patients receive a medical evaluation and management (E/M) service on the same day as a psychotherapy service by the same physician or other qualified health care professional. To report both E/M and psychotherapy, the two services must be significant and separately identifiable. These services are reported by using codes specific for psychotherapy when performed with evaluation and management services (90833, 90836, 90838) as add-on codes to the evaluation and management service.

►Medical symptoms and disorders inform treatment choices of psychotherapeutic interventions, and data from therapeutic communication are used to evaluate the presence, type, and severity of medical symptoms and disorders. For the purposes of reporting, the medical and psychotherapeutic components of the service may be separately identified as follows:

1. The type and level of E/M service is selected based on medical decision making.

2. Time spent on the activities of the E/M service is not included in the time used for reporting the

Medicine 90281-99607

psychotherapy service. Time may not be used as the basis of E/M code selection and prolonged services may not be reported when psychotherapy with E/M (90833, 90836, 90838) are reported.

3. A separate diagnosis is not required for the reporting of E/M and psychotherapy on the same date of service. ◄

★◀ **90832**   Psychotherapy, 30 minutes with patient

★✚◀ **90833**   Psychotherapy, 30 minutes with patient when performed with an evaluation and management service (List separately in addition to the code for primary procedure)

▶(Use 90833 in conjunction with 99202-99255, 99304-99316, 99341-99350)◄

★◀ **90834**   Psychotherapy, 45 minutes with patient

★✚◀ **90836**   Psychotherapy, 45 minutes with patient when performed with an evaluation and management service (List separately in addition to the code for primary procedure)

▶(Use 90836 in conjunction with 99202-99255, 99304-99316, 99341-99350)◄

★◀ **90837**   Psychotherapy, 60 minutes with patient

★✚◀ **90838**   Psychotherapy, 60 minutes with patient when performed with an evaluation and management service (List separately in addition to the code for primary procedure)

▶(Use 90838 in conjunction with 99202-99255, 99304-99316, 99341-99350)◄

(Use 90785 in conjunction with 90832, 90833, 90834, 90836, 90837, 90838 when psychotherapy includes interactive complexity services)

Rationale

In accordance with the changes to the guidelines for reporting E/M services using either time or medical decision making, the Psychotherapy subsection guidelines have been revised to reflect these changes.

Refer to the codebook and the Rationale for the E/M Services Guidelines for a full discussion of these changes.

In accordance with the deletion of codes 99318, 99324-99328, and 99334-99337, the inclusionary parenthetical notes following codes 90833, 90836, and 90838 have been revised to reflect these changes.

Refer to the codebook and the Rationale for codes 99318, 99324-99328, and 99334-99337 for a full discussion of these changes.

Other Psychiatric Services or Procedures

(For electronic analysis with programming, when performed, of vagal nerve neurostimulators, see 95970, 95976, 95977)

★✚ **90863**   Pharmacologic management, including prescription and review of medication, when performed with psychotherapy services (List separately in addition to the code for primary procedure)

(Use 90863 in conjunction with 90832, 90834, 90837)

▶(For pharmacologic management with psychotherapy services performed by a physician or other qualified health care professional who may report evaluation and management codes, use the appropriate evaluation and management codes 99202-99255, 99281-99285, 99304, 99305, 99306, 99307, 99308, 99309, 99310, 99341-99350 and the appropriate psychotherapy with evaluation and management service 90833, 90836, 90838)◄

(Do not count time spent on providing pharmacologic management services in the time used for selection of the psychotherapy service)

90867   Therapeutic repetitive transcranial magnetic stimulation (TMS) treatment; initial, including cortical mapping, motor threshold determination, delivery and management

(Report only once per course of treatment)

(Do not report 90867 in conjunction with 90868, 90869, 95860, 95870, 95928, 95929, 95939)

▶(For peripheral nerve transcutaneous magnetic stimulation, see 0766T, 0767T, 0768T, 0769T)◄

Rationale

In accordance with the deletion of codes 99318, 99324-99328, and 99334-99337, the inclusionary parenthetical note following code 90863 has been revised to reflect these changes.

Refer to the codebook and the Rationale for codes 99318, 99324-99328, and 99334-99337 for a full discussion of these changes.

In accordance with the establishment of Category III codes 0766T-0769T, a cross-reference parenthetical note has been added following code 90867 to reflect these changes.

Refer to the codebook and the Rationale for codes 0766T-0769T for a full discussion of these changes.

Dialysis

Hemodialysis

▶Codes 90935, 90937 are reported to describe the hemodialysis procedure with all evaluation and management services related to the patient's renal disease on the day of the hemodialysis procedure. These codes are used for inpatient end-stage renal disease (ESRD) and non-ESRD procedures or for outpatient non-ESRD dialysis services. Code 90935 is reported if only one evaluation of the patient is required related to that hemodialysis procedure. Code 90937 is reported when patient re-evaluation(s) is required during a hemodialysis procedure. Use modifier 25 with evaluation and management codes, including new or established patient office or other outpatient services (99202-99215), office or other outpatient consultations (99242, 99243, 99244, 99245), hospital inpatient or observation care including admission and discharge (99234, 99235, 99236), initial and subsequent hospital inpatient or observation care (99221, 99222, 99223, 99231, 99232, 99233), hospital inpatient or observation discharge services (99238, 99239), new or established patient emergency department services (99281-99285), critical care services (99291, 99292), inpatient neonatal intensive care services and pediatric and neonatal critical care services (99466-99480), nursing facility services (99304, 99305, 99306, 99307, 99308, 99309, 99310, 99315, 99316), and home or residence services (99341-99350), for separately identifiable services unrelated to the dialysis procedure or renal failure that cannot be rendered during the dialysis session.◀

(For home visit hemodialysis services performed by a non-physician health care professional, use 99512)

(For cannula declotting, see 36831, 36833, 36860, 36861)

(For declotting of implanted vascular access device or catheter by thrombolytic agent, use 36593)

(For collection of blood specimen from a partially or completely implantable venous access device, use 36591)

▶(For prolonged attendance by a physician or other qualified health care professional, use 99360)◀

90935   Hemodialysis procedure with single evaluation by a physician or other qualified health care professional

Rationale

In accordance with the deletion of codes 99217, 99218-99220, 99224-99226, 99241, 99318, 99324-99328, and 99334-99337, the Hemodialysis subsection guidelines have been revised to reflect these changes.

Refer to the codebook and the Rationale for codes 99217, 99218-99220, 99224-99226, 99241, 99318, 99324-99328, and 99334-99337 for a full discussion of these changes.

In accordance with the deletion of codes 99354-99357, the cross-reference parenthetical note directing users to the appropriate codes for prolonged attendance by a physician or other QHP has been revised to reflect these changes.

Refer to the codebook and the Rationale for codes 99354-99357 for a full discussion of these changes.

Miscellaneous Dialysis Procedures

▶Codes 90945, 90947 describe dialysis procedures other than hemodialysis (eg, peritoneal dialysis, hemofiltration or continuous renal replacement therapies), and all evaluation and management services related to the patient's renal disease on the day of the procedure. Code 90945 is reported if only one evaluation of the patient is required related to that procedure. Code 90947 is reported when patient re-evaluation(s) is required during a procedure. Use modifier 25 with evaluation and management codes, including office or other outpatient services (99202-99215), office or other outpatient consultations (99242, 99243, 99244, 99245), hospital inpatient or observation care including admission and discharge (99234, 99235, 99236), initial and subsequent hospital inpatient or observation care (99221, 99222, 99223, 99231, 99232, 99233), hospital inpatient or observation discharge services (99238, 99239), new or established patient emergency department services (99281-99285), critical care services (99291, 99292), inpatient neonatal intensive care services and pediatric and neonatal critical care services (99466-99480), nursing facility services (99304, 99305, 99306, 99307, 99308, 99309, 99310, 99315, 99316), and home or residence services (99341-99350) for separately identifiable services unrelated to the procedure or the renal failure that cannot be rendered during the dialysis session.◀

(For percutaneous insertion of intraperitoneal tunneled catheter, use 49418. For open insertion of tunneled intraperitoneal catheter, use 49421)

▶(For prolonged attendance by a physician or other qualified health care professional, use 99360)◀

90945   Dialysis procedure other than hemodialysis (eg, peritoneal dialysis, hemofiltration, or other continuous renal replacement therapies), with single evaluation by a physician or other qualified health care professional

(For home infusion of peritoneal dialysis, use 99601, 99602)

Rationale

In accordance with the deletion of codes 99217, 99218-99220, 99224-99226, 99241, 99318, 99324-99328, and 99334-99337, the Miscellaneous Dialysis Procedures subsection guidelines have been revised to reflect these changes.

Refer to the codebook and the Rationale for codes 99217, 99218-99220, 99224-99226, 99241, 99318, 99324-99328, and 99334-99337 for a full discussion of these changes.

In accordance with the deletion of codes 99354-99357, the cross-reference parenthetical note directing users to the appropriate codes for prolonged attendance by a physician or other QHP has been revised to reflect these changes.

Refer to the codebook and the Rationale for codes 99354-99357 for a full discussion of these changes.

Gastroenterology

Other Procedures

91299	Unlisted diagnostic gastroenterology procedure
91305	Code is out of numerical sequence. See 90473-90477
91306	Code is out of numerical sequence. See 90473-90477
91307	Code is out of numerical sequence. See 90473-90477
91308	Code is out of numerical sequence. See 90473-90477
91309	Code is out of numerical sequence. See 90473-90477
91310	Code is out of numerical sequence. See 90473-90477
91311	Code is out of numerical sequence. See 90473-90477

Ophthalmology

Special Ophthalmological Services

▲ **92065** Orthoptic training; performed by a physician or other qualified health care professional

▶(Do not report 92065 in conjunction with 92066, 0687T, 0688T, when performed on the same day)◀

● **92066**   under supervision of a physician or other qualified health care professional

▶(Do not report 92066 in conjunction with 92065, 0687T, 0688T, when performed on the same day)◀

Rationale

Code 92065 has been revised and new code 92066 has been added to delineate the individual providing the orthoptic training.

Code 92065 has been revised as a new parent code to code 92066 to specify that the service is performed by a physician or other QHP. Child code 92066 has been added to report the service being performed "under supervision of a physician or other qualified health care professional." Previously, code 92065 identified orthoptic training only and did not differentiate who was performing the service.

Two exclusionary parenthetical notes following codes 92065 and 92066 have been added. The first parenthetical note following code 92065 has been added to restrict reporting code 92065 in conjunction with codes 92066, 0687T, and 0688T, when performed on the same day. The second parenthetical note following code 92066 has been added to restrict reporting code 92066 in conjunction with codes 92065, 0687T, and 0688T, when performed on the same day.

Clinical Example (92065)

A 25-year-old female is referred for orthoptic training by a physician or other QHP to address convergence insufficiency issues after a concussion.

Description of Procedure (92065)

Position patient before specialized instruments that allow the systematic application of lenses, prisms, and angular disparity designed to address the ocular motor defect and to treat the dysfunction. Prescribed treatment regimens include a series of interventions during the treatment period, including convergence exercises using an accommodative target of letters, numbers, or pictures; vergence exercises with applied base in or base out prism; jump to near convergence training on a brock string; stereogram convergence exercises; and three-dimensional (3D) vergence demand exercises applied with an interactive video display. The patient demonstrates understanding to the physician or other QHP by proper performance of each of the prescribed exercises.

| 92132 | Scanning computerized ophthalmic diagnostic imaging, anterior segment, with interpretation and report, unilateral or bilateral |

▶(Do not report 92132 in conjunction with 0730T)◀

(For specular microscopy and endothelial cell analysis, use 92286)

(For tear film imaging, use 0330T)

Rationale

In accordance with the establishment of Category III code 0730T, an exclusionary parenthetical note has been added following code 92132 restricting reporting with code 0730T.

Refer to the codebook and the Rationale for code 0730T for a full discussion of this change.

Ophthalmoscopy

★ **92227** Imaging of retina for detection or monitoring of disease; with remote clinical staff review and report, unilateral or bilateral

(Do not report 92227 in conjunction with 92133, 92134, 92228, 92229, 92250)

★ **92228** with remote physician or other qualified health care professional interpretation and report, unilateral or bilateral

(Do not report 92228 in conjunction with 92133, 92134, 92227, 92229, 92250)

▲ **92229** point-of-care autonomous analysis and report, unilateral or bilateral

(Do not report 92229 in conjunction with 92133, 92134, 92227, 92228, 92250)

Rationale

Code 92229 has been editorially revised by removing the term "automated" and adding "autonomous." This revision aligns with Appendix S, which provides guidance for classifying various artificial intelligence (AI) medical procedures.

As stated in Appendix S, the work performed by the machine for the physician or other QHP is autonomous when the machine automatically interprets data and independently generates clinically meaningful conclusions without concurrent physician or other QHP involvement. Autonomous medical services and procedures include interrogating and analyzing data. The work of the algorithm may or may not include acquisition, preparation, and/or transmission of data. The clinically meaningful conclusion may be a characterization of data (eg, likelihood of pathophysiology) that may be used to establish a diagnosis or to implement a therapeutic intervention.

Other Specialized Services

▶For prescription, fitting, and/or medical supervision of ocular prosthetic (artificial eye) adaptation by a physician, see evaluation and management services, including office or other outpatient services (99202-99215), office or other outpatient consultations (99242, 99243, 99244, 99245), or general ophthalmological service codes (92002-92014).◀

Electroretinography (ERG) is used to evaluate function of the retina and optic nerve of the eye, including photoreceptors and ganglion cells. A number of techniques are used which target different areas of the eye, including full field (flash and flicker) (92273) for a global response of photoreceptors of the retina, multifocal (92274) for photoreceptors in multiple separate locations in the retina including the macula, and pattern (0509T) for retinal ganglion cells. Multiple additional terms and techniques are used to describe various types of ERG. If the technique used is not specifically named in the code descriptors for 92273, 92274, or 0509T, use the unlisted procedure code 92499.

92265 Needle oculoelectromyography, 1 or more extraocular muscles, 1 or both eyes, with interpretation and report

92283 Color vision examination, extended, eg, anomaloscope or equivalent

(Color vision testing with pseudoisochromatic plates [such as HRR or Ishihara] is not reported separately. It is included in the appropriate general or ophthalmological service, or 99172)

▲ **92284** Diagnostic dark adaptation examination with interpretation and report

Rationale

In accordance with the deletion of code 99241, the Other Specialized Services subsection guidelines have been revised to reflect this change.

Refer to the codebook and the Rationale for code 99241 for a full discussion of this change.

Also, code 92284 has been revised. Because the service described in code 92284 is diagnostic in nature, the term "diagnostic" has been added to the descriptor to clarify that this is a diagnostic service and to reflect current clinical practice.

Clinical Example (92284)

A 55-year-old female with poor night vision has no identifiable cause on examination. Dark adaptation testing is performed to assess retinal function.

Medicine 90281-99607

Description of Procedure (92284)

Review the test results for each eye to determine reliability and interocular consistency. Interpret results, correlating the dark adaptation plot with age-adjusted norms, physical findings, and prior test results. Prepare a report and include in the medical record.

Special Otorhinolaryngologic Services

Diagnostic or treatment procedures that are reported as evaluation and management services (eg, otoscopy, anterior rhinoscopy, tuning fork test, removal of non-impacted cerumen) are not reported separately.

▶Special otorhinolaryngologic services are those diagnostic and treatment services not included in an evaluation and management service, including office or other outpatient services (99202-99215) or office or other outpatient consultations (99242, 99243, 99244, 99245).◀

Codes 92507, 92508, 92520, 92521, 92522, 92523, 92524, and 92526 are used to report evaluation and treatment of speech sound production, receptive language, and expressive language abilities, voice and resonance production, speech fluency, and swallowing. Evaluations may include examination of speech sound production, articulatory movements of oral musculature, oral-pharyngeal swallowing function, qualitative analysis of voice and resonance, and measures of frequency, type, and duration of stuttering. Evaluations may also include the patient's ability to understand the meaning and intent of written and verbal expressions, as well as the appropriate formulation and utterance of expressive thought.

(For laryngoscopy with stroboscopy, use 31579)

Rationale

In accordance with the deletion of code 99241, the Special Otorhinolaryngologic Services subsection guidelines have been revised to reflect this change.

Refer to the codebook and the Rationale for code 99241 for a full discussion of this change.

Vestibular Function Tests, Without Electrical Recording

92532 Positional nystagmus test

▶(Do not report 92531, 92532 with evaluation and management services, including office or other outpatient services [99202-99215], hospital inpatient or observation care services including admission and discharge [99234-99236], hospital inpatient or observation care services [99221-99223, 99231-99233], office or other outpatient consultations [99242, 99243, 99244, 99245], nursing facility services [99304-99316])◀

Rationale

In accordance with the deletion of codes 99217, 99218-99220, 99224-99226, 99241, 99318, 99324-99328, and 99334-99337, the exclusionary parenthetical note following code 92532 has been revised to reflect these changes.

Refer to the codebook and the Rationale for codes 99217, 99218-99220, 99224-99226, 99241, 99318, 99324-99328, and 99334-99337 for a full discussion of these changes.

Evaluative and Therapeutic Services

★ **92601** Diagnostic analysis of cochlear implant, patient younger than 7 years of age; with programming

★ **92602** subsequent reprogramming

(Do not report 92602 in addition to 92601)

(For aural rehabilitation services following cochlear implant, including evaluation of rehabilitation status, see 92626-92627, 92630-92633)

★ **92603** Diagnostic analysis of cochlear implant, age 7 years or older; with programming

★ **92604** subsequent reprogramming

(Do not report 92604 in addition to 92603)

▶(For initial and subsequent diagnostic analysis and programming of vestibular implant, see 0728T, 0729T)◀

Rationale

In accordance with the establishment of Category III codes 0728T and 0729T, a cross-reference parenthetical note directing users to the new codes has been added following code 92604.

Refer to the codebook and the Rationale for codes 0728T and 0729T for a full discussion of these changes.

★ = Telemedicine   ◀ = Audio-only   ✛ = Add-on code   ✗ = FDA approval pending   # = Resequenced code   ⊘ = Modifier 51 exempt

Cardiovascular

Therapeutic Services and Procedures

Coronary Therapeutic Services and Procedures

▶Codes 92920-92944 describe percutaneous revascularization services performed for occlusive disease of the coronary vessels (major coronary arteries, coronary artery branches, or coronary artery bypass grafts). These percutaneous coronary intervention (PCI) codes are built on progressive hierarchies with more intensive services inclusive of lesser intensive services. These PCI codes all include the work of accessing and selectively catheterizing the vessel, traversing the lesion, radiological supervision and interpretation directly related to the intervention(s) performed, closure of the arteriotomy when performed through the access sheath, and imaging performed to document completion of the intervention in addition to the intervention(s) performed. These codes include angioplasty (eg, balloon, cutting balloon, wired balloons, cryoplasty), atherectomy (eg, directional, rotational, laser), and stenting (eg, balloon expandable, self-expanding, bare metal, drug eluting, covered). Each code in this family includes balloon angioplasty, when performed. Diagnostic coronary angiography may be reported separately under specific circumstances. Percutaneous transluminal coronary lithotripsy may be reported using 0715T in conjunction with 92920, 92924, 92928, 92933, 92937, 92941, 92943, 92975, as appropriate.◀

Diagnostic coronary angiography codes (93454-93461) and injection procedure codes (93563-93564) should not be used with percutaneous coronary revascularization services (92920-92944) to report:

1. Contrast injections, angiography, roadmapping, and/or fluoroscopic guidance for the coronary intervention,

2. Vessel measurement for the coronary intervention, **or**

3. Post-coronary angioplasty/stent/atherectomy angiography, as this work is captured in the percutaneous coronary revascularization services codes (92920-92944).

Diagnostic angiography performed at the time of a coronary interventional procedure may be separately reportable if:

1. No prior catheter-based coronary angiography study is available, and a full diagnostic study is performed, and a decision to intervene is based on the diagnostic angiography, **or**

2. A prior study is available, but as documented in the medical record:

a. The patient's condition with respect to the clinical indication has changed since the prior study, **or**

b. There is inadequate visualization of the anatomy and/or pathology, **or**

c. There is a clinical change during the procedure that requires new evaluation outside the target area of intervention.

Diagnostic coronary angiography performed at a separate session from an interventional procedure is separately reportable.

Major coronary arteries: The major coronary arteries are the left main, left anterior descending, left circumflex, right, and ramus intermedius arteries. All PCI procedures performed in all segments (proximal, mid, distal) of a single major coronary artery through the native coronary circulation are reported with one code. When one segment of a major coronary artery is treated through the native circulation and treatment of another segment of the same artery requires access through a coronary artery bypass graft, the intervention through the bypass graft is reported separately.

Coronary artery branches: Up to two coronary artery branches of the left anterior descending (diagonals), left circumflex (marginals), and right (posterior descending, posterolaterals) coronary arteries are recognized. The left main and ramus intermedius coronary arteries do not have recognized branches for reporting purposes. All PCI(s) performed in any segment (proximal, mid, distal) of a coronary artery branch is reported with one code. PCI is reported for up to two branches of a major coronary artery. Additional PCI in a third branch of the same major coronary artery is not separately reportable.

Coronary artery bypass grafts: Each coronary artery bypass graft represents a coronary vessel. A sequential bypass graft with more than one distal anastomosis represents only one graft. A branching bypass graft (eg, Y graft) represents a coronary vessel for the main graft, and each branch off the main graft constitutes an additional coronary vessel. PCI performed on major coronary arteries or coronary artery branches by access through a bypass graft is reported using the bypass graft PCI codes. All bypass graft PCI codes include the use of coronary artery embolic protection devices when performed.

Only one base code from this family may be reported for revascularization of a major coronary artery and its recognized branches. Only one base code should be reported for revascularization of a coronary artery bypass graft, its subtended coronary artery, and recognized branches of the subtended coronary artery. If one segment of a major coronary artery and its recognized branches is treated through the native circulation, and treatment of another segment of the same vessel requires access through a coronary artery bypass graft, an additional base code is reported to describe the intervention performed through the bypass graft. The

Medicine 90281-99607

PCI base codes are 92920, 92924, 92928, 92933, 92937, 92941, and 92943. The PCI base code that includes the most intensive service provided for the target vessel should be reported. The hierarchy of these services is built on an intensity of service ranked from highest to lowest as 92943 = 92941 = 92933 > 92924 > 92937 = 92928 > 92920.

PCI performed during the same session in additional recognized branches of the target vessel should be reported using the applicable add-on code(s). The add-on codes are 92921, 92925, 92928, 92934, 92938, and 92944 and follow the same principle in regard to reporting the most intensive service provided. The intensity of service is ranked from highest to lowest as 92944 = 92938 > 92934 > 92925 > 92929 > 92921.

PCI performed during the same session in additional major coronary or in additional coronary artery bypass grafts should be reported using the applicable additional base code(s). PCI performed during the same session in additional coronary artery branches should be reported using the applicable additional add-on code(s).

If a single lesion extends from one target vessel (major coronary artery, coronary artery bypass graft, or coronary artery branch) into another target vessel, but can be revascularized with a single intervention bridging the two vessels, this PCI should be reported with a single code despite treating more than one vessel. For example, if a left main coronary lesion extends into the proximal left circumflex coronary artery and a single stent is placed to treat the entire lesion, this PCI should be reported as a single vessel stent (92928). In this example, a code for additional vessel treatment (92929) would not be additionally reported.

When bifurcation lesions are treated, PCI is reported for both vessels treated. For example, when a bifurcation lesion involving the left anterior descending artery and the first diagonal artery is treated by stenting both vessels, 92928 and 92929 are both reported.

Target vessel PCI for acute myocardial infarction is inclusive of all balloon angioplasty, atherectomy, stenting, manual aspiration thrombectomy, distal protection, and intracoronary rheolytic agent administration performed. Mechanical thrombectomy is reported separately.

Chronic total occlusion of a coronary vessel is present when there is no antegrade flow through the true lumen, accompanied by suggestive angiographic and clinical criteria (eg, antegrade "bridging" collaterals present, calcification at the occlusion site, no current presentation with ST elevation or Q wave acute myocardial infarction attributable to the occluded target lesion). Current presentation with ST elevation or Q wave acute myocardial infarction attributable to the occluded target lesion, subtotal occlusion, and occlusion with dye staining at the site consistent with fresh thrombus are not considered chronic total occlusion.

▶Codes 92973 (percutaneous transluminal coronary thrombectomy, mechanical), 92974 (coronary brachytherapy), 92978 and 92979 (intravascular ultrasound/optical coherence tomography), 93571 and 93572 (intravascular Doppler velocity and/or pressure [fractional flow reserve {FFR} or coronary flow reserve {CFR}]), and 0715T (percutaneous transluminal coronary lithotripsy), are add-on codes for reporting procedures performed in addition to coronary and bypass graft diagnostic and interventional services, unless included in the base code. Non-mechanical, aspiration thrombectomy is not reported with 92973, and is included in the PCI code for acute myocardial infarction (92941), when performed.◀

(To report transcatheter placement of radiation delivery device for coronary intravascular brachytherapy, use 92974)

(For intravascular radioelement application, see 77770, 77771, 77772)

(For nonsurgical septal reduction therapy [eg, alcohol ablation], use 93799)

92920 Percutaneous transluminal coronary angioplasty; single major coronary artery or branch

▶(For percutaneous transluminal coronary lithotripsy, use 0715T)◀

#+ 92921 each additional branch of a major coronary artery (List separately in addition to code for primary procedure)

(Use 92921 in conjunction with 92920, 92924, 92928, 92933, 92937, 92941, 92943)

92924 Percutaneous transluminal coronary atherectomy, with coronary angioplasty when performed; single major coronary artery or branch

▶(For percutaneous transluminal coronary lithotripsy, use 0715T)◀

#+ 92925 each additional branch of a major coronary artery (List separately in addition to code for primary procedure)

(Use 92925 in conjunction with 92924, 92928, 92933, 92937, 92941, 92943)

92928 Percutaneous transcatheter placement of intracoronary stent(s), with coronary angioplasty when performed; single major coronary artery or branch

▶(For percutaneous transluminal coronary lithotripsy, use 0715T)◀

#+ 92929 each additional branch of a major coronary artery (List separately in addition to code for primary procedure)

(Use 92929 in conjunction with 92928, 92933, 92937, 92941, 92943)

92933 Percutaneous transluminal coronary atherectomy, with intracoronary stent, with coronary angioplasty when performed; single major coronary artery or branch

★ = Telemedicine   ◀ = Audio-only   + = Add-on code   ✔ = FDA approval pending   # = Resequenced code   ⊘ = Modifier 51 exempt

▶(For percutaneous transluminal coronary lithotripsy, use 0715T)◀

#+ 92934   each additional branch of a major coronary artery (List separately in addition to code for primary procedure)

(Use 92934 in conjunction with 92933, 92937, 92941, 92943)

 # 92937   Percutaneous transluminal revascularization of or through coronary artery bypass graft (internal mammary, free arterial, venous), any combination of intracoronary stent, atherectomy and angioplasty, including distal protection when performed; single vessel

▶(For percutaneous transluminal coronary lithotripsy, use 0715T)◀

#+ 92938   each additional branch subtended by the bypass graft (List separately in addition to code for primary procedure)

(Use 92938 in conjunction with 92937)

 # 92941   Percutaneous transluminal revascularization of acute total/subtotal occlusion during acute myocardial infarction, coronary artery or coronary artery bypass graft, any combination of intracoronary stent, atherectomy and angioplasty, including aspiration thrombectomy when performed, single vessel

(For additional vessels treated, see 92920-92938, 92943, 92944)

(For transcatheter intra-arterial hyperoxemic reperfusion/supersaturated oxygen therapy [SSO$_2$], use 0659T)

▶(For percutaneous transluminal coronary lithotripsy, use 0715T)◀

 # 92943   Percutaneous transluminal revascularization of chronic total occlusion, coronary artery, coronary artery branch, or coronary artery bypass graft, any combination of intracoronary stent, atherectomy and angioplasty; single vessel

▶(For percutaneous transluminal coronary lithotripsy, use 0715T)◀

#+ 92944   each additional coronary artery, coronary artery branch, or bypass graft (List separately in addition to code for primary procedure)

(Use 92944 in conjunction with 92924, 92928, 92933, 92937, 92941, 92943)

(To report transcatheter placement of radiation delivery device for coronary intravascular brachytherapy, use 92974)

(For intravascular radioelement application, see 77770, 77771, 77772)

#+ 92973   Percutaneous transluminal coronary thrombectomy mechanical (List separately in addition to code for primary procedure)

(Use 92973 in conjunction with 92920, 92924, 92928, 92933, 92937, 92941, 92943, 92975, 93454-93461, 93563, 93564)

(Do not report 92973 for aspiration thrombectomy)

#+ 92974   Transcatheter placement of radiation delivery device for subsequent coronary intravascular brachytherapy (List separately in addition to code for primary procedure)

(Use 92974 in conjunction with 92920, 92924, 92928, 92933, 92937, 92941, 92943, 93454-93461)

(For intravascular radioelement application, see 77770, 77771, 77772)

 # 92975   Thrombolysis, coronary; by intracoronary infusion, including selective coronary angiography

▶(For percutaneous transluminal coronary lithotripsy, use 0715T)◀

 # 92977   by intravenous infusion

(For thrombolysis of vessels other than coronary, see 37211-37214)

(For cerebral thrombolysis, use 37195)

Rationale

The introductory guidelines in the Coronary Therapeutic Services and Procedures subsection have been revised with instructions about which codes should be used in conjunction with new code 0715T (percutaneous transluminal coronary lithotripsy).

In addition, parenthetical notes have been established following codes 92920, 92924, 92928, 92933, 92937, 92941, 92943, and 92975 to instruct users to use code 0715T for percutaneous transluminal coronary lithotripsy.

Refer to the codebook and the Rationale for code 0715T for a full discussion of these changes.

Cardiography

93000   Electrocardiogram, routine ECG with at least 12 leads; with interpretation and report

93005   tracing only, without interpretation and report

93010   interpretation and report only

▶(For ECG monitoring, use 99418)◀

(Do not report 93000, 93005, 93010 in conjunction with, 0525T, 0526T, 0527T, 0528T, 0529T, 0530T, 0531T, 0532T)

▲=Revised code   ●=New code   ▶◀=Contains new or revised text   ✖=Duplicate PLA test   ⇅=Category I PLA   American Medical Association   **189**

Medicine 90281-99607

Rationale

In accordance with the deletion of codes 99354-99357 and the establishment of code 99418, the cross-reference parenthetical note following code 93010 has been revised to reflect these changes.

Refer to the codebook and the Rationale for codes 99354-99357 and 99418 for a full discussion of these changes.

Cardiovascular Monitoring Services

 # 93241 External electrocardiographic recording for more than 48 hours up to 7 days by continuous rhythm recording and storage; includes recording, scanning analysis with report, review and interpretation

 # 93242 recording (includes connection and initial recording)

 # 93243 scanning analysis with report

 # 93244 review and interpretation

▶(Do not report 93241, 93242, 93243, 93244 in conjunction with 93224, 93225, 93226, 93227, 93228, 93229, 93245, 93246, 93247, 93248, 93268, 93270, 93271, 93272, 99091, 99453, 99454, for the same monitoring period)◀

 # 93245 External electrocardiographic recording for more than 7 days up to 15 days by continuous rhythm recording and storage; includes recording, scanning analysis with report, review and interpretation

 # 93246 recording (includes connection and initial recording)

 # 93247 scanning analysis with report

 # 93248 review and interpretation

▶(Do not report 93245, 93246, 93247, 93248 in conjunction with 93224, 93225, 93226, 93227, 93228, 93229, 93241, 93242, 93243, 93244, 93268, 93270, 93271, 93272, 99091, 99453, 99454, for the same monitoring period)◀

Rationale

In accordance with the deletion of Category III codes 0497T-0498T, exclusionary parenthetical notes following codes 93244 and 93248 have been revised with the removal of these codes.

Refer to the codebook and the Rationale for codes 0497T-0498T for a full discussion of the changes.

Cardiac Catheterization

Cardiac catheterization is a diagnostic medical procedure which includes introduction, positioning and repositioning, when necessary, of catheter(s), within the vascular system, recording of intracardiac and/or intravascular pressure(s), and final evaluation and report of procedure. There are two code families for cardiac catheterization: one for congenital heart disease and one for all other conditions. For cardiac catheterization for congenital heart defects (93593, 93594, 93595, 93596, 93597, 93598), see the **Medicine/Cardiovascular/ Cardiac Catheterization for Congenital Heart Defects** subsection. The following guidelines apply to cardiac catheterization performed for indications other than the evaluation of congenital heart defects.

Right heart catheterization for indications other than the evaluation of congenital heart defects (93453, 93456, 93457, 93460, 93461): includes catheter placement in one or more right-sided cardiac chamber(s) or structures (ie, the right atrium, right ventricle, pulmonary artery, pulmonary wedge), obtaining blood samples for measurement of blood gases, and cardiac output measurements (Fick or other method), when performed. For placement of a flow directed catheter (eg, Swan-Ganz) performed for hemodynamic monitoring purposes not in conjunction with other catheterization services, use 93503. Do not report 93503 in conjunction with other diagnostic cardiac catheterization codes. Right heart catheterization does not include right ventricular or right atrial angiography (93566).

Codes for catheter placement(s) in native coronary arteries (93454-93461), and bypass graft(s) (93455, 93457, 93459, 93461) include intraprocedural injection(s) for coronary/bypass graft angiography, imaging supervision, and interpretation, except when these catheter placements are performed during cardiac catheterization for the evaluation of congenital heart defects. Do not report 93563-93565 in conjunction with 93452-93461.

▶For right ventricular or right atrial angiography performed in conjunction with right heart catheterization for noncongenital heart disease (93451, 93453, 93456, 93457, 93460, 93461) or for the evaluation of congenital heart defects (93593, 93594, 93596, 93597), use 93566. For reporting purposes, angiography of the morphologic right ventricle or morphologic right atrium is reported with 93566, whether these structures are in the standard prepulmonic position or in a systemic (subaortic) position. Left heart catheterization performed for noncongenital heart disease (93452, 93453, 93458, 93459, 93460, 93461) includes left ventriculography, when performed. For reporting purposes, angiography of the morphologic left ventricle or morphologic left atrium is reported with 93565, whether these structures are in the standard systemic (subaortic) position or in a

Medicine 90281-99607

prepulmonic position. Do not report 93565 in conjunction with 93452, 93453, 93454, 93455, 93456, 93457, 93458, 93459, 93460, 93461. For cardiac catheterization performed for the evaluation of congenital heart defects, left ventriculography is separately reported with 93565. For cardiac catheterization for both congenital and noncongenital heart defects, supravalvular aortography is reported with 93567. For cardiac catheterization for both congenital and noncongenital heart defects, pulmonary arterial angiography or selective pulmonary venous angiography is reported with the appropriate pulmonary angiography code(s) (93568, 93569, 93573, 93574, 93575) plus the appropriate cardiac catheterization code.

When contrast injection(s) are performed in conjunction with cardiac catheterization for congenital heart disease (93593, 93594, 93595, 93596, 93597), see 93563, 93564, 93565, 93566, 93567, 93568, 93569, 93573, 93574, 93575. Injection procedures 93563, 93564, 93565, 93566, 93567, 93568, 93569, 93573, 93574, 93575 represent separate identifiable services and may be reported in conjunction with one another when appropriate. Codes 93563, 93564, 93565, 93566, 93567, 93568, 93569, 93573, 93574, 93575 include imaging supervision, interpretation, and report.

For angiography of noncoronary and nonpulmonary arteries and veins, performed as a distinct service, use appropriate codes from the Radiology section and the Vascular Injection Procedures subsection in the Surgery/Cardiovascular System section.

For nonselective pulmonary arterial angiography, use 93568. For selective unilateral or bilateral pulmonary arterial angiography, see 93569, 93573. For selective pulmonary venous angiography, use 93574 for each distinct vessel. For selective pulmonary arterial angiography of major aortopulmonary collateral arteries (MAPCAs) arising off the aorta or its systemic branches, use 93575 for each distinct vessel.

Injection procedures 93574, 93575 represent selective venous and arterial angiography, respectively, for each distinct vessel. Codes 93574, 93575 require evaluation of a distinct, named vessel (eg, right upper pulmonary vein, left lower pulmonary vein, left pulmonary artery via Blalock-Taussig [BT] shunt access, major aortopulmonary collateral artery [MAPCA] vessel #1 from underside of aortic arch) and may be reported for each distinct, named vessel evaluated.

Selective pulmonary angiography codes for cardiac catheterization (93569, 93573, 93574, 93575) include selective angiographic catheter positioning, injection, and radiologic supervision and interpretation).

Adjunctive hemodynamic assessments: when cardiac catheterization is combined with pharmacologic agent administration with the specific purpose of repeating hemodynamic measurements to evaluate hemodynamic

response, use 93463 in conjunction with 93451-93453 and 93456-93461, 93593, 93594, 93595, 93596, 93597. Do not report 93463 for intracoronary administration of pharmacologic agents during percutaneous coronary interventional procedures, during intracoronary assessment of coronary pressure, flow or resistance, or during intracoronary imaging procedures. Do not report 93463 in conjunction with 92920-92944, 92975, 92977.◄

When cardiac catheterization is combined with exercise (eg, walking or arm or leg ergometry protocol) with the specific purpose of repeating hemodynamic measurements to evaluate hemodynamic response, report 93464 in conjunction with 93451-93453, 93456-93461, 93593, 93594, 93595, 93596, 93597.

Contrast injection to image the access site(s) for the specific purpose of placing a closure device is inherent to the catheterization procedure and not separately reportable. Closure device placement at the vascular access site is inherent to the catheterization procedure and not separately reportable.

93451   Right heart catheterization including measurement(s) of oxygen saturation and cardiac output, when performed

(Do not report 93451 in conjunction with 33289, 93453, 93456, 93457, 93460, 93461, 0613T, 0632T)

(Do not report 93451 in conjunction with 33418, 0345T, 0483T, 0484T, 0544T, 0545T, 0643T, for diagnostic right heart catheterization procedures intrinsic to the valve repair, annulus reconstruction procedure, or left ventricular restoration device implantation)

93503   Insertion and placement of flow directed catheter (eg, Swan-Ganz) for monitoring purposes

(Do not report 93503 in conjunction with 0632T)

►(For subsequent monitoring, use 99418)◄

(Use 93563 in conjunction with 33741, 33745, 93582, 93593, 93594, 93595, 93596, 93597)

+▲ 93568   for nonselective pulmonary arterial angiography (List separately in addition to code for primary procedure)

►(Use 93568 in conjunction with 33361, 33362, 33363, 33364, 33365, 33366, 33418, 33419, 33477, 33741, 33745, 33894, 33895, 33900, 33901, 33902, 33903, 33904, 37187, 37188, 37236, 37237, 37238, 37246, 37248, 92997, 92998, 93451, 93453, 93456, 93457, 93460, 93461, 93580, 93581, 93582, 93583, 93593, 93594, 93595, 93596, 93597)◄

(Do not report 93568 in conjunction with 0632T)

►(For selective unilateral or bilateral pulmonary arterial angiography, use 93569, 93573, which include catheter placement, injection, and radiologic supervision and interpretation)◄

Medicine 90281-99607

+● 93569   for selective pulmonary arterial angiography, unilateral (List separately in addition to code for primary procedure)

#+● 93573   for selective pulmonary arterial angiography, bilateral (List separately in addition to code for primary procedure)

►(Use 93569, 93573 in conjunction with 33361, 33362, 33363, 33364, 33365, 33366, 33418, 33419, 33477, 33741, 33745, 37236, 37237, 37238, 37246, 37248, 33894, 33895, 33900, 33901, 33902, 33903, 33904, 37187, 37188, 92997, 92998, 93451, 93453, 93456, 93457, 93460, 93461, 93505, 93580, 93581, 93582, 93583, 93593, 93594, 93595, 93596, 93597)◄

#+● 93574   for selective pulmonary venous angiography of each distinct pulmonary vein during cardiac catheterization (List separately in addition to code for primary procedure)

►(Use 93574 in conjunction with 33361, 33362, 33363, 33364, 33365, 33366, 33418, 33419, 33477, 33741, 33745, 37236, 37237, 37238, 37246, 37248, 33894, 33895, 33900, 33901, 33902, 33903, 33904, 37187, 37188, 92997, 92998, 93451, 93453, 93456, 93457, 93460, 93461, 93505, 93580, 93581, 93582, 93583, 93593, 93594, 93595, 93596, 93597)◄

#+● 93575   for selective pulmonary angiography of major aortopulmonary collateral arteries (MAPCAs) arising off the aorta or its systemic branches, during cardiac catheterization for congenital heart defects, each distinct vessel (List separately in addition to code for primary procedure)

►(Use 93575 in conjunction with 33361, 33362, 33363, 33364, 33365, 33366, 33418, 33419, 33477, 33741, 33745, 37236, 37237, 37238, 37246, 37248, 33894, 33895, 33900, 33901, 33902, 33903, 33904, 37187, 37188, 92997, 92998, 93451, 93453, 93456, 93457, 93460, 93461, 93505, 93580, 93581, 93582, 93583, 93593, 93594, 93595, 93596, 93597)◄

►(93569, 93573, 93574, 93575 include the selective introduction and positioning of the angiographic catheter, injection, and radiologic supervision and interpretation)◄

+ 93572   each additional vessel (List separately in addition to code for primary procedure)

(Use 93572 in conjunction with 93571)

(Do not report 93572 in conjunction with 0523T)

(Intravascular distal coronary blood flow velocity measurements include all Doppler transducer manipulations and repositioning within the specific vessel being examined, during coronary angiography or therapeutic intervention [eg, angioplasty])

(For unlisted cardiac catheterization procedure, use 93799)

93573   Code is out of numerical sequence. See 93567-93572

93574   Code is out of numerical sequence. See 93567-93572

93575   Code is out of numerical sequence. See 93567-93572

Rationale

Add-on codes 93569 and 93573-93575 have been established, add-on code 93568 has been revised, and the Cardiac Catheterization subsection guidelines have been revised.

Prior to 2023, code 93568 described pulmonary angiography and did not distinguish between the work involved in angiography performed on pulmonary arteries vs on pulmonary veins. Pulmonary arteries are right-heart structures and pulmonary veins are left-heart structures. Different approaches are utilized to perform the procedures in the right heart vs the left heart.

Effective in 2023, code 93568 has been revised and codes 93569 and 93573-93575 have been established to accurately reflect angiography procedures performed on pulmonary arteries and pulmonary veins. Code 93568 now describes the injection procedure specifically for nonselective pulmonary arterial angiography during cardiac catheterization. Codes 93569 and 93573 describe injection procedures for pulmonary arterial angiography during cardiac catheterization. Code 93569 is reported for a unilateral procedure, and code 93573 is reported for a bilateral procedure. Code 93574 describes the injection procedure for pulmonary *venous* angiography of each distinct pulmonary vein during cardiac catheterization. Code 93575 describes the injection procedure for pulmonary angiography of major aortopulmonary collateral arteries (MAPCAs) arising off the aorta or its systemic branches during cardiac catheterization for congenital heart defects. Codes 93569 and 93573-93575 include the selective introduction and positioning of the angiographic catheter, injection, and radiologic supervision and interpretation. An instructional parenthetical note has been added to indicate this following code 93575.

The procedures described by codes 93568, 93569, and 93573-93575 are add-on procedures performed with primary transcatheter procedures, including cardiac valve procedures, stent repair of coarctation of the aorta, pulmonary artery revascularization, venous mechanical thrombectomy, intravascular stent placement, balloon angioplasty, cardiac catheterization procedures, cardiac catheterization for congenital heart defects, and structural heart defect repair. Inclusionary parenthetical notes have been added listing the specific primary procedure codes with which codes 93569 and 93573-93575 should be reported. The existing inclusionary parenthetical note following code 93568 has been revised with additional primary procedure codes with which it may be reported.

The Cardiac Catheterization subsection guidelines have been revised and parenthetical notes have been added to provide instruction on the appropriate use of codes 93568, 93569, and 93573-93575.

★=Telemedicine   ◀=Audio-only   +=Add-on code   ✚=FDA approval pending   #=Resequenced code   ⊘=Modifier 51 exempt

In accordance with the deletion of codes 99356 and 99357, the cross-reference parenthetical note for subsequent monitoring following code 93503 has been revised to reflect these changes.

Refer to the codebook and the Rationale for codes 99356 and 99357 for a full discussion of these changes.

Clinical Example (93568)

A 40-year-old female with dyspnea and echocardiographic findings of a dilated right ventricle undergoes a diagnostic right heart catheterization during a diagnostic cardiac catheterization. During the procedure, nonselective pulmonary arterial angiography is performed. [**Note:** This is an add-on code. Only consider the additional work related to the nonselective pulmonary artery angiogram.]

Description of Procedure (93568)

(Note that diagnostic congenital or non-congenital catheterization codes include the work of passing a catheter into the main pulmonary artery. The work of code 93568 begins when the catheter is attached to a power injector with careful removal of air from the tubing.) Use fluoroscopic guidance to ensure proper catheter position. Then perform power injection in appropriate angiographic views to fully opacify the pulmonary artery, allowing evaluation of pulmonary valve regurgitation, branch pulmonary blood flow, and other vessel abnormalities. Disconnect the power injector from the catheter, re-attach the catheter to the manifold, and again remove any air. Continuously monitor patient's arterial pressure, electrocardiogram (ECG), and oxygen saturation throughout the procedure. Review all images and describe them in the procedure report. Per routine, monitor any contrast injection afterward for complications of allergic reaction, arrhythmia, hemodynamic instability, and contrast-induced nephropathy.

Clinical Example (93569)

A 2-year-old female, who has a prior history of repaired tetralogy of Fallot, has selective branch pulmonary artery angiograms to evaluate for branch stenosis during a diagnostic right heart cardiac catheterization. [**Note:** This is an add-on code. Only consider the additional work related to the nonselective pulmonary artery angiogram.]

Description of Procedure (93569)

(Note that diagnostic cardiac catheterization for both congenital and noncongenital indications includes the work of passing a diagnostic catheter into the main pulmonary artery. The work of code 93569 begins when a wire is introduced through the diagnostic catheter to a more distal segmental pulmonary artery branch for selective catheterization. Then the diagnostic catheter is either advanced over the wire and the wire removed for a selective hand injection, or the diagnostic catheter is exchanged over the wire for an angiographic catheter to perform an angiogram with a power injector.) Use fluoroscopic guidance to confirm proper catheter position before angiography. Based on the findings from the initial imaging, additional angles may need to be acquired for better definition of suspected defects, and an angiographic injection is repeated. Continuously monitor patient's arterial pressure, ECG, and oxygen saturation throughout the procedure. Review all images and describe in the procedure report. Per routine, monitor any contrast injection afterward for complications of allergic reaction, arrhythmia, hemodynamic instability, and contrast-induced nephropathy.

Clinical Example (93573)

A 2-year-old female, who has a prior history of repaired tetralogy of Fallot, has selective branch pulmonary artery angiograms to evaluate for branch stenosis during a diagnostic right heart cardiac catheterization. [**Note:** This is an add-on code. Only consider the additional work related to the nonselective pulmonary artery angiogram.]

Description of Procedure (93573)

(Note that diagnostic cardiac catheterization for both congenital and noncongenital indications includes the work of passing a diagnostic catheter into the main pulmonary artery. The work of code 93573 begins when a wire is introduced through the diagnostic catheter to further select a more distal segmental pulmonary artery branch for selective catheterization. The diagnostic catheter is then either advanced over the wire and the wire removed for a selective hand injection, or the diagnostic catheter is exchanged over the wire for an angiographic catheter to perform an angiogram with a power injector.) Use fluoroscopic guidance to confirm proper catheter position before angiography. Based on the findings from the initial imaging, additional angles may need to be acquired for better definition of suspected defects, and an angiographic injection is repeated. Using the same or a differently shaped catheter, re-insert a wire and use to enter the contralateral branch pulmonary artery and selectively position the catheter into another segmental pulmonary artery branch. Repeat the above process for contrast injection of the contralateral branch pulmonary artery. Continuously monitor patient's arterial pressure, ECG, and oxygen saturation throughout the procedure. Review all images and describe in the procedure report. Per routine, monitor any contrast injection afterward for complications of allergic reaction, arrhythmia, hemodynamic instability, and contrast-induced nephropathy.

Clinical Example (93574)

A 6-month-old male with Down syndrome, who is status post-atrioventricular (AV) canal repair with new pulmonary hypertension, undergoes multiple selective pulmonary venous angiograms to evaluate for presence of any pulmonary vein stenosis during a diagnostic cardiac catheterization. [**Note:** This is an add-on code. Only consider the additional work related to each additional distinct pulmonary vein angiogram.]

Description of Procedure (93574)

(Note that diagnostic cardiac catheterization for both congenital and noncongenital indications includes the work of passing a diagnostic catheter into the pulmonary venous atrium. The work of code 93574 begins after diagnostic catheterization and after achieving catheter position in the pulmonary venous atrium.) Use an end-hole catheter and wire to selectively enter a single pulmonary vein ostium. Once a pulmonary vein is securely engaged with the catheter, remove the wire, observing appropriate de-airing of the catheter. Perform a hand injection angiogram within the vein and review in real time for any abnormalities. After pressure pullback from the pulmonary vein to the atrium, disconnect the catheter from the transducer and re-insert the guidewire to repeat the process by probing for a different pulmonary vein ostium. Once a second vein is selectively engaged, repeat angiography to evaluate this vein for any abnormalities. This process may be repeated as many as 4 to 5 times, selectively entering each distinct pulmonary vein that directly enters the pulmonary venous atrium. Each distinct vessel is additionally reportable. Continuously monitor patient's arterial pressure, ECG, and oxygen saturation throughout the procedure. Review all images and describe in the procedure report. Per routine, monitor any contrast injection afterward for complications of allergic reaction, arrhythmia, hemodynamic instability, and contrast-induced nephropathy.

Clinical Example (93575)

A 1-week-old female with pulmonary valve atresia, ventricular septal defect (VSD), and major aortopulmonary collateral arteries (MAPCAs), undergoes several selective angiograms of MAPCA vessels supplying pulmonary blood flow from the aorta during a diagnostic cardiac catheterization. [**Note:** This is an add-on service. Only consider the additional work related to each selective pulmonary artery angiogram from an arterial (left heart) approach.]

Description of Procedure (93575)

(Note that diagnostic cardiac catheterization for both congenital and noncongenital indications includes the work of passing a diagnostic catheter into the aorta. The work of code 93575 begins after diagnostic catheterization.) Pass an end-hole catheter with the aid of a guidewire from the arterial system and use to probe for and selectively catheterize individual pulmonary arteries, arterial collaterals, or surgical shunts supplying pulmonary blood flow from the aorta. Once the catheter is securely within one of the target vessels, remove the wire and de-air the catheter. Perform a hand-injection angiogram within the vessel and review in real time for any abnormalities. Record a pressure as needed. Withdraw the catheter into the aorta and re-insert the guidewire to repeat the process by probing for a different target vessel. Once a second target vessel is selectively engaged, repeat angiography to evaluate this vessel for any abnormalities. Repeat this entire process as many times as needed until all suspected vessels supplying flow from the aorta to the pulmonary circulation are identified. Each distinct named vessel is additionally reportable. Continuously monitor patient's arterial pressure, ECG, and oxygen saturation throughout the procedure. Review all images and describe in the procedure report. Per routine, monitor any contrast injection afterward for complications of allergic reaction, arrhythmia, hemodynamic instability, and contrast-induced nephropathy.

Repair of Structural Heart Defect

93582   Percutaneous transcatheter closure of patent ductus arteriosus

(93582 includes congenital right and left heart catheterization, catheter placement in the aorta, and aortic arch angiography, when performed)

(Do not report 93582 in conjunction with 36013, 36014, 36200, 75600, 75605, 93451, 93453, 93456, 93457, 93458, 93459, 93460, 93461, 93567, 93593, 93594, 93595, 93596, 93597, 93598)

▶(For other cardiac angiographic procedures performed at the time of transcatheter PDA closure, see 93563, 93564, 93565, 93566, 93568, 93569, 93573, 93574, 93575 as appropriate)◀

(For repair of patent ductus arteriosus by ligation, see 33820, 33822, 33824)

(For intracardiac echocardiographic services performed at the time of transcatheter PDA closure, use 93662. Other echocardiographic services provided by a separate individual are reported using the appropriate echocardiography service codes, 93315, 93316, 93317)

Medicine 90281-99607

93583 Percutaneous transcatheter septal reduction therapy (eg, alcohol septal ablation) including temporary pacemaker insertion when performed

(93583 includes insertion of temporary pacemaker, when performed, and left heart catheterization)

(Do not report 93583 in conjunction with 33210, 93452, 93453, 93458, 93459, 93460, 93461, 93565, 93595, 93596, 93597)

(93583 includes left anterior descending coronary angiography for the purpose of roadmapping to guide the intervention. Do not report 93454, 93455, 93456, 93457, 93458, 93459, 93460, 93461, 93563 for coronary angiography performed during alcohol septal ablation for the purpose of roadmapping, guidance of the intervention, vessel measurement, and completion angiography)

▶(Diagnostic cardiac catheterization procedures may be separately reportable when no prior catheter-based diagnostic study of the treatment zone is available, the prior diagnostic study is inadequate, or the patient's condition with respect to the clinical indication has changed since the prior study or during the intervention. Use the appropriate codes from 93451, 93454, 93455, 93456, 93457, 93563, 93564, 93566, 93567, 93568, 93593, 93594, 93598, 93569, 93573, 93574, 93575)◀

(Do not report 93583 in conjunction with 33210, 33211)

(Do not report 93463 for the injection of alcohol for this procedure)

(For intracardiac echocardiographic services performed at the time of alcohol septal ablation, use 93662)

(Other echocardiographic services provided by a separate physician are reported using the appropriate echocardiography services codes, 93312, 93313, 93314, 93315, 93316, 93317)

(For surgical ventriculomyotomy [-myectomy] for idiopathic hypertrophic subaortic stenosis, use 33416)

Rationale

In accordance with the establishment of codes 93569 and 93573-93575, the cross-reference parenthetical note following code 93582 regarding other cardiac angiographic procedures performed at the time of transcatheter patent ductus arteriosus (PDA) closure and the instructional parenthetical note following code 93583 have been revised to reflect these changes.

Refer to the codebook and the Rationale for codes 93569 and 93573-93575 for a full discussion of these changes.

Cardiac Catheterization for Congenital Heart Defects

Cardiac catheterization for the evaluation of congenital heart defect(s) is reported with 93593, 93594, 93595, 93596, 93597, 93598. Cardiac catheterization services for anomalous coronary arteries arising from the aorta or off of other coronary arteries, patent foramen ovale, mitral valve prolapse, and bicuspid aortic valve, in the absence of other congenital heart defects, are reported with 93451-93464, 93566, 93567, 93568. However, when these conditions exist in conjunction with other congenital heart defects, 93593, 93594, 93595, 93596, 93597 may be reported. Evaluation of anomalous coronary arteries arising from the pulmonary arterial system is reported with the cardiac catheterization for congenital heart defects codes.

▶For additional guidance on reporting cardiac catheterization services for congenital heart defects versus non-congenital indications, see Cardiac Catheterization guidelines.◀

Right heart catheterization for congenital heart defects (93593, 93594, 93596, 93597): includes catheter placement in one or more right-sided cardiac chamber(s) or structures (ie, the right atrium, right ventricle, pulmonary artery, pulmonary wedge), obtaining blood samples for measurement of blood gases, and Fick cardiac output measurements, when performed. While the morphologic right atrium and morphologic right ventricle are typically the right heart structures supplying blood flow to the pulmonary artery, in congenital heart disease the subpulmonic ventricle may be a morphologic left ventricle and the subpulmonic atrium may be a morphologic left atrium. For reporting purposes, when the morphologic left ventricle or left atrium is in a subpulmonic position due to congenital heart disease, catheter placement in either of these structures is considered part of right heart catheterization and does not constitute left heart catheterization. Right heart catheterization for congenital cardiac anomalies does not typically involve thermodilution cardiac output assessments. When thermodilution cardiac output is performed in this setting, it may be separately reported using add-on code 93598. Right heart catheterization does not include right ventricular or right atrial angiography. When right ventricular or right atrial angiography is performed, use 93566. For reporting purposes, angiography of the morphologic right ventricle or morphologic right atrium is reported with 93566, whether these structures are in the standard pre-pulmonic position or in a systemic (subaortic) position. For placement of a flow directed catheter (eg, Swan-Ganz) performed for hemodynamic monitoring purposes not in conjunction with other catheterization services, use 93503. Do not report 93503 in conjunction with 93453, 93456, 93457, 93460, 93461, 93593, 93594, 93595, 93596, 93597.

Catheter placement and injection procedures: The work of imaging guidance, including fluoroscopy and ultrasound guidance for vascular access and to guide catheter placement for hemodynamic evaluation, is included in the cardiac catheterization for congenital heart defects codes, when performed by the same operator.

For cardiac catheterization for congenital heart defects, injection procedures are separately reportable due to the marked variability in the cardiovascular anatomy encountered.

▶When contrast injection(s) is performed in conjunction with cardiac catheterization for congenital heart defects, see injection procedure codes 93563, 93564, 93565, 93566, 93567, 93568, 93569, 93573, 93574, 93575, or use appropriate codes from the Radiology section and the Vascular Injection Procedures subsection in the Surgery/ Cardiovascular System section. Codes 93563, 93564, 93565, 93566, 93567, 93568 include imaging supervision, interpretation, and report.

Injection procedures 93563, 93564, 93565, 93566, 93567, 93568, 93569, 93573, 93574, 93575 represent separate, identifiable services and may be reported in conjunction with one another, when appropriate. For angiography of noncoronary and nonpulmonary arteries and veins, performed as a distinct service, use appropriate codes from the Radiology section and the Vascular Injection Procedures subsection in the Surgery/ Cardiovascular System section.◀

Angiography of the native coronary arteries or bypass grafts during cardiac catheterization for congenital heart defects is reported with 93563, 93564. Catheter placement(s) in coronary artery(ies) or bypass grafts involves selective engagement of the origins of the native coronary artery(ies) or bypass grafts for the purpose of coronary angiography.

▶(Selective pulmonary angiography codes for cardiac catheterization [93569, 93573, 93574, 93575] include selective catheter positioning of the angiographic catheter, injection, and radiologic supervision and interpretation)◀

93593 Right heart catheterization for congenital heart defect(s) including imaging guidance by the proceduralist to advance the catheter to the target zone; normal native connections

93594 abnormal native connections

93595 Left heart catheterization for congenital heart defect(s) including imaging guidance by the proceduralist to advance the catheter to the target zone, normal or abnormal native connections

93596 Right and left heart catheterization for congenital heart defect(s) including imaging guidance by the proceduralist to advance the catheter to the target zone(s); normal native connections

93597 abnormal native connections

+ 93598 Cardiac output measurement(s), thermodilution or other indicator dilution method, performed during cardiac catheterization for the evaluation of congenital heart defects (List separately in addition to code for primary procedure)

(Use 93598 in conjunction with 93593, 93594, 93595, 93596, 93597)

(Do not report 93598 in conjunction with 93451-93461)

(For pharmacologic agent administration during cardiac catheterization for congenital heart defect[s], use 93463)

(For physiological exercise study with cardiac catheterization for congenital heart defect[s], use 93464)

(For indicator dilution studies such as thermodilution for cardiac output measurement during cardiac catheterization for congenital heart defect[s], use 93598)

▶(For contrast injections during cardiac catheterization for congenital heart defect[s], see 93563, 93564, 93565, 93566, 93567, 93568, 93569, 93573, 93574, 93575)◀

(For angiography or venography not described in the 90000 series code section, see appropriate codes from the Radiology section and the Vascular Injection Procedures subsection in the Surgery/Cardiovascular System section)

(For transseptal or transapical access of the left atrium during cardiac catheterization for congenital heart defect[s], use 93462 in conjunction with 93595, 93596, 93597, as appropriate)

Rationale

The Cardiac Catheterization for Congenital Heart Defects subsection guidelines have been revised to distinguish between cardiac catheterization services for congenital heart defects and cardiac catheterization for non-congenital indications.

Also, in accordance with the establishment of codes 93569 and 93573-93575, a parenthetical note following code 93598 and the Cardiac Catheterization for Congenital Heart Defects subsection guidelines have been revised to reflect these changes. An instructional parenthetical note indicating the procedures included in cardiac catheterization codes 93569 and 93573-93575 has been added.

Refer to the codebook and the Rationale for codes 93569 and 93573-93575 for a full discussion of these changes.

★ = Telemedicine ◀ = Audio-only ✛ = Add-on code ✗ = FDA approval pending # = Resequenced code ⊘ = Modifier 51 exempt

Intracardiac Electrophysiological Procedures/Studies

+ 93613   Intracardiac electrophysiologic 3-dimensional mapping (List separately in addition to code for primary procedure)

(Use 93613 in conjunction with 93620)

(Do not report 93613 in conjunction with 93609, 93654)

▶(For noninvasive arrhythmia localization and mapping, use 0745T)◀

93620   Comprehensive electrophysiologic evaluation including insertion and repositioning of multiple electrode catheters with induction or attempted induction of arrhythmia; with right atrial pacing and recording, right ventricular pacing and recording, His bundle recording

(Do not report 93620 in conjunction with 93600, 93602, 93603, 93610, 93612, 93618, 93619, 93653, 93654, 93655, 93656, 93657)

+ 93621   with left atrial pacing and recording from coronary sinus or left atrium (List separately in addition to code for primary procedure)

(Use 93621 in conjunction with 93620)

(Do not report 93621 in conjunction with 93656)

+ 93622   with left ventricular pacing and recording (List separately in addition to code for primary procedure)

(Use 93622 in conjunction with 93620, 93653, 93656)

(Do not report 93622 in conjunction with 93654)

▶(For noninvasive arrhythmia localization and mapping, use 0745T)◀

Rationale

In accordance with the establishment of Category III code 0745T, cross-reference parenthetical notes directing users to the new code have been added following codes 93613 and 93622.

Refer to the codebook and the Rationale for code 0745T for a full discussion of this change.

Peripheral Arterial Disease Rehabilitation

▶Peripheral arterial disease (PAD) rehabilitative physical exercise consists of a series of sessions, lasting 45-60 minutes per session, involving use of either a motorized treadmill or a track to permit each patient to achieve symptom-limited claudication. Each session is supervised by an exercise physiologist or nurse. The supervising provider monitors the individual patient's claudication threshold and other cardiovascular limitations for

adjustment of workload. During this supervised rehabilitation program, the development of new arrhythmias, symptoms that might suggest angina or the continued inability of the patient to progress to an adequate level of exercise may require review and examination of the patient by a physician or other qualified health care professional. These services would be separately reported with an appropriate level E/M service code, including office or other outpatient services (99202-99215), initial hospital inpatient or observation care (99221-99223), subsequent hospital inpatient or observation care (99231-99233), critical care services (99291-99292).◀

93668   Peripheral arterial disease (PAD) rehabilitation, per session

Rationale

In accordance with the revision of codes 99221-99233, the Peripheral Arterial Disease Rehabilitation subsection guidelines have been revised to reflect these changes.

Refer to the codebook and the Rationale for codes 99221-99233 for a full discussion of these changes.

Home and Outpatient International Normalized Ratio (INR) Monitoring Services

93793   Anticoagulant management for a patient taking warfarin, must include review and interpretation of a new home, office, or lab international normalized ratio (INR) test result, patient instructions, dosage adjustment (as needed), and scheduling of additional test(s), when performed

▶(Do not report 93793 in conjunction with 99202, 99203, 99204, 99205, 99211, 99212, 99213, 99214, 99215, 99242, 99243, 99244, 99245)◀

(Report 93793 no more than once per day, regardless of the number of tests reviewed)

Rationale

In accordance with the deletion of code 99241, the exclusionary parenthetical note following code 93793 has been revised to reflect this change.

Refer to the codebook and the Rationale for code 99241 for a full discussion of this change.

Pulmonary

Ventilator Management

94005 Home ventilator management care plan oversight of a patient (patient not present) in home, domiciliary or rest home (eg, assisted living) requiring review of status, review of laboratories and other studies and revision of orders and respiratory care plan (as appropriate), within a calendar month, 30 minutes or more

> ►(Do not report 94005 in conjunction with 99374-99378, 99424, 99425, 99437, 99491)◄

> ►(Ventilator management care plan oversight is reported separately from home or domiciliary, rest home [eg, assisted living] services. A physician or other qualified health care professional may report 94005, when performed, including when a different individual reports 99374-99378, 99424, 99425, 99437, 99491, for the same 30 days)◄

Rationale

In accordance with the deletion of codes 99339 and 99340, the parenthetical notes following code 94005 have been revised to reflect these changes.

Refer to the codebook and the Rationale for codes 99339 and 99340 for a full discussion of these changes.

Pulmonary Diagnostic Testing, Rehabilitation, and Therapies

►Codes 94010-94799 include laboratory procedure(s) and interpretation of test results. If a separate identifiable evaluation and management service is performed, the appropriate E/M service code, including new or established patient office or other outpatient services (99202-99215), office or other outpatient consultations (99242, 99243, 99244, 99245), emergency department services (99281-99285), nursing facility services (99304-99316), and home or residence services (99341-99350), may be reported in addition to 94010-94799.◄

Spirometry (94010) measures expiratory airflow and volumes and forms the basis of most pulmonary function testing. When spirometry is performed before and after administration of a bronchodilator, report 94060. Measurement of vital capacity (94150) is a component of spirometry and is only reported when performed alone. The flow-volume loop (94375) is used to identify patterns of inspiratory and/or expiratory obstruction in central or peripheral airways. Spirometry (94010, 94060) includes maximal breathing capacity (94200) and flow-volume loop (94375), when performed.

Measurement of lung volumes may be performed using plethysmography, helium dilution or nitrogen washout. Plethysmography (94726) is utilized to determine total lung capacity, residual volume, functional residual capacity, and airway resistance. Nitrogen washout or helium dilution (94727) may be used to measure lung volumes, distribution of ventilation and closing volume. Oscillometry (94728) assesses airway resistance and may be reported in addition to gas dilution techniques. Spirometry (94010, 94060) and bronchial provocation (94070) are not included in 94726 and 94727 and may be reported separately.

Diffusing capacity (94729) is most commonly performed in conjunction with lung volumes or spirometry and is an add-on code to 94726-94728, 94010, 94060, 94070, and 94375.

Pulmonary function tests (94011-94013) are reported for measurements in infants and young children through 2 years of age.

Pulmonary function testing measurements are reported as actual values and as a percent of predicted values by age, gender, height, and race.

Chest wall manipulation for the mobilization of secretions and improvement in lung function can be performed using manual (94667, 94668) or mechanical (94669) methods. Manual techniques include cupping, percussing, and use of a hand-held vibration device. A mechanical technique is the application of an external vest or wrap that delivers mechanical oscillation.

94010 Spirometry, including graphic record, total and timed vital capacity, expiratory flow rate measurement(s), with or without maximal voluntary ventilation

Rationale

In accordance with the deletion of codes 99241, 99318, and 99324-99337, the Pulmonary Diagnostic Testing, Rehabilitation, and Therapies subsection guidelines have been revised to reflect these changes.

Refer to the codebook and the Rationale for codes 99241, 99318, and 99324-99337 for a full discussion of these changes.

Allergy and Clinical Immunology

Definitions

Immunotherapy (desensitization, hyposensitization): is the parenteral administration of allergenic extracts as antigens at periodic intervals, usually on an increasing dosage scale to a dosage which is maintained as maintenance therapy. Indications for immunotherapy are determined by appropriate diagnostic procedures coordinated with clinical judgment and knowledge of the natural history of allergic diseases.

Other therapy: for medical conferences on the use of mechanical and electronic devices (precipitators, air conditioners, air filters, humidifiers, dehumidifiers), climatotherapy, physical therapy, occupational and recreational therapy, see Evaluation and Management services.

▶Do not report evaluation and management (E/M) services for test interpretation and report. If a significant separately identifiable E/M service is performed, the appropriate E/M service code, which may include new or established patient office or other outpatient services (99202-99215), hospital inpatient or observation care (99221-99223, 99231-99233), consultations (99242, 99243, 99244, 99245, 99252, 99253, 99254, 99255), emergency department services (99281-99285), nursing facility services (99304-99316), home or residence services (99341-99350), or preventive medicine services (99381-99429), should be reported using modifier 25.◀

Rationale

In accordance with the deletion of codes 99217-99220, 99224-99226, 99241, 99318, and 99324-99337, the Allergy and Clinical Immunology subsection guidelines have been revised to reflect these changes.

Refer to the codebook and the Rationale for codes 99217-99220, 99224-99226, 99241, 99318, and 99324-99337 for a full discussion of these changes.

Neurology and Neuromuscular Procedures

▶Neurologic services are typically consultative, and any of the levels of consultation (99242, 99243, 99244, 99245, 99252, 99253, 99254, 99255) may be appropriate.◀

In addition, services and skills outlined under **Evaluation and Management** levels of service appropriate to neurologic illnesses should be reported similarly.

The electroencephalogram (EEG), video electroencephalogram (VEEG), autonomic function, evoked potential, reflex tests, electromyography (EMG), nerve conduction velocity (NCV), and magnetoencephalography (MEG) services (95700-95726, 95812-95829, and 95860-95967) include recording, interpretation, and report by a physician or other

qualified health care professional. For interpretation only, use modifier 26 with 95812-95829, 95860-95967. For interpretation only for long-term EEG services, report 95717, 95718, 95719, 95720, 95721, 95722, 95723, 95724, 95725, 95726.

Codes 95700-95726 and 95812-95822 use EEG/VEEG recording time as a basis for code use. Recording time is when the recording is underway and diagnostic EEG data is being collected. Recording time excludes set up and take down time. If diagnostic EEG recording is disrupted, recording time stops until diagnostic EEG recording is resumed. Codes 95961-95962 use physician or other qualified health care professional attendance time as a basis for code use.

(Do not report codes 95860-95875 in addition to 96000-96004)

Rationale

In accordance with the deletion of code 99241, the Neurology and Neuromuscular Procedures subsection guidelines have been revised to reflect this change.

Refer to the codebook and the Rationale for code 99241 for a full discussion of this change.

Electromyography

#+ 95885   Needle electromyography, each extremity, with related paraspinal areas, when performed, done with nerve conduction, amplitude and latency/velocity study; limited (List separately in addition to code for primary procedure)

#+ 95886   complete, five or more muscles studied, innervated by three or more nerves or four or more spinal levels (List separately in addition to code for primary procedure)

(Use 95885, 95886 in conjunction with 95907-95913)

(Do not report 95885, 95886 in conjunction with 95860-95864, 95870, 95905)

▶(Do not report 95885, 95886 for noninvasive nerve conduction guidance used in conjunction with 0766T, 0768T)◀

#+ 95887   Needle electromyography, non-extremity (cranial nerve supplied or axial) muscle(s) done with nerve conduction, amplitude and latency/velocity study (List separately in addition to code for primary procedure)

(Use 95887 in conjunction with 95907-95913)

(Do not report 95887 in conjunction with 95867-95870, 95905)

▶(Do not report 95887 for noninvasive nerve conduction guidance used in conjunction with 0766T, 0768T)◀

Medicine 90281-99607

Rationale

In accordance with the establishment of Category III codes 0766T and 0768T, exclusionary parenthetical notes have been added following codes 95886 and 95887 to reflect these changes.

Refer to the codebook and the Rationale for codes 0766T and 0768T for a full discussion of these changes.

Nerve Conduction Tests

95907 Nerve conduction studies; 1-2 studies

95908   3-4 studies

95909   5-6 studies

95910   7-8 studies

95911   9-10 studies

95912   11-12 studies

95913   13 or more studies

▶(Do not report 95905, 95907, 95908, 95909, 95910, 95911, 95912, 95913 for noninvasive nerve conduction guidance used in conjunction with 0766T, 0768T)◀

Rationale

In accordance with the establishment of Category III codes 0766T and 0768T, an exclusionary parenthetical note has been added following code 95913 to reflect these changes.

Refer to the codebook and the Rationale for codes 0766T and 0768T for a full discussion of these changes.

Autonomic Function Tests

The purpose of autonomic nervous system function testing is to determine the presence of autonomic dysfunction, the site of autonomic dysfunction, and the various autonomic subsystems that may be disordered.

Code 95924 should be reported only when both the parasympathetic function and the adrenergic function are tested together with the use of a tilt table.

● **95919**   Quantitative pupillometry with physician or other qualified health care professional interpretation and report, unilateral or bilateral

Rationale

New code 95919 has been established to report quantitative pupillometry. A parenthetical note has been updated to accommodate the revision.

Code 95919 is reported for quantitative pupillometry, performed unilaterally or bilaterally, and includes the work involved in the interpretation and generation of a report. The procedure involves the rapid, noninvasive measurement of autonomic nervous system function via assessment of the pupil's response to light. This allows for objective documentation of pupillometry-specific autonomic deficit, as well as objective measures of the pupil's response to light.

A related cross-reference parenthetical note in the Category III section following code 0339T has been updated to direct use of new code 95919, instead of the unlisted ophthalmological services or procedure code 92499.

Clinical Example (95919)

A 14-year-old male playing football got tackled and developed a concussion. He now requires a comprehensive neurologic examination to assess for vestibular, balance, and vision problems. To assess the concussion severity, he requires cranial imaging tests, such as MRI or CT, along with quantitative pupillometry to assess pupillary response to light as an early indicator of increased intracranial pressure.

Description of Procedure (95919)

The physician or other QHP reviews the measurements and waveforms from both right and left eyes in the context of the patient's condition and compares them to published normative values by age, as well as to prior pupillometry measurements in the same patient.

95921   Testing of autonomic nervous system function; cardiovagal innervation (parasympathetic function), including 2 or more of the following: heart rate response to deep breathing with recorded R-R interval, Valsalva ratio, and 30:15 ratio

Health Behavior Assessment and Intervention

96158   Health behavior intervention, individual, face-to-face; initial 30 minutes

+ 96159   each additional 15 minutes (List separately in addition to code for primary service)

★ = Telemedicine ◀ = Audio-only ✛ = Add-on code ✗ = FDA approval pending # = Resequenced code ⊘ = Modifier 51 exempt

(Use 96159 in conjunction with 96158)

▶(Do not report 96158, 96159 for service time reported in conjunction with 98975, 98978)◀

Rationale

In accordance with the addition of code 98978, the exclusionary parenthetical note following code 96159 has been revised to include code 98978.

Refer to the codebook and the Rationale for code 98978 for a full discussion of these changes.

▶Behavior Management Services◀

▶Behavior modification is defined as the process of altering human-behavior patterns over a long-term period using various motivational techniques, namely, consequences and rewards. More simply, behavior modification is the method of changing the way a person reacts either physically or mentally to a given stimulus.

Behavior modification treatment is based on the principles of operant conditioning. The intended clinical outcome for this treatment approach is to replace unwanted or problematic behaviors with more positive, desirable behaviors through the use of evidence-based techniques and methods.

The purpose of the group-based behavioral management/ modification training services is to teach the parent(s)/ guardian(s)/caregiver(s) interventions that they can independently use to effectively manage the identified patient's illness(es) or disease(s). Codes 96202, 96203 are used to report the total duration of face-to-face time spent by the physician or other qualified health care professional providing group-based parent(s)/ guardian(s)/caregiver(s) behavioral management/ modification training services. This service involves behavioral treatment training provided to a multiple-family group of parent(s)/guardian(s)/caregiver(s), without the patient present. These services emphasize active engagement and involvement of the parent(s)/ guardian(s)/caregiver(s) in the treatment of a patient with a mental or physical health diagnosis. These services do not represent preventive medicine counseling and risk factor reduction interventions.

During these sessions, the parent(s)/guardian(s)/ caregiver(s) are trained, using verbal instruction, video and live demonstrations, and feedback from physician or other qualified health care professional or other parent(s)/ guardian(s)/caregiver(s) in group sessions, to use skills and strategies to address behaviors impacting the patient's

mental or physical health diagnosis. These skills and strategies help to support compliance with the identified patient's treatment and the clinical plan of care.

For counseling and education provided by a physician or other qualified health care professional to a patient and/ or family, see the appropriate evaluation and management codes, including office or other outpatient services (99202, 99203, 99204, 99205, 99211, 99212, 99213, 99214, 99215), hospital inpatient and observation care services (99221, 99222, 99223, 99231, 99232, 99233, 99234, 99235, 99236), new or established patient office or other outpatient consultations (99242, 99243, 99244, 99245), inpatient or observation consultations (99252, 99253, 99254, 99255), emergency department services (99281, 99282, 99283, 99284, 99285), nursing facility services (99304, 99305, 99306, 99307, 99308, 99309, 99310, 99315, 99316), home or residence services (99341, 99342, 99344, 99345, 99347, 99348, 99349, 99350), and counseling risk factor reduction and behavior change intervention (99401-99429). See also **Instructions for Use of the CPT Codebook** for definition of reporting qualifications.

Counseling risk factor reduction and behavior change intervention codes (99401, 99402, 99403, 99404, 99406, 99407, 99408, 99409, 99411, 99412) are included and may not be separately reported on the same day as parent(s)/guardian(s)/caregiver(s) training services codes 96202, 96203 by the same provider.

Medical nutrition therapy (97802, 97803, 97804) provided to the identified patient may be reported on the same date of service as parent(s)/guardian(s)/caregiver(s) training service.◀

▶(For health behavior assessment and intervention that is not part of a standardized curriculum, see 96156, 96158, 96159, 96164, 96165, 96167, 96168, 96170, 96171)◀

▶(For educational services that use a standardized curriculum provided to patients with an established illness/disease, see 98960, 98961, 98962)◀

▶(For education provided as genetic counseling services, use 96040. For education to a group regarding genetic risks, see 98961, 98962)◀

● **96202**   Multiple-family group behavior management/ modification training for parent(s)/guardian(s)/ caregiver(s) of patients with a mental or physical health diagnosis, administered by physician or other qualified health care professional (without the patient present), face-to-face with multiple sets of parent(s)/guardian(s)/ caregiver(s); initial 60 minutes

▶(Do not report 96202 for behavior management services to the patient and the parent[s]/guardian[s]/ caregiver[s] during the same session)◀

▶(Do not report 96202 for less than 31 minutes of service)◀

+● 96203   each additional 15 minutes (List separately in addition to code for primary service)

▶(Use 96203 in conjunction with 96202)◀

▶(Do not report 96202, 96203 in conjunction with 97151, 97152, 97153, 97154, 97155, 97156, 97157, 97158, 0362T, 0373T)◀

▶(For educational services [eg, prenatal, obesity, or diabetic instructions] rendered to patients in a group setting, use 99078)◀

▶(For counseling and/or risk factor reduction intervention provided by a physician or other qualified health care professional to patient[s] without symptoms or established disease, see 99401, 99402, 99403, 99404, 99406, 99407, 99408, 99409, 99411, 99412)◀

Rationale

A new subsection, Behavior Management Services, new guidelines, new parenthetical notes, and two new codes have been established for behavior management services within the Medicine section.

The new subsection and codes 96202 and 96203 have been established to report physician- and other QHP-administered multifamily group behavior management or modification training for parent(s)/guardian(s)/caregiver(s) of patients with a mental or physical health diagnosis. The codes identify the efforts of the physicians or other QHPs to train the caregivers of patients regarding intervention methods that they may use to manage a patient's disease(s)/illness(es). The disease(s)/illness(es) may be portrayed or expressed via an objectionable, problematic, or disagreeable behavior exchange that requires action. The physicians or other QHPs train the caregivers regarding how to respond to these circumstances with more positive, desirable behaviors through the use of evidence-based techniques and methods. The service is intended to be provided in a multifamily group setting.

To help users understand what these services are and how the codes are intended to be used, extensive language has been included within the code descriptors, guidelines, and parenthetical notes. The guidelines provide intuitive insight regarding the service (including a specific definition to differentiate it from other related behavioral services), the purpose of the service (ie, for training in modification techniques), who provides it, the circumstances in which it is provided (ie, face-to-face with the caregiver[s] in a multifamily setting for a specific period of time), what is commonly involved to accomplish the training, and what codes to report for other counseling, education services, and other services that do not utilize these techniques. The code descriptors

reiterate much of the same information by specifying the components that are important for use of these codes (ie, face-to-face, multifamily training session provided to the parent[s]/guardians[s]/caregiver[s] for patients who have a mental or physical health diagnosis without patient presence and reported as an initial service of 60 minutes [96202] with additional 15-minute segments [96203] as necessary). The parenthetical notes provide additional instruction regarding services that are excluded (such as use of these codes to report service provided to the patient and the parent[s]/guardian[s]/caregiver[s] during the same session, restrictions for reporting time [ie, exclusion of reporting code 96202 for less than 31 minutes of initial service]) and the codes to use for other related services.

Clinical Example (96202)

Psychiatry/Psychology: A 7-year-old male presents with attention-deficit/hyperactivity disorder and oppositional defiant disorder. Patient's symptoms of inattention, hyperactivity, and impulsiveness result in difficulties in social and psychological functioning. Patient's parent(s)/caregiver(s) is referred for group-based behavior management/modification training to learn strategies and techniques to improve monitoring and management of patient's behaviors, facilitate positive behavior changes, improve parent–child interactions, and improve overall symptom management and functioning.

Dieticians: The parent(s)/caregiver(s) of a 10-year-old male with obesity, limited variety of food intake, limited physical activity, and a family history of type 2 diabetes are referred for group-based behavior management/modification training.

Description of Procedure (96202)

Initiate or continue the multifamily group-based session of behavior training intervention for parent(s)/caregiver(s), training them on behavioral strategies and interventions they can use independently outside of treatment, and helping them develop new skills to improve functioning and better manage/reduce the patient's challenging behaviors that result from or affect the patient's diagnosis. Parent(s)/caregiver(s) is taught to engage via verbal instruction (didactic discussion and Socratic questioning), video and live demonstrations, role-playing, and feedback sessions to learn how to set realistic and age-appropriate expectations for the patient's behavior; reinforce positive/healthy behaviors to improve social and psychological functioning and physical health; and reduce or modify negative behaviors that impair function and treatment progress. Completely assess patient's progress toward treatment goals.

★ = Telemedicine   ◀ = Audio-only   + = Add-on code   𝒩 = FDA approval pending   # = Resequenced code   ⦸ = Modifier 51 exempt

Clinical Example (96203)

Patient 1: The parent(s)/caregiver(s) of a 7-year-old male, who has attention-deficit/hyperactivity disorder and oppositional defiant disorder, received training on monitoring and coping with his symptoms of inattention, hyperactivity and impulsiveness, and facilitating positive behavior changes during group-based behavior management/modification training. An additional 15 minutes, beyond the first 60 minutes, was required to complete group behavior management/modification training on improving overall symptom management and functioning. [**Note:** This is an add-on code. Only consider the additional physician or other QHP work beyond the work separately reported with code 96202.]

Patient 2: The parent(s)/caregiver(s) of a 10-year-old male with obesity, limited variety of food intake, limited physical activity, and a family history of type 2 diabetes received training during the group-based behavior management/modification training. An additional 15 minutes was required. [**Note:** This is an add-on code. Only consider the additional physician or other QHP work beyond the work separately reported with code 96202.]

Description of Procedure (96203)

Continue multifamily group-based session of behavior training intervention for parent(s)/caregiver(s), including verbal instruction (didactic discussion and Socratic questioning), video and live demonstrations, role-playing, and feedback sessions to learn how to set realistic and age-appropriate expectations for the patient's behavior; reinforce positive/healthy behaviors to improve social and psychological functioning and physical health; and reduce or modify negative behaviors that impair function and treatment progress.

Hydration, Therapeutic, Prophylactic, Diagnostic Injections and Infusions, and Chemotherapy and Other Highly Complex Drug or Highly Complex Biologic Agent Administration

Physician or other qualified health care professional work related to hydration, injection, and infusion services predominantly involves affirmation of treatment plan and direct supervision of staff.

▶Codes 96360-96379, 96401, 96402, 96409-96425, 96521-96523 are not intended to be reported by the physician in the facility setting. If a significant, separately identifiable office or other outpatient evaluation and management (E/M) service is performed, the appropriate E/M service (99202-99215, 99242, 99243, 99244, 99245) should be reported using modifier 25, in addition to 96360-96549. For same day E/M service, a different diagnosis is not required.◀

Rationale

In accordance with the deletion of codes 99241, 99354, and 99355, the Hydration, Therapeutic, Prophylactic, Diagnostic Injections and Infusions, and Chemotherapy and Other Highly Complex Drug or Highly Complex Biologic Agent Administration subsection guidelines have been revised to reflect these changes.

Refer to the codebook and the Rationale for codes 99241, 99354, and 99355 for a full discussion of these changes.

Therapeutic, Prophylactic, and Diagnostic Injections and Infusions (Excludes Chemotherapy and Other Highly Complex Drug or Highly Complex Biologic Agent Administration)

96372　Therapeutic, prophylactic, or diagnostic injection (specify substance or drug); subcutaneous or intramuscular

▶(For administration of vaccines/toxoids, see 90460, 90461, 90471, 90472, 0001A, 0002A, 0003A, 0004A, 0011A, 0012A, 0013A, 0021A, 0022A, 0031A, 0034A, 0041A, 0042A, 0051A, 0052A, 0053A, 0054A, 0064A, 0071A, 0072A, 0073A, 0074A, 0081A, 0082A, 0083A, 0094A, 0104A, 0111A, 0112A)◀

(Report 96372 for non-antineoplastic hormonal therapy injections)

Rationale

To accommodate the new codes for COVID-19 vaccination products and administrations, codes 0003A, 0004A, 0013A, 0034A, 0051A-0054A, 0064A, 0071A-0074A, 0081A-0083A, 0094A, 0104A, 0111A, and 0112A have been added to the existing parenthetical note following code 96372 to direct users to these codes.

Refer to the codebook and the Rationale for codes 0003A-0112A for a full discussion of these changes.

Physical Medicine and Rehabilitation

Modalities

Supervised

97010   Application of a modality to 1 or more areas; hot or cold packs

97012   traction, mechanical

97014   electrical stimulation (unattended)

(For acupuncture with electrical stimulation, see 97813, 97814)

▶(For peripheral nerve transcutaneous magnetic stimulation, see 0766T, 0767T, 0768T, 0769T)◀

Rationale

In accordance with the establishment of Category III codes 0766T-0769T, a cross-reference parenthetical note has been added following code 97014 to reflect these changes.

Refer to the codebook and the Rationale for these codes for a full discussion of these changes.

Constant Attendance

97032   Application of a modality to 1 or more areas; electrical stimulation (manual), each 15 minutes

(For transcutaneous electrical modulation pain reprocessing [TEMPR/scrambler therapy], use 0278T)

▶(For peripheral nerve transcutaneous magnetic stimulation, see 0766T, 0767T, 0768T, 0769T)◀

Rationale

In accordance with the establishment of Category III codes 0766T-0769T, a cross-reference parenthetical note has been added following code 97032 to reflect these changes.

Refer to the codebook and the Rationale for codes 0766T-0769T for a full discussion of these changes.

Therapeutic Procedures

A manner of effecting change through the application of clinical skills and/or services that attempt to improve function.

▶Physician or other qualified health care professional (eg, therapist) is required to have direct, one-on-one patient contact, except for group therapeutic procedure (97150) and work hardening/conditioning (97545, 97546) that require direct patient contact, but not one-on-one contact.◀

★ **97110**   Therapeutic procedure, 1 or more areas, each 15 minutes; therapeutic exercises to develop strength and endurance, range of motion and flexibility

97150   Therapeutic procedure(s), group (2 or more individuals)

(Report 97150 for each member of group)

▶(Group therapy procedures involve constant attendance of the physician or other qualified health care professional [eg, therapist], but by definition do not require one-on-one patient contact by the same physician or other qualified health care professional)◀

(For manipulation under general anesthesia, see appropriate anatomic section in **Musculoskeletal System**)

(For osteopathic manipulative treatment [OMT], see 98925-98929)

(Do not report 97150 in conjunction with 97154, 97158)

Rationale

The Therapeutic Procedures subsection's introductory guidelines have been revised to clarify group therapy and work hardening/conditioning services. A parenthetical note following code 97150 has also been revised.

Prior to 2023, the introductory guidelines stated that the physician or other QHP were required to have direct (one-on-one) patient contact. However, the codes for group therapeutic procedures (97150) and work hardening/conditioning (97545 and 97546) in this section differ in that one-on-one contact is not required. Therefore, the guidelines have been revised to specifically indicate that codes 97150, 97545, and 97546 do require direct patient contact but not one-on-one contact. Also, in both the guidelines and the parenthetical note following code 97150, the term "ie" has been replaced with "eg" in reference to the therapist performing the service.

★ = Telemedicine   ◀ = Audio-only   ✚ = Add-on code   ✗ = FDA approval pending   # = Resequenced code   ⊘ = Modifier 51 exempt

Medicine 90281-99607

Acupuncture

Acupuncture is reported based on 15-minute increments of personal (face-to-face) contact with the patient, not the duration of acupuncture needle(s) placement.

If no electrical stimulation is used during a 15-minute increment, use 97810, 97811. If electrical stimulation of any needle is used during a 15-minute increment, use 97813, 97814.

Only one code may be reported for each 15-minute increment. Use either 97810 or 97813 for the initial 15-minute increment. Only one initial code is reported per day.

▶Evaluation and management services may be reported in addition to acupuncture procedures, when performed by physicians or other health care professionals who may report evaluation and management (E/M) services, including new or established patient office or other outpatient services (99202-99215), hospital inpatient or observation care (99221-99223, 99231-99233), office or other outpatient consultations (99242, 99243, 99244, 99245), inpatient or observation consultations (99252, 99253, 99254, 99255), critical care services (99291, 99292), inpatient neonatal intensive care services and pediatric and neonatal critical care services (99466-99480), emergency department services (99281-99285), nursing facility services (99304-99316), and home or residence services (99341-99350), separately using modifier 25 if the patient's condition requires a significant, separately identifiable E/M service above and beyond the usual preservice and postservice work associated with the acupuncture services. The time of the E/M service is not included in the time of the acupuncture service.◀

For needle insertion(s) without injection(s) (eg, dry needling, trigger point acupuncture), see 20560, 20561.

97810   Acupuncture, 1 or more needles; without electrical stimulation, initial 15 minutes of personal one-on-one contact with the patient

(Do not report 97810 in conjunction with 97813)

Rationale

In accordance with the deletion of codes 99217-99220, 99224-99226, 99241, 99251, 99318, and 99324-99337, the Acupuncture subsection guidelines have been revised to reflect these changes.

Refer to the codebook and the Rationale for codes 99217-99220, 99224-99226, 99241, 99251, 99318, and 99324-99337 for a full discussion of these changes.

Osteopathic Manipulative Treatment

Osteopathic manipulative treatment (OMT) is a form of manual treatment applied by a physician or other qualified health care professional to eliminate or alleviate somatic dysfunction and related disorders. This treatment may be accomplished by a variety of techniques.

▶Evaluation and management (E/M) services, including new or established patient office or other outpatient services (99202-99215), initial and subsequent hospital inpatient or observation care (99221-99223, 99231-99233), critical care services (99291, 99292), hospital inpatient or observation care services (including admission and discharge services 99234-99236), office or other outpatient consultations (99242, 99243, 99244, 99245), emergency department services (99281-99285), nursing facility services (99304-99316), and home or residence services (99341-99350), may be reported separately using modifier 25 if the patient's condition requires a significant, separately identifiable E/M service above and beyond the usual preservice and postservice work associated with the procedure. The E/M service may be caused or prompted by the same symptoms or condition for which the OMT service was provided. As such, different diagnoses are not required for the reporting of the OMT and E/M service on the same date.◀

Body regions referred to are: head region; cervical region; thoracic region; lumbar region; sacral region; pelvic region; lower extremities; upper extremities; rib cage region; abdomen and viscera region.

98925   Osteopathic manipulative treatment (OMT); 1-2 body regions involved

Rationale

In accordance with the deletion of codes 99217-99220, 99224-99226, 99241, 99318, and 99324-99337, the Osteopathic Manipulative Treatment subsection guidelines have been revised to reflect these changes.

Refer to the codebook and the Rationale for codes 99217-99220, 99224-99226, 99241, 99318, and 99324-99337 for a full discussion of these changes.

Chiropractic Manipulative Treatment

Chiropractic manipulative treatment (CMT) is a form of manual treatment to influence joint and neurophysiological function. This treatment may be accomplished using a variety of techniques.

▶The chiropractic manipulative treatment codes include a pre-manipulation patient assessment. Additional evaluation and management (E/M) services, including office or other outpatient services (99202-99215), subsequent hospital inpatient or observation care (99231-99233), office or other outpatient consultations (99242, 99243, 99244, 99245), subsequent nursing facility services (99307-99310), and home or residence services (99341-99350), may be reported separately using modifier 25 if the patient's condition requires a significant, separately identifiable E/M service above and beyond the usual preservice and postservice work associated with the procedure. The E/M service may be caused or prompted by the same symptoms or condition for which the CMT service was provided. As such, different diagnoses are not required for the reporting of the CMT and E/M service on the same date.◀

For purposes of CMT, the five spinal regions referred to are: cervical region (includes atlanto-occipital joint); thoracic region (includes costovertebral and costotransverse joints); lumbar region; sacral region; and pelvic (sacro-iliac joint) region. The five extraspinal regions referred to are: head (including temporomandibular joint, excluding atlanto-occipital) region; lower extremities; upper extremities; rib cage (excluding costotransverse and costovertebral joints) and abdomen.

98940   Chiropractic manipulative treatment (CMT); spinal, 1-2 regions

Rationale

In accordance with the deletion of codes 99224-99226, 99241, and 99324-99337, the Chiropractic Manipulative Treatment subsection guidelines have been revised to reflect these changes.

Refer to the codebook and the Rationale for codes 99224-99226, 99241, and 99324-99337 for a full discussion of these changes.

Education and Training for Patient Self-Management

The following codes are used to report educational and training services prescribed by a physician or other qualified health care professional and provided by a qualified, nonphysician health care professional using a standardized curriculum to an individual or a group of patients for the treatment of established illness(s)/disease(s) or to delay comorbidity(s). Education and training for patient self-management may be reported with these codes only when using a standardized curriculum as described below. This curriculum may be modified as necessary for the clinical needs, cultural norms and health literacy of the individual patient(s).

The purpose of the educational and training services is to teach the patient (may include caregiver[s]) how to effectively self-manage the patient's illness(s)/disease(s) or delay disease comorbidity(s) in conjunction with the patient's professional healthcare team. Education and training related to subsequent reinforcement or due to changes in the patient's condition or treatment plan are reported in the same manner as the original education and training. The type of education and training provided for the patient's clinical condition will be identified by the appropriate diagnosis code(s) reported.

The qualifications of the nonphysician healthcare professionals and the content of the educational and training program must be consistent with guidelines or standards established or recognized by a physician society, nonphysician healthcare professional society/association, or other appropriate source.

▶(For counseling and education provided by a physician to an individual, see the appropriate evaluation and management codes, including office or other outpatient services [99202-99215], initial and subsequent hospital inpatient or observation care [99221-99223, 99231-99233, 99234, 99235, 99236], new or established patient office or other outpatient consultations [99242, 99243, 99244, 99245], inpatient or observation consultations [99252, 99253, 99254, 99255], emergency department services [99281-99285], nursing facility services [99304-99316], home or residence services [99341-99350], and counseling risk factor reduction and behavior change intervention [99401-99429]. See also **Instructions for Use of the CPT Codebook** for definition of reporting qualifications)◀

(For counseling and education provided by a physician to a group, use 99078)

(For counseling and/or risk factor reduction intervention provided by a physician to patient[s] without symptoms or established disease, see 99401-99412)

(For medical nutrition therapy, see 97802-97804)

★ = Telemedicine   ◀ = Audio-only   ✚ = Add-on code   ⅄ = FDA approval pending   # = Resequenced code   ⊘ = Modifier 51 exempt

(For health behavior assessment and intervention that is not part of a standardized curriculum, see 96156, 96158, 96159, 96164, 96165, 96167, 96168, 96170, 96171)

(For education provided as genetic counseling services, use 96040. For education to a group regarding genetic risks, see 98961, 98962)

Rationale

In accordance with the deletion of codes 99217-99220, 99224-99226, 99241, 99251, 99318, and 99324-99337, the cross-reference parenthetical note following the Education and Training for Patient Self-Management subsection guidelines has been revised to reflect these changes.

Refer to the codebook and the Rationale for codes 99217-99220, 99224-99226, 99241, 99251, 99318, and 99324-99337 for a full discussion of these changes.

Non-Face-to-Face Nonphysician Services

Qualified Nonphysician Health Care Professional Online Digital Assessment and Management Service

98970   Qualified nonphysician health care professional online digital assessment and management, for an established patient, for up to 7 days, cumulative time during the 7 days; 5-10 minutes

98971   11-20 minutes

98972   21 or more minutes

(Report 98970, 98971, 98972 once per 7-day period)

(Do not report online digital E/M services for cumulative visit time less than 5 minutes)

(Do not count 98970, 98971, 98972 time otherwise reported with other services)

(Do not report 98970, 98971, 98972 for home and outpatient INR monitoring when reporting 93792, 93793)

▶(Do not report 98970, 98971, 98972 when using 99091, 99374, 99375, 99377, 99378, 99379, 99380, 99426, 99427, 99437, 99439, 99487, 99489, 99490, 99491, for the same communication[s])◀

Rationale

In accordance with the deletion of codes 99339 and 99340, an exclusionary parenthetical note following code 98972 has been revised to reflect these changes.

Refer to the codebook and the Rationale for codes 99339 and 99340 for a full discussion of these changes.

Remote Therapeutic Monitoring Services

▶Remote therapeutic monitoring services (eg, musculoskeletal system status, respiratory system status, cognitive behavioral therapy, therapy adherence, therapy response) represent the review and monitoring of data related to signs, symptoms, and functions of a therapeutic response. These data may represent objective device-generated integrated data or subjective inputs reported by a patient. These data are reflective of therapeutic responses that provide a functionally integrative representation of patient status.

Codes 98976, 98977, 98978 are used to report remote therapeutic monitoring services during a 30-day period. To report 98975, 98976, 98977, 98978, the service(s) must be ordered by a physician or other qualified health care professional. Code 98975 may be used to report the set-up and patient education on the use of any device(s) utilized for therapeutic data collection. Codes 98976, 98977, 98978 may be used to report supply of the device for scheduled (eg, daily) recording(s) and/or programmed alert(s) transmissions. To report 98975, 98976, 98977, 98978, the device used must be a medical device as defined by the FDA. Codes 98975, 98976, 98977, 98978 are not reported if monitoring is less than 16 days. Do not report 98975, 98976, 98977, 98978 with other physiologic monitoring services (eg, 95250 for continuous glucose monitoring requiring a minimum of 72 hours of monitoring or 99453, 99454 for remote monitoring of physiologic parameter[s]).◀

Code 98975 is reported for each episode of care. For reporting remote therapeutic monitoring parameters, an episode of care is defined as beginning when the remote therapeutic monitoring service is initiated and ends with attainment of targeted treatment goals.

▲ **98975**   Remote therapeutic monitoring (eg, therapy adherence, therapy response); initial set-up and patient education on use of equipment

(Do not report 98975 more than once per episode of care)

(Do not report 98975 for monitoring of less than 16 days)

▲ **98976**   device(s) supply with scheduled (eg, daily) recording(s) and/or programmed alert(s) transmission to monitor respiratory system, each 30 days

▲ **98977**   device(s) supply with scheduled (eg, daily) recording(s) and/or programmed alert(s) transmission to monitor musculoskeletal system, each 30 days

Rationale

Codes 98975-98977 have been revised by removing "respiratory system status" and "musculoskeletal system status" from the example in the descriptor. These have been removed to avoid redundancy, because there are specific codes for reporting these services.

● **98978**   device(s) supply with scheduled (eg, daily) recording(s) and/or programmed alert(s) transmission to monitor cognitive behavioral therapy, each 30 days

▶(Do not report 98975, 98976, 98977, 98978 in conjunction with codes for more specific physiologic parameters [93296, 94760, 99453, 99454])◀

▶(Do not report 98976, 98977, 98978 for monitoring of less than 16 days)◀

(For therapeutic monitoring treatment management services, use 98980)

(For remote physiologic monitoring, see 99453, 99454)

(For physiologic monitoring treatment management services, use 99457)

(For self-measured blood pressure monitoring, see 99473, 99474)

Rationale

Code 98978 to report remote therapeutic monitoring of cognitive behavioral therapy has been added as a child code to parent code 98975 in the Remote Therapeutic Monitoring Services subsection.

Code 98978 is intended to report a 30-day device supply with scheduled recordings and/or programmed alert transmission to monitor cognitive behavioral therapy. The guidelines in this subsection have been revised to include this code and to provide clarity on the reporting of these codes.

Code 98978 describes the cost of the device supplied to the patient. This family of codes has been designed to accommodate additional technology and devices that may have variable costs, depending on the therapeutic approach taken by the physician and/or other QHP.

The Digitally Stored Data Services/Remote Physiologic Monitoring subsection guidelines have also been revised to include code 98978. Parenthetical notes throughout the code set have also been revised to include code 98978, accordingly.

Clinical Example (98978)

A 43-year-old female presents to the physician's or other QHP's office and is diagnosed with substance use disorder. Following the visit, the physician or other QHP initiates a cognitive behavioral therapy–based digital remote therapeutic monitoring program as an adjunct to outpatient treatment for a specified duration to enable data collection, monitoring, and support therapeutic management of the patient's behavioral condition.

Description of Procedure (98978)

N/A

Remote Therapeutic Monitoring Treatment Management Services

▶Remote therapeutic monitoring treatment management services are provided when a physician or other qualified health care professional uses the results of remote therapeutic monitoring to manage a patient under a specific treatment plan. To report remote therapeutic monitoring, the service must be ordered by a physician or other qualified health care professional. To report 98980, 98981, any device used must be a medical device as defined by the FDA. Do not use 98980, 98981 for time that can be reported using codes for more specific monitoring services. Codes 98980, 98981 may be reported during the same service period as chronic care management services (99439, 99487, 99489, 99490, 99491), transitional care management services (99495, 99496), principal care management services (99424, 99425, 99426, 99427), behavioral health integration services (99484), and psychiatric collaborative care services (99492, 99493, 99494). However, time spent performing these services should remain separate and no time should be counted toward the required time for both services in a single month. Codes 98980, 98981 require at least one interactive communication with the patient or caregiver. The interactive communication contributes to the total time, but it does not need to represent the entire cumulative reported time of the treatment management service. For the first completed 20 minutes of physician or other qualified health care professional time in a calendar month, report 98980, and report 98981 for each additional completed 20 minutes. Do not report 98980, 98981 for services of less than 20 minutes. Report 98980 once, regardless of the number of therapeutic monitoring modalities performed in a given calendar month.

★ = Telemedicine   ◀ = Audio-only   ✦ = Add-on code   ✗ = FDA approval pending   # = Resequenced code   ⊘ = Modifier 51 exempt

Medicine 90281-99607

Do not count any time on a day when the physician or other qualified health care professional reports an E/M service (office or other outpatient services [99202, 99203, 99204, 99205, 99211, 99212, 99213, 99214, 99215], home or residence services [99341, 99342, 99344, 99345, 99347, 99348, 99349, 99350], inpatient or observation care services [99221, 99222, 99223, 99231, 99232, 99233, 99234, 99235, 99236], inpatient consultations [99252, 99253, 99254, 99255]).◄

Rationale

In accordance with the addition of code 98978, the Remote Therapeutic Monitoring Treatment Management Services subsection guidelines have been revised by adding the subsection heading, Psychiatric Collaborative Care Services, to the guidelines to accurately identify the psychiatric collaborative care services codes (99492, 99493, 99494) that can be reported with codes 98980 and 98981 during the same service period.

Refer to the codebook and the Rationale for code 98978 for a full discussion of these changes.

The guidelines have also been revised in accordance with the deletion of codes 99324-99337, 99343, and 99251.

Refer to the codebook and the Rationale for codes 99324-99337, 99343, and 99251 for a full discussion of these changes.

Home Health Procedures/ Services

►These codes are used by non-physician health care professionals. Physicians should utilize the home or residence services codes 99341-99350 and utilize CPT codes other than 99500-99600 for any additional procedure/service provided to a patient living in a home or residence.

The following codes are used to report services provided in a patient's home or residence (including assisted living facility, group home, custodial care facility, nontraditional private homes, or schools).◄

Health care professionals who are authorized to use Evaluation and Management (E/M) Home Visit codes (99341-99350) may report 99500-99600 in addition to 99341-99350 if both services are performed. E/M services may be reported separately, using modifier 25, if the patient's condition requires a significant separately identifiable E/M service, above and beyond the home health service(s)/procedure(s) codes 99500-99600.

99500   Home visit for prenatal monitoring and assessment to include fetal heart rate, non-stress test, uterine monitoring, and gestational diabetes monitoring

Rationale

In accordance with the revision of codes 99341-99350, the Home Health Procedures/Services subsection guidelines have been revised to reflect these changes.

Refer to the codebook and the Rationale for codes 99341-99350 for a full discussion of these changes.

Notes

Category III Codes

Summary of Additions, Deletions, and Revisions

The summary of changes shows the actual changes that have been made to the code descriptors.

New codes appear with a bullet (●) and are indicated as "Code added." Revised codes are preceded with a triangle (▲). Within revised codes, or if a code symbol has been deleted, the deleted language and code symbol appear with a ~~strikethrough~~, while new text appears underlined.

The ✗ symbol is used to identify codes for vaccines that are pending FDA approval. The # symbol is used to identify codes that have been resequenced. CPT add-on codes are annotated by the ✚ symbol. The ⊘ symbol is used to identify codes that are exempt from the use of modifier 51. The ★ symbol is used to identify codes that may be used for reporting telemedicine services. The ✕ symbol is used to identify a proprietary laboratory analyses (PLA) test that has an identical descriptor as another PLA test. A PLA code that satisfies Category I code criteria and has been accepted by the CPT Editorial Panel is annotated with the ↑↓ symbol. The ◀ symbol is used to identify codes that may be used to report audio-only telemedicine services when appended by modifier 93 (see Appendix T).

Code	Description
0163T	~~Total disc arthroplasty (artificial disc), anterior approach, including discectomy to prepare interspace (other than for decompression), each additional interspace, lumbar (List separately in addition to code for primary procedure)~~
0312T	~~Vagus nerve blocking therapy (morbid obesity); laparoscopic implantation of neurostimulator electrode array, anterior and posterior vagal trunks adjacent to esophagogastric junction (EGJ), with implantation of pulse generator, includes programming~~
0313T	~~laparoscopic revision or replacement of vagal trunk neurostimulator electrode array, including connection to existing pulse generator~~
0314T	~~laparoscopic removal of vagal trunk neurostimulator electrode array and pulse generator~~
0315T	~~removal of pulse generator~~
0316T	~~replacement of pulse generator~~
0317T	~~neurostimulator pulse generator electronic analysis, includes reprogramming when performed~~
▲0402T	Collagen cross-linking of cornea, including removal of the corneal epithelium, when performed, and intraoperative pachymetry, when performed ~~(Report medication separately)~~
#●0714T	Code added
0470T	~~Optical coherence tomography (OCT) for microstructural and morphological imaging of skin, image acquisition, interpretation, and report; first lesion~~
0471T	~~each additional lesion (List separately in addition to code for primary procedure)~~
0475T	~~Recording of fetal magnetic cardiac signal using at least 3 channels; patient recording and storage, data scanning with signal extraction, technical analysis and result, as well as supervision, review, and interpretation of report by a physician or other qualified health care professional~~
0476T	~~patient recording, data scanning, with raw electronic signal transfer of data and storage~~
0477T	~~signal extraction, technical analysis, and result~~

▲=Revised code   ●=New code   ▶ ◀=Contains new or revised text   ✕=Duplicate PLA test   ↑↓=Category I PLA   American Medical Association   211

Category III 0042T–0713T

Code	Description
0478T	review, interpretation, report by physician or other qualified health care professional
0487T	Biomechanical mapping, transvaginal, with report
0491T	Ablative laser treatment, non-contact, full field and fractional ablation, open wound, per day, total treatment surface area; first 20 sq cm or less
0492T	each additional 20 sq cm, or part thereof (List separately in addition to code for primary procedure)
0493T	Contact near-infrared spectroscopy studies of lower extremity wounds (eg, for oxyhemoglobin measurement)
0497T	External patient-activated, physician- or other qualified health care professional-prescribed, electrocardiographic rhythm derived event recorder without 24-hour attended monitoring; in-office connection
0498T	review and interpretation by a physician or other qualified health care professional per 30 days with at least one patient-generated triggered event
0499T	Cystourethroscopy, with mechanical dilation and urethral therapeutic drug delivery for urethral stricture or stenosis, including fluoroscopy, when performed
0514T	Intraoperative visual axis identification using patient fixation (List separately in addition to code for primary procedure)
0702T	Remote therapeutic monitoring of a standardized online digital cognitive behavioral therapy program ordered by a physician or other qualified health care professional; supply and technical support, per 30 days
0703T	management services by physician or other qualified health care professional, per calendar month
✚●0715T	Code added
●0716T	Code added
●0717T	Code added
●0718T	Code added
●0719T	Code added
●0720T	Code added
●0721T	Code added
✚●0722T	Code added
●0723T	Code added
✚●0724T	Code added
●0725T	Code added
●0726T	Code added
●0727T	Code added
●0728T	Code added
●0729T	Code added
●0730T	Code added
●0731T	Code added
●0732T	Code added

★ = Telemedicine   ◀ = Add-on code   ✚ = Add-on code   ⚕ = FDA approval pending   # = Resequenced code   ⃠ = Modifier 51 exempt

Code	Description
▲0733T	Remote real-time, motion capture–based neurorehabilitative ~~body and limb kinematic measurement-based~~ therapy ordered by a physician or other qualified health care professional; supply and technical support, per 30 days
▲0734T	treatment management services by a physician or other qualified health care professional, per calendar month
+●0735T	Code added
●0736T	Code added
●0737T	Code added
●0738T	Code added
●0739T	Code added
●0740T	Code added
●0741T	Code added
+●0742T	Code added
●0743T	Code added
#●0749T	Code added
#●0750T	Code added
●0744T	Code added
●0745T	Code added
●0746T	Code added
●0747T	Code added
●0748T	Code added
+●0751T	Code added
+●0752T	Code added
+●0753T	Code added
+●0754T	Code added
+●0755T	Code added
+●0756T	Code added
+●0757T	Code added
+●0758T	Code added
+●0759T	Code added
+●0760T	Code added
+●0761T	Code added
+●0762T	Code added
+●0763T	Code added
+●0764T	Code added

Code	Description
●0765T	Code added
●0766T	Code added
➕●0767T	Code added
●0768T	Code added
➕●0769T	Code added
➕●0770T	Code added
●0771T	Code added
➕●0772T	Code added
●0773T	Code added
➕●0774T	Code added
●0775T	Code added
●0776T	Code added
➕●0777T	Code added
●0778T	Code added
●0779T	Code added
●0780T	Code added
●0781T	Code added
●0782T	Code added
●0783T	Code added

★ = Telemedicine   ◀ = Add-on code   ➕ = Add-on code   ✚ = FDA approval pending   # = Resequenced code   ⊘ = Modifier 51 exempt

Category III Codes

►(0163T has been deleted)◄

►(To report total disc arthroplasty [artificial disc], anterior approach, lumbar, see 22857, 22860)◄

+ 0164T Removal of total disc arthroplasty, (artificial disc), anterior approach, each additional interspace, lumbar (List separately in addition to code for primary procedure)

(Use 0164T in conjunction with 22865)

+ 0165T Revision including replacement of total disc arthroplasty (artificial disc), anterior approach, each additional interspace, lumbar (List separately in addition to code for primary procedure)

(Use 0165T in conjunction with 22862)

►(Do not report 0164T, 0165T in conjunction with 22853, 22854, 22859, 49010, when performed at the same level)◄

(For decompression, see 63001-63048)

Rationale

Code 0163T has been deleted from the Category III section and parenthetical notes have been added and revised to accommodate the addition of code 22860.

Refer to the codebook and the Rationale for code 22860 for a full discussion of these changes.

0278T Transcutaneous electrical modulation pain reprocessing (eg, scrambler therapy), each treatment session (includes placement of electrodes)

►(For peripheral nerve transcutaneous magnetic stimulation, see 0766T, 0767T, 0768T, 0769T)◄

Rationale

In accordance with the establishment of codes 0766T-0769T, a cross-reference parenthetical note has been added following code 0278T to reflect these changes.

Refer to the codebook and the Rationale for codes 0766T-0769T for a full discussion of these changes.

►(0312T, 0313T, 0314T, 0315T, 0316T, 0317T have been deleted)◄

►(For laparoscopic implantation, revision, replacement, or removal of vagus nerve blocking neurostimulator electrode array and/or pulse generator at the esophagogastric junction, use 64999)◄

Rationale

In accordance with CPT guidelines for archiving Category III codes, codes 0312T-0317T have been deleted with instructions added to report code 64999, *Unlisted procedure, nervous system,* if laparoscopic implantation, revision, replacement, or removal of vagus nerve blocking neurostimulator electrode array and/or pulse generator at the esophagogastric junction is performed. A cross-reference parenthetical note has been added to reflect these changes.

In accordance with the deletion of Category III codes 0312T-0317T, parenthetical notes in the Surgery and Medicine sections that reference these codes have also been deleted.

0338T Transcatheter renal sympathetic denervation, percutaneous approach including arterial puncture, selective catheter placement(s) renal artery(ies), fluoroscopy, contrast injection(s), intraprocedural roadmapping and radiological supervision and interpretation, including pressure gradient measurements, flush aortogram and diagnostic renal angiography when performed; unilateral

0339T bilateral

(Do not report 0338T, 0339T in conjunction with 36251, 36252, 36253, 36254)

►(For quantitative pupillometry with interpretation and report, unilateral or bilateral, use 95919)◄

Rationale

To accommodate the addition of code 95919 to report quantitative pupillometry, a parenthetical note following code 0339T has been revised to reflect this change.

Refer to the codebook and the Rationale for code 95919 for a full discussion of this change.

▲ 0402T Collagen cross-linking of cornea, including removal of the corneal epithelium, when performed, and intraoperative pachymetry, when performed

►(Report medication separately)◄

(Do not report 0402T in conjunction with 65435, 69990, 76514)

Rationale

Category III code 0402T has been revised to more accurately describe the removal of corneal epithelium. Code 0402T describes collagen cross-linking of the cornea and intraoperative pachymetry, when performed. Prior to 2023, code 0402T also described removal of the corneal epithelium. However, removal of the corneal epithelium is not always performed, but it is included when performed. Effective in 2023, code 0402T has been revised to clarify that removal of corneal epithelium is included, when performed. In addition, code 0402T has been revised with the removal of the parenthetical phrase "Report medication separately," and included in a new parenthetical note following code 0402T, instead.

Clinical Example (0402T)

A 25-year-old male with progressive keratoconus in both eyes over the past 10 years is unable to perform activities of daily living with eyeglasses or contact lenses, even after multiple lens changes. To avoid penetrating keratoplasty at this time, transepithelial collagen cross-linking of the cornea is recommended starting with the right eye.

Description of Procedure (0402T)

Administer topical anesthesia to the eye. Administer blow-by oxygen to the cornea, either with the epithelium on the cornea or off the cornea. Administer specially formulated riboflavin (vitamin B2) eyedrops to the eye for about 30 minutes at frequent intervals to saturate the corneal stroma. Then administer ultraviolet light (UVA) to the cornea to create the cross-linking. Patch the eye and give the patient discharge instructions.

0419T Destruction of neurofibroma, extensive (cutaneous, dermal extending into subcutaneous); face, head and neck, greater than 50 neurofibromas

(For excision of neurofibroma, use 64792)

(Report 0419T once per session regardless of the number of lesions treated)

0420T trunk and extremities, extensive, greater than 100 neurofibromas

(For excision of neurofibroma, use 64792)

(Report 0420T once per session regardless of the number of lesions treated)

#● 0714T Transperineal laser ablation of benign prostatic hyperplasia, including imaging guidance

Rationale

Category III code 0714T has been established to report transperineal laser ablation of benign prostatic hyperplasia. This procedure is an alternative to surgical excision and describes a minimally invasive intervention that includes imaging guidance as an inclusive service.

Clinical Example (0714T)

A 68-year-old male presents with a two-year history of progressive voiding symptoms, including difficulty urinating, due to bladder outlet obstruction caused by benign prostatic hyperplasia (BPH), with international prostate symptom score (IPSS) of 21 and uroflowmetry of 10 cc/sec. Digital rectal examination reveals a benign, enlarged prostate. His symptoms have failed to improve while on medical therapy. After discussion of treatment options, he elects to undergo ultrasound-guided transperineal laser ablation of the prostate.

Description of Procedure (0714T)

Position the patient in the lithotomy position, administer local anesthesia or conscious sedation, if required (separately reported), and antibiotics. Insert Foley catheter. Monitor vital signs. Localize target lesion(s) with transrectal ultrasound guidance to position the transperineal laser applicator. Place one or more introducer needles in the deeper portion of the target lesion, guided by real-time ultrasound imaging. Insert optical fibers into the introducer needle(s). Deliver laser energy to the target lesion(s). Evaluate progress of ablation of target lesion using ultrasound imaging. Once the target lesion is completely ablated, withdraw optical fibers and introducer needle(s). Remove catheter 12 to 48 hours after the procedure.

+ 0437T Implantation of non-biologic or synthetic implant (eg, polypropylene) for fascial reinforcement of the abdominal wall (List separately in addition to code for primary procedure)

▶(For implantation of absorbable mesh or other prosthesis for delayed closure of defect[s] [ie, external genitalia, perineum, abdominal wall] due to soft tissue infection or trauma, use 15778)◀

▶(For implantation of mesh or other prosthesis for anterior abdominal hernia[s] repair or parastomal hernia repair, see 49591-49622)◀

★ = Telemedicine   ◀ = Add-on code   ✚ = Add-on code   �унктF = FDA approval pending   # = Resequenced code   ⊘ = Modifier 51 exempt

Rationale

In accordance with the deletion of codes 49560-49590 and 49652-49657 and the establishment of new hernia repair codes 49591-49622 and add-on code 49623, two parenthetical notes following code 0437T have been deleted. Two new parenthetical notes have been established to instruct users on reporting of implantation of mesh or other prosthesis for anterior abdominal hernia repair and for delayed closure of defects due to soft tissue infection or trauma.

Refer to the codebook and the Rationale for codes 49591-49622 for a full discussion of these changes.

▶(0470T, 0471T have been deleted)◀

▶(For optical coherence tomography [OCT] for microstructural and morphological imaging of skin, use 96999)◀

Rationale

In accordance with CPT guidelines for archiving Category III codes, codes 0470T and 0471T have been deleted with instructions added to report code 96999, *Unlisted special dermatological service or procedure,* if optical coherence tomography for microstructural and morphological imaging of skin is performed. A cross-reference parenthetical note has been added to reflect these changes.

▶(0475T, 0476T, 0477T, 0478T have been deleted)◀

▶(For recording of fetal magnetic cardiac signal, data scanning, transfer data, signal extraction, review, and interpretation and report, use 93799)◀

Rationale

In accordance with CPT guidelines for archiving Category III codes, codes 0475T-0478T have been deleted with instructions added to report code 93799, *Unlisted cardiovascular service or procedure,* for recording of fetal magnetic cardiac signal, data scanning, transfer data, signal extraction, review, and interpretation and report. A cross-reference parenthetical note has been added to reflect these changes.

▶(0487T has been deleted)◀

▶(For transvaginal biomechanical mapping, use 58999)◀

Rationale

In accordance with CPT guidelines for archiving Category III codes, code 0487T has been deleted with instructions added to report code 58999, *Unlisted procedure, female genital system (nonobstetrical),* for transvaginal biomechanical mapping. A cross-reference parenthetical note has been added to reflect these changes.

▶(0491T, 0492T have been deleted)◀

▶(For non-contact full-field and fractional ablative laser treatment of an open wound, use 17999)◀

Rationale

In accordance with CPT guidelines for archiving Category III codes, codes 0491T and 0492T have been deleted with instructions added to report code 17999, *Unlisted procedure, skin, mucous membrane and subcutaneous tissue,* for noncontact full-field and fractional ablative laser treatment of an open wound. A cross-reference parenthetical note has been added to reflect these changes.

▶(0493T has been deleted)◀

▶(For transcutaneous oxyhemoglobin measurement in a lower extremity wound by near-infrared spectroscopy, use 93998)◀

(For noncontact near-infrared spectroscopy studies, see 0640T, 0641T, 0642T)

▶Near-infrared spectroscopy is used to measure cutaneous vascular perfusion. Codes 0640T, 0641T, 0642T describe noncontact near-infrared spectroscopy of skin flaps or wounds for measurement of cutaneous vascular perfusion that does not require direct contact of the spectrometer sensors with the patient's skin.◀

Rationale

In accordance with CPT guidelines for archiving Category III codes, code 0493T has been deleted and introductory guidelines have been revised by removing reference to this code. An instructional parenthetical note has been added to report code 93998, *Unlisted noninvasive vascular diagnostic study,* for transcutaneous oxyhemoglobin measurement in a lower extremity wound by near-infrared spectroscopy. A cross-reference parenthetical note has been added to reflect these changes.

Category III 0042T-0713T

0640T Noncontact near-infrared spectroscopy studies of flap or wound (eg, for measurement of deoxyhemoglobin, oxyhemoglobin, and ratio of tissue oxygenation [StO_2]); image acquisition, interpretation and report, each flap or wound

0641T   image acquisition only, each flap or wound

(Do not report 0641T in conjunction with 0640T, 0642T)

0642T   interpretation and report only, each flap or wound

(Do not report 0642T in conjunction with 0640T, 0641T)

▶(0497T, 0498T have been deleted)◀

▶ (For in-office connection or review and interpretation of an external patient-activated electrocardiographic rhythm–derived event recorder without 24-hour attended monitoring, use 93799)◀

Rationale

In accordance with CPT guidelines for archiving Category III codes, codes 0497T and 0498T have been deleted with instructions added to report code 93799, *Unlisted cardiovascular service or procedure*, for in-office connection or review and interpretation of an external patient-activated electrocardiographic rhythm derived– event recorder without 24-hour attending monitoring. A cross-reference parenthetical note has been added to reflect these changes.

▶(0499T has been deleted)◀

▶(For cystourethroscopy with urethral therapeutic drug delivery, use 53899)◀

Rationale

In accordance with CPT guidelines for archiving Category III codes, code 0499T has been deleted with instructions added to report code 53899, *Unlisted procedure, urinary system*, for cystourethroscopy with urethral therapeutic drug delivery. A cross-reference parenthetical note has been added to reflect these changes.

▶(0514T has been deleted)◀

Rationale

Category III code 0514T, *Intraoperative visual axis identification using patient fixation (List separately in addition to code for primary procedure)*, has been deleted. Code 0514T was established in 2019. However, it had very low utilization because there is no significant need for the procedure. A parenthetical note has been added to indicate that code 0514T has been deleted.

0554T Bone strength and fracture risk using finite element analysis of functional data and bone-mineral density utilizing data from a computed tomography scan; retrieval and transmission of the scan data, assessment of bone strength and fracture risk and bone-mineral density, interpretation and report

(Do not report 0554T in conjunction with 0555T, 0556T, 0557T)

0555T   retrieval and transmission of the scan data

0556T   assessment of bone strength and fracture risk and bone-mineral density

0557T   interpretation and report

▶(Do not report 0554T, 0555T, 0556T, 0557T in conjunction with 0691T, 0743T)◀

Rationale

In accordance with the establishment of code 0743T, the exclusionary parenthetical note following code 0557T has been revised to reflect this change.

Refer to the codebook and the Rationale for code 0743T for a full discussion of this change.

Health and Well-Being Coaching

▶Health and well-being coaching is a patient-centered approach wherein patients determine their goals, use self-discovery or active learning processes together with content education to work toward their goals, and self-monitor behaviors to increase accountability, all within the context of an interpersonal relationship with a coach. The health and well-being coach is qualified to perform health and well-being coaching by education, training, national examination and, when applicable, licensure/ regulation, and has completed a training program in health and well-being coaching whose content meets standards established by an applicable national credentialing organization. The training includes behavioral change theory, motivational strategies, communication techniques, health education and

★ = Telemedicine   ◀ = Add-on code   ✚ = Add-on code   ⟋ = FDA approval pending   # = Resequenced code   ⊘ = Modifier 51 exempt

promotion theories, which are used to assist patients to develop intrinsic motivation and obtain skills to create sustainable change for improved health and well-being.◄

0591T Health and well-being coaching face-to-face; individual, initial assessment

0592T individual, follow-up session, at least 30 minutes

(Do not report 0592T in conjunction with 96156, 96158, 96159, 98960, 0488T, 0591T)

(For medical nutrition therapy, see 97802, 97803, 97804)

0593T group (2 or more individuals), at least 30 minutes

(Do not report 0593T in conjunction with 96164, 96165, 97150, 98961, 98962, 0403T)

Rationale

The Health and Well-Being Coaching subsection guidelines have been revised with the removal of mention of certification by the National Board of Health and Wellness Coaching and National Commission for Health Education Credentialing, Inc. These changes reflect the need to allow any qualified health coach to perform health and well-being services.

0619T Cystourethroscopy with transurethral anterior prostate commissurotomy and drug delivery, including transrectal ultrasound and fluoroscopy, when performed

►(Do not report 0619T in conjunction with 52000, 52441, 52442, 52450, 52500, 52601, 52630, 52640, 52647, 52648, 52649, 53850, 53852, 53854, 76872)◄

Rationale

In accordance with the deletion of Category III code 0499T, the exclusionary parenthetical note following code 0619T has been revised with the removal of this code.

Refer to the codebook and the Rationale for code 0499T for a full discussion of this change.

0621T Trabeculostomy ab interno by laser;

0622T with use of ophthalmic endoscope

►(Do not report 0621T, 0622T in conjunction with 92020, 0730T)◄

Rationale

In accordance with the establishment of code 0730T, the exclusionary parenthetical note following code 0622T has been revised to reflect this change.

Refer to the codebook and the Rationale for code 0730T for a full discussion of this change.

0640T Code is out of numerical sequence. See 0489T-0495T

0641T Code is out of numerical sequence. See 0489T-0495T

0642T Code is out of numerical sequence. See 0489T-0495T

0691T Automated analysis of an existing computed tomography study for vertebral fracture(s), including assessment of bone density when performed, data preparation, interpretation, and report

►(Do not report 0691T in conjunction with 71250, 71260, 71270, 71271, 71275, 72125, 72126, 72127, 72128, 72129, 72130, 72131, 72132, 72133, 72191, 72192, 72193, 72194, 74150, 74160, 74170, 74174, 74175, 74176, 74177, 74178, 74261, 74262, 74263, 75571, 75572, 75573, 75574, 75635, 78814, 78815, 78816, 0554T, 0555T, 0556T, 0557T, 0558T, 0743T)◄

Rationale

In accordance with the establishment of code 0743T, the exclusionary parenthetical note following code 0691T has been revised to reflect this change.

Refer to the codebook and the Rationale for code 0743T for a full discussion of this change.

►(0702T, 0703T have been deleted)◄

►(For remote therapeutic monitoring of a standardized online digital cognitive behavioral therapy program, use 98978)◄

Rationale

In accordance with the deletion of codes 0702T and 0703T and the addition of code 98978, two parenthetical notes have been added. These include a parenthetical note indicating the deletion of codes 0702T and 0703T, as well as an instructional parenthetical note referring users to code 98978 when remote therapeutic monitoring of a standardized online digital cognitive behavioral therapy program is performed.

Refer to the codebook and the Rationale for code 98978 for a full discussion of these changes.

▲ = Revised code   ● = New code   ►◄ = Contains new or revised text   ✖ = Duplicate PLA test   ↕ = Category I PLA   American Medical Association   **219**

Category III 0042T-0713T

0714T   Code is out of numerical sequence. See 0419T-0422T

➕⬤ **0715T**   Percutaneous transluminal coronary lithotripsy (List separately in addition to code for primary procedure)

▶(Use 0715T in conjunction with 92920, 92924, 92928, 92933, 92937, 92941, 92943, 92975)◀

Rationale

Category III add-on code 0715T has been established to report percutaneous transluminal coronary lithotripsy. In addition, an instructional parenthetical note following code 0715T has been added to instruct users on the correct use of the code.

To support the addition of add-on code 0715T, the Coronary Therapeutic Services and Procedures subsection guidelines have been revised by instructing users which codes should be used in conjunction with code 0715T. In addition, parenthetical notes have been established following codes 92920, 92924, 92928, 92933, 92937, 92941, 92943, and 92975 to instruct using code 0715T for percutaneous transluminal coronary lithotripsy.

Clinical Example (0715T)

A 72-year-old male presents with unstable angina consistent with acute coronary syndrome. Coronary arteriography demonstrates a 24-mm long, calcified, 80% stenosis in the circumflex coronary artery. During the intracoronary stent procedure, additional treatment of the lesion is necessary. The patient undergoes percutaneous coronary intervention (PCI) coronary lithotripsy followed by coronary stenting. [**Note:** This is an add-on code. Consider only the work associated with percutaneous transluminal coronary lithotripsy.]

Description of Procedure (0715T)

During coronary angiography, observe the presence of severe coronary artery calcium (CAC) in the target lesion(s). Use standard techniques and practices for PCI to prepare patient, gain arterial access, place a sheath, insert a guiding catheter, and engage the guide in the right or left coronary artery (reported with codes 92920, 92924, 92928, 92933, 92937, 92941, 92943, 92975). Advance a standard guidewire across the lesion(s). Select the appropriate diameter coronary intravascular lithotripsy (IVL) catheter. Insert the coronary IVL catheter over the standard guidewire and advance to the first target location and place under fluoroscopy using marker bands. Due to the complexity of the typical calcific lesions, delivery of the IVL catheter often requires predilation of the target treatment site with a balloon(s) or placement of a guide extension or exchange for a different guidewire through a microcatheter. Once the coronary IVL catheter is placed, inflate the

integrated balloon to 4 atm, or enough pressure to make contact with the vessel wall. Then deliver the first lithotripsy cycle of pulses. Once the cycle is complete, inflate the integrated balloon to its nominal pressure of 6 atm. Then deflate the balloon. Perform several cycles of therapy at each location. If dilation is adequate, advance the coronary IVL catheter to the next portion of the lesion and perform lithotripsy cycles and inflations in similar fashion. Typically, 8 separate cycles of therapy are delivered throughout the treatment zone. Exchange out the IVL catheter over a wire and perform a completion angiography to assess for perforation, dissection, or distal embolization. After IVL therapy is complete, perform coronary stenting or other coronary interventional procedures as appropriate to complete treatment of the target lesion(s), remove the equipment, and close the arterial access site (reported with codes 92920, 92924, 92928, 92933, 92937, 92941, 92943, 92975).

⬤ **0716T**   Cardiac acoustic waveform recording with automated analysis and generation of coronary artery disease risk score

Clinical Example (0716T)

A 42-year-old female presents with shortness of breath, fatigue, and atypical chest discomfort.

Description of Procedure (0716T)

Locate the fourth left intercostal space (IC4-L) position (approximately 2 cm of the sternum bone) and mark for sensor placement. Place the sensor on IC4-L. Observe the patient at rest for at least 5 minutes to ensure hemodynamic balance before doing the coronary artery disease (CAD) scoring. Each recording loop has two phases. Four recording loops are performed with 18 seconds of normal abdominal breathing and 8 seconds with breathing paused. The patient does not talk while breathing is paused. The main heart-sound recording phase lasts approximately 2 minutes. After the heart-sound recording has ended, evaluate the sound file for errors and calculate a CAD score.

⬤ **0717T**   Autologous adipose-derived regenerative cell (ADRC) therapy for partial thickness rotator cuff tear; adipose tissue harvesting, isolation and preparation of harvested cells, including incubation with cell dissociation enzymes, filtration, washing, and concentration of ADRCs

▶(Do not report 0717T in conjunction with 15769, 15771, 15772, 15773, 15774, 15876, 15877, 15878, 15879, 20610, 20611, 76942, 77002, 0232T, 0481T, 0489T, 0565T)◀

⬤ **0718T**   injection into supraspinatus tendon including ultrasound guidance, unilateral

►(Do not report 0718T in conjunction with 20610, 20611, 76942, 77002, 0232T, 0481T, 0490T, 0566T)◄

Rationale

Two Category III codes (0717T, 0718T) have been established to report autologous adipose-derived regenerative cell (ADRC) therapy for partial-thickness rotator cuff tear. In addition, exclusionary parenthetical notes have been added to direct users regarding the appropriate use of codes 0717T and 0718T.

This procedure, which had not been previously described in the CPT code set, is performed in patients with a partial-thickness rotator cuff tear. The procedure includes injecting the supraspinatus tendon defect and surrounding area with a preparation of autologous regenerative cell mixture from acquired adipose tissue.

Clinical Example (0717T)

A 58-year-old female presents with chronic right shoulder pain with a positive external rotation test and supraspinatus weakness test. Magnetic resonance imaging (MRI) or ultrasound reveals a partial rotator cuff tear. There has been no improvement with physical therapy and oral steroids. Injection of autologous adipose-derived regenerative cells (ADRC) into the supraspinatus tendon defect and surrounding area is recommended.

Description of Procedure (0717T)

Mark the area where adipose tissue is to be extracted. Make puncture incisions, insert the infiltration cannula, and inject the tumescent solution throughout the subcutaneous adipose tissue. Once the skin appears visibly blanched from vasoconstriction, place the collection cannula in the subcutaneous space and advance and withdraw in a fanning motion while monitoring to avoid injury. Allow the harvested lipoaspirate to rest until phase separation of adipose tissue and tumescent solution has occurred. Add saline solution and an enzymatic reagent to the adipose tissue and process through multiple steps including filtering, washing, and centrifugation until the cell pellet is extracted.

Clinical Example (0718T)

A 60-year-old male presents with chronic right shoulder pain with a positive external rotation test and supraspinatus weakness test. MRI or ultrasound reveals a partial rotator cuff tear. There has been no improvement with physical therapy and oral steroids. Injection of ADRC into the supraspinatus tendon defect and surrounding area is recommended.

Description of Procedure (0718T)

Using aseptic technique and a 25- to 31-gauge needle, inject the suspended cell mixture into the supraspinatus tendon defect and surrounding area under ultrasound guidance. After cell delivery is completed, place a dressing on the injection site.

● **0719T**   Posterior vertebral joint replacement, including bilateral facetectomy, laminectomy, and radical discectomy, including imaging guidance, lumbar spine, single segment

►(Do not report 0719T in conjunction with 22840, 63005, 63012, 63017, 63030, 63042, 63047, 63056, 76000, 76496)◄

Rationale

A new Category III code (0719T) has been established to report posterior vertebral joint replacement. This service is designed to treat conditions such as lumbar degenerative disease. As indicated in the code descriptor, posterior vertebral joint replacement also includes bilateral facetectomy, laminectomy, and radical discectomy and imaging guidance (lumbar spine, single segment), which are bundled together as part of the service.

To support accurate coding, a parenthetical note has been added to indicate that code 0719T should not be reported with codes 22840, 63005, 63012, 63030, 63042, 63047, 63056, 76000, and 76496.

Clinical Example (0719T)

A 55-year-old male presents with bilateral lower extremity and low-back pain, refractory to conservative management. MRI reveals L4-L5 spinal stenosis. The patient is referred for consideration of posterior decompression with facetectomy and posterior vertebral total joint replacement.

Description of Procedure (0719T)

Indicate areas surrounding skin incision to be prepared and draped. Perform a time out with operating surgical team and anesthesia team. Make a posterior midline incision down to the level of the lumbodorsal fascia. Perform subperiosteal dissection. Perform decompression via laminectomy, bilateral total facetectomy, and complete discectomy at the involved level. Release the exiting nerve root tethering ligaments and mobilize the exiting nerve root. Mobilize the segment using sequential bilateral dilation. Determine the construct height and length using trials. Make a bony resection per the preoperative plan to re-establish lumbar lordosis and sagittal plane balance. Using anteroposterior and lateral plane fluoroscopy, confirm the trial is appropriately sized and located. Perform left and right compartment soft tissue balancing. Perform additional bone preparation for initial fixation along the axis of the pedicle followed by insertion of the biomechanical device, including screw fixation. Obtain final biplanar fluoroscopic confirmation of the positioning of the device and bone fixation.

● **0720T**   Percutaneous electrical nerve field stimulation, cranial nerves, without implantation

Rationale

Category III code 0720T has been established to report percutaneous electrical nerve field stimulation for cranial nerves. This procedure involves placement of a noninvasive device that delivers percutaneous electrical nerve field stimulation (PENFS) to the external ear. As noted in the code descriptor, stimulation is applied to the cranial nerve region on the ventral/dorsal side of the ear lobe. After visualization of the cranial and occipital neurovascular bundles, needle arrays are placed behind the patient's ear, activated, and secured in place with adhesives.

PENFS may be used in the treatment of pediatric patients with disorders such as functional abdominal pain disorder.

Clinical Example (0720T)

A 16-year-old female with a two-year history of chronic abdominal pain associated with irritable bowel syndrome, who has not responded to changes in diet, lifestyle, over-the-counter therapies, and off-label medications, is referred for placement of a percutaneous electrical nerve field stimulator.

Description of Procedure (0720T)

Examine the skin behind the ear. Perform transillumination of the ventral and dorsal aspects of the external ear to visualize the cranial and occipital neurovascular bundles. Place the needle arrays on the ventral/dorsal side of the ear lobe. Position the electrical nerve field stimulator behind the patient's ear, activate, and secure in place with adhesives.

● **0721T**   Quantitative computed tomography (CT) tissue characterization, including interpretation and report, obtained without concurrent CT examination of any structure contained in previously acquired diagnostic imaging

▶(Do not report 0721T in conjunction with 70450, 70460, 70470, 70480, 70481, 70482, 70486, 70487, 70488, 70490, 70491, 70492, 71250, 71260, 71270, 71271, 72125, 72126, 72127, 72128, 72129, 72130, 72131, 72132, 72133, 72192, 72193, 72194, 73200, 73201, 73202, 73700, 73701, 73702, 74150, 74160, 74170, 74176, 74177, 74178, 74261, 74262, 74263, 75571, 75572, 75573, 76497, 0722T, when performed on the same anatomy)◀

✚● **0722T**   Quantitative computed tomography (CT) tissue characterization, including interpretation and report, obtained with concurrent CT examination of any structure contained in the concurrently acquired diagnostic imaging dataset (List separately in addition to code for primary procedure)

▶(Use 0722T in conjunction with 70450, 70460, 70470, 70480, 70481, 70482, 70486, 70487, 70488, 70490, 70491, 70492, 71250, 71260, 71270, 71271, 72125, 72126, 72127, 72128, 72129, 72130, 72131, 72132, 72133, 72192, 72193, 72194, 73200, 73201, 73202, 73700, 73701, 73702, 74150, 74160, 74170, 74176, 74177, 74178, 74261, 74262, 74263, 75571, 75572, 75573, 76497, 0721T)◀

Rationale

Two Category III codes (0721T, 0722T) have been established to report quantitative computed tomography (CT) tissue characterization. Additional guidance, such as inclusionary and exclusionary parenthetical notes, have been provided for when to report and when not to report these procedures in conjunction with other services.

Code 0721T is used to report quantitative CT tissue characterization, which includes interpretation and report, that is obtained without concurrent CT examination of any structure contained in previously acquired diagnostic imaging. This is different from quantitative ultrasound tissue characterization.

Code 0722T is an add-on code used to report quantitative CT tissue characterization, which includes interpretation and report. The tissue is obtained with concurrent CT examination of any structure contained in the concurrently acquired diagnostic imaging dataset. If quantitative CT tissue characterization is performed with CT examination of the same anatomy on the same date of service, then code 0722T would be reported on the same date of service.

Clinical Example (0721T)

A 57-year-old female had a recent chest computed tomography (CT) scan for an abnormality discovered on chest X ray. The primary care physician now requests quantitative CAC characterization utilizing the original CT dataset.

★ = Telemedicine   ◀ = Add-on code   ✚ = Add-on code   ✒ = FDA approval pending   # = Resequenced code   ⊘ = Modifier 51 exempt

Description of Procedure (0721T)

The referring physician requests performance of quantitative CAC characterization to be performed from a pre-existing CT dataset. Load the original dataset to the processing servers for coronary calcium quantification. Return a quantitative analysis to the physician or other qualified health care professional (QHP). The physician or other QHP reviews the computer output, makes any necessary modification to account for any computer-generated errors or artifacts, and dictates a report.

Clinical Example (0722T)

A 67-year-old male with a known pulmonary nodule is planned for a follow-up CT scan of a known lung nodule. The primary physician requests concurrent quantitative CAC characterization to be performed utilizing the CT data from this examination. [**Note:** This is an add-on code for the additional work related to quantitative CT tissue characterization. The work related to the associated CT of the same anatomy is reported separately and not related to the work of the add-on procedure.]

Description of Procedure (0722T)

The referring physician requests quantitative CAC characterization to be performed during a scheduled upcoming chest CT scan (reported separately). Once performed, load the CT dataset to the processing servers for coronary calcium quantification. Return a quantitative analysis to the physician or other QHP. The physician or other QHP reviews the computer output, makes any necessary modification to account for any computer-generated errors or artifacts, and incorporates the quantitative CAC characterization into the chest CT report.

● **0723T**　Quantitative magnetic resonance cholangiopancreatography (QMRCP), including data preparation and transmission, interpretation and report, obtained without diagnostic magnetic resonance imaging (MRI) examination of the same anatomy (eg, organ, gland, tissue, target structure) during the same session

　　▶(Do not report 0723T in conjunction with 74181, 74182, 74183, 76376, 76377, 0724T, when also evaluating same organ, gland, tissue, or target structure)◀

+● **0724T**　Quantitative magnetic resonance cholangiopancreatography (QMRCP), including data preparation and transmission, interpretation and report, obtained with diagnostic magnetic resonance imaging (MRI) examination of the same anatomy (eg, organ, gland, tissue, target structure) (List separately in addition to code for primary procedure)

　　▶(Use 0724T in conjunction with 74181, 74182, 74183, when also evaluating same organ, gland, tissue, or target structure)◀

　　▶(Do not report 0724T in conjunction with 76376, 76377, 0723T)◀

Rationale

Category III codes 0723T and 0724T have been established to report quantitative magnetic resonance cholangiopancreatography (QMRCP) procedures. In addition, new parenthetical notes have been added to guide users in the appropriate reporting for these new procedures.

QMRCP is a new diagnostic procedure that is not previously included in the CPT code set. These new procedures provide the ability to quantitatively evaluate pancreatobiliary structure anatomy from MRI by producing quantitative metrics of the biliary tree and pancreatic ducts.

Code 0723T is reported for QMRCP, including data preparation and transmission, interpretation and report, obtained without diagnostic MRI examination of the same anatomy.

Code 0724T describes QMRCP, including data preparation and transmission, interpretation and report, obtained with diagnostic MRI examination of the same anatomy.

To assist in the appropriate reporting of these new services, three parenthetical notes have been added. The first exclusionary parenthetical note has been added following code 0723T to restrict reporting code 0723T with codes 74181-74183, 76376, 76377, and 0724T, when also evaluating the same organ, gland, tissue, or target structure.

The second inclusionary parenthetical note has been added following code 0724T to instruct that code 0724T can be used with codes 74181-74183, when also evaluating the same organ, gland, tissue, or target structure.

Lastly, an exclusionary parenthetical note has been added to restrict reporting code 0724T with codes 76376, 76377, and 0723T.

Clinical Example (0723T)

A 47-year-old male presents with a recent abnormal MRI and magnetic resonance cholangiopancreatography (MRCP), suggesting a diagnosis of primary sclerosing cholangitis. Quantitative MRCP (QMRCP) is requested from the pre-existing MRCP dataset to quantify total intrahepatic biliary tree volume prior to initiation of therapy for primary sclerosing cholangitis.

▲ = Revised code　● = New code　▶ ◀ = Contains new or revised text　✕ = Duplicate PLA test　↕ = Category I PLA　　American Medical Association　**223**

Category III　0042T-0713T

Description of Procedure (0723T)

The physician reviews the request for service to clarify indications for procedure and determine the clinical questions that need to be answered by QMRCP. Review previously obtained three-dimensional (3D) MRCP sequences to check for motion or banding artifacts. The data are processed through an algorithm that generates quantitative biliary tree metrics. Manually obtain post-processed metrics of total biliary tree and gallbladder volume, ducts maximum, median, and minimum width, and interquartile range. The physician reviews and interprets all data output resulting from the QMRCP. Compare data to all pertinent available prior examinations. Prepare and dictate a report and document in the patient's record. Communicate study results to the referring physician to facilitate appropriate patient management.

Clinical Example (0724T)

A 32-year-old female presents with fatigue, itching, yellow eyes and skin, 12-pound weight loss, and abdominal pain. An abdominal ultrasound shows dilation of the biliary tree. Laboratory tests show elevated alkaline phosphatase (ALP), aspartate transaminase (AST), alanine aminotransferase (ALT), and bilirubin. The patient is referred for QMRCP in conjunction with abdominal MRI and MRCP for assessment. [**Note:** This is an add-on code for the additional work related to QMRCP performed utilizing a pre-existing abdominal MRI dataset acquired during a separate imaging session. The work related to the abdominal MRI examination is reported separately and not related to the work of the add-on procedure.]

Description of Procedure (0724T)

The physician reviews the request for service to clarify indications for procedure and determine the clinical questions that need to be answered by QMRCP. 3D MRCP sequences obtained with an abdominal MRI (separately reported with codes 74181, 74182, or 74183) are reviewed to check for motion or banding artifacts. The data are processed through an algorithm that generates quantitative biliary tree metrics. Manually obtain post-processed metrics of total biliary tree and gallbladder volume, ducts maximum, median, and minimum width, and interquartile range.

The physician then reviews and interprets all sequences and data output resulting from the abdominal MRI examination and the QMRCP. Compare data to all pertinent available prior examinations. Prepare and dictate a report and document in the patient's record. Communicate study results to the referring physician to facilitate appropriate patient management.

● **0725T** Vestibular device implantation, unilateral

▶(Do not report 0725T in conjunction with 69501, 69502, 69505, 69511, 69601, 69602, 69603, 69604)◀

● **0726T** Removal of implanted vestibular device, unilateral

▶(Do not report 0726T in conjunction with 69501, 69502, 69505, 69511, 69601, 69602, 69603, 69604)◀

● **0727T** Removal and replacement of implanted vestibular device, unilateral

▶(Do not report 0727T in conjunction with 69501, 69502, 69505, 69511, 69601, 69602, 69603, 69604)◀

▶(For cochlear device implantation, with or without mastoidectomy, use 69930)◀

● **0728T** Diagnostic analysis of vestibular implant, unilateral; with initial programming

● **0729T** with subsequent programming

▶(For initial and subsequent diagnostic analysis and programming of cochlear implant, see 92601, 92602, 92603, 92604)◀

Rationale

Five Category III codes (0725T-0729T) have been established for reporting vestibular device procedures. A vestibular device stimulates the vestibular nerve to imitate the inner ear labyrinth for proper function of gaze- and posture-stabilizing reflexes. Vestibular devices are implanted in patients with disorders such as vestibular hypofunction.

Code 0725T describes unilateral vestibular device implantation. Code 0726T describes the removal of an implanted vestibular device. Code 0727T describes the removal and replacement of an implanted vestibular device. Code 0728T describes diagnostic analysis of a vestibular implant with initial programming. Code 0729T describes diagnostic analysis of a vestibular implant with subsequent programming. The procedures described in all five codes are unilateral procedures. Exclusionary parenthetical notes have been added restricting the use of codes 0725T-0729T with codes 69501, 69502, 69505, 69511, and 69601-69604. Cross-reference parenthetical notes have been added following code 0727T, directing users to code 69930 for cochlear device implantation with or without mastoidectomy, and code 0729T, directing users to codes 92601-92604 for initial and subsequent diagnostic analysis and programming of cochlear implant.

★ = Telemedicine ◀ = Add-on code ✚ = Add-on code ✗ = FDA approval pending # = Resequenced code ⊘ = Modifier 51 exempt

Category III 0042T-0713T

Clinical Example (0725T)

A 60-year-old female presents with bilateral vestibular hypofunction. She has failed vestibular rehabilitation therapy. The patient undergoes surgical implantation of a vestibular implant receiver/stimulator.

Description of Procedure (0725T)

Place the patient under general endotracheal anesthesia. Make a post-auricular incision and elevate a periosteal flap to expose mastoid and external auditory canal. Develop a subperiosteal pocket posterior and superior to the incision and drill a bone well to accommodate the implant. Perform a complete canal-wall-up mastoidectomy using an otologic drill. Identify all three semicircular canals and expose using a blue-lining technique. Make openings into each of the three canals' ampullae and optionally into the common crus. Drill channels in cortical bone to guide electrode arrays toward these entry points. Insert the receiver/stimulator into the subperiosteal pocket and position and secure its electrode lead. Insert the three ampullary electrode arrays in the ampullotomies and secure with pieces of fascia and bone. Insert the reference electrode. Close the wound in layers and apply a mastoid dressing.

Clinical Example (0726T)

A 60-year-old female with a previously implanted vestibular receiver/stimulator develops an infection at the implant site and is scheduled for implant removal.

Description of Procedure (0726T)

Place the patient under general endotracheal anesthesia. Make a postauricular incision and elevate a periosteal flap to expose the implant. Dissect the tissue as needed to free the receiver/stimulator and electrode lead, which are then removed. Either close the wound in layers or pack and apply a mastoid dressing.

Clinical Example (0727T)

A 62-year-old male with a previously implanted vestibular receiver/stimulator has an implant failure and is referred for replacement of the implant.

Description of Procedure (0727T)

Place the patient under general endotracheal anesthesia. Make a postauricular incision and elevate a periosteal flap to expose the implant. After dissection as needed, remove the receiver/stimulator and electrode leads. Enlarge the subperiosteal pocket as needed to accommodate a new implant. Identify all three semicircular canals and ampullotomies. Modify channels as necessary by drilling in cortical bone to guide electrode arrays to their entry points. Insert the receiver/stimulator into the

subperiosteal pocket. Insert its ampullary electrode arrays in the ampullotomies and secure with pieces of fascia and bone. Insert the reference electrode. Close the wound in layers and apply a mastoid dressing.

Clinical Example (0728T)

A 60-year-old male with bilateral vestibular hypofunction undergoes surgical implantation of a vestibular implant receiver/stimulator. The device was implanted at the time of surgery but not yet activated. The device is activated and programmed based on the patient's response.

Description of Procedure (0728T)

Fit and adjust the external components for secure fit. Test the integrity of each electrode. Adjust the vestibular implant to determine thresholds of motion perception and maximum comfort levels. Then activate stimulation and adjust stimulus parameters based on the patient's perception and responses to changes in stimulus pulse rate and amplitude.

Clinical Example (0729T)

A 60-year-old male with bilateral vestibular hypofunction presents with a need for adjustment of stimulus parameters 6 months after undergoing surgical implantation of a vestibular implant receiver/stimulator. The device was activated and programmed after surgery but needs to be reprogrammed.

Description of Procedure (0729T)

Fit and adjust the external components for secure fit. Test the integrity of each electrode. Adjust the vestibular implant to determine thresholds of motion perception and maximum comfort levels. Then reprogram the electrodes and adjust stimulus parameters based on the patient's perception and responses to changes in stimulus pulse rate and amplitude.

● **0730T**   Trabeculotomy by laser, including optical coherence tomography (OCT) guidance

▶(Do not report 0730T in conjunction with 65850, 65855, 92132, 0621T, 0622T)◀

Category III 0042T–0713T

Rationale

Category III code 0730T has been established to report laser trabeculotomy, including optical coherence tomography (OCT) guidance. This nonsurgical procedure employs a laser beam directed by OCT guidance to the trabecular meshwork, allowing drainage of aqueous humor. The laser trabeculotomy creates an additional channel for drainage in the trabecular meshwork as a means to relieve intraocular pressure. An exclusionary parenthetical note has been added restricting the use of code 0730T with codes 65850, 65855, 92132, 0621T, and 0622T.

Clinical Example (0730T)

A 68-year-old female with uncontrolled open-angle glaucoma has an elevated intraocular pressure (IOP) on maximally tolerated medical therapy. Optical coherence tomography (OCT)–guided femtosecond laser trabeculotomy is planned to reduce IOP.

Description of Procedure (0730T)

Instill topical anesthetic drops and preoperative IOP-lowering or angle-opening medications in the operative eye. Lay the patient horizontally, and to stabilize the globe, place the optical patient interface on the eye and affix using suction. Insert the integrated gonioscopic camera device into the patient interface to perform an initial investigation of the iridocorneal angle and determine the best 90° segment for treatment. Remove the gonioscopic camera device and dock the laser system to the patient interface. Direct a scan of the selected segment with the OCT beam to identify the optimal location in the trabecular meshwork (TM) for the drainage channel(s). Use the aiming beam to adjust the surgical depth and the azimuthal and circumferential positioning of the treatment target. Repeat OCT imaging to confirm the treatment target. Apply the femtosecond laser to the TM target, scanning across a preprogrammed pattern, while treatment progress is monitored on the integrated display screen. Use OCT imaging to confirm treatment success. Separate the patient interface from the delivery system and remove from the eye. Irrigate the surface of the eye to remove the coupling gel and then remove the speculum. Instill additional topical anti-inflammatory drops and measure IOP. If IOP is elevated, instill additional anti-glaucoma medications as needed or administer orally.

● **0731T**   Augmentative AI-based facial phenotype analysis with report

Rationale

Category III code 0731T has been established to report augmentative artificial intelligence (AI)–based facial phenotype analysis. Facial phenotype refers to an individual's observable facial traits (eg, shape of chin, eyes, cheeks). This service employs AI to obtain a patient's facial phenotype, which is then compared with a database of facial images of rare-disease patients to assist in identification of a genetic cause of a patient's symptoms. Code 0731T includes the creation of a report.

Clinical Example (0731T)

A 12-month-old female with failure to thrive is referred for facial phenotyping.

Description of Procedure (0731T)

Obtain a frontal facial photo of the patient. Upload the photo into the facial phenotyping platform. Annotate clinical features.

● **0732T**   Immunotherapy administration with electroporation, intramuscular

Rationale

A new Category III code (0732T) has been established to report immunotherapy administration with electroporation. As indicated in the code descriptor, code 0732T is intended to describe intramuscular immunotherapy administration with electroporation. This procedure uses electroporation alongside injection of DNA plasmids to enhance cellular uptake, which may be used for the treatment of disorders such as cervical cancer.

Similar procedures in the CPT code set describe other approaches, such as code 96373, *Therapeutic prophylactic, or diagnostic injection (specify substance or drug); intra-arterial*, or code 96374, *Therapeutic prophylactic, or diagnostic injection (specify substance or drug); intravenous push, single or initial substance/drug*. However, these procedures do not describe the intramuscular injection and electroporation aspects of DNA-based drug administration.

★ = Telemedicine   ◀ = Add-on code   ✛ = Add-on code   ✗ = FDA approval pending   # = Resequenced code   ⊘ = Modifier 51 exempt

Category III 0042T–0713T

Clinical Example (0732T)

A 30-year-old female presents with high-grade cervical dysplasia caused by the human papillomavirus (HPV) type 16 and/or 18. The physician has determined that surgical excision of the diseased cervical tissue or immunotherapy are recommended. The patient wishes to avoid surgical excision, and the physician determines that immunotherapy is appropriate.

Description of Procedure (0732T)

The physician or other QHP inspects the drug cartridge for any damage and verifies expiration date. Set the needle depth on the handset based on the system's recommendation and clinical judgment. Prepare the sterile, single-use device array by inserting the drug cartridge. Then lift the handset off the base station and attach the assembled array and drug cartridge to the handset. A second QHP positions the patient so that she is appropriately braced for treatment. The physician braces the patient by placing a hand firmly on the person's injection limb to limit limb movement during treatment. The physician applies the array to the anatomic administration site to initiate the procedure. Once the dose is completely administered, withdraw and discard the array and return the handset to its docking station. The physician or other QHP conducts post-procedural observation and provides appropriate instructions regarding immediate care.

▲ **0733T**   Remote real-time, motion capture–based neurorehabilitative therapy ordered by a physician or other qualified health care professional; supply and technical support, per 30 days

▲ **0734T**   treatment management services by a physician or other qualified health care professional, per calendar month

Rationale

Category III codes 0733T and 0734T were early released to the AMA website January 1, 2022, and effective July 1, 2022. These codes were established to report remote therapeutic dynamic activities without direct patient contact.

Prior to publication in the *CPT 2023* codebook, the descriptors have been revised to more clearly describe the technology involved in the service. These codes describe neurorehabilitative therapy utilizing measurements based on body-motion capture through optical markerless technology. This technology captures compensation metrics that provide the patient with real-time feedback on their quality of movement.

Code 0733T describes the supply and technical support of the service. Code 0734T describes remote real-time, motion capture–based neurorehabilitative treatment management services by a physician or other QHP and is reported once per calendar month.

Clinical Example (0733T)

A 58-year-old male with Parkinson's disease, who can maintain movement on his own, is referred for neurorehabilitation to improve activities of daily living (ADLs) and function of affected limbs.

Description of Procedure (0733T)

A physician or other QHP defines a therapy plan for the patient, where measures of impairment are used to automatically adjust difficulty of the exercises. The body motion capture system that includes dynamic activities, compensation metrics, and/or remote strength assessment, and/or kinematic assessment of limb function, is supplied to the patient. The patient selects the prescribed therapy plan and is sequentially presented with calibration steps as needed, followed by the exercises prescribed for the chosen session. Once the therapy session has been completed, data associated with the patient's performance are uploaded to the web portal.

Clinical Example (0734T)

A 58-year-old male with Parkinson's disease, who can maintain movement on his own, is referred for neurorehabilitation to improve ADLs and function of affected limbs.

Description of Procedure (0734T)

Access the portal to review the patient's training performance. Based on the patient's performance in the training session(s) and their rehabilitation goals, the physician or other QHP adjusts the therapy plan for the patient's subsequent training session(s).

+● **0735T**   Preparation of tumor cavity, with placement of a radiation therapy applicator for intraoperative radiation therapy (IORT) concurrent with primary craniotomy (List separately in addition to code for primary procedure)

▶(Use 0735T in conjunction with 61510, 61512, 61518, 61519, 61521)◀

Category III 0042T-0713T

Rationale

Category III code 0735T has been established to report the preparation of a cavity left by the removal of a tumor for placement of a radiation therapy applicator for intraoperative radiation therapy (IORT) that is performed concurrently with a craniotomy. Tumor cavity preparation, as described by code 0735T, is performed following the removal of a brain tumor, and the tumor bed is prepared for placement of the IORT applicator. Code 0735T is an add-on code that should be reported in conjunction with the appropriate craniotomy code. An inclusionary parenthetical note listing the craniotomy codes that may be reported with code 0735T has been added.

Clinical Example (0735T)

A 63-year-old male's brain-tumor cavity is prepared and an appropriately sized applicator to deliver intraoperative radiation therapy (IORT) is placed at the treatment site, following a craniectomy (separately reported) to remove his brain tumor. [**Note:** This is an add-on code for the additional work related to preparing the tumor cavity with intraoperative placement of a radiation therapy applicator. The craniotomy, removal of tumor, and closure are reported separately as the primary procedure and not included in the work of this add-on code.]

Description of Procedure (0735T)

Following maximal safe tumor resection (reported separately), examine the resection cavity for active egress of cerebrospinal fluid from the ventricular space with direct repair as required. Take measurements from the closest distance of the cavity wall to the brain stem and optic apparatus (ipsilateral optic nerve; optic chiasm, ipsilateral optic tract) using neuronavigation or intraoperative imaging (MRI, CT) to ensure safe distance from organs at risk and aid in appropriate radiation therapy dose calculation. Then take intracavity measurements of the diameter in three planes using direct assessment with a sterile ruler and select and place an appropriate IORT applicator for trial confirmation of direct apposition of the applicator surface to the wall of the resection cavity. After confirmation of correct size, remove the applicator from the cavity and affix with a sterile drape to the radiation treatment device for sterile final insertion. Roll the stand and sterilely draped arm to the operative site and engage the electromagnetic clutches to facilitate placement of radiation source into the tumor cavity. Conduct a final verification to ensure intracranial close approximation of tumor cavity to the applicator. Drape sterile saline-soaked gauze around the applicator and craniotomy site to keep soft tissue protected and moist during IORT treatment. Drape a radiation barrier around the applicator and the patient's head. Then start IORT delivery for the appropriate period of time based on target surface dose (reported separately). Upon completion of the treatment, remove the draping and applicator from the cavity under direct visualization. Re-inspect the cavity for active egress of cerebrospinal fluid and bleeding with corrective action taken as needed.

● **0736T**   Colonic lavage, 35 or more liters of water, gravity-fed, with induced defecation, including insertion of rectal catheter

Rationale

Category III code 0736T has been established to report colonic lavage. As described by the code descriptor, code 0736T is intended to describe a gravity-fed colonic lavage with induced defecation using 35 or more liters of water.

Gravity-fed, colonic lavage induces defecation and may be used in the management of patients with constipation who have not responded to dietary changes, exercise, and medication. The service is performed by clinical staff, under physician supervision.

Clinical Example (0736T)

A 51-year-old female with chronic functional constipation, who remains symptomatic despite pharmacologic therapies, is referred for gravity-fed colonic lavage with induced defecation for therapeutic management.

Description of Procedure (0736T)

Insert a sterile, disposable rectal catheter approximately 3 cm into the rectum. A slow stream of warm, filtered (UV + gravel) water (without any additives), drained by gravity (PSI approximately 1), flows into the bowel loosening the stool, inducing natural colonic peristalsis and defecation. At the conclusion of the procedure, remove the rectal catheter.

● **0737T**   Xenograft implantation into the articular surface

▶(Use 0737T once per joint)◀

▶(Do not report 0737T in conjunction with 27415, 27416)◀

Rationale

Code 0737T has been established to report xenograft implantation into the articular surface. This procedure places a xenograft scaffold for osteochondral regeneration.

Codes 27415 and 27416 are intended for osteochondral knee grafts and are split between autografts and allografts and between open procedures and arthroscopic procedures. Parenthetical notes have been added following codes 27415 and 27416 to preclude the reporting of these codes with code 0737T. Code 0737T may be reported for each graft implanted in different joints during the same operative session (eg, right and left knees) but may only be reported once per joint.

Clinical Example (0737T)

A 58-year-old male presents with medial right knee pain of nine months duration. The patient has been treated with anti-inflammatory medicines and physical therapy without improvement. Physical examination demonstrates normal alignment, a small joint effusion, medial joint line tenderness, and no knee instability. Imaging studies reveal early stages of osteoarthritis, International Cartilage Regeneration & Joint Preservation Society grade III lesions present. Because of failure to respond to conservative therapies, a xenograft scaffold for osteochondral regeneration is implanted through an open incision.

Description of Procedure (0737T)

With the patient under general anesthesia, perform a medial or lateral para-patellar arthrotomy to allow exposure of the entire compartment to visualize arthritic surfaces. Confirm and/or complete appropriate debridement of the lesion. Carefully size and mark the defect. Prepare the defect for graft implantation using customized instrumentation to develop a donor site to accept the xenograft. Place the graft appropriately using a press fit technique into the prepared defect. Then bring the knee through a range of motion to assure proper fixation and alignment of the xenograft graft with the native medial femoral condyle. Close the incision in layers.

● **0738T** Treatment planning for magnetic field induction ablation of malignant prostate tissue, using data from previously performed magnetic resonance imaging (MRI) examination

   ▶(Do not report 0738T in conjunction with 0739T on the same date of service)◀

● **0739T** Ablation of malignant prostate tissue by magnetic field induction, including all intraprocedural, transperineal needle/catheter placement for nanoparticle installation and intraprocedural temperature monitoring, thermal dosimetry, bladder irrigation, and magnetic field nanoparticle activation

   ▶(Do not report 0739T in conjunction with 51700, 51702, 72192, 72193, 72194, 72195, 72196, 72197, 74176, 74177, 74178, 76497, 76498, 76856, 76857, 76872, 76873, 76940, 76942, 76998, 76999, 77011, 77012, 77013, 77021, 77022, 77600, 77605, 77610, 77615, 77620)◀

Rationale

Category III codes 0738T and 0739T have been established to report services related to ablation of malignant prostate tissue by magnetic field induction. Code 0738T is reported for ablation treatment planning and code 0739T is reported for the ablation procedure.

New parenthetical notes have been added to provide instructions on the appropriate reporting of codes 0738T and 0739T.

The ablation procedure involves the introduction of magnetic nanoparticles into malignant prostate tissue where the nanoparticles are heated in an alternating magnetic field, which results in ablating the malignant prostate tissue.

Clinical Example (0738T)

A 66-year-old male presents with a history of increasing prostate-specific antigen (PSA) levels. A multiparametric MRI of the prostate reveals a focal lesion, and lesion-directed biopsy reveals Gleason 3+4 prostate cancer. The decision is made to ablate the tumor by magnetic field induction. Detailed treatment planning is necessary prior to performing the ablation procedure.

Description of Procedure (0738T)

The physician uses a recent and previously reported MRI to map regions of interest within the prostate for nanoparticle injections, to calculate the appropriate nanoparticle volume for each region of interest, and to plan the placement of temperature sensors for procedure monitoring.

Clinical Example (0739T)

A 66-year-old male presents with a history of increasing PSA levels. A multiparametric MRI of the prostate reveals a focal lesion, and lesion-directed biopsy reveals Gleason 3+4 prostate cancer. The decision is made to ablate the tumor by magnetic field induction. Using the

▲=Revised code   ●=New code   ▶◀=Contains new or revised text   ✘=Duplicate PLA test   ↕=Category I PLA   American Medical Association   **229**

Category III 0042T-0713T

detailed treatment plan developed by the physician in a separately reported procedure, the ablation by magnetic field induction procedure is performed.

Description of Procedure (0739T)

Use a previously performed and separately reported treatment plan to guide the procedure. Use anesthesia or conscious sedation at the physician's discretion during catheter placement and nanoparticle infusion. The physician uses the planning-MRI, fusing-images real-time prostatic ultrasound for guiding transperineal placement of catheters, which will be used to hold temperature sensors to monitor procedure safety and efficacy. Initiate continuous bladder irrigation to protect the bladder and urethra. Inject a suspension of magnetic nanoparticles via the perineum through needles placed into targeted prostate regions of interest that were previously confirmed to be prostate cancer. Use CT to assess nanoparticle placement and volume, which may be adjusted through further injection. Terminate bladder irrigation when instillation is complete and there is no detectable nanoparticle residue in the urethra. Then place temperature sensors in the catheters to monitor temperatures in the tumor and in surrounding tissues during the activation phase of the procedure. Expose the patient to an alternating magnetic field for a treatment period of approximately one hour. Adjust the strength of the magnetic field throughout to keep temperatures within the planned target range. The patient is conscious during this phase to allow reporting of sensation and comfort level.

● **0740T** Remote autonomous algorithm-based recommendation system for insulin dose calculation and titration; initial set-up and patient education

▶(Do not report 0740T in conjunction with 95249, 95250, 95251, 98975, 99453)◀

● **0741T** provision of software, data collection, transmission, and storage, each 30 days

▶(Do not report 0741T in conjunction with 95249, 95250, 95251, 99091, 99454)◀

▶(Do not report 0741T for data collection less than 16 days)◀

Rationale

Category III codes 0740T and 0741T have been established to report remote autonomous algorithm-based insulin dose calculation and titration.

Code 0740T describes the education of a patient on the technology/process of the remote, autonomous insulin dose calculation and titration recommendation system,

which takes inputs, including the physiologic parameters and intermittent glucose reading(s), and utilizes autonomous technology (algorithm) to provide the patient the appropriate adjusted insulin dose (per prescribed regimen) in real-time. An exclusionary parenthetical note has been added to preclude the reporting of code 0740T with codes 95249-95251, 98975, and 99453.

Code 0741T describes the provision of software, data collection, transmission, and storage. Code 0741T should not be reported for data collection of less than 16 days in a 30-day time period. An exclusionary parenthetical note has been added to preclude the reporting of code 0740T with codes 95249-95251, 99091, and 99454.

Clinical Example (0740T)

A 62-year-old male with type 2 diabetes for 22 years, who has required insulin injections for the past 7 years, has poor control of his diabetes with increasing hemoglobin A1c levels despite multiple daily injections of insulin. A remote autonomous algorithm-based insulin dose calculation and titration recommendation system is recommended to improve control of diabetes.

Description of Procedure (0740T)

A QHP uploads the autonomous algorithm-based insulin dose calculation and titration recommendation system to the patient's smart device and configures the system based on the patient's diabetes clinical history and medication profile. The patient is instructed on the use of the system.

Clinical Example (0741T)

A 62-year-old male with type 2 diabetes for 22 years, who has required insulin injections for the past 7 years, has poor control of his diabetes with increasing hemoglobin A1c levels despite multiple daily injections of insulin. A remote autonomous algorithm-based insulin dose calculation and titration recommendation system is recommended to improve control of diabetes.

Description of Procedure (0741T)

Provide the autonomous algorithm-based insulin dose calculation and titration recommendation system software, data collection, transmission, and storage for 30 days.

+● **0742T** Absolute quantitation of myocardial blood flow (AQMBF), single-photon emission computed tomography (SPECT), with exercise or pharmacologic stress, and at rest, when performed (List separately in addition to code for primary procedure)

▶(Use 0742T in conjunction with 78451, 78452)◀

▶(For absolute quantification of myocardial blood flow [AQMBF] with positron emission tomography [PET], use 78434)◀

Rationale

Category III add-on code 0742T has been established to report absolute quantitation of myocardial blood flow (AQMBF) single-photon emission computed tomography (SPECT). In 2020, code 78434 was established to report AQMBF positron emission tomography (PET). The procedure described by code 0742T uses SPECT rather than PET. AQMBF SPECT is performed with stress and, sometimes, at rest. Code 0742T is an add-on code reported in conjunction with SPECT codes 78451 and 78452. Accordingly, an inclusionary parenthetical note has been added following code 0742T. A cross-reference parenthetical note has been added directing users to code 78434 for AQMBF PET.

Clinical Example (0742T)

A 67-year-old female, who is without known coronary artery disease, has symptoms of chest pain is being evaluated for regional relative perfusion defects suggestive of myocardial ischemia, during a stress/rest single-photon emission computed tomography (SPECT) myocardial perfusion imaging study. An absolute quantitation of myocardial blood flow is also requested because more specific physiological assessment of absolute myocardial blood flow and coronary flow reserve is desired. [**Note:** This is an add-on code. Only consider the additional work related to the absolute quantitation myocardial blood flow.]

Description of Procedure (0742T)

During a SPECT myocardial perfusion imaging study, a nuclear medicine/nuclear cardiology technologist acquires images in a manner that will allow for quantitation of absolute quantitation myocardial blood flow (AQMBF). The data are then separately organized to allow AQMBF and the dataset is reviewed in a dedicated computer/software program for AQMBF. In addition to the usual myocardial perfusion imaging processing, the technologist then processes the separately organized data for AQMBF using a separate software program. The technologist imports the data into a computerized control software program for analysis of data quality. The processed dataset and quality control information are transferred to the interpreting physician. The physician then reviews the quality control information for AQMBF (for example, the bolus duration, peak, and plateau waveforms) and, if quality is acceptable, reviews the numeric output of AQMBF in mL/g/min for stress or stress and rest, studies, and the

indexed/reserve flow for each coronary bed and for the entire left ventricle. The physician also reviews the interactive polar map display. The AQMBF data are then integrated with the static perfusion image data, attenuation maps, and clinical data, and an overall report is generated.

● **0743T**   Bone strength and fracture risk using finite element analysis of functional data and bone mineral density (BMD), with concurrent vertebral fracture assessment, utilizing data from a computed tomography scan, retrieval and transmission of the scan data, measurement of bone strength and BMD and classification of any vertebral fractures, with overall fracture-risk assessment, interpretation and report

▶(Do not report 0743T in conjunction with 0554T, 0555T, 0556T, 0557T, 0691T)◀

Rationale

Category III code 0743T has been established to report bone strength and fracture-risk assessment using finite element analysis of functional data and bone mineral density (BMD) with concurrent vertebral fracture assessment. The service uses data from a CT scan. Retrieval and transmission of the CT scan data and measurement of bone strength and BMD are performed. Any vertebral fractures that are present are classified and overall fracture risk is assessed. Code 0743T includes interpretation and report. An exclusionary parenthetical note has been added following code 0743T restricting its use with codes 0554T-0557T and 0691T.

Clinical Example (0743T)

A 68-year-old female has not had a bone mass measurement in the previous 5 years. Her primary care physician notes she had a recent CT scan for gastrointestinal distress and orders a test for biomechanical CT analysis (BCT) with vertebral fracture assessment (VFA).

Description of Procedure (0743T)

The technical staff at the appropriate radiology facility identify and retrieve the patient's CT scan and transmit it to the centralized laboratory for analysis. The technical staff at the laboratory then performs the BCT analysis and VFA procedure, using specialized analysis software and advanced engineering computation. All results from the BCT and VFA procedure, including any relevant images, are included in a results report. The results report is then sent to a QHP for review and interpretation. The QHP considers all data in the results report and dictates a medical report.

Category III 0042T-0713T

#● **0749T**   Bone strength and fracture-risk assessment using digital X-ray radiogrammetry-bone mineral density (DXR-BMD) analysis of bone mineral density (BMD) utilizing data from a digital X ray, retrieval and transmission of digital X-ray data, assessment of bone strength and fracture risk and BMD, interpretation and report;

▶(When the data from a concurrently performed wrist or hand X ray obtained for another purpose is used for the DXR-BMD analysis, use the appropriate X-ray code in conjunction with 0749T. If a single-view digital X ray of the hand is used as a data source, use 0750T)◀

#● **0750T**   with single-view digital X-ray examination of the hand taken for the purpose of DXR-BMD

Rationale

Category III codes 0749T and 0750T have been established to report bone strength and fracture-risk assessment using digital X-ray radiogrammetry-BMD (DXR-BMD) analysis.

Code 0749T describes DXR-BMD analysis of an available appropriate digital X ray (eg, hand/wrist) to assess bone strength, fracture risk, and BMD. If the X ray is taken concurrently (eg, for other purposes such as a fracture), then the X-ray code may be separately reported in addition to 0749T.

Code 0750T is reported if an appropriate digital X ray is not available and a single digital X-ray view of the hand is taken specifically to be used for DXR-BMD analysis. In this instance, because there are no current CPT codes for a single view of the hand, the work related to obtaining the X ray is included in code 0750T.

An instructional parenthetical note has been added following code 0749T to further specify to users when to report a separate X-ray code as noted in code 0749T and when to report a single code in code 0750T.

Clinical Example (0749T)

A 72-year-old female, who is suspected of having osteopenia, has a recently performed digital wrist/hand X ray analyzed using digital X-ray radiogrammetry-bone mineral density (DXR-BMD).

Description of Procedure (0749T)

The interpreting physician or other QHP at the request of the patient's treating physician selects a recent digital X ray for evaluation. Transmit the digital image to a server where the automated DXR-BMD analytic services are performed. Analyze the bone strength, bone mineral density (BMD), and fracture risk. Return the data generated, including graphic representation of BMD and listing of the patient's T-score and Z-score, to the interpreting physician or other QHP for interpretation and report.

Clinical Example (0750T)

A 67-year-old female has a digital, single-view X ray of her hand obtained solely for the purpose of BMD evaluation, which is analyzed using DXR-BMD.

Description of Procedure (0750T)

Obtain a single-view digital X ray of the hand for the purpose of DXR-BMD. Transmit this image to a server where the automated DXR-BMD analytic services are performed. Analyze the bone strength, BMD, and fracture risk. Return the data generated, including graphic representation of BMD and listing of the patient's T-score and Z-score, to the interpreting physician or other QHP for interpretation and report.

● **0744T**   Insertion of bioprosthetic valve, open, femoral vein, including duplex ultrasound imaging guidance, when performed, including autogenous or nonautogenous patch graft (eg, polyester, ePTFE, bovine pericardium), when performed

▶(Do not report 0744T in conjunction with 34501, 34510, 76998, 93971)◀

Rationale

Category III code 0744T has been established to report insertion of a bioprosthetic valve in the femoral vein via an open approach. Bioprosthetic valves in the femoral vein are used to treat conditions such as chronic deep vein insufficiency, reflux in the deep venous system, or leg ulcers. Code 0744T includes imaging guidance using duplex ultrasound, when performed, and placement of an autogenous or nonautogenous patch graft, when performed. An exclusionary parenthetical note has been added following code 0744T restricting its use with codes 34501, 34510, 76998, and 93971.

Clinical Example (0744T)

A 68-year-old female has chronic lower leg ulcers, pain, and uncontrolled leg swelling. She is diagnosed with lower limb C6 chronic deep vein insufficiency due to reflux in the deep venous system.

Description of Procedure (0744T)

Following general or regional anesthesia, make an incision in the mid to upper thigh. Once the femoral vein is exposed, use vessel loops to mobilize the vein and control blood flow. Following intravenous heparin anticoagulation, use atraumatic vascular clamps to stop blood flow through the exposed area of the femoral vein. Make a longitudinal venotomy in the vein between the clamps. Temporarily open the inflow clamp to allow the

★ = Telemedicine   ◀ = Add-on code   ✚ = Add-on code   ✗ = FDA approval pending   # = Resequenced code   ⊘ = Modifier 51 exempt

insertion of a 9-mm Bakes dilator to size the vein. Place the appropriately sized device in sterile saline where it should remain until implanted. Remove the tag with the serial number attached to the inflow stabilization ring of the device. Insert the bioprosthetic valve into the vein through the venotomy with the base or apex of the "V" of the bioprosthetic valve frame pointing towards the patient's foot (the direction of inflow). Tack the inflow stabilization ring of the bioprosthetic valve frame to the native vein. Close the venotomy with running 6.0 or 5.0 polypropylene suture. A bovine patch can be used to assist in closing the venotomy. Remove the clamps to restore blood flow. Then compress the calf muscle to ensure that the closed venotomy does not leak under pressure and that blood flows through the bioprosthetic valve. Then apply pressure to the groin area to ensure that the bioprosthetic valve leaflet deploys and reduces the backwards flow of blood. Duplex ultrasound may be used to evaluate valve function. Once proper functioning of the bioprosthetic valve is confirmed, close the wound.

● **0745T**   Cardiac focal ablation utilizing radiation therapy for arrhythmia; noninvasive arrhythmia localization and mapping of arrhythmia site (nidus), derived from anatomical image data (eg, CT, MRI, or myocardial perfusion scan) and electrical data (eg, 12-lead ECG data), and identification of areas of avoidance

▶(For catheter-based electrophysiologic evaluation, see 93609, 93619, 93620, 93621, 93622)◀

● **0746T**   conversion of arrhythmia localization and mapping of arrhythmia site (nidus) into a multidimensional radiation treatment plan

● **0747T**   delivery of radiation therapy, arrhythmia

Rationale

Category III codes 0745T, 0746T, and 0747T have been established to report cardiac focal ablation utilizing radiation therapy for arrhythmia. Cardiac focal ablation is a noninvasive procedure used to treat arrhythmias such as ventricular tachycardia (VT). The procedures involved in this treatment are described by the three separate Category III codes. First, data about the arrhythmia are obtained. This work is reported with code 0745T, which describes noninvasive arrhythmia localization and mapping of the arrhythmia site derived from anatomical image data and electrical data and identification of areas of avoidance. Next, the obtained data are converted into a treatment plan. This is reported with code 0746T, which describes conversion of the arrhythmia localization and mapping of the arrhythmia site into a multidimensional radiation treatment plan. Finally, the radiation treatment is delivered and reported with code 0747T, which

describes delivery of radiation therapy to treat an arrhythmia. A cross-reference parenthetical note has been added following code 0745T directing users to codes 93609 and 93619-93622 for catheter-based electrophysiologic evaluation.

Clinical Example (0745T)

A 62-year-old female presents with recurrent episodes of sustained monomorphic VT despite two prior catheter ablations for VT and taking the maximum dose of amiodarone daily.

Description of Procedure (0745T)

The electrophysiologist reviews the relevant cardiac imaging for noninvasive arrhythmia localization, including scar imaging (eg, CT, MRI, myocardial perfusion, ultrasound, catheter maps) and electrical imaging (eg, 12-lead electrocardiography [ECG], catheter maps, noninvasive mapping). For scar imaging, the electrophysiologist may determine the precise location of the myocardial scarring in the heart (eg, regions or segments affected), the depth of the scar process (eg, endocardial, midmyocardial, epicardial), locations within the scar more likely to harbor VT circuits (eg, myocardial channels through scar), and the likely cause of the pattern of scar (eg, ischemic cardiomyopathy, cardiac sarcoidosis, valvular cardiomyopathy). For electrical data, the electrophysiologist will interpret images (eg, 12-lead ECG of VT, catheter maps, noninvasive mapping) to determine the most likely region or segment of the heart that corresponds to the initiation of the VT beat (exit site), the diastolic corridor/isthmus of the VT circuit, or prior catheter ablation locations. Using targeting software as an aid to decision making, the electrophysiologist combines information from all selected studies to determine which location in the heart (eg, segments) to include as the ablation target. The electrophysiologist identifies adjacent cardiac and noncardiac structures for specific consideration by the radiation oncologist in developing the radiation therapy treatment plan to reduce potential injury to these structures.

Clinical Example (0746T)

A 62-year-old female presents with recurrent episodes of sustained monomorphic VT despite two prior catheter ablations for VT and taking the maximum dose of amiodarone daily.

Description of Procedure (0746T)

The radiation oncologist identifies the arrhythmia localization and mapping of arrhythmia site data for treatment planning and delineates the left and right ventricles and other structures of interest (eg, aorta, stomach, liver, lungs, etc). The radiation oncologist reviews the delineated structures and exports the resulting dataset, along with the patient's identifier and demographic information, to the targeting software. Using the treatment planning system, the radiation oncologist retrieves targeting information from the targeting software tool, assesses target motion, and finalizes the respiratory/cardiac motion management strategy (eg, motion management technique and image guidance). The radiation oncologist also defines internal target volume (ITV) and planning target volume (PTV) margins. The radiation oncologist creates a treatment plan that is highly customized and with a high degree of accuracy. The radiation oncologist reviews the adjacent cardiac and noncardiac structures identified by the electrophysiologist for specific consideration in developing the radiation therapy treatment plan to reduce potential injury to these structures. Particular attention is paid to plan optimization that can be particularly challenging due to motion and the proximity of organs at risk (OAR), such as the spinal cord, esophagus, stomach, liver, and lungs. The radiation oncologist performs a final review of the treatment plan that includes a review of the planned dose distribution to ensure that target volume and OAR dose goals have been met.

Clinical Example (0747T)

A 62-year-old female presents with recurrent episodes of sustained monomorphic VT despite two prior catheter ablations for VT and taking the maximum dose of amiodarone daily.

Description of Procedure (0747T)

Bring the patient to the linear accelerator and set up according to radiation treatment and motion management plan. Perform imaging to ensure current position of patient; heart and nidus are exactly targeted as in the treatment plan. Once exact location is verified, deliver the prescribed dose according to the final radiation treatment plan with the radiation oncologist present.

● **0748T**   Injections of stem cell product into perianal perifistular soft tissue, including fistula preparation (eg, removal of setons, fistula curettage, closure of internal openings)

▶(Report 0748T once per session)◀

▶(Report stem cell product separately)◀

▶(Do not report 0748T in conjunction with 46030, 46940, 46942)◀

Rationale

Category III code 0748T has been established to report perianal tissue injection. New parenthetical notes have been added to provide instructions on the appropriate reporting of code 0748T.

Code 0748T describes the work involved for the perianal intra-tissue drug administration procedure. This fistula treatment procedure involves injecting stem cell product into the patient's perianal perifistular soft tissue. Work related to fistula preparation is included and may not be separately reported.

Clinical Example (0748T)

A 40-year-old female with Crohn's disease presents with perianal pain, swelling, and discharge. After physician clinical examination, the patient is diagnosed with a perianal fistula. Once the Crohn's disease is controlled, the patient is recommended for fistula treatment with a stem cell product.

Description of Procedure (0748T)

Bring the patient into the operating room and place under general anesthesia. The physician prepares the fistula for injection (eg, removing setons performing fistula curettage and closing internal openings) (do not report separately). The physician inserts a needle through the patient's anus to administer stem cell product into the perianal perifistular soft tissues around each internal fistula opening, making several small blebs. Half of the dose of stem cell product should be divided equally for injection into the tissues surrounding each internal opening(s). Administer the remaining half of stem cell product dose into the soft tissue along the length of the fistula tract(s) divided equally among the external opening(s). Once full dose of stem cell product has been injected, the physician then softly massages the area around the external opening(s) for 20 to 30 seconds and covers the external opening(s) with a sterile bandage to complete the procedure.

0749T   Code is out of numerical sequence. See 0742T-0745T

0750T   Code is out of numerical sequence. See 0742T-0745T

▶Digital Pathology Digitization Procedures◀

▶Digital pathology is a dynamic, image-based environment that enables the acquisition, management, and interpretation of pathology information generated from digitized glass microscope slides.

Glass microscope slides are scanned by clinical staff, and captured images (either in real-time or stored in a computer server or cloud-based digital image archival and communication system) are used for digital examination for pathologic diagnosis distinct from direct visualization through a microscope.

Digitization of glass microscope slides enables remote examination by the pathologist and/or in conjunction with the use of artificial intelligence (AI) algorithms. Category III add-on codes 0751T-0763T may be reported in addition to the appropriate Category I service code when the digitization procedure of glass microscope slides is performed and reported in conjunction with the Category I code for the primary service.

Do not report the Category III codes in this subsection solely for archival purposes (eg, after the Category I service has already been performed and reported), solely for educational purposes (eg, when services are not used for individual patient reporting), solely for developing a database for training or validation of AI algorithms, or solely for clinical conference presentations (eg, tumor board interdisciplinary conferences).◀

+● **0751T**　Digitization of glass microscope slides for level II, surgical pathology, gross and microscopic examination (List separately in addition to code for primary procedure)

　　　▶(Use 0751T in conjunction with 88302)◀

+● **0752T**　Digitization of glass microscope slides for level III, surgical pathology, gross and microscopic examination (List separately in addition to code for primary procedure)

　　　▶(Use 0752T in conjunction with 88304)◀

+● **0753T**　Digitization of glass microscope slides for level IV, surgical pathology, gross and microscopic examination (List separately in addition to code for primary procedure)

　　　▶(Use 0753T in conjunction with 88305)◀

+● **0754T**　Digitization of glass microscope slides for level V, surgical pathology, gross and microscopic examination (List separately in addition to code for primary procedure)

　　　▶(Use 0754T in conjunction with 88307)◀

+● **0755T**　Digitization of glass microscope slides for level VI, surgical pathology, gross and microscopic examination (List separately in addition to code for primary procedure)

　　　▶(Use 0755T in conjunction with 88309)◀

+● **0756T**　Digitization of glass microscope slides for special stain, including interpretation and report, group I, for microorganisms (eg, acid fast, methenamine silver) (List separately in addition to code for primary procedure)

　　　▶(Use 0756T in conjunction with 88312)◀

+● **0757T**　Digitization of glass microscope slides for special stain, including interpretation and report, group II, all other (eg, iron, trichrome), except stain for microorganisms, stains for enzyme constituents, or immunocytochemistry and immunohistochemistry (List separately in addition to code for primary procedure)

　　　▶(Use 0757T in conjunction with 88313)◀

+● **0758T**　Digitization of glass microscope slides for special stain, including interpretation and report, histochemical stain on frozen tissue block (List separately in addition to code for primary procedure)

　　　▶(Use 0758T in conjunction with 88314)◀

+● **0759T**　Digitization of glass microscope slides for special stain, including interpretation and report, group III, for enzyme constituents (List separately in addition to code for primary procedure)

　　　▶(Use 0759T in conjunction with 88319)◀

+● **0760T**　Digitization of glass microscope slides for immunohistochemistry or immunocytochemistry, per specimen, initial single antibody stain procedure (List separately in addition to code for primary procedure)

　　　▶(Use 0760T in conjunction with 88342)◀

+● **0761T**　Digitization of glass microscope slides for immunohistochemistry or immunocytochemistry, per specimen, each additional single antibody stain procedure (List separately in addition to code for primary procedure)

　　　▶(Use 0761T in conjunction with 88341)◀

+● **0762T**　Digitization of glass microscope slides for immunohistochemistry or immunocytochemistry, per specimen, each multiplex antibody stain procedure (List separately in addition to code for primary procedure)

　　　▶(Use 0762T in conjunction with 88344)◀

+● **0763T**　Digitization of glass microscope slides for morphometric analysis, tumor immunohistochemistry (eg, Her-2/neu, estrogen receptor/progesterone receptor), quantitative or semiquantitative, per specimen, each single antibody stain procedure, manual (List separately in addition to code for primary procedure)

　　　▶(Use 0763T in conjunction with 88360)◀

Category III 0042T–0713T

Rationale

Thirteen Category III add-on codes (0751T-0763T) have been established to report additional clinical staff work and service requirements associated with digitizing glass microscope slides for primary diagnosis. A new heading "Digital Pathology Digitization Procedures" and its associated guidelines have also been established to define digital pathology and to outline the appropriate reporting of these codes.

Digital pathology refers to systems in which slides are scanned into a computer so that slides can be examined digitally, rather than directly visualized through a microscope. Digitization of glass microscope slides facilitates/enables remote examination by the pathologist. Add-on codes (0751T-0763T) may be reported in addition to the appropriate Category I service when the digitization of glass microscope slides is performed.

Codes 0751T-0763T capture additional service requirements associated with digitizing glass microscope slides for primary diagnosis (surgical pathology microscopic examination services [88302, 88304, 88305, 88307, 88309] and digitizing glass microscope slides for ancillary services described as special stain services [88312-88314, 88319], immunohistochemistry and immunocytochemistry services [88341, 88342, 88344], and morphometric analysis, tumor immunohistochemistry services [88360]).

Category I surgical pathology services codes 88302, 88304, 88305, 88307, and 88309 include accession, gross and microscopic examination, and reporting. Specific Category III add-on codes (0751T-0755T) have been established to report in addition to the appropriate Category I service when the digitization of glass microscope slides is performed. Instructional parenthetical notes following each Category I code have been added to direct users to the specific Category III code to report.

Category I pathology services codes 88312-88314 and 88319 include the special stain, interpretation, and reporting. Specific Category III add-on codes (0756T-0759T) have been established to report in addition to the appropriate Category I service when the digitization of glass microscope slides is performed. Instructional parenthetical notes following each Category I code have been added to direct users to the specific Category III code to report.

Category I pathology services codes 88341, 88342, and 88344 include the immunohistochemistry or immunocytochemistry antibody stain procedure, interpretation, and reporting. Specific Category III add-on codes (0760T-0762T) have been established to report in addition to the appropriate Category I service when the digitization of glass

microscope slides is performed. Instructional parenthetical notes following each Category I code have been added to direct users to the specific Category III code to report.

Category I pathology service code 88360 includes morphometric analysis, tumor immunohistochemistry quantitative or semiquantitative, antibody stain procedure, interpretation, and reporting. A specific Category III add-on code (0763T) has been established to report in addition to the appropriate Category I service when the digitization of glass microscope slides is performed. Instructional parenthetical notes following each Category I code have been added to direct users to the specific Category III code to report.

Clinical Example (0751T)

A 48-year-old female's ventral hernia specimen is examined. Glass microscope slide digitization is performed. [**Note:** This is an add-on code. Only consider the additional work related to 0751T glass microscope slide digitization.]

Description of Procedure (0751T)

Scan glass microscope slides using a digital slide imaging system and store the images.

Clinical Example (0752T)

A 50-year-old male's 5-cm subcutaneous lipoma thigh excision specimen is examined. Glass microscope slide digitization is performed. [**Note:** This is an add-on code. Only consider the additional work related to 0752T glass microscope slide digitization.]

Description of Procedure (0752T)

Scan glass microscope slides using a digital slide imaging system and store the images.

Clinical Example (0753T)

A 35-year-old female's 1-cm pigmented skin lesion with irregular borders excision specimen is examined. Glass microscope slide digitization is performed. [**Note:** This is an add-on code. Only consider the additional work related to 0753T glass microscope slide digitization.]

Description of Procedure (0753T)

Scan glass microscope slides using a digital slide imaging system and store the images.

Clinical Example (0754T)

A 55-year-old female's 5-cm breast lumpectomy specimen following needle localization of microcalcifications requiring assessment of margins is examined. Glass microscope slide digitization is performed. [**Note:** This is an add-on code. Only consider the additional work related to 0754T glass microscope slide digitization.]

Description of Procedure (0754T)

Scan glass microscope slides using a digital slide imaging system and store the images.

Clinical Example (0755T)

A 67-year-old male presents with rectal bleeding. He undergoes low anterior resection of an adenocarcinoma of the rectum. Glass microscope slide digitization is performed. [**Note:** This is an add-on code. Only consider the additional work related to 0755T glass microscope slide digitization.]

Description of Procedure (0755T)

Scan glass microscope slides using a digital slide imaging system and store the images.

Clinical Example (0756T)

A 70-year-old male with gastritis undergoes stomach biopsy. A Warthin-Starry (WS) stain performed on stomach biopsy specimen is examined. Glass microscope slide digitization is performed. [**Note:** This is an add-on code. Only consider the additional work related to 0756T glass microscope slide digitization.]

Description of Procedure (0756T)

Scan glass microscope slides using a digital slide imaging system and store the images.

Clinical Example (0757T)

A 75-year-old male with monoclonal gammopathy undergoes bone marrow biopsy. A Congo red stain performed on a bone marrow biopsy specimen is examined. Glass microscope slide digitization is performed. [**Note:** This is an add-on code. Only consider the additional work related to 0757T glass microscope slide digitization.]

Description of Procedure (0757T)

Scan glass microscope slides using a digital slide imaging system and store the images.

Clinical Example (0758T)

A 30-year-old male with muscular dystrophy undergoes skeletal muscle biopsy. An oil red O (ORO) stain performed on a frozen skeletal muscle biopsy specimen is examined. Glass microscope slide digitization is performed. [**Note:** This is an add-on code. Only

consider the additional work related to 0758T glass microscope slide digitization.]

Description of Procedure (0758T)

Scan glass microscope slides using a digital slide imaging system and store the images.

Clinical Example (0759T)

A 30-year-old male with muscular dystrophy undergoes skeletal muscle biopsy. A nicotinamide adenosine dinucleotide-tetrazolium reductase (NADH-TR) stained slide performed on a skeletal muscle biopsy specimen is examined. Glass microscope slide digitization is performed. [**Note:** This is an add-on code. Only consider the additional work related to 0759T glass microscope slide digitization.]

Description of Procedure (0759T)

Scan glass microscope slides using a digital slide imaging system and store the images.

Clinical Example (0760T)

A 25-year-old male presents with suspected Hodgkin lymphoma. A CD15 immunohistochemical antibody stain performed on a lymph node specimen is examined. Glass microscope slide digitization is performed. [**Note:** This is an add-on code. Only consider the additional work related to 0760T glass microscope slide digitization.]

Description of Procedure (0760T)

Scan glass microscope slides using a digital slide imaging system and store the images.

Clinical Example (0761T)

A 25-year-old male presents with suspected Hodgkin lymphoma. After the CD15 immunohistochemical stain performed on a lymph node specimen is examined, a CD45 immunohistochemical antibody stain performed on a lymph node specimen is examined. Glass microscope slide digitization is performed. [**Note:** This is an add-on code. Only consider the additional work related to 0761T glass microscope slide digitization.]

Description of Procedure (0761T)

Scan glass microscope slides using a digital slide imaging system and store the images.

Clinical Example (0762T)

A 66-year-old male presents with elevated prostate-specific antigen (PSA) levels. An immunohistochemical cocktail of P504S and HMWK (34ßE12) performed on a prostate needle core biopsy specimen is examined. Glass microscope slide digitization is performed. [**Note:** This is an add-on code. Only consider the additional work related to 0762T glass microscope slide digitization.]

Description of Procedure (0762T)

Scan glass microscope slides using a digital slide imaging system and store the images.

Clinical Example (0763T)

A 54-year-old female has invasive ductal carcinoma of the breast diagnosed on needle biopsy. Estrogen receptor-stained slides from the patient's specimen and reference positive and negative samples are examined to determine if the staining process is interpretable. The estrogen receptor stain is positive, and a semiquantitative or quantitative interpretation is manually performed. Glass microscope slide digitization is performed. [**Note:** This is an add-on code. Only consider the additional work related to 0763T glass microscope slide digitization.]

Description of Procedure (0763T)

Scan glass microscope slides using a digital slide imaging system and store the images.

+● **0764T**   Assistive algorithmic electrocardiogram risk-based assessment for cardiac dysfunction (eg, low-ejection fraction, pulmonary hypertension, hypertrophic cardiomyopathy); related to concurrently performed electrocardiogram (List separately in addition to code for primary procedure)

▶(Use 0764T in conjunction with 93000, 93010)◀

▶(Use 0764T only once for each unique, concurrently performed electrocardiogram tracing)◀

● **0765T**   related to previously performed electrocardiogram

▶(Use 0765T only once for each unique, previously performed electrocardiogram tracing)◀

Rationale

Two new Category III codes (0764T, 0765T) have been established to report assistive algorithmic electrocardiogram risk assessment for cardiac dysfunction. These codes capture the application of assistive algorithms to ECG data for possible detection and autonomous generation of clinical conclusions and aid in diagnosis, which requires no physician or other QHP review and interpretation.

Codes 0764T and 0765T are designed to capture different clinical situations in which the AI may be ran (archived or new 12-lead ECG data) and to allow ECG data to be sent to another location for the AI analysis. Current CPT codes for ECG (93000, 93010) do not include autonomous AI analysis.

Code 0764T is an add-on code that is intended to be reported for assistive algorithmic ECG risk-based assessment for cardiac dysfunction. This code may be reported in conjunction with electrocardiogram codes (93000, 93010), as stated in the instructional parenthetical note. However, code 0764T should only be reported once for each unique, concurrently performed ECG tracing.

Code 0765T is a child code to 0764T and may be reported for assistive algorithmic ECG risk-based assessment for cardiac dysfunction that is related to previously performed ECG. Code 0765T should only be reported once for each unique, previously performed ECG tracing.

Clinical Example (0764T)

A 64-year-old female hypertensive patient with a previous history of dyspnea and palpitations and medications to control the heart rate returns to her cardiologist with new cardiac symptoms. A 12-lead electrocardiogram (ECG) is obtained. [**Note:** This is an add-on code. Only consider the additional work related to 93000, 93010.]

Description of Procedure (0764T)

Perform a 12-lead ECG (reported separately). Concurrently, analyze the waveform via artificial intelligence (AI) software. A report is automatically generated and returned to the physician for review.

Clinical Example (0765T)

A 58-year-old male presents to his primary care physician's office with a complaint of intermittent palpitations. Assistive algorithmic electrocardiogram risk-based assessment for cardiac dysfunction is performed on 12-lead ECG that had been performed at a previous visit.

Description of Procedure (0765T)

Upload the digital ECG waveform from a previously performed 12-lead ECG to the cloud via an application programming interface. Analyze the waveform via AI software. A result is automatically generated and returned to the physician for review.

►Codes 0766T, 0767T, 0768T, 0769T describe transcutaneous magnetic stimulation that is performed to treat chronic nerve pain and provided by a physician or other qualified health care professional. The injured nerve is localized using magnetic stimulation at the time of the initial treatment, the skin is marked (with photographic record) to facilitate rapid localization of the correct site for subsequent treatments, and the appropriate amplitude of magnetic stimulation is defined. Noninvasive electroneurography (nerve conduction) may be used as guidance to confirm the precise localization of the injured nerve and, when performed, should not be separately reported as a diagnostic study. A separate diagnostic nerve conduction study performed prior to the decision to treat with transcutaneous magnetic stimulation may be separately reported.◄

● **0766T** Transcutaneous magnetic stimulation by focused low-frequency electromagnetic pulse, peripheral nerve, initial treatment, with identification and marking of the treatment location, including noninvasive electroneurographic localization (nerve conduction localization), when performed; first nerve

+● **0767T** each additional nerve (List separately in addition to code for primary procedure)

► (Use 0767T in conjunction with 0766T)◄

► (Do not report 0766T, 0767T in conjunction with 95885, 95886, 95887, 95905, 95907, 95908, 95909, 95910, 95911, 95912, 95913, for nerve conduction used as guidance for transcutaneous magnetic stimulation therapy)◄

► (Do not report 0766T, 0767T in conjunction with 64566, 90867, 90868, 90869, 97014, 97032, 0278T, for the same nerve)◄

● **0768T** Transcutaneous magnetic stimulation by focused low-frequency electromagnetic pulse, peripheral nerve, subsequent treatment, including noninvasive electroneurographic localization (nerve conduction localization), when performed; first nerve

+● **0769T** each additional nerve (List separately in addition to code for primary procedure)

► (Use 0769T in conjunction with 0768T)◄

► (Do not report 0768T, 0769T in conjunction with 95885, 95886, 95887, 95905, 95907, 95908, 95909, 95910, 95911, 95912, 95913, for nerve conduction used as guidance for transcutaneous magnetic stimulation therapy)◄

► (Do not report 0768T, 0769T in conjunction with 64566, 90867, 90868, 90869, 97014, 97032, 0278T, for the same nerve)◄

► (For posterior tibial neurostimulation, percutaneous needle electrode, use 64566)◄

► (For therapeutic repetitive transcranial magnetic stimulation [TMS] treatment, see 90867, 90868, 90869)◄

► (For application of a modality to one or more areas, electrical stimulation [unattended], use 97014)◄

► (For application of a modality to one or more areas, electrical stimulation [manual], each 15 minutes, use 97032)◄

► (For transcutaneous electrical modulation pain reprocessing [eg, scrambler therapy], each treatment session [includes placement of electrodes], use 0278T)◄

Rationale

Category III codes 0766T-0769T are used to report transcutaneous magnetic stimulation of a peripheral nerve by focused, low-frequency electromagnetic pulse with noninvasive electroneurographic localization, when performed. Guidelines and parenthetical notes have been added to provide guidance on the appropriate use of these codes.

This new technology is used in the management of chronic pain following a traumatic injury. The treatment is repeated over a period of months. Codes 0766T and 0767T describe the initial treatment and include identification and marking of the treatment location. Codes 0768T and 0769T are reported for subsequent treatments. The codes are reported per peripheral nerve treated. Codes 0766T and 0768T are reported for the first nerve treated and add-on codes 0767T and 0769T are reported for each additional nerve treated.

Codes 0766T-0769T should not be reported with code 64566, 90867-90869, 97014, 97032, or 0278T for the same nerve. Codes 0766T-0769T should not be reported with code 95885-95887, 95905, or 95907-95913 for nerve conduction used as guidance for transcutaneous magnetic stimulation therapy.

Clinical Example (0766T)

A 62-year-old male, who is 5 years post-inguinal hernia repair surgery, presents with left groin pain (continuous, throbbing, worse with activity, and 7 out of 10 on a 0-to-10 pain scale). The patient is diagnosed with left groin neuroma based on a palpable neuroma (1.5 x 1 cm) and paresthesia in the distribution of the genital branch of the left genitofemoral nerve. A CT scan showed no hernia recurrence. Previous pain management therapies have failed.

Description of Procedure (0766T)

The physician or other QHP identifies the exact point of nerve pain proximal to the neuroma or nerve trauma and further localized by applying low-amplitude electromagnetic impulses to the focus of pain, sequentially moving the coil head over the area, applying impulse until the patient identifies that the exact spot is being stimulated. Noninvasive electroneurography (nerve conduction) may be used for guidance to identify the exact target spot for treatment. Identify the treatment amplitude for the specific site by gradually increasing the amplitude of stimulation to the nerve until sensory threshold is reached and the patient acknowledges a very strong sensation of relief per pulse. Mark the position of the coil head with permanent ink on the patient's skin to ensure accurate positioning for future treatments, and take and save a photograph of the site with the coil head in position for reference for subsequent treatments. Then treat the nerve by application of magnetic stimulation by focused, low-frequency electromagnetic pulse for approximately 15 minutes.

Clinical Example (0767T)

A 51-year-old female with history of Crohn's disease and multiple abdominal surgeries presents with right lower quadrant pain along a surgical incision site that is rated as 5 out of 10 on a 0-to-10 pain scale. Two neuromas (1.5 x 1.25 cm and 1.5 x 1.0 cm) are palpable. Tactile allodynia to light stroking is present. [**Note:** This is an add-on code. Only consider the additional service specific to localizing, defining the treatment parameters and treatment of the second neuroma.]

Description of Procedure (0767T)

A separate nerve is targeted for therapy after the initial nerve is identified and treated (separately reported). The physician or other QHP identifies the exact point of nerve pain proximal to the neuroma or nerve trauma and further localized by applying low-amplitude electromagnetic impulses to the focus of pain, sequentially moving the coil head over the area, applying impulses until the patient identifies that the exact spot is being stimulated. Noninvasive electroneurography (nerve conduction) may be used for guidance to identify the exact target spot for treatment. Identify the treatment amplitude for the specific site by gradually increasing the amplitude of stimulation to the nerve until sensory threshold is reached and the patient acknowledges a very strong sensation of relief per pulse. Mark the position of the coil head with permanent ink on the patient's skin to ensure accurate positioning for future treatments, and take and save a photograph of the site with the coil head in position for reference for subsequent treatments. Then treat the nerve by application of magnetic stimulation by focused, low-frequency electromagnetic pulse for approximately 15 minutes.

Clinical Example (0768T)

A 62-year-old male, who is 5 years post-inguinal hernia repair surgery, presents with left groin pain (continuous, throbbing, worse with activity, and 7 out of 10 on a 0-to-10 pain scale). The patient is diagnosed with left groin neuroma based on palpable neuroma (1.5 x 1 cm) and paresthesia in the distribution of the genital branch of the left genitofemoral nerve. A CT scan showed no hernia recurrence. Previous pain management therapies have failed.

Description of Procedure (0768T)

Identify characteristics on the patient's skin from notes and photos of earlier treatment. Electroneurography (nerve conduction) may be used to help accurately identify the exact site of treatment. Position the coil head over the point of the injured nerve. Confirm the correct positioning of the coil head by application of stimulus, moving the head as needed and gradually increasing the amplitude until the desired patient reaction is achieved. Then treat the nerve by transcutaneous magnetic stimulation by focused, low-frequency electromagnetic pulse for approximately 15 minutes.

Clinical Example (0769T)

A 51-year-old female with a history of Crohn's disease and multiple abdominal surgeries presents with right lower quadrant pain along a surgical incision site that is rated as 5 out of 10 on a 0-to-10 pain scale. Two neuromas (1.5 x 1.25 cm and 1.5 x 1.0 cm) are palpable. Tactile allodynia to light stroking was present prior to the intervention. [**Note:** This is an add-on code. Only consider the additional work of treating the second neuroma.]

Description of Procedure (0769T)

A separate nerve is targeted for subsequent therapy after the initial nerve is identified and treated (separately reported). Identify the characteristics for the additional nerve treatment site on the patient's skin from notes and photos of earlier treatment. Position the coil head over the point of the injured nerve. Confirm the correct positioning of the coil head by application of stimulus, moving the head as needed and gradually increasing the amplitude until the desired patient reaction is achieved. Noninvasive electroneurography (nerve conduction) may also be used to accurately identify the target treatment point. Then treat the nerve by transcutaneous magnetic stimulation by focused, low-frequency electromagnetic pulse for approximately 15 minutes.

★ = Telemedicine   ◀ = Add-on code   ✚ = Add-on code   ✒ = FDA approval pending   # = Resequenced code   ⊘ = Modifier 51 exempt

Category III 0042T-0713T

▶Virtual reality (VR) technology may be integrated into multiple types of patient therapy as an adjunct to the base therapy. Code 0770T is an add-on code that represents the practice expense for the software used for the VR technology and may be reported for each session for which the VR technology is used. VR technology is incorporated into the base therapy session and is used to enhance the training or teaching of a skill upon which the therapy is focused. Code 0770T does not incur any additional reported therapist time beyond that already reported with the base therapy code.◀

+● 0770T   Virtual reality technology to assist therapy (List separately in addition to code for primary procedure)

> ▶(Use 0770T only in conjunction with 90832, 90833, 90834, 90836, 90837, 90838, 90847, 90849, 90853, 92507, 92508, 96158, 96159, 96164, 96165, 96167, 96168, 96170, 96171, 97110, 97112, 97129, 97150, 97153, 97154, 97155, 97158, 97530, 97533, 97535, 97537)◀

> ▶(Do not report 0770T more than once per session)◀

Rationale

A new Category III add-on code 0770T has been established to report virtual reality (VR) technology to assist therapy. Introductory guidelines have also been added to describe VR and the use of code 0770T.

VR-mediated therapy may be used as an adjunct to the base therapy service and is typically used for skill-building for social communication, emotional regulation, and daily functional skills in people with neurodevelopmental and mental health disorders (such as autism spectrum disorder). Code 0770T is for practice expense only. The therapy time and professional time may be reported as part of the therapy and not additionally reported for the use of the VR-mediated aspects of the therapy. Code 0770T may not be reported more than once per session.

An instructional parenthetical note has been added to identify the services that may be reported in conjunction with code 0770T.

Clinical Example (0770T)

A 6-year-old male with autism spectrum disorder and accompanying language impairment requiring very substantial support receives treatment from a behavior analyst. In the course of applied-behavior analysis therapy sessions, the treating provider uses virtual reality (VR) lessons directly with the child to build joint attention, imitation, and gesture skills to assist in improving the patient's social communication skills.

Description of Procedure (0770T)

During an applied-behavior analysis session (separately reported), VR technology is used to engage the child and to work on social communication skills. The applied-behavior analysis therapist introduces the VR headset and instructs the patient on what will transpire while using VR technology. The therapist begins the software module and follows the patient's interactions on the therapist's own computer or tablet, interacting or intervening as needed to help the patient complete the tasks as required. Various modules of the VR sessions may be used several times per week or month. [**Note:** This is a practice-expense only code. The therapist's time is reported using therapy codes.]

▶Virtual Reality Patient Procedural Dissociation◀

▶Virtual reality (VR) procedural dissociation is a VR-based state of altered consciousness that supports and optimizes the patient's comfort, increases procedural tolerance, and decreases the patient's pain during the associated procedure. VR procedural dissociation establishes a computer-generated audio, visual, and proprioceptive immersive environment in which patients respond purposefully to verbal commands and stimuli, either alone or accompanied by light tactile stimulation. VR procedural dissociation does not involve interventions to maintain cardiovascular function, patent airway, or spontaneous ventilation.

VR procedural dissociation codes 0771T, 0772T, 0773T, 0774T are not used to report administration of medications for pain control, minimal sedation (anxiolysis), moderate sedation (99151, 99152, 99153, 99155, 99156, 99157), deep sedation, or monitored anesthesia care (00100-01999). Time spent administering VR procedural dissociation cannot be used to report moderate sedation or anesthesia services. VR procedural dissociation is not reported for patients younger than 5 years of age.

For 0771T, 0772T, the independent, trained observer is an individual who is qualified to monitor the patient during the procedure and has no other duties (eg, assisting at surgery) during the procedure. This individual has undergone training in immersive technologies and can adjust the technology under the supervision of the physician or other qualified health care professional who is performing the procedure. If the physician or other qualified health care professional who provides the VR also performs the procedure supported by VR (0771T, 0772T), the physician or other qualified health care professional will supervise and direct the independent, trained observer who will assist in monitoring the patient's level of consciousness, procedural disassociation, and physiological status throughout the procedure.

Intraservice time is used to determine the appropriate code to report VR procedural dissociation and is defined as:

- beginning with administration of the immersive VR technology, which at a minimum, includes audio, video, and proprioceptive feedback;

- requiring continuous face-to-face attendance of the physician or other qualified health care professional. Once continuous face-to-face time with the patient has ended, additional face-to-face time with the patient is not added to the intraservice time;

- ending when the procedure and the administration of the VR technology ends and the physician or other qualified health care professional is no longer continuously face-to-face with the patient;

- requiring monitoring patient response to the VR procedural dissociation, including;

  - periodic assessment of the patient;

  - monitoring of procedural tolerance, oxygen saturation, heart rate, pain, neurological status, and global anxiety;

  - altering of and/or adjustment of the VR program to optimize the dissociated state based on patient tolerance of the associated.

  - Optimization techniques include:

    o changing the VR baseline software program and/or adjustment of program volume;

    o adjusting the visual virtual environment;

    o altering the visual virtual position of the VR program to enable patient repositioning;

    o changing an embedded video programming in the virtual environment to maintain the dissociated state; and

    o utilizing and adjusting a proprioception, olfactory, or tactile feedback loop that corresponds to the VR program to achieve a proper and/or deeper dissociated state.

Preservice work and time are not reported separately and include the initial ordering and selecting of the VR program, describing VR procedural dissociation to the patient and/or family, and applying the VR device to the patient prior to starting the procedure. Postservice work and time is not reported separately and begins with the end of the procedure, the termination of the VR technology, and when the physician or other qualified health care professional is no longer continuously face-to-face with the patient. ◀

● **0771T** Virtual reality (VR) procedural dissociation services provided by the same physician or other qualified health care professional performing the diagnostic or therapeutic service that the VR procedural dissociation supports, requiring the presence of an independent, trained observer to assist in the monitoring of the patient's level of dissociation or consciousness and physiological status; initial 15 minutes of intraservice time, patient age 5 years or older

+● **0772T** each additional 15 minutes intraservice time (List separately in addition to code for primary service)

▶(Use 0772T in conjunction with 0771T)◀

Total Intraservice Time for VR Procedural Dissociation	Patient Age	▶Virtual reality (VR) procedural dissociation by physician or other qualified health care professional (same physician or other qualified health care professional performing the procedure the VR is supporting) Code(s)	Virtual reality (VR) procedural dissociation by different physician or other qualified health care professional (not the physician or other qualified health care professional who is performing the procedure the VR is supporting) Code(s)
Less than 10 minutes	< 5 years	Not reported separately	Not reported separately
	5 years or older	Not reported separately	Not reported separately
10-22 minutes	5 years or older	0771T	0773T
23-37 minutes	5 years or older	0771T+ 0772T X 1	0773T + 0774T X 1
38-52 minutes	5 years or older	0771T + 0772T X 2	0773T + 0774T X 2
53-67 minutes	5 years or older	0771T + 0772T X 3	0773T + 0774T X 3◀

★=Telemedicine ◀=Add-on code ✚=Add-on code ✗=FDA approval pending #=Resequenced code ⊘=Modifier 51 exempt

● **0773T**   Virtual reality (VR) procedural dissociation services provided by a physician or other qualified health care professional other than the physician or other qualified health care professional performing the diagnostic or therapeutic service that the VR procedural dissociation supports; initial 15 minutes of intraservice time, patient age 5 years or older

+● **0774T**   each additional 15 minutes intraservice time (List separately in addition to code for primary service)

▶(Use 0774T in conjunction with 0773T)◀

Rationale

Four Category III codes (0771T, 0772T, 0773T, 0774T) have been created to report virtual reality (VR) procedural dissociation services. A new Category III subheading with guidelines and a table that outlines patient age and duration of the service and identifies who is performing the service has also been added.

VR technology allows for the implementation of VR procedural dissociation to avoid anesthesia during painful and anxiety-provoking medical, surgical, and radiological procedures. This technology has been used as an anesthesia replacement for adult and pediatric patients with severe burns, rehabilitation, radiological interventional procedures, gastroenterology procedures, orthopedic procedures, oncology therapies, dermatologic procedures, otolaryngology endoscopy, and intravenous placement. VR procedures are typically performed with a wide variety of diagnostic, therapeutic, and interventional services.

Codes 0771T and 0772T include an independently trained observer who is qualified to monitor the patient during the procedure and has no other duties (eg, assisting at surgery) during the procedure. This individual has undergone training in immersive technologies and can adjust the technology under the supervision of the physician or other QHP who is performing the procedure.

If the physician or other QHP who provides the VR also performs the procedure supported by VR (0771T, 0772T), the physician or other QHP will supervise and direct the independently trained observer who will assist in monitoring the patient's level of consciousness, procedural disassociation, and physiological status throughout the procedure. Codes 0773T and 0774T are reported for VR dissociation services when provided by a physician or other QHP other than the physician or other QHP who is performing the service being supported by the VR procedural dissociation.

Intraservice time is used to determine the appropriate code to report VR procedural dissociation. Preservice work and time are not reported separately and include the initial ordering and selecting of the VR program, describing VR procedural dissociation to the patient and/or family, and applying the VR device to the patient prior to start of the procedure.

Postservice work and time are not reported separately and begin with the end of the procedure, the termination of the VR technology, and when the physician or other QHP is no longer continuously face-to-face with the patient.

The introductory guidelines provide specific details on the preservice work, intraservice time, and postservice work.

A table has been included to assist users in selecting the appropriate code combination to report the VR procedural dissociation by physician or other QHP (same physician or other QHP performing the procedure VR is supporting) or VR procedural dissociation by a different physician or other QHP (not the physician or other QHP who is performing the procedure VR is supporting). The table displays ranges of time taken for VR procedural dissociation. The rows in the table illustrate the time taken to perform the VR procedural dissociation (as a range); the age of the patient; and the appropriate code(s) to report based on the time within that range. To make the table user friendly, minutes have been captured in the left column to identify the time. The table specifies that sedation less than 10 minutes for a patient of any age is not separately reported.

Clinical Example (0771T)

An 8-year-old male patient undergoes a procedure that requires virtual reality (VR) procedural dissociation.

Description of Procedure (0771T)

The physician or other QHP performs patient assessment prior to initiation of VR procedural dissociation; supervises or personally provides VR procedural dissociation; and supervises an independent, trained observer who monitors the patient's level of consciousness and physiologic status throughout the procedure. Assess the patient continuously throughout the procedure to achieve an effective and safe level of procedural dissociation. The physician orders or provides adjustment of VR procedural dissociation as needed. The physician orders additional administration of VR procedural dissociation as needed to maintain the desired level of procedural dissociation for the supported procedure. The physician's intraservice time ends when the procedure is complete, the patient is physiologically stable, and face-to-face physician time is no longer required.

Clinical Example (0772T)

A 15-year-old male undergoes a procedure that requires VR procedural dissociation. [**Note:** This is an add-on service. Only consider the additional work related to 0771T.]

Category III 0042T-0713T

Description of Procedure (0772T)

After the initial 15 minutes of VR procedural dissociation (reported separately with 0771T), provide additional VR procedural dissociation to complete the supported procedure. The physician performing the procedure, who is also administering VR procedural dissociation, monitors the patient closely and delivers additional VR procedural dissociation as needed.

Clinical Example (0773T)

A 5-year-old female undergoes a procedure that requires VR procedural dissociation performed by a separate physician or other QHP.

Description of Procedure (0773T)

A physician or other QHP (separate from the physician performing the supported procedure) performs patient assessment prior to the initiation of VR procedural dissociation, personally provides the VR procedural dissociation and supervises the patient's level of consciousness and physiologic status throughout the procedure. The physician provides adjustment and additional administration of VR procedural dissociation as needed to maintain the achieved level of procedural dissociation for the supported procedure. The physician's intraservice time ends when the procedure is complete, the patient is physiologically stable, and face-to-face physician time is no longer required.

Clinical Example (0774T)

A 16-year-old female undergoes a procedure that requires VR procedural dissociation performed by a separate physician or other QHP. [**Note:** This is an add-on service. Only consider the additional work related to 0773T.]

Description of Procedure (0774T)

After the initial 15 minutes of VR procedural dissociation (reported separately with 0773T), perform additional VR procedural dissociation to complete the supported procedure. The physician performing the VR procedural dissociation closely monitors the patient and provides additional VR procedural dissociation as needed.

►Code 27279 describes percutaneous arthrodesis of the sacroiliac joint using a minimally invasive technique to place an internal fixation device(s) that passes through the ilium, across the sacroiliac joint, and into the sacrum, thus transfixing the sacroiliac joint. Report 0775T for the percutaneous placement of an intra-articular stabilization device into the sacroiliac joint using a minimally invasive technique that does not transfix the sacroiliac joint. For percutaneous arthrodesis of the

sacroiliac joint utilizing both a transfixation device and intra-articular implant(s), use 27299.◄

● **0775T** Arthrodesis, sacroiliac joint, percutaneous, with image guidance, includes placement of intra-articular implant(s) (eg, bone allograft[s], synthetic device[s])

►(Do not report 0775T in conjunction with 27279, 27280)◄

►(For percutaneous arthrodesis, sacroiliac joint, with transfixation device, use 27279)◄

►(For removal or replacement of sacroiliac intra-articular implant[s], use 27299)◄

►(For bilateral procedure, report 0775T with modifier 50)◄

Rationale

Code 0775T has been established to allow separate reporting for percutaneous/minimally invasive arthrodesis transfixation of the sacroiliac joint (27279) vs percutaneous arthrodesis of the sacroiliac joint via placement of an intra-articular implant (0775T). In addition, guidelines and parenthetical notes have been added and revised to provide instruction and further exemplify the intent of use for these procedure codes. An editorial revision has also been made to code 27280.

The descriptor for code 27279 includes language that may be misconstrued for reporting any type of percutaneous or minimally invasive arthrodesis of the sacroiliac joint. This code is intended to identify any percutaneous sacroiliac fusion procedure in which fusion is accomplished via transfixation of the sacroiliac joint—ie, fusing the ilium to the sacrum (such as by use of pins passed through the joint to "transfix" both bones that constitute the joint). Decortication (ie, removal of the outer layer of bone to accommodate the fusion) in the joint is done to facilitate fusion of the bones. As is noted in the descriptor, grafting (and obtaining the graft material) may be utilized to accomplish the fusion and is inherently included as part of the procedure (ie, not separately reportable). The fusion may also be accomplished using allograft. Language within the descriptor for code 27279 notes that the approach for the procedure is performed using minimal or percutaneous access of the joint to accomplish the procedure (thus differentiating it from the open procedure described in 27280). In addition, the approach is also lateral.

To eliminate confusion regarding intent for use, code 0775T has been added to the CPT code set. This code is specifically intended to identify a unique method of stabilizing the sacroiliac joint via use of a distracting intra-articular implant placed between the two boney surfaces of the iliac and sacral bones. "Tensioning" accomplishes the stabilization of the joint with different work, a

★=Telemedicine ◀=Add-on code ✚=Add-on code ✗=FDA approval pending #=Resequenced code ⊘=Modifier 51 exempt

Category III 0042T-0713T

different directional approach (posterior), and a different method from that identified within the procedure represented by code 27279.

Guidelines have been placed within the Pelvis and Hip Joint/Arthrodesis subsection where codes 27279 and 27280 reside and in the Category III section prior to the listing of code 0775T. The guidelines are identical and provide instructions regarding: (1) intent for use of 27279; (2) intent for use of 0775T; and (3) instructions regarding how to report procedures that incorporate use of both techniques (ie, use of a spacer implant AND struts that transfix the sacroiliac joint—code 27299). Parenthetical notes have also been placed (or updated) throughout both sections: (1) to restrict use of code 27279 in conjunction with 0775T as well as to reciprocally restrict use of 0775T in conjunction with 27279 and 27280; (2) as a cross-reference to direct users to the appropriate code to report when both the spacer and transfixation techniques are both used in the same procedure (27299); (3) to direct users to the correct code to report for fusion accomplished by transfixation (27279) or by intra-articular implant(s) (0775T). Parenthetical notes have also been established to provide instruction regarding how to report removal of a sacroiliac intra-articular implant (27299) and how to report code 0775T for a bilateral procedure (0775T appended with modifier 50).

Code 27280 was editorially revised to match the CPT code convention for descriptor language.

Clinical Example (0775T)

A 50-year-old female has chronic low-back, buttock, and thigh pain. She has been diagnosed with sacroiliac joint pain and has not responded to nonsurgical management. Physical examination provocative maneuvers have confirmed that the sacroiliac joint is the pain generator. A diagnostic injection has confirmed pain relief. The patient elects to undergo a minimally invasive arthrodesis of the sacroiliac joint with an intra-articular implant.

Description of Procedure (0775T)

Place the patient on the operating room table and induce general anesthesia. Then place the patient in the prone position and prepare and drape her for the procedure. Rotate the fluoroscope in a medial to lateral oblique orientation until the posterior and anterior sacroiliac joint lines become superimposed. Place a pin(s) into the sacroiliac joint under fluoroscopic guidance. Insert a retraction guide over the pin. Decorticate the sacroiliac joint by using a joint decorticator and/or surgical drill through the guide retraction tube. Then place demineralized bone matrix and the cortical allograft(s) within the sacroiliac joint. Close and dress the wound(s).

● **0776T** Therapeutic induction of intra-brain hypothermia, including placement of a mechanical temperature-controlled cooling device to the neck over carotids and head, including monitoring (eg, vital signs and sport concussion assessment tool 5 [SCAT5]), 30 minutes of treatment

► (Do not report 0776T more than once per day) ◄

► (For initiation of selective head or total body hypothermia in the critically ill neonate, use 99184) ◄

Rationale

Category III code 0776T has been established to report mechanical hypothermia management. New parenthetical notes have been added to provide instructions on the appropriate reporting of code 0776T.

This procedure is for intra-brain hypothermic/cooling therapy. The device garment is placed over the carotids and head and delivers a precise yet constant temperature to induce therapeutic intra-brain hypothermia. This treatment is typically for patients who have suffered from or are recovering from a concussion or traumatic brain injury.

Clinical Example (0776T)

An 18-year-old male diagnosed with a mild traumatic brain injury based on a sports concussion assessment tool receives an intra-brain cooling session using a mechanical cooling garment on the head and carotid arteries.

Description of Procedure (0776T)

Clinical staff places and fits the garment for hypothermic treatment. The chiller is set to the "cool down" mode for approximately 10 to 12 minutes, providing the subject with the optimal temperature acclimation period (6°C). Once the desired treatment temperature is reached, the device initiates treatment and an onboard clock begins to track total treatment time of 30 minutes. Remove the device garment and take the vital signs.

+● **0777T** Real-time pressure-sensing epidural guidance system (List separately in addition to code for primary procedure)

► (Use 0777T in conjunction with 62320, 62321, 62322, 62323, 62324, 62325, 62326, 62327) ◄

▲ = Revised code   ● = New code   ► ◄ = Contains new or revised text   ✕ = Duplicate PLA test   ↕ = Category I PLA   American Medical Association   **245**

Category III   0042T-0713T

Rationale

A new Category III add-on code (0777T) has been established to report real-time pressure sensing epidural guidance system.

The services described in code 0777T integrate artificial intelligence (AI) to place an epidural needle. It is typically utilized during analgesic epidural needle placement in patients. It is real-time software to assist the physician by transmitting key data points. The sensor interprets epidural pressures, details anatomical needle placement, and measures precise saline volume via software facilitating data transmission to an epidural system console screen. The software analyzes the data allowing the practitioner to place the epidural spinal needle.

An instructional parenthetical note has been added following code 0777T to support the accurate reporting of this service in conjunction with codes 62320-62327.

Clinical Example (0777T)

A 52-year-old male with intractable lower back pain presents for epidural injection treatment. [**Note:** This is an add-on code. Only consider the additional work related to 62320, 62321, 62322, 62323, 62324, 62325, 62326, 62327.]

Description of Procedure (0777T)

Perform patient pain assessment. Place the patient in the lateral decubitus position on a table with the dorsal spine exposed. Cleanse the epidural injection site and administer a local anesthetic. Prepare the epidural software system. The proceduralist verifies the existence of power to the epidural console and attaches one end of the epidural catheter to the console pressure sensor while the other end of the catheter is inserted into the epidural or subarachnoid needle. Introduce the needle into the epidural or subarachnoid space through a paramedian interlaminar method, with additional guidance as indicated (ie, fluoroscopy or CT). The software is used to analyze epidural pressure and needle location during the epidural needle placement. The epidural console display is a liquid crystal display (LCD) screen that provides pressure indicators and location information with a touch screen interface for entering parameters into the system. The pressure sensor will transmit to the screen allowing the proceduralist to confirm the location of the needle confirming proper needle placement.

▶Office-Based Measurement of Mechanomyography and Inertial Measurement Units◀

▶Code 0778T represents the measurement and recording of dynamic joint motion and muscle function that includes the incorporation of multiple inertial measurement unit (IMU) with concurrent surface mechanomyography (sMMG) sensors. Code 0778T is not a remote service and measurements are obtained in the office setting while the patient is physically present.

The IMU sensors contain an accelerometer that measures acceleration and velocity of the body during movement, a gyroscope that measures the positioning, rotation, and orientation of the body during movement, and a magnetometer that measures the strength and direction of the magnetic field to orient the body position during movement relative to the earth's magnetic north field. The sMMG sensors measure muscle function by quantifying muscle activation and contraction amplitude and duration by recording high-sensitivity volumetric change.

A combination of the sensors is used to dynamically record multi-joint motion and muscle function bilaterally and concurrently during functional movement. Data collected from the wireless-enabled IMUs and sMMGs are then uploaded to a secure, Health Insurance Portability and Accountability Act (HIPAA)-compliant cloud-based processing platform. The cloud-based application immediately processes the data and produces an automated report with digestible chronological data to assist in serial tracking improvement, decline, or plateau of progress during the episode of care. When 0778T is performed on the same day as another therapy, assessment, or evaluation services, those services may be reported separately and in addition to 0778T.◀

● **0778T** Surface mechanomyography (sMMG) with concurrent application of inertial measurement unit (IMU) sensors for measurement of multi-joint range of motion, posture, gait, and muscle function

▶(Do not report 0778T in conjunction with 96000, 96004, 98975, 98977, 98980, 98981)◀

Rationale

Code 0778T has been established to report measurement and recording of dynamic joint motion and muscle function, which includes the incorporation of multiple inertial measurement units (IMUs) with concurrent surface mechanomyography (sMMG) sensors. A new subheading and guidelines preceding the code have also been established to describe the use of this code.

Code 0778T is not a remote service, and measurements are obtained in the office setting while the patient is physically present. This code is intended to capture the measurement and recording of dynamic joint motion and muscle function, which includes the incorporation of IMUs with concurrent sMMG sensors.

The purpose of this technology is to increase the accuracy of measuring and recording joint motion of the axial and appendicular skeleton as well as record muscle function in a standardized fashion, and to decrease the variability and bias of recording such, by the spectrum of providers who treat musculoskeletal conditions.

In the context of injury, code 0778T may be used serially, at regular intervals (typically biweekly or monthly, depending on the severity of injury), to record evolving functional status during the episode of care.

An exclusionary parenthetical note has been added to preclude the reporting of code 0778T with codes 96000, 96004, 98975, 98977, 98980, and 98981.

Clinical Example (0778T)

A 54-year-old male stock worker presents with acute low-back pain and difficulty standing for long periods of time. There are no neurologic findings on physical examination and no comorbidities. Standard radiographs of lumbosacral spine demonstrate mild degenerative changes. The patient was prescribed over-the-counter oral analgesics and referred for physical therapy. A physician or other QHP reviews the patient history, identifies the injury area of interest, and determines that the patient would benefit from a standardized high-accuracy musculoskeletal assessment. The care plan includes concurrent surface mechanomyography (sMMG) with concurrent application of inertial measurement unit (IMU) sensors for measurement of multi-joint range of motion, posture, gait, and muscle function.

Description of Procedure (0778T)

The evaluation consists of a multi-sensor technology that quantifies joint motion and muscle function and includes calibration of the sensors, set-up and placement over bony landmarks and specific muscle groups, and augmentative measurement and processing of joint motion and muscle function during functional activities (eg, sit to stand to sit, gait). Upon completion of the testing session, the physician or other QHP removes the sensors and syncs the data within the secure platform. A report is generated and accessible to the physician or other QHP through a web portal by utilizing secure login credentials.

● **0779T**   Gastrointestinal myoelectrical activity study, stomach through colon, with interpretation and report

▶(Do not report 0779T in conjunction with 91020, 91022, 91112, 91117, 91122, 91132, 91133)◀

Rationale

Category III code 0779T has been established to report gastrointestinal (GI) myoelectrical activity study from the stomach through the colon. GI myoelectrical activity study is a noninvasive procedure that assesses motility in the GI tract from the stomach through the colon. The study may be performed over several days. This assessment is performed for GI symptoms such as gastrointestinal pain, bloating, and distension. An exclusionary parenthetical note has been added following code 0779T, restricting its use with codes 91020, 91022, 91112, 91117, 91122, 91132, and 91133.

Clinical Example (0779T)

A 35-year-old female presents with gastrointestinal pain, bloating, distension, and change in bowel habits that have failed to improve despite pharmacologic measures. Measurement of gastrointestinal myoelectrical activity is recommended to guide further management.

Description of Procedure (0779T)

Prepare the abdominal skin. Apply the patches for measuring myoelectric activity to the skin. Turn on the battery power to the patches and confirm that the remote monitoring application is communicating with the patches. Instruct the patient on proper care of the patches and use of the remote monitoring application. Data are continually uploaded to the cloud, where algorithms process the data. At the conclusion of the procedure, the physician reviews and interprets the data and generates a report.

● **0780T**   Instillation of fecal microbiota suspension via rectal enema into lower gastrointestinal tract

▶(Do not report 0780T in conjunction with 44705, 44799, 45999, 74283)◀

Rationale

A new Category III code 0780T has been established to report the instillation of fecal microbiota suspension via rectal enema into the GI tract. In addition, inclusionary and cross-reference parenthetical notes have been added in the Surgery, Digestive System and Category III sections to clarify the appropriate reporting of this new service. The exclusionary parenthetical note following code 44705 has been revised to include code 0780T. A cross-reference parenthetical note has been added following code 44705 to direct users to report the appropriate new code. Note that it is not appropriate to report codes 44705, 44799, 45999, and 74283 with the new code 0780T. This is a therapeutic procedure to assist in the treatment of diseases such as Clostridium difficile infection.

Clinical Example (0780T)

A 64-year-old female with two prior episodes of Clostridium difficile infection has completed antibiotic therapy for the most recent infection more than 24 hours ago. Evaluation by her physician or other QHP indicates that she is an appropriate candidate for fecal microbiota transplantation.

Description of Procedure (0780T)

Review the patient's medical/treatment history to verify appropriateness of the planned fecal microbiota instillation therapy. Instruct the patient to empty bladder and bowel, if possible. Position the patient in either a left-side or knee-chest position on a stable, comfortable surface to facilitate proper administration. In a non-surgical environment, insert a lubricated delivery tube ~12 cm (5 inches) into the patient's rectum and the tube is connected to a gravity flow instillation bag containing a suspension of fecal microbiota. Raise the bag so the product is instilled via gravity flow. Once all product has been instilled, remove the delivery tube from the patient's rectum. The patient can remain in the administration position for up to 15 minutes to help minimize any cramping; after which, discharge the patient.

● **0781T**   Bronchoscopy, rigid or flexible, with insertion of esophageal protection device and circumferential radiofrequency destruction of the pulmonary nerves, including fluoroscopic guidance when performed; bilateral mainstem bronchi

● **0782T**   unilateral mainstem bronchus

▶(Use 0781T, 0782T only once, regardless of the number of treatments per bronchus)◀

▶(Do not report 0781T, 0782T in conjunction with 31622-31638, 31640, 31641, 31643, 31645, 31646, 31647, 31648, 31649, 31651, 31652, 31653, 31654, 31660, 31661)◀

▶(For bronchial thermoplasty, see 31660, 31661)◀

Rationale

Two new Category III codes (0781T, 0782T) have been established to describe bronchoscopy, rigid or flexible, with insertion of esophageal protection device and circumferential radiofrequency destruction of the pulmonary nerves, including fluoroscopic guidance when performed. Code 0781T is intended to be reported for bilateral mainstem bronchi, and code 0782T is intended to be reported for unilateral mainstem bronchus. In addition, inclusionary, exclusionary, instructional, and cross-reference parenthetical notes have been added in the Surgery/Respiratory System and Category III sections to clarify the appropriate reporting of this new service. A cross-reference parenthetical note has been added following code 31661 to direct users to report the appropriate new code.

In addition, an instructional parenthetical note has been added following code 0782T to indicate that codes 0781T and 0782T should only be reported once, regardless of the number of treatments per bronchus. In addition, an exclusionary parenthetical note has been added to restrict reporting bronchoscopy procedures with new codes 0781T and 0782T. A cross-reference parenthetical note has been added following code 0782T. Codes 0781T and 0782T have been added to describe a procedure that may aid in the treatment of chronic obstructive pulmonary disease (COPD).

Clinical Example (0781T)

A 64-year-old male with chronic obstructive pulmonary disease (COPD) has had several moderate COPD exacerbations in the past 12 months resulting in multiple supplemental prescriptions in addition to his routine COPD inhaler therapy and is recommended for targeted lung denervation.

Description of Procedure (0781T)

The anesthesia team drapes the patient, places appropriate intravenous (IV) lines, and administers general anesthesia. The proceduralist affixes an electrode pad to the patient's skin to complete the electrical circuit required for the procedure and places an esophageal device for esophageal protection. Insert a standard flexible bronchoscope through the nose or mouth for access to the lung. Perform a detailed inspection of the proximal airway of the lung. Insert a cooling balloon-radiofrequency catheter electrode assembly and advance to the first treatment site. Coolant flows to unfold the electrode and inflate the balloon. A trained technician operates the console to start and stop energy delivery and inflate or deflate the treatment catheter balloon per physician instruction, measuring the distance between the radio-opaque catheter electrode and the esophagus via fluoroscopy prior to each energy activation. Deliver radiofrequency energy to ablate the vagal nerves surrounding each bronchus. Once energy delivery is complete, deflate the balloon before repositioning the patient. The process of balloon inflation, thermal energy delivery, and balloon deflation is typically repeated in each of four quadrant positions to achieve circumferential treatment in the proximal bronchus of each lung. Full circumferential treatment (four activations) may not always be possible, principally due to the anatomical proximity to the esophagus. When treatment of both lungs is complete, remove the esophageal protection device, the cooling balloon-radiofrequency catheter electrode assembly, and the bronchoscope. Perform a post-bronchoscopy visual inspection of the airways to ascertain that no complications have occurred. Discharge the patient home the same day of the procedure.

Clinical Example (0782T)

A 64-year-old male with COPD has had several moderate COPD exacerbations in the past 12 months resulting in multiple supplemental prescriptions in addition to his routine COPD inhaler therapy and is recommended for targeted lung denervation.

Description of Procedure (0782T)

The anesthesia team drapes the patient, places appropriate IV lines, and administers general anesthesia. The proceduralist affixes an electrode pad to the patient's skin to complete the electrical circuit required for the procedure and places an esophageal device for esophageal protection. Insert a standard flexible bronchoscope through the nose or mouth for access to the lung. Perform a detailed inspection of the proximal airway of the lung. Insert a cooling balloon-radiofrequency catheter electrode assembly and advance to the first treatment site. Coolant flows to unfold the electrode and inflate the balloon. A trained technician operates the console to start and stop energy delivery and inflate or deflate the treatment catheter balloon per physician instruction, measuring the distance between the radio-opaque catheter electrode and the esophagus via fluoroscopy prior to each energy activation. Deliver radiofrequency energy to ablate the vagal nerves surrounding each bronchus. Once energy delivery is complete, deflate the balloon before repositioning the patient. The process of balloon inflation, thermal energy delivery, and balloon deflation is typically repeated in each of four quadrant positions to achieve circumferential treatment in the proximal bronchus of the lung. Full circumferential treatment (four activations) may not always be possible, principally due to anatomical proximity to the esophagus. When treatment of the lung is complete, remove the esophageal protection device, the cooling balloon-radiofrequency

catheter electrode assembly, and the bronchoscope. Perform a post-bronchoscopy visual inspection of the airways to ascertain that no complications have occurred. Discharge the patient home the same day of the procedure.

● **0783T**   Transcutaneous auricular neurostimulation, set-up, calibration, and patient education on use of equipment

Rationale

Category III code 0783T has been established to report transcutaneous auricular neurostimulation. This procedure involves electrical stimulation transcutaneously to vagus and trigeminal nerves and may be used to aid in the relief of opioid-withdrawal symptoms.

Clinical Example (0783T)

A 32-year-old male with a repeat history of opioid addiction seeks treatment. A physician writes a treatment plan and includes a prescription for transcutaneous auricular neurostimulation in conjunction with the current standard of care.

Description of Procedure (0783T)

Prescribe transcutaneous auricular neurostimulation and have the patient come to the office. The physician, other QHP, or other clinical staff sets up the device, shows the patient how it functions and how to operate it. The physician, other QHP, or clinical staff then connects the device to the patient controller and programs the parameters for patient use. The physician, other QHP, or clinical staff teaches the patient how to apply the earpiece, secure the wires at the correct location over the trigeminal and vagus nerve points, and shows the patient how to use the controller to adjust the neurostimulation for comfort and efficacy. The patient is instructed on how often to replace the earpiece and who to contact for assistance, if needed. Provide supplemental information packet for home use.

Category III 0042T–0713T

Notes

Appendix A

Summary of Additions, Deletions, and Revisions

The summary of changes shows the actual changes that have been made to the code descriptors.

New codes appear with a bullet (●) and are indicated as "Code added." Revised codes are preceded with a triangle (▲). Within revised codes, or if a code symbol has been deleted, the deleted language and code symbol appear with a ~~strikethrough~~, while new text appears <u>underlined</u>.

The ✗ symbol is used to identify codes for vaccines that are pending FDA approval. The # symbol is used to identify codes that have been resequenced. CPT add-on codes are annotated by the ✚ symbol. The ⊘ symbol is used to identify codes that are exempt from the use of modifier 51. The ★ symbol is used to identify codes that may be used for reporting telemedicine services. The ✤ symbol is used to identify a proprietary laboratory analyses (PLA) test that has an identical descriptor as another PLA test. A PLA code that satisfies Category I code criteria and has been accepted by the CPT Editorial Panel is annotated with the ↑↓ symbol. The ◀ symbol is used to identify codes that may be used to report audio-only telemedicine services when appended by modifier 93 (**see Appendix T**).

Modifier	Modifier Descriptor
63	▶**Procedure Performed on Infants less than 4 kg**: Procedures performed on neonates and infants up to a present body weight of 4 kg may involve significantly increased complexity and physician or other qualified health care professional work commonly associated with these patients. This circumstance may be reported by adding modifier 63 to the procedure number. **Note:** Unless otherwise designated, this modifier may only be appended to procedures/services listed in the 20100-69990 code series and 92920, 92928, 92953, 92960, 92986, 92987, 92990, 92997, 92998, 93312, 93313, 93314, 93315, 93316, 93317, 93318, 93452, 93505, 93563, 93564, 93568, <u>93569, 93573, 93574, 93575,</u> 93580, <u>93581,</u> 93582, 93590, 93591, 93592, 93593, 93594, 93595, 93596, 93597, 93598, 93615, 93616 from the Medicine/Cardiovascular section. Modifier 63 should not be appended to any CPT codes listed in the **Evaluation and Management Services, Anesthesia, Radiology, Pathology**~~/~~<u> and **Laboratory,**</u> or **Medicine** sections (other than those identified above from the Medicine/Cardiovascular section).◀
93	▶<u>**Synchronous Telemedicine Service Rendered Via Telephone or Other Real-Time Interactive Audio-Only Telecommunications System**: Synchronous telemedicine service is defined as a real-time interaction between a physician or other qualified health care professional and a patient who is located away at a distant site from the physician or other qualified health care professional. The totality of the communication of information exchanged between the physician or other qualified health care professional and the patient during the course of the synchronous telemedicine service must be of an amount and nature that is sufficient to meet the key components and/or requirements of the same service when rendered via a face-to-face interaction.</u>◀

Appendix A

Modifiers

63 ►**Procedure Performed on Infants less than 4 kg:**
Procedures performed on neonates and infants up to a
present body weight of 4 kg may involve significantly
increased complexity and physician or other qualified
health care professional work commonly associated with
these patients. This circumstance may be reported by
adding modifier 63 to the procedure number. **Note:** Unless
otherwise designated, this modifier may only be appended
to procedures/services listed in the 20100-69990 code series
and 92920, 92928, 92953, 92960, 92986, 92987, 92990,
92997, 92998, 93312, 93313, 93314, 93315, 93316,
93317, 93318, 93452, 93505, 93563, 93564, 93568,
93569, 93573, 93574, 93575, 93580, 93581, 93582,
93590, 93591, 93592, 93593, 93594, 93595, 93596,
93597, 93598, 93615, 93616 from the Medicine/
Cardiovascular section. Modifier 63 should not be
appended to any CPT codes listed in the **Evaluation and
Management Services, Anesthesia, Radiology, Pathology
and Laboratory,** or **Medicine** sections (other than those
identified above from the Medicine/Cardiovascular
section).◄

Rationale

The guidelines for modifier 63, *Procedures Performed on
Infants less than 4 kg,* have been revised with the addition
of new codes 93569, 93573-93575, and 93581 to the
listing of codes with which modifier 63 may be reported.
Codes 93569, 93573-93575, and 93581 describe
procedures that may be performed on an infant weighing
less than 4 kilograms.

Refer to the codebook and the Rationale for codes 93569,
93573-93575, and 93581 for a full discussion of these
changes.

93 ►**Synchronous Telemedicine Service Rendered Via
Telephone or Other Real-Time Interactive Audio-Only
Telecommunications System:** Synchronous telemedicine
service is defined as a real-time interaction between a
physician or other qualified health care professional and a
patient who is located away at a distant site from the
physician or other qualified health care professional. The
totality of the communication of information exchanged
between the physician or other qualified health care
professional and the patient during the course of the
synchronous telemedicine service must be of an amount
and nature that is sufficient to meet the key components
and/or requirements of the same service when rendered via
a face-to-face interaction.◄

Rationale

Modifier 93 has been established to allow the reporting of
medical services that are provided via real-time
interaction between the physician or other qualified
health care professional and a patient through audio-only
technology. The use of this modifier has been in effect
since January 1, 2022.

In addition, a new Appendix T was created and has been
effective since April 1, 2022. This appendix is a listing of
CPT codes that may be used for reporting audio-only
services when appended with modifier 93. The codes
listed in Appendix T have been identified with the ◄
symbol in the CPT 2023 code set.

Refer to the codebook and the Rationale for Appendix T
for a full discussion of these changes.

★ = Telemedicine　◄ = Audio-only　✚ = Add-on code　𝒩 = FDA approval pending　# = Resequenced code　⊘ = Modifier 51 exempt

Appendix C

Clinical Examples

▶The clinical examples for CPT evaluation and management (E/M) services codes (formerly Appendix C) have been removed from the CPT code set. For information or guidance on reporting E/M services, refer to the E/M Guidelines.◀

Rationale

In accordance with the change in the structure of the evaluation and management (E/M) level-based codes, Appendix C, Clinical Examples, has been deleted from the CPT code set. The clinical examples in Appendix C reflect the former structure of the E/M level-based codes that required specific levels of history and examination and medical decision making. Because the E/M codes no longer follow this structure, Appendix C has been removed from the CPT code set.

Notes

Appendix O

Summary of Additions, Deletions, and Revisions

The summary of changes shows the actual changes that have been made to the code descriptors.

New codes appear with a bullet (●) and are indicated as "Code added." Revised codes are preceded with a triangle (▲). Within revised codes, or if a code symbol has been deleted, the deleted language and code symbol appear with a ~~strikethrough~~, while new text appears <u>underlined</u>.

The ✓ symbol is used to identify codes for vaccines that are pending FDA approval. The # symbol is used to identify codes that have been resequenced. CPT add-on codes are annotated by the ✚ symbol. The ⊘ symbol is used to identify codes that are exempt from the use of modifier 51. The ★ symbol is used to identify codes that may be used for reporting telemedicine services. The ✕ symbol is used to identify a proprietary laboratory analyses (PLA) test that has an identical descriptor as another PLA test. A PLA code that satisfies Category I code criteria and has been accepted by the CPT Editorial Panel is annotated with the ↕ symbol. The ◀ symbol is used to identify codes that may be used to report audio-only telemedicine services when appended by modifier 93 (see Appendix T).

Proprietary Name and Clinical Laboratory or Manufacturer	Alpha-Numeric Code	Code Descriptor
Administrative Codes for Multianalyte Assays with Algorithmic Analyses (MAAA)		
Decipher Bladder ~~TURBT®; Decipher Biosciences, Inc,~~ <u>Veracyte Labs SD</u>	▲0016M	Oncology (bladder), mRNA, microarray gene expression profiling of ~~209~~ <u>219</u> genes, utilizing formalin-fixed paraffin-embedded tissue, algorithm reported as molecular subtype (luminal, luminal infiltrated, basal, basal claudin-low, neuroendocrine-like)
Category I Codes for Multianalyte Assays with Algorithmic Analyses (MAAA)		
Proprietary Laboratory Analyses (PLA)		
~~MatePair Targeted Rearrangements, Congenital, Mayo Clinic~~	~~0012U~~	~~Germline disorders, gene rearrangement detection by whole genome next-generation sequencing, DNA, whole blood, report of specific gene rearrangement(s)~~
~~MatePair Targeted Rearrangements, Oncology, Mayo Clinic~~	~~0013U~~	~~Oncology (solid organ neoplasia), gene rearrangement detection by whole genome next-generation sequencing, DNA, fresh or frozen tissue or cells, report of specific gene rearrangement(s)~~
~~MatePair Targeted Rearrangements, Hematologic, Mayo Clinic~~	~~0014U~~	~~Hematology (hematolymphoid neoplasia), gene rearrangement detection by whole genome next-generation sequencing, DNA, whole blood or bone marrow, report of specific gene rearrangement(s)~~
Oncomine™ Dx Target Test, Thermo Fisher Scientific<u>, Thermo Fisher Scientific</u>	▲0022U	Targeted genomic sequence analysis panel, <u>cholangiocarcinoma and</u> non-small cell lung neoplasia, DNA and RNA analysis, <u>1-</u>23 genes, interrogation for sequence variants and rearrangements, reported as presence/absence of variants and associated therapy(ies) to consider

(Continued on page 256)

▲ = Revised code   ● = New code   ▶ ◀ = Contains new or revised text   ✕ = Duplicate PLA test   ↕ = Category I PLA   American Medical Association   **255**

Proprietary Name and Clinical Laboratory or Manufacturer	Alpha-Numeric Code	Code Descriptor
~~MatePair Acute Myeloid Leukemia Panel, Mayo Clinic, Laboratory Developed Test~~	~~0056U~~	~~Hematology (acute myelogenous leukemia), DNA, whole genome next-generation sequencing to detect gene rearrangement(s), blood or bone marrow, report of specific gene rearrangement(s)~~
myPath® Melanoma, ~~Myriad Genetic Laboratories~~Castle Biosciences, Inc	▲0090U	Oncology (cutaneous melanoma), mRNA gene expression profiling by RT-PCR of 23 genes (14 content and 9 housekeeping), utilizing formalin-fixed paraffin-embedded (FFPE) tissue, algorithm reported as a categorical result (ie, benign, intermediate~~indeterminate~~, malignant)
~~BioFire® FilmArray® Gastrointestinal (GI) Panel, BioFire® Diagnostics~~	~~0097U~~	~~Gastrointestinal pathogen, multiplex reverse transcription and multiplex amplified probe technique, multiple types or subtypes, 22 targets (Campylobacter [C. jejuni/C. coli/C. upsaliensis], Clostridium difficile [C. difficile] toxin A/B, Plesiomonas shigelloides, Salmonella, Vibrio [V. parahaemolyticus/V. vulnificus/V. cholerae], including specific identification of Vibrio cholerae, Yersinia enterocolitica, Enteroaggregative Escherichia coli [EAEC], Enteropathogenic Escherichia coli [EPEC], Enterotoxigenic Escherichia coli [ETEC] lt/st, Shiga-like toxin-producing Escherichia coli [STEC] stx1/ stx2 [including specific identification of the E. coli O157 serogroup within STEC], Shigella/ Enteroinvasive Escherichia coli [EIEC], Cryptosporidium, Cyclospora cayetanensis, Entamoeba histolytica, Giardia lamblia [also known as G. intestinalis and G. duodenalis], adenovirus F 40/41, astrovirus, norovirus GI/GII, rotavirus A, sapovirus [Genogroups I, II, IV, and V])~~
~~BioFire® FilmArray® Pneumonia Panel, BioFire® Diagnostics, BioFire® Diagnostics~~	~~0151U~~	~~Infectious disease (bacterial or viral respiratory tract infection), pathogen specific nucleic acid (DNA or RNA), 33 targets, real-time semi-quantitative PCR, bronchoalveolar lavage, sputum, or endotracheal aspirate, detection of 33 organismal and antibiotic resistance genes with limited semi-quantitative results~~
~~Afirma Medullary Thyroid Carcinoma (MTC) Classifier, Veracyte, Inc, Veracyte, Inc~~	~~0208U~~	~~Oncology (medullary thyroid carcinoma), mRNA, gene expression analysis of 108 genes, utilizing fine needle aspirate, algorithm reported as positive or negative for medullary thyroid carcinoma~~
Colvera®, Clinical Genomics Pathology Inc	▲0229U	*BCAT1 (Branched chain amino acid transaminase 1)* ~~or~~ and *IKZF1 (IKAROS family zinc finger 1)* (eg, colorectal cancer) promoter methylation analysis
Versiti™ Inherited Thrombocytopenia Panel, Versiti™ Diagnostic Laboratories, Versiti™	▲0276U	Hematology (inherited thrombocytopenia), genomic sequence analysis of ~~23~~ 42 genes, blood, buccal swab, or amniotic fluid
	●0285U	Code added
	●0286U	Code added
	●0287U	Code added

★=Telemedicine ◀=Audio-only ✚=Add-on code ✒=FDA approval pending #=Resequenced code ⊘=Modifier 51 exempt

Proprietary Name and Clinical Laboratory or Manufacturer	Alpha-Numeric Code	Code Descriptor
	●0288U	Code added
	●0289U	Code added
	●0290U	Code added
	●0291U	Code added
	●0292U	Code added
	●0293U	Code added
	●0294U	Code added
	●0295U	Code added
	●0296U	Code added
	●0297U	Code added
	●0298U	Code added
	●0299U	Code added
	●0300U	Code added
	●0301U	Code added
	●0302U	Code added
	●0303U	Code added
	●0304U	Code added
	●0305U	Code added
	●0306U	Code added
	●0307U	Code added
	●0308U	Code added
	●0309U	Code added
	●0310U	Code added
	●0311U	Code added
	●0312U	Code added
	●0313U	Code added
	●0314U	Code added
	●0315U	Code added
	●0316U	Code added
	●0317U	Code added
	●0318U	Code added
	●0319U	Code added
	●0320U	Code added
	●0321U	Code added
	●0322U	Code added
	●0323U	Code added
	●0324U	Code added
	●0325U	Code added
	●0326U	Code added
	●0327U	Code added
	●0328U	Code added

(Continued on page 258)

▲ = Revised code   ● = New code   ▶ ◀ = Contains new or revised text   ✕ = Duplicate PLA test   ↑↓ = Category I PLA   American Medical Association   **257**

Proprietary Name and Clinical Laboratory or Manufacturer	Alpha-Numeric Code	Code Descriptor
	●0329U	Code added
	●0330U	Code added
	●0331U	Code added
	●0332U	Code added
	●0333U	Code added
	●0334U	Code added
	●0335U	Code added
	●0336U	Code added
	●0337U	Code added
	●0338U	Code added
	●0339U	Code added
	●0340U	Code added
	●0341U	Code added
	●0342U	Code added
	●0343U	Code added
	●0344U	Code added
	●0345U	Code added
	●0346U	Code added
	●0347U	Code added
	●0348U	Code added
	●0349U	Code added
	●0350U	Code added
	●0351U	Code added
	●0352U	Code added
	●0353U	Code added
	●0354U	Code added

★ = Telemedicine   ◀ = Audio-only   ✚ = Add-on code   ✗ = FDA approval pending   # = Resequenced code   ⊘ = Modifier 51 exempt

Appendix O

Multianalyte Assays with Algorithmic Analyses and Proprietary Laboratory Analyses

The following list includes three types of CPT codes:

1. Multianalyte assays with algorithmic analyses (MAAA) administrative codes
2. Category I MAAA codes
3. Proprietary laboratory analyses (PLA) codes

1. Multianalyte assays with algorithmic analyses (MAAAs) are procedures that utilize multiple results derived from assays of various types, including molecular pathology assays, fluorescent in situ hybridization assays and non-nucleic acid based assays (eg, proteins, polypeptides, lipids, carbohydrates). Algorithmic analysis using the results of these assays as well as other patient information (if used) is then performed and reported typically as a numeric score(s) or as a probability. MAAAs are typically unique to a single clinical laboratory or manufacturer. The results of individual component procedure(s) that are inputs to the MAAAs may be provided on the associated laboratory report, however these assays are not reported separately using additional codes. MAAAs, by nature, are typically unique to a single clinical laboratory or manufacturer.

The list includes a proprietary name and clinical laboratory or manufacturer in the first column, an alpha-numeric code in the second column and code descriptor in the third column. The format for the code descriptor usually includes (in order):

- Disease type (eg, oncology, autoimmune, tissue rejection),
- Chemical(s) analyzed (eg, DNA, RNA, protein, antibody),
- Number of markers (eg, number of genes, number of proteins),
- Methodology(s) (eg, microarray, real-time [RT]-PCR, in situ hybridization [ISH], enzyme linked immunosorbent assays [ELISA]),
- Number of functional domains (if indicated),
- Specimen type (eg, blood, fresh tissue, formalin-fixed paraffin-embedded),
- Algorithm result type (eg, prognostic, diagnostic),
- Report (eg, probability index, risk score).

MAAA procedures that have been assigned a Category I code are noted in the list below and additionally listed in the Category I MAAA section (81500-81599). The Category I MAAA section introductory language and associated parenthetical instruction(s) should be used to govern the appropriate use for Category I MAAA codes. If a specific MAAA procedure has not been assigned a Category I code, it is indicated as a four-digit number followed by the letter M.

When a specific MAAA procedure is not included in either the list below or in the Category I MAAA section, report the analysis using the Category I MAAA unlisted code (81599). The codes below are specific to the assays identified in Appendix O by proprietary name. In order to report an MAAA code, the analysis performed must fulfill the code descriptor **and**, if proprietary, must be the test represented by the proprietary name listed in Appendix O. When an analysis is performed that may potentially fall within a specific descriptor, however the proprietary name is not included in the list below, the MAAA unlisted code (81599) should be used.

Additions in this section may be released tri-annually (or quarterly for PLA codes) via the AMA CPT website to expedite dissemination for reporting. See the Introduction section of the CPT code set for a complete list of the dates of release and implementation.

These administrative codes encompass all analytical services required for the algorithmic analysis (eg, cell lysis, nucleic acid stabilization, extraction, digestion, amplification, hybridization and detection) in addition to the algorithmic analysis itself, when applicable. Procedures that are required prior to cell lysis (eg, microdissection, codes 88380 and 88381) should be reported separately.

The codes in this list are provided as an administrative coding set to facilitate accurate reporting of MAAA services. The minimum standard for inclusion in this list is that an analysis is generally available for patient care. The AMA has not reviewed procedures in the administrative coding set for clinical utility. The list is not a complete list of all MAAA procedures.

1. Category I MAAA codes are included below along with their proprietary names. These codes are also listed in the Pathology and Laboratory section of the CPT code set (81490-81599).

2. PLA codes created in response to the Protecting Access to Medicare Act (PAMA) of 2014 are listed along with their proprietary names. These codes are also located at the end of the Pathology and Laboratory section of the CPT code set. In some instances, the descriptor language of PLA codes may be identical, which are differentiated only by the listed propriety names.

The accuracy of a PLA code is to be maintained by the original applicant, or the current owner of the test kit or laboratory performing the proprietary test.

A new PLA code is required when:

1. Additional nucleic acid (DNA or RNA) and/or protein analysis(es) are added to the current PLA test, or

2. The name of the PLA test has changed in association with changes in test performance or test characteristics.

The addition or modification of the therapeutic applications of the test require submission of a code change application, but it may not require a new code number.

Proprietary Name and Clinical Laboratory or Manufacturer	Alpha-Numeric Code	Code Descriptor
Administrative Codes for Multianalyte Assays with Algorithmic Analyses (MAAA)		
ASH FibroSURE™, BioPredictive S.A.S	0002M	Liver disease, ten biochemical assays (ALT, A2-macroglobulin, apolipoprotein A-1, total bilirubin, GGT, haptoglobin, AST, glucose, total cholesterol and triglycerides) utilizing serum, prognostic algorithm reported as quantitative scores for fibrosis, steatosis and alcoholic steatohepatitis (ASH)
NASH FibroSURE™, BioPredictive S.A.S	0003M	Liver disease, ten biochemical assays (ALT, A2-macroglobulin, apolipoprotein A-1, total bilirubin, GGT, haptoglobin, AST, glucose, total cholesterol and triglycerides) utilizing serum, prognostic algorithm reported as quantitative scores for fibrosis, steatosis and nonalcoholic steatohepatitis (NASH)
ScoliScore™ Transgenomic	0004M	Scoliosis, DNA analysis of 53 single nucleotide polymorphisms (SNPs), using saliva, prognostic algorithm reported as a risk score
HeproDX™, GoPath Laboratories, LLC	0006M	Oncology (hepatic), mRNA expression levels of 161 genes, utilizing fresh hepatocellular carcinoma tumor tissue, with alpha-fetoprotein level, algorithm reported as a risk classifier
NETest, Wren Laboratories, LLC	0007M	Oncology (gastrointestinal neuroendocrine tumors), real-time PCR expression analysis of 51 genes, utilizing whole peripheral blood, algorithm reported as a nomogram of tumor disease index
NeoLAB™ Prostate Liquid Biopsy, NeoGenomics Laboratories	0011M	Oncology, prostate cancer, mRNA expression assay of 12 genes (10 content and 2 housekeeping), RT-PCR test utilizing blood plasma and urine, algorithms to predict high-grade prostate cancer risk

★=Telemedicine ◀=Audio-only +=Add-on code ✗=FDA approval pending #=Resequenced code ⊘=Modifier 51 exempt

Proprietary Name and Clinical Laboratory or Manufacturer	Alpha-Numeric Code	Code Descriptor
Cxbladder™ Detect, Pacific Edge Diagnostics USA, Ltd	0012M	Oncology (urothelial), mRNA, gene expression profiling by real-time quantitative PCR of five genes *(MDK, HOXA13, CDC2 [CDK1], IGFBP5,* and *CXCR2)*, utilizing urine, algorithm reported as a risk score for having urothelial carcinoma
Cxbladder™ Monitor, Pacific Edge Diagnostics USA, Ltd	0013M	Oncology (urothelial), mRNA, gene expression profiling by real-time quantitative PCR of five genes *(MDK, HOXA13, CDC2 [CDK1], IGFBP5,* and *CXCR2)*, utilizing urine, algorithm reported as a risk score for having recurrent urothelial carcinoma
Enhanced Liver Fibrosis™ (ELF™) Test, Siemens Healthcare Diagnostics Inc/Siemens Healthcare Laboratory LLC	0014M	Liver disease, analysis of 3 biomarkers (hyaluronic acid [HA], procollagen III amino terminal peptide [PIIINP], tissue inhibitor of metalloproteinase 1 [TIMP-1]), using immunoassays, utilizing serum, prognostic algorithm reported as a risk score and risk of liver fibrosis and liver-related clinical events within 5 years
Adrenal Mass Panel, 24 Hour, Urine, Mayo Clinic Laboratories (MCL), Mayo Clinic	0015M	Adrenal cortical tumor, biochemical assay of 25 steroid markers, utilizing 24-hour urine specimen and clinical parameters, prognostic algorithm reported as a clinical risk and integrated clinical steroid risk for adrenal cortical carcinoma, adenoma, or other adrenal malignancy
▶Decipher Bladder, Veracyte Labs SD◀	▲0016M	▶Oncology (bladder), mRNA, microarray gene expression profiling of 219 genes, utilizing formalin-fixed paraffin-embedded tissue, algorithm reported as molecular subtype (luminal, luminal infiltrated, basal, basal claudin-low, neuroendocrine-like)◀
Lymph2Cx, Mayo Clinic Arizona Molecular Diagnostics Laboratory	0017M	Oncology (diffuse large B-cell lymphoma [DLBCL]), mRNA, gene expression profiling by fluorescent probe hybridization of 20 genes, formalin-fixed paraffin-embedded tissue, algorithm reported as cell of origin (Do not report 0017M in conjunction with 0120U)
Pleximark™, Plexision, Inc	0018M	Transplantation medicine (allograft rejection, renal), measurement of donor and third-party-induced CD154+T-cytotoxic memory cells, utilizing whole peripheral blood, algorithm reported as a rejection risk score (Do not report 0018M in conjunction with 81560, 85032, 86353, 86821, 88184, 88185, 88187, 88230, 88240, 88241)
Category I Codes for Multianalyte Assays with Algorithmic Analyses (MAAA)		
Vectra® DA, Crescendo Bioscience, Inc	81490	Autoimmune (rheumatoid arthritis), analysis of 12 biomarkers using immunoassays, utilizing serum, prognostic algorithm reported as a disease activity score (Do not report 81490 in conjunction with 86140)

(Continued on page 262)

Proprietary Name and Clinical Laboratory or Manufacturer	Alpha-Numeric Code	Code Descriptor
AlloMap®, CareDx, Inc	#81595	Cardiology (heart transplant), mRNA, gene expression profiling by real-time quantitative PCR of 20 genes (11 content and 9 housekeeping), utilizing subfraction of peripheral blood, algorithm reported as a rejection risk score
Corus® CAD, CardioDx, Inc	81493	Coronary artery disease, mRNA, gene expression profiling by real-time RT-PCR of 23 genes, utilizing whole peripheral blood, algorithm reported as a risk score
PreDx Diabetes Risk Score™, Tethys Clinical Laboratory	81506	Endocrinology (type 2 diabetes), biochemical assays of seven analytes (glucose, HbA1c, insulin, hs-CRP, adiponectin, ferritin, interleukin 2-receptor alpha), utilizing serum or plasma, algorithm reporting a risk score

(Do not report 81506 in conjunction with constituent components [ie, 82728, 82947, 83036, 83525, 86141], 84999 [for adopectin], and 83520 [for interleukin 2-receptor alpha]) |
| Harmony™ Prenatal Test, Ariosa Diagnostics | 81507 | Fetal aneuploidy (trisomy 21, 18, and 13) DNA sequence analysis of selected regions using maternal plasma, algorithm reported as a risk score for each trisomy

(Do not report 81228, 81229, 88271 when performing genomic sequencing procedures or other molecular multianalyte assays for copy number analysis) |

★ = Telemedicine ◀ = Audio-only ✚ = Add-on code ✔ = FDA approval pending # = Resequenced code ⊘ = Modifier 51 exempt

Proprietary Name and Clinical Laboratory or Manufacturer	Alpha-Numeric Code	Code Descriptor
No proprietary name and clinical laboratory or manufacturer. Maternal serum screening procedures are well-established procedures and are performed by many laboratories throughout the country. The concept of prenatal screens has existed and evolved for over 10 years and is not exclusive to any one facility.	81508	Fetal congenital abnormalities, biochemical assays of two proteins (PAPP-A, hCG [any form]), utilizing maternal serum, algorithm reported as a risk score (Do not report 81508 in conjunction with 84163, 84702)
	81509	Fetal congenital abnormalities, biochemical assays of three proteins (PAPP-A, hCG [any form], DIA), utilizing maternal serum, algorithm reported as a risk score (Do not report 81509 in conjunction with 84163, 84702, 86336)
	81510	Fetal congenital abnormalities, biochemical assays of three analytes (AFP, uE3, hCG [any form]), utilizing maternal serum, algorithm reported as a risk score (Do not report 81510 in conjunction with 82105, 82677, 84702)
	81511	Fetal congenital abnormalities, biochemical assays of four analytes (AFP, uE3, hCG [any form], DIA) utilizing maternal serum, algorithm reported as a risk score (may include additional results from previous biochemical testing) (Do not report 81511 in conjunction with 82105, 82677, 84702, 86336)
	81512	Fetal congenital abnormalities, biochemical assays of five analytes (AFP, uE3, total hCG, hyperglycosylated hCG, DIA) utilizing maternal serum, algorithm reported as a risk score (Do not report 81512 in conjunction with 82105, 82677, 84702, 86336)
Aptima® BV Assay, Hologic, Inc	81513	Infectious disease, bacterial vaginosis, quantitative real-time amplification of RNA markers for Atopobium vaginae, Gardnerella vaginalis, and Lactobacillus species, utilizing vaginal-fluid specimens, algorithm reported as a positive or negative result for bacterial vaginosis
BD MAX™ Vaginal Panel, Becton Dickson and Company	81514	Infectious disease, bacterial vaginosis and vaginitis, quantitative real-time amplification of DNA markers for Gardnerella vaginalis, Atopobium vaginae, Megasphaera type 1, Bacterial Vaginosis Associated Bacteria-2 (BVAB-2), and Lactobacillus species (L. crispatus and L. jensenii), utilizing vaginal-fluid specimens, algorithm reported as a positive or negative for high likelihood of bacterial vaginosis, includes separate detection of Trichomonas vaginalis and/or Candida species (C. albicans, C. tropicalis, C. parapsilosis, C. dubliniensis), Candida glabrata, Candida krusei, when reported (Do not report 81514 in conjunction with 87480, 87481, 87482, 87510, 87511, 87512, 87660, 87661)

(Continued on page 264)

Proprietary Name and Clinical Laboratory or Manufacturer	Alpha-Numeric Code	Code Descriptor
HCV FibroSURE™, FibroTest™, BioPredictive S.A.S.	#81596	Infectious disease, chronic hepatitis C virus (HCV) infection, six biochemical assays (ALT, A2-macroglobulin, apolipoprotein A-1, total bilirubin, GGT, and haptoglobin) utilizing serum, prognostic algorithm reported as scores for fibrosis and necroinflammatory activity in liver
Breast Cancer Index, Biotheranostics, Inc	81518	Oncology (breast), mRNA, gene expression profiling by real-time RT-PCR of 11 genes (7 content and 4 housekeeping), utilizing formalin-fixed paraffin-embedded tissue, algorithms reported as percentage risk for metastatic recurrence and likelihood of benefit from extended endocrine therapy
EndoPredict®, Myriad Genetic Laboratories, Inc	#81522	Oncology (breast), mRNA, gene expression profiling by RT-PCR of 12 genes (8 content and 4 housekeeping), utilizing formalin-fixed paraffin-embedded tissue, algorithm reported as recurrence risk score
Oncotype DX®, Genomic Health	81519	Oncology (breast), mRNA, gene expression profiling by real-time RT-PCR of 21 genes, utilizing formalin-fixed paraffin-embedded tissue, algorithm reported as recurrence score
Prosigna® Breast Cancer Assay, NanoString Technologies, Inc	81520	Oncology (breast), mRNA gene expression profiling by hybrid capture of 58 genes (50 content and 8 housekeeping), utilizing formalin-fixed paraffin-embedded tissue, algorithm reported as a recurrence risk score
MammaPrint®, Agendia, Inc	81521	Oncology (breast), mRNA, microarray gene expression profiling of 70 content genes and 465 housekeeping genes, utilizing fresh frozen or formalin-fixed paraffin-embedded tissue, algorithm reported as index related to risk of distant metastasis

(Do not report 81521 in conjunction with 81523 for the same specimen) |
| MammaPrint®, Agendia, Inc | 81523 | Oncology (breast), mRNA, next-generation sequencing gene expression profiling of 70 content genes and 31 housekeeping genes, utilizing formalin-fixed paraffin-embedded tissue, algorithm reported as index related to risk to distant metastasis

(Do not report 81523 in conjunction with 81521 for the same specimen) |
| Oncotype DX® Colon Cancer Assay, Genomic Health | 81525 | Oncology (colon), mRNA, gene expression profiling by real-time RT-PCR of 12 genes (7 content and 5 housekeeping), utilizing formalin-fixed paraffin-embedded tissue, algorithm reported as a recurrence score |

★ = Telemedicine   ◀ = Audio-only   ✛ = Add-on code   ✍ = FDA approval pending   # = Resequenced code   ⃠ = Modifier 51 exempt

Proprietary Name and Clinical Laboratory or Manufacturer	Alpha-Numeric Code	Code Descriptor
Cologuard™, Exact Sciences, Inc	81528	Oncology (colorectal) screening, quantitative real-time target and signal amplification of 10 DNA markers (*KRAS* mutations, promoter methylation of *NDRG4* and *BMP3*) and fecal hemoglobin, utilizing stool, algorithm reported as a positive or negative result (Do not report 81528 in conjunction with 81275, 82274)
DecisionDx® Melanoma, Castle Biosciences, Inc	81529	Oncology (cutaneous melanoma), mRNA, gene expression profiling by real-time RT-PCR of 31 genes (28 content and 3 housekeeping), utilizing formalin-fixed paraffin-embedded tissue, algorithm reported as recurrence risk, including likelihood of sentinel lymph node metastasis
ChemoFX®, Helomics, Corp	81535	Oncology (gynecologic), live tumor cell culture and chemotherapeutic response by DAPI stain and morphology, predictive algorithm reported as a drug response score; first single drug or drug combination
	+81536	each additional single drug or drug combination (List separately in addition to code for primary procedure) (Use 81536 in conjunction with 81535)
VeriStrat, Biodesix, Inc	81538	Oncology (lung), mass spectrometric 8-protein signature, including amyloid A, utilizing serum, prognostic and predictive algorithm reported as good versus poor overall survival
Risk of Ovarian Malignancy Algorithm (ROMA)™, Fujirebio Diagnostics	#81500	Oncology (ovarian), biochemical assays of two proteins (CA-125 and HE4), utilizing serum, with menopausal status, algorithm reported as a risk score (Do not report 81500 in conjunction with 86304, 86305)
OVA1™, Vermillion, Inc	#81503	Oncology (ovarian), biochemical assays of five proteins (CA-125, apolipoprotein A1, beta-2 microglobulin, transferrin, and pre-albumin), utilizing serum, algorithm reported as a risk score (Do not report 81503 in conjunction with 82172, 82232, 84134, 84466, 86304)
4Kscore test, OPKO Health, Inc	81539	Oncology (high-grade prostate cancer), biochemical assay of four proteins (Total PSA, Free PSA, Intact PSA, and human kallikrein-2 [hK2]), utilizing plasma or serum, prognostic algorithm reported as a probability score
Prolaris®, Myriad Genetic Laboratories, Inc	81541	Oncology (prostate), mRNA gene expression profiling by real-time RT-PCR of 46 genes (31 content and 15 housekeeping), utilizing formalin-fixed paraffin-embedded tissue, algorithm reported as a disease-specific mortality risk score

(*Continued on page 266*)

Appendix O

Proprietary Name and Clinical Laboratory or Manufacturer	Alpha-Numeric Code	Code Descriptor
Decipher® Prostate, Decipher® Biosciences	81542	Oncology (prostate), mRNA, microarray gene expression profiling of 22 content genes, utilizing formalin-fixed paraffin-embedded tissue, algorithm reported as metastasis risk score
—	(81545 has been deleted)	—
ConfirmMDx® for Prostate Cancer, MDxHealth, Inc	81551	Oncology (prostate), promoter methylation profiling by real-time PCR of 3 genes (GSTP1, APC, RASSF1), utilizing formalin-fixed paraffin-embedded tissue, algorithm reported as a likelihood of prostate cancer detection on repeat biopsy
Afirma® Genomic Sequencing Classifier, Veracyte, Inc	#81546	Oncology (thyroid), mRNA, gene expression analysis of 10,196 genes, utilizing fine needle aspirate, algorithm reported as a categorical result (eg, benign or suspicious)
Tissue of Origin Test Kit-FFPE, Cancer Genetics, Inc	#81504	Oncology (tissue of origin), microarray gene expression profiling of > 2000 genes, utilizing formalin-fixed paraffin-embedded tissue, algorithm reported as tissue similarity scores
CancerTYPE ID, bioTheranostics, Inc	#81540	Oncology (tumor of unknown origin), mRNA, gene expression profiling by real-time RT-PCR of 92 genes (87 content and 5 housekeeping) to classify tumor into main cancer type and subtype, utilizing formalin-fixed paraffin-embedded tissue, algorithm reported as a probability of a predicted main cancer type and subtype
DecisionDx®-UM test, Castle Biosciences, Inc	81552	Oncology (uveal melanoma), mRNA, gene expression profiling by real-time RT-PCR of 15 genes (12 content and 3 housekeeping), utilizing fine needle aspirate or formalin-fixed paraffin-embedded tissue, algorithm reported as risk of metastasis
Envisia® Genomic Classifier, Veracyte, Inc	81554	Pulmonary disease (idiopathic pulmonary fibrosis [IPF]), mRNA, gene expression analysis of 190 genes, utilizing transbronchial biopsies, diagnostic algorithm reported as categorical result (eg, positive or negative for high probability of usual interstitial pneumonia [UIP])
Pleximmune™, Plexision, Inc	81560	Transplantation medicine (allograft rejection, pediatric liver and small bowel), measurement of donor and third-party-induced CD154+T-cytotoxic memory cells, utilizing whole peripheral blood, algorithm reported as a rejection risk score (Do not report 81560 in conjunction with 85032, 86353, 86821, 88184, 88185, 88187, 88230, 88240, 88241, 0018M)
—	81599	Unlisted multianalyte assay with algorithmic analysis (Do not use 81599 for multianalyte assays with algorithmic analyses listed in Appendix O)

★ = Telemedicine   ◀ = Audio-only   ✚ = Add-on code   ✗ = FDA approval pending   # = Resequenced code   ⦸ = Modifier 51 exempt

Proprietary Name and Clinical Laboratory or Manufacturer	Alpha-Numeric Code	Code Descriptor
Proprietary Laboratory Analyses (PLA)		
PreciseType® HEA Test, Immucor, Inc	0001U	Red blood cell antigen typing, DNA, human erythrocyte antigen gene analysis of 35 antigens from 11 blood groups, utilizing whole blood, common RBC alleles reported
PolypDX™, Atlantic Diagnostic Laboratories, LLC, Metabolomic Technologies, Inc	0002U	Oncology (colorectal), quantitative assessment of three urine metabolites (ascorbic acid, succinic acid and carnitine) by liquid chromatography with tandem mass spectrometry (LC-MS/MS) using multiple reaction monitoring acquisition, algorithm reported as likelihood of adenomatous polyps
Overa (OVA1 Next Generation), Aspira Labs, Inc, Vermillion, Inc	0003U	Oncology (ovarian) biochemical assays of five proteins (apolipoprotein A-1, CA 125 II, follicle stimulating hormone, human epididymis protein 4, transferrin), utilizing serum, algorithm reported as a likelihood score
ExosomeDx® Prostate (IntelliScore), Exosome Diagnostics, Inc, Exosome Diagnostics, Inc	0005U	Oncology (prostate) gene expression profile by real-time RT-PCR of 3 genes (*ERG, PCA3,* and *SPDEF*), urine, algorithm reported as risk score
—	(0006U has been deleted)	—
ToxProtect, Genotox Laboratories LTD	0007U	Drug test(s), presumptive, with definitive confirmation of positive results, any number of drug classes, urine, includes specimen verification including DNA authentication in comparison to buccal DNA, per date of service
AmHPR® H. pylori Antibiotic Resistance Panel, American Molecular Laboratories, Inc	0008U	Helicobacter pylori detection and antibiotic resistance, DNA, 16S and 23S rRNA, gyrA, pbp1, rdxA and rpoB, next generation sequencing, formalin-fixed paraffin-embedded or fresh tissue or fecal sample, predictive, reported as positive or negative for resistance to clarithromycin, fluoroquinolones, metronidazole, amoxicillin, tetracycline, and rifabutin
DEPArray™ HER2, PacificDx	0009U	Oncology (breast cancer), *ERBB2* (HER2) copy number by FISH, tumor cells from formalin-fixed paraffin-embedded tissue isolated using image-based dielectrophoresis (DEP) sorting, reported as *ERBB2* gene amplified or non-amplified
Bacterial Typing by Whole Genome Sequencing, Mayo Clinic	0010U	Infectious disease (bacterial), strain typing by whole genome sequencing, phylogenetic-based report of strain relatedness, per submitted isolate
Cordant CORE™, Cordant Health Solutions	0011U	Prescription drug monitoring, evaluation of drugs present by LC-MS/MS, using oral fluid, reported as a comparison to an estimated steady-state range, per date of service including all drug compounds and metabolites
—	▶(0012U has been deleted)◀	—
—	▶(0013U has been deleted)◀	—

(Continued on page 268)

▲ = Revised code   ● = New code   ▶ ◀ = Contains new or revised text   ✖ = Duplicate PLA test   ↕ = Category I PLA   American Medical Association   **267**

Appendix O

Proprietary Name and Clinical Laboratory or Manufacturer	Alpha-Numeric Code	Code Descriptor
—	▶(0014U has been deleted)◀	—
BCR-ABL1 major and minor breakpoint fusion transcripts, University of Iowa, Department of Pathology, Asuragen	0016U	Oncology (hematolymphoid neoplasia), RNA, *BCR/ABL1* major and minor breakpoint fusion transcripts, quantitative PCR amplification, blood or bone marrow, report of fusion not detected or detected with quantitation
JAK2 Mutation, University of Iowa, Department of Pathology	0017U	Oncology (hematolymphoid neoplasia), *JAK2* mutation, DNA, PCR amplification of exons 12-14 and sequence analysis, blood or bone marrow, report of *JAK2* mutation not detected or detected
ThyraMIR™, Interpace Diagnostics	0018U	Oncology (thyroid), microRNA profiling by RT-PCR of 10 microRNA sequences, utilizing fine needle aspirate, algorithm reported as a positive or negative result for moderate to high risk of malignancy
OncoTarget/OncoTreat, Columbia University Department of Pathology and Cell Biology, Darwin Health	0019U	Oncology, RNA, gene expression by whole transcriptome sequencing, formalin-fixed paraffin-embedded tissue or fresh frozen tissue, predictive algorithm reported as potential targets for therapeutic agents
Apifiny®, Armune BioScience, Inc	0021U	Oncology (prostate), detection of 8 autoantibodies (ARF 6, NKX3-1, 5'-UTR-BMI1, CEP 164, 3'-UTR-Ropporin, Desmocollin, AURKAIP-1, CSNK2A2), multiplexed immunoassay and flow cytometry serum, algorithm reported as risk score
Oncomine™ Dx Target Test, Thermo Fisher Scientific, ▶Thermo Fisher Scientific◀	▲0022U	▶Targeted genomic sequence analysis panel, cholangiocarcinoma and non-small cell lung neoplasia, DNA and RNA analysis, 1-23 genes, interrogation for sequence variants and rearrangements, reported as presence/absence of variants and associated therapy(ies) to consider◀
LeukoStrat® CDx *FLT3* Mutation Assay, LabPMM LLC, an Invivoscribe Technologies, Inc Company, Invivoscribe Technologies, Inc	0023U	Oncology (acute myelogenous leukemia), DNA, genotyping of internal tandem duplication, p.D835, p.I836, using mononuclear cells, reported as detection or non-detection of *FLT3* mutation and indication for or against the use of midostaurin
GlycA, Laboratory Corporation of America, Laboratory Corporation of America	0024U	Glycosylated acute phase proteins (GlycA), nuclear magnetic resonance spectroscopy, quantitative
UrSure Tenofovir Quantification Test, Synergy Medical Laboratories, UrSure Inc	0025U	Tenofovir, by liquid chromatography with tandem mass spectrometry (LC-MS/MS), urine, quantitative
Thyroseq Genomic Classifier, CBLPath, Inc, University of Pittsburgh Medical Center	0026U	Oncology (thyroid), DNA and mRNA of 112 genes, next-generation sequencing, fine needle aspirate of thyroid nodule, algorithmic analysis reported as a categorical result ("Positive, high probability of malignancy" or "Negative, low probability of malignancy")
JAK2 Exons 12 to 15 Sequencing, Mayo Clinic, Mayo Clinic	0027U	*JAK2 (Janus kinase 2)* (eg, myeloproliferative disorder) gene analysis, targeted sequence analysis exons 12-15

★=Telemedicine ◀=Audio-only ✚=Add-on code ✗=FDA approval pending #=Resequenced code ⊘=Modifier 51 exempt

Proprietary Name and Clinical Laboratory or Manufacturer	Alpha-Numeric Code	Code Descriptor
Focused Pharmacogenomics Panel, Mayo Clinic, Mayo Clinic	0029U	Drug metabolism (adverse drug reactions and drug response), targeted sequence analysis (ie, *CYP1A2, CYP2C19, CYP2C9, CYP2D6, CYP3A4, CYP3A5, CYP4F2, SLCO1B1, VKORC1* and rs12777823)
Warfarin Response Genotype, Mayo Clinic, Mayo Clinic	0030U	Drug metabolism (warfarin drug response), targeted sequence analysis (ie, *CYP2C9, CYP4F2, VKORC1,* rs12777823)
Cytochrome P450 1A2 Genotype, Mayo Clinic, Mayo Clinic	0031U	*CYP1A2 (cytochrome P450 family 1, subfamily A, member 2)* (eg, drug metabolism) gene analysis, common variants (ie, *1F, *1K, *6, *7)
Catechol-O-Methyltransferase (*COMT*) Genotype, Mayo Clinic, Mayo Clinic	0032U	*COMT (catechol-O-methyltransferase)* (eg, drug metabolism) gene analysis, c.472G>A (rs4680) variant
Serotonin Receptor Genotype (*HTR2A* and *HTR2C*), Mayo Clinic, Mayo Clinic	0033U	*HTR2A (5-hydroxytryptamine receptor 2A), HTR2C (5-hydroxytryptamine receptor 2C)* (eg, citalopram metabolism) gene analysis, common variants (ie, *HTR2A* rs7997012 [c.614-2211T>C], *HTR2C* rs3813929 [c.-759C>T] and rs1414334 [c.551-3008C>G])
Thiopurine Methyltransferase (*TPMT*) and Nudix Hydrolase (*NUDT15*) Genotyping, Mayo Clinic, Mayo Clinic	0034U	*TPMT (thiopurine S-methyltransferase), NUDT15 (nudix hydroxylase 15)* (eg, thiopurine metabolism) gene analysis, common variants (ie, *TPMT* *2, *3A, *3B, *3C, *4, *5, *6, *8, *12; *NUDT15* *3, *4, *5)
Real-time quaking-induced conversion for prion detection (RT-QuIC), National Prion Disease Pathology Surveillance Center	0035U	Neurology (prion disease), cerebrospinal fluid, detection of prion protein by quaking-induced conformational conversion, qualitative
EXaCT-1 Whole Exome Testing, Lab of Oncology-Molecular Detection, Weill Cornell Medicine-Clinical Genomics Laboratory	0036U	Exome (ie, somatic mutations), paired formalin-fixed paraffin-embedded tumor tissue and normal specimen, sequence analyses
FoundationOne CDx™ (F1CDx), Foundation Medicine, Inc, Foundation Medicine, Inc	0037U	Targeted genomic sequence analysis, solid organ neoplasm, DNA analysis of 324 genes, interrogation for sequence variants, gene copy number amplifications, gene rearrangements, microsatellite instability and tumor mutational burden
Sensieva™ Droplet 25OH Vitamin D2/D3 Microvolume LC/MS Assay, InSource Diagnostics, InSource Diagnostics	0038U	Vitamin D, 25 hydroxy D2 and D3, by LC-MS/MS, serum microsample, quantitative
Anti-dsDNA, High Salt/Avidity, University of Washington, Department of Laboratory Medicine, Bio-Rad	0039U	Deoxyribonucleic acid (DNA) antibody, double stranded, high avidity
MRDx BCR-ABL Test, MolecularMD, MolecularMD	0040U	*BCR/ABL1 (t(9;22))* (eg, chronic myelogenous leukemia) translocation analysis, major breakpoint, quantitative
Lyme ImmunoBlot IgM, IGeneX Inc, ID-FISH Technology Inc (ASR) (Lyme ImmunoBlot IgM Strips Only)	0041U	Borrelia burgdorferi, antibody detection of 5 recombinant protein groups, by immunoblot, IgM

(Continued on page 270)

Proprietary Name and Clinical Laboratory or Manufacturer	Alpha-Numeric Code	Code Descriptor
Lyme ImmunoBlot IgG, IGeneX Inc, ID-FISH Technology Inc (ASR) (Lyme ImmunoBlot IgG Strips Only)	0042U	Borrelia burgdorferi, antibody detection of 12 recombinant protein groups, by immunoblot, IgG
Tick-Borne Relapsing Fever (TBRF) Borrelia ImmunoBlots IgM Test, IGeneX Inc, ID-FISH Technology (Provides TBRF ImmunoBlot IgM Strips)	0043U	Tick-borne relapsing fever Borrelia group, antibody detection to 4 recombinant protein groups, by immunoblot, IgM
Tick-Borne Relapsing Fever (TBRF) Borrelia ImmunoBlots IgG Test, IGeneX Inc, ID-FISH Technology Inc (Provides TBRF ImmunoBlot IgG Strips)	0044U	Tick-borne relapsing fever Borrelia group, antibody detection to 4 recombinant protein groups, by immunoblot, IgG
The Oncotype DX® Breast DCIS Score™ Test, Genomic Health, Inc, Genomic Health, Inc	0045U	Oncology (breast ductal carcinoma in situ), mRNA, gene expression profiling by real-time RT-PCR of 12 genes (7 content and 5 housekeeping), utilizing formalin-fixed paraffin-embedded tissue, algorithm reported as recurrence score
FLT3 ITD MRD by NGS, LabPMM LLC, an Invivoscribe Technologies, Inc Company	0046U	*FLT3 (fms-related tyrosine kinase 3)* (eg, acute myeloid leukemia) internal tandem duplication (ITD) variants, quantitative
Oncotype DX Genomic Prostate Score, Genomic Health, Inc, Genomic Health, Inc	0047U	Oncology (prostate), mRNA, gene expression profiling by real-time RT-PCR of 17 genes (12 content and 5 housekeeping), utilizing formalin-fixed paraffin-embedded tissue, algorithm reported as a risk score
MSK-IMPACT (Integrated Mutation Profiling of Actionable Cancer Targets), Memorial Sloan Kettering Cancer Center	0048U	Oncology (solid organ neoplasia), DNA, targeted sequencing of protein-coding exons of 468 cancer-associated genes, including interrogation for somatic mutations and microsatellite instability, matched with normal specimens, utilizing formalin-fixed paraffin-embedded tumor tissue, report of clinically significant mutation(s)
NPM1 MRD by NGS, LabPMM LLC, an Invivoscribe Technologies, Inc Company	0049U	*NPM1 (nucleophosmin)* (eg, acute myeloid leukemia) gene analysis, quantitative
MyAML NGS Panel, LabPMM LLC, an Invivoscribe Technologies, Inc Company	0050U	Targeted genomic sequence analysis panel, acute myelogenous leukemia, DNA analysis, 194 genes, interrogation for sequence variants, copy number variants or rearrangements
UCompliDx, Elite Medical Laboratory Solutions, LLC, Elite Medical Laboratory Solutions, LLC (LDT)	0051U	Prescription drug monitoring, evaluation of drugs present by liquid chromatography tandem mass spectrometry (LC-MS/MS), urine or blood, 31 drug panel, reported as quantitative results, detected or not detected, per date of service
VAP Cholesterol Test, VAP Diagnostics Laboratory, Inc, VAP Diagnostics Laboratory, Inc	0052U	Lipoprotein, blood, high resolution fractionation and quantitation of lipoproteins, including all five major lipoprotein classes and subclasses of HDL, LDL, and VLDL by vertical auto profile ultracentrifugation

★ = Telemedicine   ◀ = Audio-only   ✦ = Add-on code   ✗ = FDA approval pending   # = Resequenced code   ⊘ = Modifier 51 exempt

Proprietary Name and Clinical Laboratory or Manufacturer	Alpha-Numeric Code	Code Descriptor
Prostate Cancer Risk Panel, Mayo Clinic, Laboratory Developed Test	0053U	Oncology (prostate cancer), FISH analysis of 4 genes (*ASAP1, HDAC9, CHD1* and *PTEN*), needle biopsy specimen, algorithm reported as probability of higher tumor grade
AssuranceRx Micro Serum, Firstox Laboratories, LLC, Firstox Laboratories, LLC	0054U	Prescription drug monitoring, 14 or more classes of drugs and substances, definitive tandem mass spectrometry with chromatography, capillary blood, quantitative report with therapeutic and toxic ranges, including steady-state range for the prescribed dose when detected, per date of service
myTAIHEART, TAI Diagnostics, Inc, TAI Diagnostics, Inc	0055U	Cardiology (heart transplant), cell-free DNA, PCR assay of 96 DNA target sequences (94 single nucleotide polymorphism targets and two control targets), plasma
—	▶(0056U has been deleted)◀	—
Merkel SmT Oncoprotein Antibody Titer, University of Washington, Department of Laboratory Medicine	0058U	Oncology (Merkel cell carcinoma), detection of antibodies to the Merkel cell polyoma virus oncoprotein (small T antigen), serum, quantitative
Merkel Virus VP1 Capsid Antibody, University of Washington, Department of Laboratory Medicine	0059U	Oncology (Merkel cell carcinoma), detection of antibodies to the Merkel cell polyoma virus capsid protein (VP1), serum, reported as positive or negative
Twins Zygosity PLA, Natera, Inc, Natera, Inc	0060U	Twin zygosity, genomic-targeted sequence analysis of chromosome 2, using circulating cell-free fetal DNA in maternal blood
Transcutaneous multispectral measurement of tissue oxygenation and hemoglobin using spatial frequency domain imaging (SFDI), Modulated Imaging, Inc, Modulated Imaging, Inc	0061U	Transcutaneous measurement of five biomarkers (tissue oxygenation [StO_2], oxyhemoglobin [$ctHbO_2$], deoxyhemoglobin [$ctHbR$], papillary and reticular dermal hemoglobin concentrations [$ctHb1$ and $ctHb2$]), using spatial frequency domain imaging (SFDI) and multi-spectral analysis
SLE-key® Rule Out, Veracis Inc, Veracis Inc	0062U	Autoimmune (systemic lupus erythematosus), IgG and IgM analysis of 80 biomarkers, utilizing serum, algorithm reported with a risk score
NPDX ASD ADM Panel I, Stemina Biomarker Discovery, Inc, Stemina Biomarker Discovery, Inc d/b/a NeuroPointDX	0063U	Neurology (autism), 32 amines by LC-MS/MS, using plasma, algorithm reported as metabolic signature associated with autism spectrum disorder
BioPlex 2200 Syphilis Total & RPR Assay, Bio-Rad Laboratories, Bio-Rad Laboratories	0064U	Antibody, Treponema pallidum, total and rapid plasma reagin (RPR), immunoassay, qualitative
BioPlex 2200 RPR Assay, Bio-Rad Laboratories, Bio-Rad Laboratories	0065U	Syphilis test, non-treponemal antibody, immunoassay, qualitative (RPR)
PartoSure™ Test, Parsagen Diagnostics, Inc, Parsagen Diagnostics, Inc, a QIAGEN Company	0066U	Placental alpha-micro globulin-1 (PAMG-1), immunoassay with direct optical observation, cervico-vaginal fluid, each specimen

(*Continued on page 272*)

▲=Revised code   ●=New code   ▶ ◀=Contains new or revised text   ✕=Duplicate PLA test   ⇅=Category I PLA   **American Medical Association   271**

Appendix O

Proprietary Name and Clinical Laboratory or Manufacturer	Alpha-Numeric Code	Code Descriptor
BBDRisk Dx™, Silbiotech, Inc, Silbiotech, Inc	0067U	Oncology (breast), immunohistochemistry, protein expression profiling of 4 biomarkers (matrix metalloproteinase-1 [MMP-1], carcinoembryonic antigen-related cell adhesion molecule 6 [CEACAM6], hyaluronoglucosaminidase [HYAL1], highly expressed in cancer protein [HEC1]), formalin-fixed paraffin-embedded precancerous breast tissue, algorithm reported as carcinoma risk score
MYCODART-PCR™ Dual Amplification Real Time PCR Panel for 6 Candida species, RealTime Laboratories, Inc/MycoDART, Inc, RealTime Laboratories, Inc	0068U	Candida species panel *(C. albicans, C. glabrata, C. parapsilosis, C. kruseii, C. tropicalis,* and *C. auris),* amplified probe technique with qualitative report of the presence or absence of each species
miR-31*now*™, GoPath Laboratories, GoPath Laboratories	0069U	Oncology (colorectal), microRNA, RT-PCR expression profiling of miR-31-3p, formalin-fixed paraffin-embedded tissue, algorithm reported as an expression score
CYP2D6 Common Variants and Copy Number, Mayo Clinic, Laboratory Developed Test	0070U	*CYP2D6 (cytochrome P450, family 2, subfamily D, polypeptide 6)* (eg, drug metabolism) gene analysis, common and select rare variants (ie, *2, *3, *4, *4N, *5, *6, *7, *8, *9, *10, *11, *12, *13, *14A, *14B, *15, *17, *29, *35, *36, *41, *57, *61, *63, *68, *83, *xN)
CYP2D6 Full Gene Sequencing, Mayo Clinic, Laboratory Developed Test	✚0071U	*CYP2D6 (cytochrome P450, family 2, subfamily D, polypeptide 6)* (eg, drug metabolism) gene analysis, full gene sequence (List separately in addition to code for primary procedure) (Use 0071U in conjunction with 0070U)
CYP2D6-2D7 Hybrid Gene Targeted Sequence Analysis, Mayo Clinic, Laboratory Developed Test	✚0072U	*CYP2D6 (cytochrome P450, family 2, subfamily D, polypeptide 6)* (eg, drug metabolism) gene analysis, targeted sequence analysis (ie, *CYP2D6-2D7* hybrid gene) (List separately in addition to code for primary procedure) (Use 0072U in conjunction with 0070U)
CYP2D7-2D6 Hybrid Gene Targeted Sequence Analysis, Mayo Clinic, Laboratory Developed Test	✚0073U	*CYP2D6 (cytochrome P450, family 2, subfamily D, polypeptide 6)* (eg, drug metabolism) gene analysis, targeted sequence analysis (ie, *CYP2D7-2D6* hybrid gene) (List separately in addition to code for primary procedure) (Use 0073U in conjunction with 0070U)
CYP2D6 trans-duplication/ multiplication non-duplicated gene targeted sequence analysis, Mayo Clinic, Laboratory Developed Test	✚0074U	*CYP2D6 (cytochrome P450, family 2, subfamily D, polypeptide 6)* (eg, drug metabolism) gene analysis, targeted sequence analysis (ie, non-duplicated gene when duplication/multiplication is trans) (List separately in addition to code for primary procedure) (Use 0074U in conjunction with 0070U)

★=Telemedicine   ◀=Audio-only   ✚=Add-on code   ✔=FDA approval pending   #=Resequenced code   ⊘=Modifier 51 exempt

Proprietary Name and Clinical Laboratory or Manufacturer	Alpha-Numeric Code	Code Descriptor
CYP2D6 5' gene duplication/ multiplication targeted sequence analysis, Mayo Clinic, Laboratory Developed Test	✚0075U	*CYP2D6 (cytochrome P450, family 2, subfamily D, polypeptide 6)* (eg, drug metabolism) gene analysis, targeted sequence analysis (ie, 5' gene duplication/ multiplication) (List separately in addition to code for primary procedure)
		(Use 0075U in conjunction with 0070U)
CYP2D6 3' gene duplication/ multiplication targeted sequence analysis, Mayo Clinic, Laboratory Developed Test	✚0076U	*CYP2D6 (cytochrome P450, family 2, subfamily D, polypeptide 6)* (eg, drug metabolism) gene analysis, targeted sequence analysis (ie, 3' gene duplication/ multiplication) (List separately in addition to code for primary procedure)
		(Use 0076U in conjunction with 0070U)
M-Protein Detection and Isotyping by MALDI-TOF Mass Spectrometry, Mayo Clinic, Laboratory Developed Test	0077U	Immunoglobulin paraprotein (M-protein), qualitative, immunoprecipitation and mass spectrometry, blood or urine, including isotype
INFINITI® Neural Response Panel, PersonalizeDx Labs, AutoGenomics Inc	0078U	Pain management (opioid-use disorder) genotyping panel, 16 common variants (ie, *ABCB1, COMT, DAT1, DBH, DOR, DRD1, DRD2, DRD4, GABA, GAL, HTR2A, HTTLPR, MTHFR, MUOR, OPRK1, OPRM1),* buccal swab or other germline tissue sample, algorithm reported as positive or negative risk of opioid-use disorder
ToxLok™, InSource Diagnostics, InSource Diagnostics	0079U	Comparative DNA analysis using multiple selected single-nucleotide polymorphisms (SNPs), urine and buccal DNA, for specimen identity verification
BDX-XL2, Biodesix®, Inc, Biodesix®, Inc	0080U	Oncology (lung), mass spectrometric analysis of galectin-3-binding protein and scavenger receptor cysteine-rich type 1 protein M130, with five clinical risk factors (age, smoking status, nodule diameter, nodule-spiculation status and nodule location), utilizing plasma, algorithm reported as a categorical probability of malignancy
NextGen Precision™ Testing, Precision Diagnostics, Precision Diagnostics LBN Precision Toxicology, LLC	0082U	Drug test(s), definitive, 90 or more drugs or substances, definitive chromatography with mass spectrometry, and presumptive, any number of drug classes, by instrument chemistry analyzer (utilizing immunoassay), urine, report of presence or absence of each drug, drug metabolite or substance with description and severity of significant interactions per date of service
Onco4D™, Animated Dynamics, Inc, Animated Dynamics, Inc	0083U	Oncology, response to chemotherapy drugs using motility contrast tomography, fresh or frozen tissue, reported as likelihood of sensitivity or resistance to drugs or drug combinations
BLOODchip® ID CORE XT™, Grifols Diagnostic Solutions Inc	0084U	Red blood cell antigen typing, DNA, genotyping of 10 blood groups with phenotype prediction of 37 red blood cell antigens
—	(0085U has been deleted)	—

(Continued on page 274)

▲ = Revised code   ● = New code   ▶ ◀ = Contains new or revised text   ✖ = Duplicate PLA test   ↑↓ = Category I PLA   American Medical Association   **273**

Appendix O

Proprietary Name and Clinical Laboratory or Manufacturer	Alpha-Numeric Code	Code Descriptor
Accelerate PhenoTest™ BC kit, Accelerate Diagnostics, Inc	0086U	Infectious disease (bacterial and fungal), organism identification, blood culture, using rRNA FISH, 6 or more organism targets, reported as positive or negative with phenotypic minimum inhibitory concentration (MIC)-based antimicrobial susceptibility
Molecular Microscope® MMDx— Heart, Kashi Clinical Laboratories	0087U	Cardiology (heart transplant), mRNA gene expression profiling by microarray of 1283 genes, transplant biopsy tissue, allograft rejection and injury algorithm reported as a probability score
Molecular Microscope® MMDx— Kidney, Kashi Clinical Laboratories	0088U	Transplantation medicine (kidney allograft rejection), microarray gene expression profiling of 1494 genes, utilizing transplant biopsy tissue, algorithm reported as a probability score for rejection
Pigmented Lesion Assay (PLA), DermTech	0089U	Oncology (melanoma), gene expression profiling by RTqPCR, *PRAME* and *LINC00518*, superficial collection using adhesive patch(es)
myPath® Melanoma, ▶Castle Biosciences, Inc◀	▲0090U	▶Oncology (cutaneous melanoma), mRNA gene expression profiling by RT-PCR of 23 genes (14 content and 9 housekeeping), utilizing formalin-fixed paraffin-embedded (FFPE) tissue, algorithm reported as a categorical result (ie, benign, intermediate, malignant)◀
FirstSight^CRC, CellMax Life	0091U	Oncology (colorectal) screening, cell enumeration of circulating tumor cells, utilizing whole blood, algorithm, for the presence of adenoma or cancer, reported as a positive or negative result
REVEAL Lung Nodule Characterization, MagArray, Inc	0092U	Oncology (lung), three protein biomarkers, immunoassay using magnetic nanosensor technology, plasma, algorithm reported as risk score for likelihood of malignancy
ComplyRX, Claro Labs	0093U	Prescription drug monitoring, evaluation of 65 common drugs by LC-MS/MS, urine, each drug reported detected or not detected
RCIGM Rapid Whole Genome Sequencing, Rady Children's Institute for Genomic Medicine (RCIGM)	0094U	Genome (eg, unexplained constitutional or heritable disorder or syndrome), rapid sequence analysis
Esophageal String Test™ (EST), Cambridge Biomedical, Inc	0095U	Inflammation (eosinophilic esophagitis), ELISA analysis of eotaxin-3 *(CCL26 [C-C motif chemokine ligand 26])* and major basic protein *(PRG2 [proteoglycan 2, pro eosinophil major basic protein])*, specimen obtained by swallowed nylon string, algorithm reported as predictive probability index for active eosinophilic esophagitis
HPV, High-Risk, Male Urine, Molecular Testing Labs	0096U	Human papillomavirus (HPV), high-risk types (ie, 16, 18, 31, 33, 35, 39, 45, 51, 52, 56, 58, 59, 66, 68), male urine
—	▶(0097U has been deleted)◀	—
—	(0098U has been deleted)	—
—	(0099U has been deleted)	—

★=Telemedicine   ◀=Audio-only   ✚=Add-on code   ⭕=FDA approval pending   #=Resequenced code   ⊘=Modifier 51 exempt

Proprietary Name and Clinical Laboratory or Manufacturer	Alpha-Numeric Code	Code Descriptor
—	(0100U has been deleted)	—
ColoNext®, Ambry Genetics®, Ambry Genetics®	0101U	Hereditary colon cancer disorders (eg, Lynch syndrome, *PTEN* hamartoma syndrome, Cowden syndrome, familial adenomatosis polyposis), genomic sequence analysis panel utilizing a combination of NGS, Sanger, MLPA, and array CGH, with mRNA analytics to resolve variants of unknown significance when indicated (15 genes [sequencing and deletion/duplication], *EPCAM* and *GREM1* [deletion/duplication only])
BreastNext®, Ambry Genetics®, Ambry Genetics®	0102U	Hereditary breast cancer-related disorders (eg, hereditary breast cancer, hereditary ovarian cancer, hereditary endometrial cancer), genomic sequence analysis panel utilizing a combination of NGS, Sanger, MLPA, and array CGH, with mRNA analytics to resolve variants of unknown significance when indicated (17 genes [sequencing and deletion/duplication])
OvaNext®, Ambry Genetics®, Ambry Genetics®	0103U	Hereditary ovarian cancer (eg, hereditary ovarian cancer, hereditary endometrial cancer), genomic sequence analysis panel utilizing a combination of NGS, Sanger, MLPA, and array CGH, with mRNA analytics to resolve variants of unknown significance when indicated (24 genes [sequencing and deletion/duplication], *EPCAM* [deletion/duplication only])
KidneyIntelX™, RenalytixAI, RenalytixAI	0105U	Nephrology (chronic kidney disease), multiplex electrochemiluminescent immunoassay (ECLIA) of tumor necrosis factor receptor 1A, receptor superfamily 2 *(TNFR1, TNFR2),* and kidney injury molecule-1 (KIM-1) combined with longitudinal clinical data, including *APOL1* genotype if available, and plasma (isolated fresh or frozen), algorithm reported as probability score for rapid kidney function decline (RKFD)
13C-Spirulina Gastric Emptying Breath Test (GEBT), Cairn Diagnostics d/b/a Advanced Breath Diagnostics, LLC, Cairn Diagnostics d/b/a Advanced Breath Diagnostics, LLC	0106U	Gastric emptying, serial collection of 7 timed breath specimens, non-radioisotope carbon-13 (^{13}C) spirulina substrate, analysis of each specimen by gas isotope ratio mass spectrometry, reported as rate of $^{13}CO_2$ excretion
Singulex Clarity C. diff toxins A/B Assay, Singulex	0107U	Clostridium difficile toxin(s) antigen detection by immunoassay technique, stool, qualitative, multiple-step method
TissueCypher® Barrett's Esophagus Assay, Cernostics, Cernostics	0108U	Gastroenterology (Barrett's esophagus), whole slide–digital imaging, including morphometric analysis, computer-assisted quantitative immunolabeling of 9 protein biomarkers (p16, AMACR, p53, CD68, COX-2, CD45RO, HIF1a, HER-2, K20) and morphology, formalin-fixed paraffin-embedded tissue, algorithm reported as risk of progression to high-grade dysplasia or cancer

(Continued on page 276)

Appendix O

Proprietary Name and Clinical Laboratory or Manufacturer	Alpha-Numeric Code	Code Descriptor
MYCODART Dual Amplification Real Time PCR Panel for 4 Aspergillus species, RealTime Laboratories, Inc/MycoDART, Inc	0109U	Infectious disease (Aspergillus species), real-time PCR for detection of DNA from 4 species (*A. fumigatus, A. terreus, A. niger,* and *A. flavus*), blood, lavage fluid, or tissue, qualitative reporting of presence or absence of each species
Oral OncolyticAssuranceRX, Firstox Laboratories, LLC, Firstox Laboratories, LLC	0110U	Prescription drug monitoring, one or more oral oncology drug(s) and substances, definitive tandem mass spectrometry with chromatography, serum or plasma from capillary blood or venous blood, quantitative report with steady-state range for the prescribed drug(s) when detected)
Praxis™ Extended RAS Panel, Illumina, Illumina	0111U	Oncology (colon cancer), targeted *KRAS* (codons 12, 13, and 61) and *NRAS* (codons 12, 13, and 61) gene analysis, utilizing formalin-fixed paraffin-embedded tissue
MicroGenDX qPCR & NGS For Infection, MicroGenDX, MicroGenDX	0112U	Infectious agent detection and identification, targeted sequence analysis (16S and 18S rRNA genes) with drug-resistance gene
MiPS (Mi-Prostate Score), MLabs, MLabs	0113U	Oncology (prostate), measurement of *PCA3* and *TMPRSS2-ERG* in urine and PSA in serum following prostatic massage, by RNA amplification and fluorescence-based detection, algorithm reported as risk score
EsoGuard™, Lucid Diagnostics, Lucid Diagnostics	0114U	Gastroenterology (Barrett's esophagus), *VIM* and *CCNA1* methylation analysis, esophageal cells, algorithm reported as likelihood for Barrett's esophagus
ePlex Respiratory Pathogen (RP) Panel, GenMark Diagnostics, Inc, GenMark Diagnostics, Inc	0115U	Respiratory infectious agent detection by nucleic acid (DNA and RNA), 18 viral types and subtypes and 2 bacterial targets, amplified probe technique, including multiplex reverse transcription for RNA targets, each analyte reported as detected or not detected
Snapshot Oral Fluid Compliance, Ethos Laboratories	0116U	Prescription drug monitoring, enzyme immunoassay of 35 or more drugs confirmed with LC-MS/MS, oral fluid, algorithm results reported as a patient-compliance measurement with risk of drug to drug interactions for prescribed medications
Foundation PI^SM, Ethos Laboratories	0117U	Pain management, analysis of 11 endogenous analytes (methylmalonic acid, xanthurenic acid, homocysteine, pyroglutamic acid, vanilmandelate, 5-hydroxyindoleacetic acid, hydroxymethylglutarate, ethylmalonate, 3-hydroxypropyl mercapturic acid (3-HPMA), quinolinic acid, kynurenic acid), LC-MS/MS, urine, algorithm reported as a pain-index score with likelihood of atypical biochemical function associated with pain
Viracor TRAC™ dd-cfDNA, Viracor Eurofins, Viracor Eurofins	0118U	Transplantation medicine, quantification of donor-derived cell-free DNA using whole genome next-generation sequencing, plasma, reported as percentage of donor-derived cell-free DNA in the total cell-free DNA

★ = Telemedicine ◀ = Audio-only ✚ = Add-on code ⟋ = FDA approval pending # = Resequenced code ⊘ = Modifier 51 exempt

Proprietary Name and Clinical Laboratory or Manufacturer	Alpha-Numeric Code	Code Descriptor
MI-HEART Ceramides, Plasma, Mayo Clinic, Laboratory Developed Test	0119U	Cardiology, ceramides by liquid chromatography–tandem mass spectrometry, plasma, quantitative report with risk score for major cardiovascular events
Lymph3Cx Lymphoma Molecular Subtyping Assay, Mayo Clinic, Laboratory Developed Test	0120U	Oncology (B-cell lymphoma classification), mRNA, gene expression profiling by fluorescent probe hybridization of 58 genes (45 content and 13 housekeeping genes), formalin-fixed paraffin-embedded tissue, algorithm reported as likelihood for primary mediastinal B-cell lymphoma (PMBCL) and diffuse large B-cell lymphoma (DLBCL) with cell of origin subtyping in the latter (Do not report 0120U in conjunction with 0017M)
Flow Adhesion of Whole Blood on VCAM-1 (FAB-V), Functional Fluidics, Functional Fluidics	0121U	Sickle cell disease, microfluidic flow adhesion (VCAM-1), whole blood
Flow Adhesion of Whole Blood to P-SELECTIN (WB-PSEL), Functional Fluidics, Functional Fluidics	0122U	Sickle cell disease, microfluidic flow adhesion (P-Selectin), whole blood
Mechanical Fragility, RBC by shear stress profiling and spectral analysis, Functional Fluidics, Functional Fluidics	0123U	Mechanical fragility, RBC, shear stress and spectral analysis profiling
—	(0124U has been deleted)	—
—	(0125U has been deleted)	—
—	(0126U has been deleted)	—
—	(0127U has been deleted)	—
—	(0128U has been deleted)	—
BRCAplus, Ambry Genetics	0129U	Hereditary breast cancer–related disorders (eg, hereditary breast cancer, hereditary ovarian cancer, hereditary endometrial cancer), genomic sequence analysis and deletion/duplication analysis panel (ATM, BRCA1, BRCA2, CDH1, CHEK2, PALB2, PTEN, and TP53)
+RNAinsight™ for ColoNext®, Ambry Genetics	+0130U	Hereditary colon cancer disorders (eg, Lynch syndrome, PTEN hamartoma syndrome, Cowden syndrome, familial adenomatosis polyposis), targeted mRNA sequence analysis panel (APC, CDH1, CHEK2, MLH1, MSH2, MSH6, MUTYH, PMS2, PTEN, and TP53) (List separately in addition to code for primary procedure) (Use 0130U in conjunction with 81435, 0101U)
+RNAinsight™ for BreastNext®, Ambry Genetics	+0131U	Hereditary breast cancer–related disorders (eg, hereditary breast cancer, hereditary ovarian cancer, hereditary endometrial cancer), targeted mRNA sequence analysis panel (13 genes) (List separately in addition to code for primary procedure) (Use 0131U in conjunction with 81162, 81432, 0102U)

(Continued on page 278)

Appendix O

Proprietary Name and Clinical Laboratory or Manufacturer	Alpha-Numeric Code	Code Descriptor
+RNAinsight™ for OvaNext®, Ambry Genetics	✚0132U	Hereditary ovarian cancer–related disorders (eg, hereditary breast cancer, hereditary ovarian cancer, hereditary endometrial cancer), targeted mRNA sequence analysis panel (17 genes) (List separately in addition to code for primary procedure) (Use 0132U in conjunction with 81162, 81432, 0103U)
+RNAinsight™ for ProstateNext®, Ambry Genetics	✚0133U	Hereditary prostate cancer–related disorders, targeted mRNA sequence analysis panel (11 genes) (List separately in addition to code for primary procedure) (Use 0133U in conjunction with 81162)
+RNAinsight™ for CancerNext®, Ambry Genetics	✚0134U	Hereditary pan cancer (eg, hereditary breast and ovarian cancer, hereditary endometrial cancer, hereditary colorectal cancer), targeted mRNA sequence analysis panel (18 genes) (List separately in addition to code for primary procedure) (Use 0134U in conjunction with 81162, 81432, 81435)
+RNAinsight™ for GYNPlus®, Ambry Genetics	✚0135U	Hereditary gynecological cancer (eg, hereditary breast and ovarian cancer, hereditary endometrial cancer, hereditary colorectal cancer), targeted mRNA sequence analysis panel (12 genes) (List separately in addition to code for primary procedure) (Use 0135U in conjunction with 81162)
+RNAinsight™ for *ATM*, Ambry Genetics	✚0136U	*ATM (ataxia telangiectasia mutated)* (eg, ataxia telangiectasia) mRNA sequence analysis (List separately in addition to code for primary procedure) (Use 0136U in conjunction with 81408)
+RNAinsight™ for *PALB2*, Ambry Genetics	✚0137U	*PALB2 (partner and localizer of BRCA2)* (eg, breast and pancreatic cancer) mRNA sequence analysis (List separately in addition to code for primary procedure) (Use 0137U in conjunction with 81307)
+RNAinsight™ for *BRCA1/2*, Ambry Genetics	✚0138U	*BRCA1 (BRCA1, DNA repair associated), BRCA2 (BRCA2, DNA repair associated)* (eg, hereditary breast and ovarian cancer) mRNA sequence analysis (List separately in addition to code for primary procedure) (Use 0138U in conjunction with 81162)
—	(0139U has been deleted)	—
ePlex® BCID Fungal Pathogens Panel, GenMark Diagnostics, Inc, GenMark Diagnostics, Inc	0140U	Infectious disease (fungi), fungal pathogen identification, DNA (15 fungal targets), blood culture, amplified probe technique, each target reported as detected or not detected

★=Telemedicine ◀=Audio-only ✚=Add-on code ✗=FDA approval pending #=Resequenced code ⊘=Modifier 51 exempt

Proprietary Name and Clinical Laboratory or Manufacturer	Alpha-Numeric Code	Code Descriptor
ePlex® BCID Gram-Positive Panel, GenMark Diagnostics, Inc, GenMark Diagnostics, Inc	0141U	Infectious disease (bacteria and fungi), gram-positive organism identification and drug resistance element detection, DNA (20 gram-positive bacterial targets, 4 resistance genes, 1 pan gram-negative bacterial target, 1 pan Candida target), blood culture, amplified probe technique, each target reported as detected or not detected
ePlex® BCID Gram-Negative Panel, GenMark Diagnostics, Inc, GenMark Diagnostics, Inc	0142U	Infectious disease (bacteria and fungi), gram-negative bacterial identification and drug resistance element detection, DNA (21 gram-negative bacterial targets, 6 resistance genes, 1 pan gram-positive bacterial target, 1 pan Candida target), amplified probe technique, each target reported as detected or not detected
CareViewRx, Newstar Medical Laboratories, LLC, Newstar Medical Laboratories, LLC	� 0143U	Drug assay, definitive, 120 or more drugs or metabolites, urine, quantitative liquid chromatography with tandem mass spectrometry (LC-MS/MS) using multiple reaction monitoring (MRM), with drug or metabolite description, comments including sample validation, per date of service (For additional PLA code with identical clinical descriptor, see 0150U. See Appendix O to determine appropriate code assignment)
CareViewRx Plus, Newstar Medical Laboratories, LLC, Newstar Medical Laboratories, LLC	0144U	Drug assay, definitive, 160 or more drugs or metabolites, urine, quantitative liquid chromatography with tandem mass spectrometry (LC-MS/MS) using multiple reaction monitoring (MRM), with drug or metabolite description, comments including sample validation, per date of service
PainViewRx, Newstar Medical Laboratories, LLC, Newstar Medical Laboratories, LLC	0145U	Drug assay, definitive, 65 or more drugs or metabolites, urine, quantitative liquid chromatography with tandem mass spectrometry (LC-MS/MS) using multiple reaction monitoring (MRM), with drug or metabolite description, comments including sample validation, per date of service
PainViewRx Plus, Newstar Medical Laboratories, LLC, Newstar Medical Laboratories, LLC	0146U	Drug assay, definitive, 80 or more drugs or metabolites, urine, by quantitative liquid chromatography with tandem mass spectrometry (LC-MS/MS) using multiple reaction monitoring (MRM), with drug or metabolite description, comments including sample validation, per date of service
RiskViewRx, Newstar Medical Laboratories, LLC, Newstar Medical Laboratories, LLC	0147U	Drug assay, definitive, 85 or more drugs or metabolites, urine, quantitative liquid chromatography with tandem mass spectrometry (LC-MS/MS) using multiple reaction monitoring (MRM), with drug or metabolite description, comments including sample validation, per date of service

(Continued on page 280)

▲ = Revised code   ● = New code   ▶ ◀ = Contains new or revised text   ✕ = Duplicate PLA test   ↿⇂ = Category I PLA   American Medical Association   **279**

Appendix O

Proprietary Name and Clinical Laboratory or Manufacturer	Alpha-Numeric Code	Code Descriptor
RiskViewRx Plus, Newstar Medical Laboratories, LLC, Newstar Medical Laboratories, LLC	0148U	Drug assay, definitive, 100 or more drugs or metabolites, urine, quantitative liquid chromatography with tandem mass spectrometry (LC-MS/MS) using multiple reaction monitoring (MRM), with drug or metabolite description, comments including sample validation, per date of service
PsychViewRx, Newstar Medical Laboratories, LLC, Newstar Medical Laboratories, LLC	0149U	Drug assay, definitive, 60 or more drugs or metabolites, urine, quantitative liquid chromatography with tandem mass spectrometry (LC-MS/MS) using multiple reaction monitoring (MRM), with drug or metabolite description, comments including sample validation, per date of service
PsychViewRx Plus, Newstar Medical Laboratories, LLC, Newstar Medical Laboratories, LLC	#0150U	Drug assay, definitive, 120 or more drugs or metabolites, urine, quantitative liquid chromatography with tandem mass spectrometry (LC-MS/MS) using multiple reaction monitoring (MRM), with drug or metabolite description, comments including sample validation, per date of service (For additional PLA code with identical clinical descriptor, see 0143U. See Appendix O to determine appropriate code assignment)
—	▶(0151U has been deleted)◀	—
Karius® Test, Karius Inc, Karius Inc	0152U	Infectious disease (bacteria, fungi, parasites, and DNA viruses), microbial cell-free DNA, plasma, untargeted next-generation sequencing, report for significant positive pathogens
Insight TNBCtype™, Insight Molecular Labs	0153U	Oncology (breast), mRNA, gene expression profiling by next-generation sequencing of 101 genes, utilizing formalin-fixed paraffin-embedded tissue, algorithm reported as a triple negative breast cancer clinical subtype(s) with information on immune cell involvement
therascreen® *FGFR* RGQ RT-PCR Kit, QIAGEN, QIAGEN GmbH	0154U	Oncology (urothelial cancer), RNA, analysis by real-time RT-PCR of the *FGFR3 (fibroblast growth factor receptor 3)* gene analysis (ie, p.R248C [c.742C>T], p.S249C [c.746C>G], p.G370C [c.1108G>T], p.Y373C [c.1118A>G], FGFR3-TACC3v1, and FGFR3-TACC3v3), utilizing formalin-fixed paraffin-embedded urothelial cancer tumor tissue, reported as *FGFR* gene alteration status
therascreen *PIK3CA* RGQ PCR Kit, QIAGEN, QIAGEN GmbH	0155U	Oncology (breast cancer), DNA, *PIK3CA (phosphatidylinositol-4,5-bisphosphate 3-kinase, catalytic subunit alpha)* (eg, breast cancer) gene analysis (ie, p.C420R, p.E542K, p.E545A, p.E545D [g.1635G>T only], p.E545G, p.E545K, p.Q546E, p.Q546R, p.H1047L, p.H1047R, p.H1047Y), utilizing formalin-fixed paraffin-embedded breast tumor tissue, reported as *PIK3CA* gene mutation status

Proprietary Name and Clinical Laboratory or Manufacturer	Alpha-Numeric Code	Code Descriptor
SMASH™, New York Genome Center, Marvel Genomics™	0156U	Copy number (eg, intellectual disability, dysmorphology), sequence analysis
CustomNext + RNA: *APC*, Ambry Genetics®, Ambry Genetics®	+0157U	*APC (APC regulator of WNT signaling pathway)* (eg, familial adenomatosis polyposis [FAP]) mRNA sequence analysis (List separately in addition to code for primary procedure) (Use 0157U in conjunction with 81201)
CustomNext + RNA: *MLH1*, Ambry Genetics®, Ambry Genetics®	+0158U	*MLH1 (mutL homolog 1)* (eg, hereditary non-polyposis colorectal cancer, Lynch syndrome) mRNA sequence analysis (List separately in addition to code for primary procedure) (Use 0158U in conjunction with 81292)
CustomNext + RNA: *MSH2*, Ambry Genetics®, Ambry Genetics®	+0159U	*MSH2 (mutS homolog 2)* (eg, hereditary colon cancer, Lynch syndrome) mRNA sequence analysis (List separately in addition to code for primary procedure) (Use 0159U in conjunction with 81295)
CustomNext + RNA: *MSH6*, Ambry Genetics®, Ambry Genetics®	+0160U	*MSH6 (mutS homolog 6)* (eg, hereditary colon cancer, Lynch syndrome) mRNA sequence analysis (List separately in addition to code for primary procedure) (Use 0160U in conjunction with 81298)
CustomNext + RNA: *PMS2*, Ambry Genetics®, Ambry Genetics®	+0161U	*PMS2 (PMS1 homolog 2, mismatch repair system component)* (eg, hereditary non-polyposis colorectal cancer, Lynch syndrome) mRNA sequence analysis (List separately in addition to code for primary procedure) (Use 0161U in conjunction with 81317)
CustomNext + RNA: Lynch *(MLH1, MSH2, MSH6, PMS2)*, Ambry Genetics®, Ambry Genetics®	+0162U	Hereditary colon cancer (Lynch syndrome), targeted mRNA sequence analysis panel *(MLH1, MSH2, MSH6, PMS2)* (List separately in addition to code for primary procedure) (Use 0162U in conjunction with 81292, 81295, 81298, 81317, 81435)
BeScreened™-CRC, Beacon Biomedical Inc, Beacon Biomedical Inc	0163U	Oncology (colorectal) screening, biochemical enzyme-linked immunosorbent assay (ELISA) of 3 plasma or serum proteins (teratocarcinoma derived growth factor-1 [TDGF-1, Cripto-1], carcinoembryonic antigen [CEA], extracellular matrix protein [ECM]), with demographic data (age, gender, CRC-screening compliance) using a proprietary algorithm and reported as likelihood of CRC or advanced adenomas
ibs-smart™, Gemelli Biotech, Gemelli Biotech	0164U	Gastroenterology (irritable bowel syndrome [IBS]), immunoassay for anti-CdtB and anti-vinculin antibodies, utilizing plasma, algorithm for elevated or not elevated qualitative results
VeriMAP™ Peanut Dx – Bead-based Epitope Assay, AllerGenis™ Clinical Laboratory, AllerGenis™ LLC	0165U	Peanut allergen-specific quantitative assessment of multiple epitopes using enzyme-linked immunosorbent assay (ELISA), blood, individual epitope results and probability of peanut allergy

(Continued on page 282)

▲ = Revised code ● = New code ▶ ◀ = Contains new or revised text ✄ = Duplicate PLA test ↕ = Category I PLA

Proprietary Name and Clinical Laboratory or Manufacturer	Alpha-Numeric Code	Code Descriptor
LiverFASt™, ▶Fibronostics◀	0166U	Liver disease, 10 biochemical assays (α2-macroglobulin, haptoglobin, apolipoprotein A1, bilirubin, GGT, ALT, AST, triglycerides, cholesterol, fasting glucose) and biometric and demographic data, utilizing serum, algorithm reported as scores for fibrosis, necroinflammatory activity, and steatosis with a summary interpretation
ADEXUSDx hCG Test, NOWDiagnostics, NOWDiagnostics	0167U	Gonadotropin, chorionic (hCG), immunoassay with direct optical observation, blood
—	(0168U has been deleted)	—
NT (*NUDT15* and *TPMT*) genotyping panel, RPRD Diagnostics	0169U	*NUDT15 (nudix hydrolase 15)* and *TPMT (thiopurine S-methyltransferase)* (eg, drug metabolism) gene analysis, common variants
Clarifi™, Quadrant Biosciences, Inc, Quadrant Biosciences, Inc	0170U	Neurology (autism spectrum disorder [ASD]), RNA, next-generation sequencing, saliva, algorithmic analysis, and results reported as predictive probability of ASD diagnosis
MyMRD® NGS Panel, Laboratory for Personalized Molecular Medicine, Laboratory for Personalized Molecular Medicine	0171U	Targeted genomic sequence analysis panel, acute myeloid leukemia, myelodysplastic syndrome, and myeloproliferative neoplasms, DNA analysis, 23 genes, interrogation for sequence variants, rearrangements and minimal residual disease, reported as presence/absence
myChoice® CDx, Myriad Genetics Laboratories, Inc, Myriad Genetics Laboratories, Inc	0172U	Oncology (solid tumor as indicated by the label), somatic mutation analysis of *BRCA1 (BRCA1, DNA repair associated), BRCA2 (BRCA2, DNA repair associated)* and analysis of homologous recombination deficiency pathways, DNA, formalin-fixed paraffin-embedded tissue, algorithm quantifying tumor genomic instability score
Psych HealthPGx Panel, RPRD Diagnostics, RPRD Diagnostics	0173U	Psychiatry (ie, depression, anxiety), genomic analysis panel, includes variant analysis of 14 genes
LC-MS/MS Targeted Proteomic Assay, OncoOmicDx Laboratory, LDT	0174U	Oncology (solid tumor), mass spectrometric 30 protein targets, formalin-fixed paraffin-embedded tissue, prognostic and predictive algorithm reported as likely, unlikely, or uncertain benefit of 39 chemotherapy and targeted therapeutic oncology agents
Genomind® Professional PGx Express™ CORE, Genomind, Inc, Genomind, Inc	0175U	Psychiatry (eg, depression, anxiety), genomic analysis panel, variant analysis of 15 genes
IB*Schek*®, Commonwealth Diagnostics International, Inc, Commonwealth Diagnostics International, Inc	0176U	Cytolethal distending toxin B (CdtB) and vinculin IgG antibodies by immunoassay (ie, ELISA)
therascreen® *PIK3CA* RGQ PCR Kit, QIAGEN, QIAGEN GmbH	0177U	Oncology (breast cancer), DNA, *PIK3CA (phosphatidylinositol-4,5-bisphosphate 3-kinase catalytic subunit alpha)* gene analysis of 11 gene variants utilizing plasma, reported as *PIK3CA* gene mutation status

★ = Telemedicine   ◀ = Audio-only   ✚ = Add-on code   ✗ = FDA approval pending   # = Resequenced code   ⊘ = Modifier 51 exempt

Appendix O

Proprietary Name and Clinical Laboratory or Manufacturer	Alpha-Numeric Code	Code Descriptor
VeriMAP™ Peanut Reactivity Threshold–Bead Based Epitope Assay, AllerGenis™ Clinical Laboratory, AllerGenis™ LLC	0178U	Peanut allergen-specific quantitative assessment of multiple epitopes using enzyme-linked immunosorbent assay (ELISA), blood, report of minimum eliciting exposure for a clinical reaction
Resolution ctDx Lung™, Resolution Bioscience, Resolution Bioscience, Inc	0179U	Oncology (non-small cell lung cancer), cell-free DNA, targeted sequence analysis of 23 genes (single nucleotide variations, insertions and deletions, fusions without prior knowledge of partner/breakpoint, copy number variations), with report of significant mutation(s)
Navigator ABO Sequencing, Grifols Immunohematology Center, Grifols Immunohematology Center	0180U	Red cell antigen (ABO blood group) genotyping (ABO), gene analysis Sanger/chain termination/ conventional sequencing, *ABO (ABO, alpha 1-3-N-acetylgalactosaminyltransferase and alpha 1-3-galactosyltransferase)* gene, including subtyping, 7 exons
Navigator CO Sequencing, Grifols Immunohematology Center, Grifols Immunohematology Center	0181U	Red cell antigen (Colton blood group) genotyping (CO), gene analysis, *AQP1 (aquaporin 1 [Colton blood group])* exon 1
Navigator CROM Sequencing, Grifols Immunohematology Center, Grifols Immunohematology Center	0182U	Red cell antigen (Cromer blood group) genotyping (CROM), gene analysis, *CD55 (CD55 molecule [Cromer blood group])* exons 1-10
Navigator DI Sequencing, Grifols Immunohematology Center, Grifols Immunohematology Center	0183U	Red cell antigen (Diego blood group) genotyping (DI), gene analysis, *SLC4A1 (solute carrier family 4 member 1 [Diego blood group])* exon 19
Navigator DO Sequencing, Grifols Immunohematology Center, Grifols Immunohematology Center	0184U	Red cell antigen (Dombrock blood group) genotyping (DO), gene analysis, *ART4 (ADP-ribosyltransferase 4 [Dombrock blood group])* exon 2
Navigator FUT1 Sequencing, Grifols Immunohematology Center, Grifols Immunohematology Center	0185U	Red cell antigen (H blood group) genotyping (FUT1), gene analysis, *FUT1 (fucosyltransferase 1 [H blood group])* exon 4
Navigator FUT2 Sequencing, Grifols Immunohematology Center, Grifols Immunohematology Center	0186U	Red cell antigen (H blood group) genotyping (FUT2), gene analysis, *FUT2 (fucosyltransferase 2)* exon 2
Navigator FY Sequencing, Grifols Immunohematology Center, Grifols Immunohematology Center	0187U	Red cell antigen (Duffy blood group) genotyping (FY), gene analysis, *ACKR1 (atypical chemokine receptor 1 [Duffy blood group])* exons 1-2
Navigator GE Sequencing, Grifols Immunohematology Center, Grifols Immunohematology Center	0188U	Red cell antigen (Gerbich blood group) genotyping (GE), gene analysis, *GYPC (glycophorin C [Gerbich blood group])* exons 1-4
Navigator GYPA Sequencing, Grifols Immunohematology Center, Grifols Immunohematology Center	0189U	Red cell antigen (MNS blood group) genotyping (GYPA), gene analysis, *GYPA (glycophorin A [MNS blood group])* introns 1, 5, exon 2
Navigator GYPB Sequencing, Grifols Immunohematology Center, Grifols Immunohematology Center	0190U	Red cell antigen (MNS blood group) genotyping (GYPB), gene analysis, *GYPB (glycophorin B [MNS blood group])* introns 1, 5, pseudoexon 3
Navigator IN Sequencing, Grifols Immunohematology Center, Grifols Immunohematology Center	0191U	Red cell antigen (Indian blood group) genotyping (IN), gene analysis, *CD44 (CD44 molecule [Indian blood group])* exons 2, 3, 6

(Continued on page 284)

Appendix O

Proprietary Name and Clinical Laboratory or Manufacturer	Alpha-Numeric Code	Code Descriptor
Navigator JK Sequencing, Grifols Immunohematology Center, Grifols Immunohematology Center	0192U	Red cell antigen (Kidd blood group) genotyping (JK), gene analysis, *SLC14A1 (solute carrier family 14 member 1 [Kidd blood group])* gene promoter, exon 9
Navigator JR Sequencing, Grifols Immunohematology Center, Grifols Immunohematology Center	0193U	Red cell antigen (JR blood group) genotyping (JR), gene analysis, *ABCG2 (ATP binding cassette subfamily G member 2 [Junior blood group])* exons 2-26
Navigator KEL Sequencing, Grifols Immunohematology Center, Grifols Immunohematology Center	0194U	Red cell antigen (Kell blood group) genotyping (KEL), gene analysis, *KEL (Kell metallo-endopeptidase [Kell blood group])* exon 8
Navigator *KLF1* Sequencing, Grifols Immunohematology Center, Grifols Immunohematology Center	0195U	*KLF1 (Kruppel-like factor 1)*, targeted sequencing (ie, exon 13)
Navigator LU Sequencing, Grifols Immunohematology Center, Grifols Immunohematology Center	0196U	Red cell antigen (Lutheran blood group) genotyping (LU), gene analysis, *BCAM (basal cell adhesion molecule [Lutheran blood group])* exon 3
Navigator LW Sequencing, Grifols Immunohematology Center, Grifols Immunohematology Center	0197U	Red cell antigen (Landsteiner-Wiener blood group) genotyping (LW), gene analysis, *ICAM4 (intercellular adhesion molecule 4 [Landsteiner-Wiener blood group])* exon 1
Navigator RHD/CE Sequencing, Grifols Immunohematology Center, Grifols Immunohematology Center	0198U	Red cell antigen (RH blood group) genotyping (RHD and RHCE), gene analysis Sanger/chain termination/conventional sequencing, *RHD (Rh blood group D antigen) exons 1-10 and RHCE (Rh blood group CcEe antigens) exon 5*
Navigator SC Sequencing, Grifols Immunohematology Center, Grifols Immunohematology Center	0199U	Red cell antigen (Scianna blood group) genotyping (SC), gene analysis, *ERMAP (erythroblast membrane associated protein [Scianna blood group])* exons 4, 12
Navigator XK Sequencing, Grifols Immunohematology Center, Grifols Immunohematology Center	0200U	Red cell antigen (Kx blood group) genotyping (XK), gene analysis, *XK (X-linked Kx blood group)* exons 1-3
Navigator YT Sequencing, Grifols Immunohematology Center, Grifols Immunohematology Center	0201U	Red cell antigen (Yt blood group) genotyping (YT), gene analysis, *ACHE (acetylcholinesterase [Cartwright blood group])* exon 2
BioFire® Respiratory Panel 2.1 (RP2.1), BioFire® Diagnostics, BioFire® Diagnostics, LLC	⅀0202U	Infectious disease (bacterial or viral respiratory tract infection), pathogen-specific nucleic acid (DNA or RNA), 22 targets including severe acute respiratory syndrome coronavirus 2 (SARS-CoV-2), qualitative RT-PCR, nasopharyngeal swab, each pathogen reported as detected or not detected (For additional PLA code with identical clinical descriptor, see 0223U. See Appendix O or the most current listing on the AMA CPT website to determine appropriate code assignment)
PredictSURE IBD™ Test, KSL Diagnostics, PredictImmune Ltd	0203U	Autoimmune (inflammatory bowel disease), mRNA, gene expression profiling by quantitative RT-PCR, 17 genes (15 target and 2 reference genes), whole blood, reported as a continuous risk score and classification of inflammatory bowel disease aggressiveness

★ = Telemedicine ◀ = Audio-only ✚ = Add-on code ⅀ = FDA approval pending # = Resequenced code ⊘ = Modifier 51 exempt

Proprietary Name and Clinical Laboratory or Manufacturer	Alpha-Numeric Code	Code Descriptor
Afirma Xpression Atlas, Veracyte, Inc, Veracyte, Inc	0204U	Oncology (thyroid), mRNA, gene expression analysis of 593 genes (including *BRAF, RAS, RET, PAX8,* and *NTRK*) for sequence variants and rearrangements, utilizing fine needle aspirate, reported as detected or not detected
Vita Risk®, Arctic Medical Laboratories, Arctic Medical Laboratories	0205U	Ophthalmology (age-related macular degeneration), analysis of 3 gene variants (2 *CFH* gene, 1 *ARMS2* gene), using PCR and MALDI-TOF, buccal swab, reported as positive or negative for neovascular age-related macular-degeneration risk associated with zinc supplements
DISCERN™, NeuroDiagnostics, NeuroDiagnostics	0206U	Neurology (Alzheimer disease); cell aggregation using morphometric imaging and protein kinase C-epsilon (PKCe) concentration in response to amylospheroid treatment by ELISA, cultured skin fibroblasts, each reported as positive or negative for Alzheimer disease
	+0207U	quantitative imaging of phosphorylated *ERK1* and *ERK2* in response to bradykinin treatment by in situ immunofluorescence, using cultured skin fibroblasts, reported as a probability index for Alzheimer disease (List separately in addition to code for primary procedure) (Use 0207U in conjunction with 0206U)
—	▶(0208U has been deleted)◀	—
CNGnome™, PerkinElmer Genomics, PerkinElmer Genomics	0209U	Cytogenomic constitutional (genome-wide) analysis, interrogation of genomic regions for copy number, structural changes and areas of homozygosity for chromosomal abnormalities
BioPlex 2200 RPR Assay – Quantitative, Bio-Rad Laboratories, Bio-Rad Laboratories	0210U	Syphilis test, non-treponemal antibody, immunoassay, quantitative (RPR)
MI Cancer Seek™ - NGS Analysis, Caris MPI d/b/a Caris Life Sciences, Caris MPI d/b/a Caris Life Sciences	0211U	Oncology (pan-tumor), DNA and RNA by next-generation sequencing, utilizing formalin-fixed paraffin-embedded tissue, interpretative report for single nucleotide variants, copy number alterations, tumor mutational burden, and microsatellite instability, with therapy association
Genomic Unity® Whole Genome Analysis – Proband, Variantyx Inc, Variantyx Inc	0212U	Rare diseases (constitutional/heritable disorders), whole genome and mitochondrial DNA sequence analysis, including small sequence changes, deletions, duplications, short tandem repeat gene expansions, and variants in non-uniquely mappable regions, blood or saliva, identification and categorization of genetic variants, proband (Do not report 0212U in conjunction with 81425)

(Continued on page 286)

▲=Revised code   ●=New code   ▶ ◀=Contains new or revised text   ✕=Duplicate PLA test   ⇅=Category I PLA   American Medical Association   **285**

Appendix O

Proprietary Name and Clinical Laboratory or Manufacturer	Alpha-Numeric Code	Code Descriptor
Genomic Unity® Whole Genome Analysis – Comparator, Variantyx Inc, Variantyx Inc	0213U	Rare diseases (constitutional/heritable disorders), whole genome and mitochondrial DNA sequence analysis, including small sequence changes, deletions, duplications, short tandem repeat gene expansions, and variants in non-uniquely mappable regions, blood or saliva, identification and categorization of genetic variants, each comparator genome (eg, parent, sibling) (Do not report 0213U in conjunction with 81426)
Genomic Unity® Exome Plus Analysis – Proband, Variantyx Inc, Variantyx Inc	0214U	Rare diseases (constitutional/heritable disorders), whole exome and mitochondrial DNA sequence analysis, including small sequence changes, deletions, duplications, short tandem repeat gene expansions, and variants in non-uniquely mappable regions, blood or saliva, identification and categorization of genetic variants, proband (Do not report 0214U in conjunction with 81415)
Genomic Unity® Exome Plus Analysis – Comparator, Variantyx Inc, Variantyx Inc	0215U	Rare diseases (constitutional/heritable disorders), whole exome and mitochondrial DNA sequence analysis, including small sequence changes, deletions, duplications, short tandem repeat gene expansions, and variants in non-uniquely mappable regions, blood or saliva, identification and categorization of genetic variants, each comparator exome (eg, parent, sibling) (Do not report 0215U in conjunction with 81416)
Genomic Unity® Ataxia Repeat Expansion and Sequence Analysis, Variantyx Inc, Variantyx Inc	0216U	Neurology (inherited ataxias), genomic DNA sequence analysis of 12 common genes including small sequence changes, deletions, duplications, short tandem repeat gene expansions, and variants in non-uniquely mappable regions, blood or saliva, identification and categorization of genetic variants
Genomic Unity® Comprehensive Ataxia Repeat Expansion and Sequence Analysis, Variantyx Inc, Variantyx Inc	0217U	Neurology (inherited ataxias), genomic DNA sequence analysis of 51 genes including small sequence changes, deletions, duplications, short tandem repeat gene expansions, and variants in non-uniquely mappable regions, blood or saliva, identification and categorization of genetic variants
Genomic Unity® DMD Analysis, Variantyx Inc, Variantyx Inc	0218U	Neurology (muscular dystrophy), *DMD* gene sequence analysis, including small sequence changes, deletions, duplications, and variants in non-uniquely mappable regions, blood or saliva, identification and characterization of genetic variants
Sentosa® SQ HIV-1 Genotyping Assay, Vela Diagnostics USA, Inc, Vela Operations Singapore Pte Ltd	0219U	Infectious agent (human immunodeficiency virus), targeted viral next-generation sequence analysis (ie, protease [PR], reverse transcriptase [RT], integrase [INT]), algorithm reported as prediction of antiviral drug susceptibility
PreciseDx™ Breast Cancer Test, PreciseDx, PreciseDx	0220U	Oncology (breast cancer), image analysis with artificial intelligence assessment of 12 histologic and immunohistochemical features, reported as a recurrence score

★ = Telemedicine ◀ = Audio-only ✛ = Add-on code ✗ = FDA approval pending # = Resequenced code ⊘ = Modifier 51 exempt

Proprietary Name and Clinical Laboratory or Manufacturer	Alpha-Numeric Code	Code Descriptor
Navigator ABO Blood Group NGS, Grifols Immunohematology Center, Grifols Immunohematology Center	0221U	Red cell antigen (ABO blood group) genotyping (ABO), gene analysis, next-generation sequencing, *ABO (ABO, alpha 1-3-N-acetylgalactosaminyltransferase and alpha 1-3-galactosyltransferase)* gene
Navigator Rh Blood Group NGS, Grifols Immunohematology Center, Grifols Immunohematology Center	0222U	Red cell antigen (RH blood group) genotyping (RHD and RHCE), gene analysis, next-generation sequencing, RH proximal promoter, exons 1-10, portions of introns 2-3
QIAstat-Dx Respiratory SARS CoV-2 Panel, QIAGEN Sciences, QIAGEN GmbH	✕0223U	Infectious disease (bacterial or viral respiratory tract infection), pathogen-specific nucleic acid (DNA or RNA), 22 targets including severe acute respiratory syndrome coronavirus 2 (SARS-CoV-2), qualitative RT-PCR, nasopharyngeal swab, each pathogen reported as detected or not detected

(For additional PLA code with identical clinical descriptor, see 0202U. See Appendix O or the most current listing on the AMA CPT website to determine appropriate code assignment) |
| COVID-19 Antibody Test, Mt Sinai, Mount Sinai Laboratory | 0224U | Antibody, severe acute respiratory syndrome coronavirus 2 (SARS-CoV-2) (coronavirus disease [COVID-19]), includes titer(s), when performed

(Do not report 0224U in conjunction with 86769) |
ePlex® Respiratory Pathogen Panel 2, GenMark Dx, GenMark Diagnostics, Inc	0225U	Infectious disease (bacterial or viral respiratory tract infection) pathogen-specific DNA and RNA, 21 targets, including severe acute respiratory syndrome coronavirus 2 (SARS-CoV-2), amplified probe technique, including multiplex reverse transcription for RNA targets, each analyte reported as detected or not detected
Tru-Immune™, Ethos Laboratories, GenScript® USA Inc	0226U	Surrogate viral neutralization test (sVNT), severe acute respiratory syndrome coronavirus 2 (SARS-CoV-2) (coronavirus disease [COVID-19]), ELISA, plasma, serum
Comprehensive Screen, Aspenti Health	0227U	Drug assay, presumptive, 30 or more drugs or metabolites, urine, liquid chromatography with tandem mass spectrometry (LC-MS/MS) using multiple reaction monitoring (MRM), with drug or metabolite description, includes sample validation
PanGIA Prostate, Genetics Institute of America, Entopsis, LLC	0228U	Oncology (prostate), multianalyte molecular profile by photometric detection of macromolecules adsorbed on nanosponge array slides with machine learning, utilizing first morning voided urine, algorithm reported as likelihood of prostate cancer
Colvera®, Clinical Genomics Pathology Inc	▲0229U	▶*BCAT1 (Branched chain amino acid transaminase 1)* and *IKZF1 (IKAROS family zinc finger 1)* (eg, colorectal cancer) promoter methylation analysis◀

(Continued on page 288)

▲ = Revised code ● = New code ▶◀ = Contains new or revised text ✕ = Duplicate PLA test ↕ = Category I PLA   American Medical Association **287**

Proprietary Name and Clinical Laboratory or Manufacturer	Alpha-Numeric Code	Code Descriptor
Genomic Unity® AR Analysis, Variantyx Inc, Variantyx Inc	0230U	*AR (androgen receptor)* (eg, spinal and bulbar muscular atrophy, Kennedy disease, X chromosome inactivation), full sequence analysis, including small sequence changes in exonic and intronic regions, deletions, duplications, short tandem repeat (STR) expansions, mobile element insertions, and variants in non-uniquely mappable regions
Genomic Unity® CACNA1A Analysis, Variantyx Inc, Variantyx Inc	0231U	*CACNA1A (calcium voltage-gated channel subunit alpha 1A)* (eg, spinocerebellar ataxia), full gene analysis, including small sequence changes in exonic and intronic regions, deletions, duplications, short tandem repeat (STR) gene expansions, mobile element insertions, and variants in non-uniquely mappable regions
Genomic Unity® CSTB Analysis, Variantyx Inc, Variantyx Inc	0232U	*CSTB (cystatin B)* (eg, progressive myoclonic epilepsy type 1A, Unverricht-Lundborg disease), full gene analysis, including small sequence changes in exonic and intronic regions, deletions, duplications, short tandem repeat (STR) expansions, mobile element insertions, and variants in non-uniquely mappable regions
Genomic Unity® FXN Analysis, Variantyx Inc, Variantyx Inc	0233U	*FXN (frataxin)* (eg, Friedreich ataxia), gene analysis, including small sequence changes in exonic and intronic regions, deletions, duplications, short tandem repeat (STR) expansions, mobile element insertions, and variants in non-uniquely mappable regions
Genomic Unity® MECP2 Analysis, Variantyx Inc, Variantyx Inc	0234U	*MECP2 (methyl CpG binding protein 2)* (eg, Rett syndrome), full gene analysis, including small sequence changes in exonic and intronic regions, deletions, duplications, mobile element insertions, and variants in non-uniquely mappable regions
Genomic Unity® PTEN Analysis, Variantyx Inc, Variantyx Inc	0235U	*PTEN (phosphatase and tensin homolog)* (eg, Cowden syndrome, PTEN hamartoma tumor syndrome), full gene analysis, including small sequence changes in exonic and intronic regions, deletions, duplications, mobile element insertions, and variants in non-uniquely mappable regions
Genomic Unity® SMN1/2 Analysis, Variantyx Inc, Variantyx Inc	0236U	*SMN1 (survival of motor neuron 1, telomeric)* and *SMN2 (survival of motor neuron 2, centromeric)* (eg, spinal muscular atrophy) full gene analysis, including small sequence changes in exonic and intronic regions, duplications, deletions, and mobile element insertions
Genomic Unity® Cardiac Ion Channelopathies Analysis, Variantyx Inc, Variantyx Inc	0237U	Cardiac ion channelopathies (eg, Brugada syndrome, long QT syndrome, short QT syndrome, catecholaminergic polymorphic ventricular tachycardia), genomic sequence analysis panel including *ANK2, CASQ2, CAV3, KCNE1, KCNE2, KCNH2, KCNJ2, KCNQ1, RYR2,* and *SCN5A,* including small sequence changes in exonic and intronic regions, deletions, duplications, mobile element insertions, and variants in non-uniquely mappable regions

★ = Telemedicine   ◀ = Audio-only   ✚ = Add-on code   ⫫ = FDA approval pending   # = Resequenced code   ⊘ = Modifier 51 exempt

Proprietary Name and Clinical Laboratory or Manufacturer	Alpha-Numeric Code	Code Descriptor
Genomic Unity® Lynch Syndrome Analysis, Variantyx Inc, Variantyx Inc	0238U	Oncology (Lynch syndrome), genomic DNA sequence analysis of *MLH1, MSH2, MSH6, PMS2,* and *EPCAM,* including small sequence changes in exonic and intronic regions, deletions, duplications, mobile element insertions, and variants in non-uniquely mappable regions
FoundationOne® Liquid CDx, Foundation Medicine Inc, Foundation Medicine Inc	0239U	Targeted genomic sequence analysis panel, solid organ neoplasm, cell-free DNA, analysis of 311 or more genes, interrogation for sequence variants, including substitutions, insertions, deletions, select rearrangements, and copy number variations
▶Xpert® Xpress CoV-2/Flu/RSV plus (SARS-CoV-2 and Flu targets)◀, Cepheid®	0240U	Infectious disease (viral respiratory tract infection), pathogen-specific RNA, 3 targets (severe acute respiratory syndrome coronavirus 2 [SARS-CoV-2], influenza A, influenza B), upper respiratory specimen, each pathogen reported as detected or not detected
▶Xpert® Xpress CoV-2/Flu/RSV plus (all targets)◀, Cepheid®	0241U	Infectious disease (viral respiratory tract infection), pathogen-specific RNA, 4 targets (severe acute respiratory syndrome coronavirus 2 [SARS-CoV-2], influenza A, influenza B, respiratory syncytial virus [RSV]), upper respiratory specimen, each pathogen reported as detected or not detected
Guardant360® CDx, Guardant Health Inc, Guardant Health Inc	0242U	Targeted genomic sequence analysis panel, solid organ neoplasm, cell-free circulating DNA analysis of 55-74 genes, interrogation for sequence variants, gene copy number amplifications, and gene rearrangements
PlGF Preeclampsia Screen, PerkinElmer Genetics, PerkinElmer Genetics, Inc	0243U	Obstetrics (preeclampsia), biochemical assay of placental-growth factor, time-resolved fluorescence immunoassay, maternal serum, predictive algorithm reported as a risk score for preeclampsia
Oncotype MAP™ Pan-Cancer Tissue Test, Paradigm Diagnostics, Inc, Paradigm Diagnostics, Inc	0244U	Oncology (solid organ), DNA, comprehensive genomic profiling, 257 genes, interrogation for single-nucleotide variants, insertions/deletions, copy number alterations, gene rearrangements, tumor-mutational burden and microsatellite instability, utilizing formalin-fixed paraffin-embedded tumor tissue
ThyGeNEXT® Thyroid Oncogene Panel, Interpace Diagnostics, Interpace Diagnostics	0245U	Oncology (thyroid), mutation analysis of 10 genes and 37 RNA fusions and expression of 4 mRNA markers using next-generation sequencing, fine needle aspirate, report includes associated risk of malignancy expressed as a percentage
PrecisionBlood™, San Diego Blood Bank, San Diego Blood Bank	0246U	Red blood cell antigen typing, DNA, genotyping of at least 16 blood groups with phenotype prediction of at least 51 red blood cell antigens
PreTRM®, Sera Prognostics, Sera Prognostics, Inc®	0247U	Obstetrics (preterm birth), insulin-like growth factor–binding protein 4 (IBP4), sex hormone–binding globulin (SHBG), quantitative measurement by LC-MS/MS, utilizing maternal serum, combined with clinical data, reported as predictive-risk stratification for spontaneous preterm birth

(Continued on page 290)

▲ = Revised code   ● = New code   ▶◀ = Contains new or revised text   ✖ = Duplicate PLA test   ↕ = Category I PLA

Proprietary Name and Clinical Laboratory or Manufacturer	Alpha-Numeric Code	Code Descriptor
3D Predict Glioma, KIYATEC®, Inc	0248U	Oncology (brain), spheroid cell culture in a 3D microenvironment, 12 drug panel, tumor-response prediction for each drug
Theralink® Reverse Phase Protein Array (RPPA), Theralink® Technologies, Inc, Theralink® Technologies, Inc	0249U	Oncology (breast), semiquantitative analysis of 32 phosphoproteins and protein analytes, includes laser capture microdissection, with algorithmic analysis and interpretative report
PGDx elio™ tissue complete, Personal Genome Diagnostics, Inc, Personal Genome Diagnostics, Inc	0250U	Oncology (solid organ neoplasm), targeted genomic sequence DNA analysis of 505 genes, interrogation for somatic alterations (SNVs [single nucleotide variant], small insertions and deletions, one amplification, and four translocations), microsatellite instability and tumor-mutation burden
Intrinsic Hepcidin IDx™ Test, IntrinsicDx, Intrinsic LifeSciences™ LLC	0251U	Hepcidin-25, enzyme-linked immunosorbent assay (ELISA), serum or plasma
POC (Products of Conception), Igenomix®, Igenomix® USA	0252U	Fetal aneuploidy short tandem–repeat comparative analysis, fetal DNA from products of conception, reported as normal (euploidy), monosomy, trisomy, or partial deletion/duplication, mosaicism, and segmental aneuploidy
ERA® (Endometrial Receptivity Analysis), Igenomix®, Igenomix® USA	0253U	Reproductive medicine (endometrial receptivity analysis), RNA gene expression profile, 238 genes by next-generation sequencing, endometrial tissue, predictive algorithm reported as endometrial window of implantation (eg, pre-receptive, receptive, post-receptive)
SMART PGT-A (Pre-implantation Genetic Testing - Aneuploidy), Igenomix®, Igenomix® USA	0254U	Reproductive medicine (preimplantation genetic assessment), analysis of 24 chromosomes using embryonic DNA genomic sequence analysis for aneuploidy, and a mitochondrial DNA score in euploid embryos, results reported as normal (euploidy), monosomy, trisomy, or partial deletion/duplication, mosaicism, and segmental aneuploidy, per embryo tested
Cap-Score™ Test, Androvia LifeSciences, Avantor Clinical Services (previously known as Therapak)	0255U	Andrology (infertility), sperm-capacitation assessment of ganglioside GM1 distribution patterns, fluorescence microscopy, fresh or frozen specimen, reported as percentage of capacitated sperm and probability of generating a pregnancy score
Trimethylamine (TMA) and TMA N-Oxide, Children's Hospital Colorado Laboratory	0256U	Trimethylamine/trimethylamine N-oxide (TMA/TMAO) profile, tandem mass spectrometry (MS/MS), urine, with algorithmic analysis and interpretive report
Very-Long Chain Acyl-CoA Dehydrogenase (VLCAD) Enzyme Activity, Children's Hospital Colorado Laboratory	0257U	Very long chain acyl-coenzyme A (CoA) dehydrogenase (VLCAD), leukocyte enzyme activity, whole blood

★=Telemedicine   ◀=Audio-only   ✚=Add-on code   ✔=FDA approval pending   #=Resequenced code   ⊘=Modifier 51 exempt

Proprietary Name and Clinical Laboratory or Manufacturer	Alpha-Numeric Code	Code Descriptor
Mind.Px, Mindera, Mindera Corporation	0258U	Autoimmune (psoriasis), mRNA, next-generation sequencing, gene expression profiling of 50-100 genes, skin-surface collection using adhesive patch, algorithm reported as likelihood of response to psoriasis biologics
GFR by NMR, Labtech™ Diagnostics	0259U	Nephrology (chronic kidney disease), nuclear magnetic resonance spectroscopy measurement of myo-inositol, valine, and creatinine, algorithmically combined with cystatin C (by immunoassay) and demographic data to determine estimated glomerular filtration rate (GFR), serum, quantitative
Augusta Optical Genome Mapping, Georgia Esoteric and Molecular (GEM) Laboratory, LLC, Bionano Genomics Inc	✣0260U	Rare diseases (constitutional/heritable disorders), identification of copy number variations, inversions, insertions, translocations, and other structural variants by optical genome mapping (For additional PLA code with identical clinical descriptor, see 0264U. See Appendix O or the most current listing on the AMA CPT website to determine appropriate code assignment)
Immunoscore®, HalioDx, HalioDx	0261U	Oncology (colorectal cancer), image analysis with artificial intelligence assessment of 4 histologic and immunohistochemical features (CD3 and CD8 within tumor-stroma border and tumor core), tissue, reported as immune response and recurrence-risk score
OncoSignal 7 Pathway Signal, Protean BioDiagnostics, Philips Electronics Nederland BV	0262U	Oncology (solid tumor), gene expression profiling by real-time RT-PCR of 7 gene pathways (*ER, AR, PI3K, MAPK, HH, TGFB,* Notch), formalin-fixed paraffin-embedded (FFPE), algorithm reported as gene pathway activity score
NPDX ASD and Central Carbon Energy Metabolism, Stemina Biomarker Discovery, Inc, Stemina Biomarker Discovery, Inc	0263U	Neurology (autism spectrum disorder [ASD]), quantitative measurements of 16 central carbon metabolites (ie, α-ketoglutarate, alanine, lactate, phenylalanine, pyruvate, succinate, carnitine, citrate, fumarate, hypoxanthine, inosine, malate, S-sulfocysteine, taurine, urate, and xanthine), liquid chromatography tandem mass spectrometry (LC-MS/MS), plasma, algorithmic analysis with result reported as negative or positive (with metabolic subtypes of ASD)
Praxis Optical Genome Mapping, Praxis Genomics LLC	✣0264U	Rare diseases (constitutional/heritable disorders), identification of copy number variations, inversions, insertions, translocations, and other structural variants by optical genome mapping (For additional PLA code with identical clinical descriptor, see 0260U. See Appendix O or the most current listing on the AMA CPT website to determine appropriate code assignment)

(Continued on page 292)

▲ = Revised code   ● = New code   ▶◀ = Contains new or revised text   ✣ = Duplicate PLA test   ⇅ = Category I PLA   American Medical Association   **291**

Appendix O

Proprietary Name and Clinical Laboratory or Manufacturer	Alpha-Numeric Code	Code Descriptor
Praxis Whole Genome Sequencing, Praxis Genomics LLC	0265U	Rare constitutional and other heritable disorders, whole genome and mitochondrial DNA sequence analysis, blood, frozen and formalin-fixed paraffin-embedded (FFPE) tissue, saliva, buccal swabs or cell lines, identification of single nucleotide and copy number variants
Praxis Transcriptome, Praxis Genomics LLC	0266U	Unexplained constitutional or other heritable disorders or syndromes, tissue-specific gene expression by whole-transcriptome and next-generation sequencing, blood, formalin-fixed paraffin-embedded (FFPE) tissue or fresh frozen tissue, reported as presence or absence of splicing or expression changes
Praxis Combined Whole Genome Sequencing and Optical Genome Mapping, Praxis Genomics LLC	0267U	Rare constitutional and other heritable disorders, identification of copy number variations, inversions, insertions, translocations, and other structural variants by optical genome mapping and whole genome sequencing
Versiti™ aHUS Genetic Evaluation, Versiti™ Diagnostic Laboratories, Versiti™	0268U	Hematology (atypical hemolytic uremic syndrome [aHUS]), genomic sequence analysis of 15 genes, blood, buccal swab, or amniotic fluid
Versiti™ Autosomal Dominant Thrombocytopenia Panel, Versiti™ Diagnostic Laboratories, Versiti™	0269U	Hematology (autosomal dominant congenital thrombocytopenia), genomic sequence analysis of 14 genes, blood, buccal swab, or amniotic fluid
Versiti™ Coagulation Disorder Panel, Versiti™ Diagnostic Laboratories, Versiti™	0270U	Hematology (congenital coagulation disorders), genomic sequence analysis of 20 genes, blood, buccal swab, or amniotic fluid
Versiti™ Congenital Neutropenia Panel, Versiti™ Diagnostic Laboratories, Versiti™	0271U	Hematology (congenital neutropenia), genomic sequence analysis of 23 genes, blood, buccal swab, or amniotic fluid
Versiti™ Comprehensive Bleeding Disorder Panel, Versiti™ Diagnostic Laboratories, Versiti™	0272U	Hematology (genetic bleeding disorders), genomic sequence analysis of 51 genes, blood, buccal swab, or amniotic fluid, comprehensive
Versiti™ Fibrinolytic Disorder Panel, Versiti™ Diagnostic Laboratories, Versiti™	0273U	Hematology (genetic hyperfibrinolysis, delayed bleeding), analysis of 9 genes (*F13A1, F13B, FGA, FGB, FGG, SERPINA1, SERPINE1, SERPINF2* by next-generation sequencing, and *PLAU* by array comparative genomic hybridization), blood, buccal swab, or amniotic fluid
Versiti™ Comprehensive Platelet Disorder Panel, Versiti™ Diagnostic Laboratories, Versiti™	0274U	Hematology (genetic platelet disorders), genomic sequence analysis of 43 genes, blood, buccal swab, or amniotic fluid
Versiti™ Heparin-Induced Thrombocytopenia Evaluation – PEA, Versiti™ Diagnostic Laboratories, Versiti™	0275U	Hematology (heparin-induced thrombocytopenia), platelet antibody reactivity by flow cytometry, serum
Versiti™ Inherited Thrombocytopenia Panel, Versiti™ Diagnostic Laboratories, Versiti™	▲0276U	▶Hematology (inherited thrombocytopenia), genomic sequence analysis of 42 genes, blood, buccal swab, or amniotic fluid◀

★=Telemedicine ◀=Audio-only ✦=Add-on code ⊬=FDA approval pending #=Resequenced code ⊘=Modifier 51 exempt

Proprietary Name and Clinical Laboratory or Manufacturer	Alpha-Numeric Code	Code Descriptor
Versiti™ Platelet Function Disorder Panel, Versiti™ Diagnostic Laboratories, Versiti™	0277U	Hematology (genetic platelet function disorder), genomic sequence analysis of 31 genes, blood, buccal swab, or amniotic fluid
Versiti™ Thrombosis Panel, Versiti™ Diagnostic Laboratories, Versiti™	0278U	Hematology (genetic thrombosis), genomic sequence analysis of 12 genes, blood, buccal swab, or amniotic fluid
Versiti™ VWF Collagen III Binding, Versiti™ Diagnostic Laboratories, Versiti™	0279U	Hematology (von Willebrand disease [VWD]), von Willebrand factor (VWF) and collagen III binding by enzyme-linked immunosorbent assays (ELISA), plasma, report of collagen III binding
Versiti™ VWF Collagen IV Binding, Versiti™ Diagnostic Laboratories, Versiti™	0280U	Hematology (von Willebrand disease [VWD]), von Willebrand factor (VWF) and collagen IV binding by enzyme-linked immunosorbent assays (ELISA), plasma, report of collagen IV binding
Versiti™ VWF Propeptide Antigen, Versiti™ Diagnostic Laboratories, Versiti™	0281U	Hematology (von Willebrand disease [VWD]), von Willebrand propeptide, enzyme-linked immunosorbent assays (ELISA), plasma, diagnostic report of von Willebrand factor (VWF) propeptide antigen level
Versiti™ Red Cell Genotyping Panel, Versiti™ Diagnostic Laboratories, Versiti™	0282U	Red blood cell antigen typing, DNA, genotyping of 12 blood group system genes to predict 44 red blood cell antigen phenotypes
Versiti™ VWD Type 2B Evaluation, Versiti™ Diagnostic Laboratories, Versiti™	0283U	von Willebrand factor (VWF), type 2B, platelet-binding evaluation, radioimmunoassay, plasma
Versiti™ VWD Type 2N Binding, Versiti™ Diagnostic Laboratories, Versiti™	0284U	von Willebrand factor (VWF), type 2N, factor VIII and VWF binding evaluation, enzyme-linked immunosorbent assays (ELISA), plasma
▶RadTox™ cfDNA test, DiaCarta Clinical Lab, DiaCarta Inc◀	●0285U	▶Oncology, response to radiation, cell-free DNA, quantitative branched chain DNA amplification, plasma, reported as a radiation toxicity score◀
▶CNT (*CEP72, TPMT* and *NUDT15*) genotyping panel, RPRD Diagnostics◀	●0286U	▶*CEP72 (centrosomal protein, 72-KDa), NUDT15 (nudix hydrolase 15)* and *TPMT (thiopurine S-methyltransferase)* (eg, drug metabolism) gene analysis, common variants◀
▶ThyroSeq® CRC, CBLPath, Inc, University of Pittsburgh Medical Center◀	●0287U	▶Oncology (thyroid), DNA and mRNA, next-generation sequencing analysis of 112 genes, fine needle aspirate or formalin-fixed paraffin-embedded (FFPE) tissue, algorithmic prediction of cancer recurrence, reported as a categorical risk result (low, intermediate, high)◀
▶DetermaRx™, Oncocyte Corporation◀	●0288U	▶Oncology (lung), mRNA, quantitative PCR analysis of 11 genes *(BAG1, BRCA1, CDC6, CDK2AP1, ERBB3, FUT3, IL11, LCK, RND3, SH3BGR, WNT3A)* and 3 reference genes *(ESD, TBP, YAP1)*, formalin-fixed paraffin-embedded (FFPE) tumor tissue, algorithmic interpretation reported as a recurrence risk score◀

(Continued on page 294)

▲=Revised code ●=New code ▶ ◀=Contains new or revised text ✕=Duplicate PLA test ⭡⭣=Category I PLA

Appendix O

Proprietary Name and Clinical Laboratory or Manufacturer	Alpha-Numeric Code	Code Descriptor
▶MindX Blood Test™ - Memory/Alzheimer's, MindX Sciences™ Laboratory, MindX Sciences™ Inc◀	●0289U	▶Neurology (Alzheimer disease), mRNA, gene expression profiling by RNA sequencing of 24 genes, whole blood, algorithm reported as predictive risk score◀
▶MindX Blood Test™ - Pain, MindX Sciences™ Laboratory, MindX Sciences™ Inc◀	●0290U	▶Pain management, mRNA, gene expression profiling by RNA sequencing of 36 genes, whole blood, algorithm reported as predictive risk score◀
▶MindX Blood Test™ - Mood, MindX Sciences™ Laboratory, MindX Sciences™ Inc◀	●0291U	▶Psychiatry (mood disorders), mRNA, gene expression profiling by RNA sequencing of 144 genes, whole blood, algorithm reported as predictive risk score◀
▶MindX Blood Test™ - Stress, MindX Sciences™ Laboratory, MindX Sciences™ Inc◀	●0292U	▶Psychiatry (stress disorders), mRNA, gene expression profiling by RNA sequencing of 72 genes, whole blood, algorithm reported as predictive risk score◀
▶MindX Blood Test™ - Suicidality, MindX Sciences™ Laboratory, MindX Sciences™ Inc◀	●0293U	▶Psychiatry (suicidal ideation), mRNA, gene expression profiling by RNA sequencing of 54 genes, whole blood, algorithm reported as predictive risk score◀
▶MindX Blood Test™ - Longevity, MindX Sciences™ Laboratory, MindX Sciences™ Inc◀	●0294U	▶Longevity and mortality risk, mRNA, gene expression profiling by RNA sequencing of 18 genes, whole blood, algorithm reported as predictive risk score◀
▶DCISionRT®, PreludeDx™, Prelude Corporation◀	●0295U	▶Oncology (breast ductal carcinoma in situ), protein expression profiling by immunohistochemistry of 7 proteins (COX2, FOXA1, HER2, Ki-67, p16, PR, SIAH2), with 4 clinicopathologic factors (size, age, margin status, palpability), utilizing formalin-fixed paraffin-embedded (FFPE) tissue, algorithm reported as a recurrence risk score◀
▶mRNA CancerDetect™, Viome Life Sciences, Inc, Viome Life Sciences, Inc◀	●0296U	▶Oncology (oral and/or oropharyngeal cancer), gene expression profiling by RNA sequencing of at least 20 molecular features (eg, human and/or microbial mRNA), saliva, algorithm reported as positive or negative for signature associated with malignancy◀
▶Praxis Somatic Whole Genome Sequencing, Praxis Genomics LLC◀	●0297U	▶Oncology (pan tumor), whole genome sequencing of paired malignant and normal DNA specimens, fresh or formalin-fixed paraffin-embedded (FFPE) tissue, blood or bone marrow, comparative sequence analyses and variant identification◀
▶Praxis Somatic Transcriptome, Praxis Genomics LLC◀	●0298U	▶Oncology (pan tumor), whole transcriptome sequencing of paired malignant and normal RNA specimens, fresh or formalin-fixed paraffin-embedded (FFPE) tissue, blood or bone marrow, comparative sequence analyses and expression level and chimeric transcript identification◀
▶Praxis Somatic Optical Genome Mapping, Praxis Genomics LLC◀	●0299U	▶Oncology (pan tumor), whole genome optical genome mapping of paired malignant and normal DNA specimens, fresh frozen tissue, blood, or bone marrow, comparative structural variant identification◀

Proprietary Name and Clinical Laboratory or Manufacturer	Alpha-Numeric Code	Code Descriptor
▶Praxis Somatic Combined Whole Genome Sequencing and Optical Genome Mapping, Praxis Genomics LLC◀	●0300U	▶Oncology (pan tumor), whole genome sequencing and optical genome mapping of paired malignant and normal DNA specimens, fresh tissue, blood, or bone marrow, comparative sequence analyses and variant identification◀
▶Bartonella ddPCR, Galaxy Diagnostics Inc◀	●0301U	▶Infectious agent detection by nucleic acid (DNA or RNA), Bartonella henselae and Bartonella quintana, droplet digital PCR (ddPCR);◀
▶Bartonella Digital ePCR™, Galaxy Diagnostics Inc◀	●0302U	▶following liquid enrichment◀
▶Hypoxic BioChip Adhesion, BioChip Labs™, BioChip Labs™◀	●0303U	▶Hematology, red blood cell (RBC) adhesion to endothelial/subendothelial adhesion molecules, functional assessment, whole blood, with algorithmic analysis and result reported as an RBC adhesion index; hypoxic◀
▶Normoxic BioChip Adhesion, BioChip Labs™, BioChip Labs™◀	●0304U	▶normoxic◀
▶Ektacytometry, BioChip Labs™, BioChip Labs™◀	●0305U	▶Hematology, red blood cell (RBC) functionality and deformity as a function of shear stress, whole blood, reported as a maximum elongation index◀
▶Invitae PCM Tissue Profiling and MRD Baseline Assay, Invitae Corporation, Invitae Corporation◀	●0306U	▶Oncology (minimal residual disease [MRD]), next-generation targeted sequencing analysis, cell-free DNA, initial (baseline) assessment to determine a patient-specific panel for future comparisons to evaluate for MRD◀ ▶(Do not report 0306U in conjunction with 0307U)◀
▶Invitae PCM MRD Monitoring, Invitae Corporation, Invitae Corporation◀	●0307U	▶Oncology (minimal residual disease [MRD]), next-generation targeted sequencing analysis of a patient-specific panel, cell-free DNA, subsequent assessment with comparison to previously analyzed patient specimens to evaluate for MRD◀ ▶(Do not report 0307U in conjunction with 0306U)◀
▶HART CADhs®, Prevencio, Inc, Prevencio, Inc◀	●0308U	▶Cardiology (coronary artery disease [CAD]), analysis of 3 proteins (high sensitivity [hs] troponin, adiponectin, and kidney injury molecule-1 [KIM-1]), plasma, algorithm reported as a risk score for obstructive CAD◀
▶HART CVE®, Prevencio, Inc, Prevencio, Inc◀	●0309U	▶Cardiology (cardiovascular disease), analysis of 4 proteins (NT-proBNP, osteopontin, tissue inhibitor of metalloproteinase-1 [TIMP-1], and kidney injury molecule-1 [KIM-1]), plasma, algorithm reported as a risk score for major adverse cardiac event◀
▶HART KD®, Prevencio, Inc, Prevencio, Inc◀	●0310U	▶Pediatrics (vasculitis, Kawasaki disease [KD]), analysis of 3 biomarkers (NTproBNP, C-reactive protein, and T-uptake), plasma, algorithm reported as a risk score for KD◀

(Continued on page 296)

▲=Revised code   ●=New code   ▶◀=Contains new or revised text   ✄=Duplicate PLA test   ⇅=Category I PLA   American Medical Association   **295**

Proprietary Name and Clinical Laboratory or Manufacturer	Alpha-Numeric Code	Code Descriptor
▶Accelerate PhenoTest® BC kit, AST configuration, Accelerate Diagnostics, Inc, Accelerate Diagnostics, Inc◀	●0311U	▶Infectious disease (bacterial), quantitative antimicrobial susceptibility reported as phenotypic minimum inhibitory concentration (MIC)–based antimicrobial susceptibility for each organism identified◀ ▶(Do not report 0311U in conjunction with 87076, 87077, 0086U)◀
▶Avise® Lupus, Exagen Inc, Exagen Inc◀	●0312U	▶Autoimmune diseases (eg, systemic lupus erythematosus [SLE]), analysis of 8 IgG autoantibodies and 2 cell-bound complement activation products using enzyme-linked immunosorbent immunoassay (ELISA), flow cytometry and indirect immunofluorescence, serum, or plasma and whole blood, individual components reported along with an algorithmic SLE-likelihood assessment◀
▶PancreaSeq® Genomic Classifier, Molecular and Genomic Pathology Laboratory, University of Pittsburgh Medical Center◀	●0313U	▶Oncology (pancreas), DNA and mRNA next-generation sequencing analysis of 74 genes and analysis of CEA (CEACAM5) gene expression, pancreatic cyst fluid, algorithm reported as a categorical result (ie, negative, low probability of neoplasia or positive, high probability of neoplasia)◀
▶DecisionDx® DiffDx™- Melanoma, Castle Biosciences, Inc, Castle Biosciences, Inc◀	●0314U	▶Oncology (cutaneous melanoma), mRNA gene expression profiling by RT-PCR of 35 genes (32 content and 3 housekeeping), utilizing formalin-fixed paraffin-embedded (FFPE) tissue, algorithm reported as a categorical result (ie, benign, intermediate, malignant)◀
▶DecisionDx®-SCC, Castle Biosciences, Inc, Castle Biosciences, Inc◀	●0315U	▶Oncology (cutaneous squamous cell carcinoma), mRNA gene expression profiling by RT-PCR of 40 genes (34 content and 6 housekeeping), utilizing formalin-fixed paraffin-embedded (FFPE) tissue, algorithm reported as a categorical risk result (ie, Class 1, Class 2A, Class 2B)◀
▶Lyme Borrelia Nanotrap® Urine Antigen Test, Galaxy Diagnostics Inc◀	●0316U	▶Borrelia burgdorferi (Lyme disease), OspA protein evaluation, urine◀
▶LungLB®, LungLife AI®, LungLife AI®◀	●0317U	▶Oncology (lung cancer), four-probe FISH (3q29, 3p22.1, 10q22.3, 10cen) assay, whole blood, predictive algorithm-generated evaluation reported as decreased or increased risk for lung cancer◀
▶EpiSign Complete, Greenwood Genetic Center◀	●0318U	▶Pediatrics (congenital epigenetic disorders), whole genome methylation analysis by microarray for 50 or more genes, blood◀
▶Clarava™, Verici Dx, Verici Dx, Inc◀	●0319U	▶Nephrology (renal transplant), RNA expression by select transcriptome sequencing, using pretransplant peripheral blood, algorithm reported as a risk score for early acute rejection◀
▶Tuteva™, Verici Dx, Verici Dx, Inc◀	●0320U	▶Nephrology (renal transplant), RNA expression by select transcriptome sequencing, using posttransplant peripheral blood, algorithm reported as a risk score for acute cellular rejection◀

★ = Telemedicine   ◀ = Audio-only   ✚ = Add-on code   ✗ = FDA approval pending   # = Resequenced code   ⃠ = Modifier 51 exempt

Proprietary Name and Clinical Laboratory or Manufacturer	Alpha-Numeric Code	Code Descriptor
▶Bridge Urinary Tract Infection Detection and Resistance Test, Bridge Diagnostics◀	●0321U	▶Infectious agent detection by nucleic acid (DNA or RNA), genitourinary pathogens, identification of 20 bacterial and fungal organisms and identification of 16 associated antibiotic-resistance genes, multiplex amplified probe technique◀
▶NPDX ASD Test Panel III, Stemina Biomarker Discovery d/b/a NeuroPointDX, Stemina Biomarker Discovery d/b/a NeuroPointDX◀	●0322U	▶Neurology (autism spectrum disorder [ASD]), quantitative measurements of 14 acyl carnitines and microbiome-derived metabolites, liquid chromatography with tandem mass spectrometry (LC-MS/MS), plasma, results reported as negative or positive for risk of metabolic subtypes associated with ASD◀
▶Johns Hopkins Metagenomic Next-Generation Sequencing Assay for Infectious Disease Diagnostics, Johns Hopkins Medical Microbiology Laboratory◀	●0323U	▶Infectious agent detection by nucleic acid (DNA and RNA), central nervous system pathogen, metagenomic next-generation sequencing, cerebrospinal fluid (CSF), identification of pathogenic bacteria, viruses, parasites, or fungi◀
▶3D Predict™ Ovarian Doublet Panel, KIYATEC® Inc◀	●0324U	▶Oncology (ovarian), spheroid cell culture, 4-drug panel (carboplatin, doxorubicin, gemcitabine, paclitaxel), tumor chemotherapy response prediction for each drug◀
▶3D Predict™ Ovarian PARP Panel, KIYATEC® Inc◀	●0325U	▶Oncology (ovarian), spheroid cell culture, poly (ADP-ribose) polymerase (PARP) inhibitors (niraparib, olaparib, rucaparib, velparib), tumor response prediction for each drug◀
▶Guardant360®, Guardant Health, Inc, Guardant Health, Inc◀	●0326U	▶Targeted genomic sequence analysis panel, solid organ neoplasm, cell-free circulating DNA analysis of 83 or more genes, interrogation for sequence variants, gene copy number amplifications, gene rearrangements, microsatellite instability and tumor mutational burden◀
▶Vasistera™, Natera, Inc, Natera, Inc◀	●0327U	▶Fetal aneuploidy (trisomy 13, 18, and 21), DNA sequence analysis of selected regions using maternal plasma, algorithm reported as a risk score for each trisomy, includes sex reporting, if performed◀
▶CareView360, Newstar Medical Laboratories, LLC, Newstar Medical Laboratories, LLC◀	●0328U	▶Drug assay, definitive, 120 or more drugs and metabolites, urine, quantitative liquid chromatography with tandem mass spectrometry (LC-MS/MS), includes specimen validity and algorithmic analysis describing drug or metabolite and presence or absence of risks for a significant patient-adverse event, per date of service◀
▶Oncomap™ ExTra, Exact Sciences, Inc, Genomic Health Inc◀	●0329U	▶Oncology (neoplasia), exome and transcriptome sequence analysis for sequence variants, gene copy number amplifications and deletions, gene rearrangements, microsatellite instability and tumor mutational burden utilizing DNA and RNA from tumor with DNA from normal blood or saliva for subtraction, report of clinically significant mutation(s) with therapy associations◀

(Continued on page 298)

▲=Revised code   ●=New code   ▶◀=Contains new or revised text   ✂=Duplicate PLA test   ↕=Category I PLA   American Medical Association   **297**

Appendix O

Proprietary Name and Clinical Laboratory or Manufacturer	Alpha-Numeric Code	Code Descriptor
▶Bridge Women's Health Infectious Disease Detection Test, Bridge Diagnostics, Thermo Fisher and Hologic Test Kit on Panther Instrument◀	●0330U	▶Infectious agent detection by nucleic acid (DNA or RNA), vaginal pathogen panel, identification of 27 organisms, amplified probe technique, vaginal swab◀
▶Augusta Hematology Optical Genome Mapping, Georgia Esoteric and Molecular Labs, Augusta University, Bionano◀	●0331U	▶Oncology (hematolymphoid neoplasia), optical genome mapping for copy number alterations and gene rearrangements utilizing DNA from blood or bone marrow, report of clinically significant alterations◀
▶EpiSwitch® CiRT (Checkpoint-inhibitor Response Test), Next Bio-Research Services, LLC, Oxford BioDynamics, PLC◀	●0332U	▶Oncology (pan-tumor), genetic profiling of 8 DNA-regulatory (epigenetic) markers by quantitative polymerase chain reaction (qPCR), whole blood, reported as a high or low probability of responding to immune checkpoint–inhibitor therapy◀
▶HelioLiver™ Test, Fulgent Genetics, LLC, Helio Health, Inc◀	●0333U	▶Oncology (liver), surveillance for hepatocellular carcinoma (HCC) in high-risk patients, analysis of methylation patterns on circulating cell-free DNA (cfDNA) plus measurement of serum of AFP/AFP-L3 and oncoprotein des-gamma-carboxy-prothrombin (DCP), algorithm reported as normal or abnormal result◀
▶Guardant360 TissueNext™, Guardant Health, Inc, Guardant Health, Inc◀	●0334U	▶Oncology (solid organ), targeted genomic sequence analysis, formalin-fixed paraffin-embedded (FFPE) tumor tissue, DNA analysis, 84 or more genes, interrogation for sequence variants, gene copy number amplifications, gene rearrangements, microsatellite instability and tumor mutational burden◀
▶IriSight™ Prenatal Analysis – Proband, Variantyx, Inc, Variantyx, Inc◀	●0335U	▶Rare diseases (constitutional/heritable disorders), whole genome sequence analysis, including small sequence changes, copy number variants, deletions, duplications, mobile element insertions, uniparental disomy (UPD), inversions, aneuploidy, mitochondrial genome sequence analysis with heteroplasmy and large deletions, short tandem repeat (STR) gene expansions, fetal sample, identification and categorization of genetic variants◀ ▶(Do not report 0335U in conjunction with 81425, 0212U)◀

★=Telemedicine ◀=Audio-only ✦=Add-on code ✗=FDA approval pending #=Resequenced code ⃠=Modifier 51 exempt

Proprietary Name and Clinical Laboratory or Manufacturer	Alpha-Numeric Code	Code Descriptor
▶IriSight™ Prenatal Analysis – Comparator, Variantyx, Inc, Variantyx, Inc◀	●0336U	▶Rare diseases (constitutional/heritable disorders), whole genome sequence analysis, including small sequence changes, copy number variants, deletions, duplications, mobile element insertions, uniparental disomy (UPD), inversions, aneuploidy, mitochondrial genome sequence analysis with heteroplasmy and large deletions, short tandem repeat (STR) gene expansions, blood or saliva, identification and categorization of genetic variants, each comparator genome (eg, parent)◀ ▶(Do not report 0336U in conjunction with 81426, 0213U)◀
▶CELLSEARCH® Circulating Multiple Myeloma Cell (CMMC) Test, Menarini Silicon Biosystems, Inc, Menarini Silicon Biosystems, Inc◀	●0337U	▶Oncology (plasma cell disorders and myeloma), circulating plasma cell immunologic selection, identification, morphological characterization, and enumeration of plasma cells based on differential CD138, CD38, CD19, and CD45 protein biomarker expression, peripheral blood◀
▶CELLSEARCH® HER2 Circulating Tumor Cell (CTC-HER2) Test, Menarini Silicon Biosystems, Inc, Menarini Silicon Biosystems, Inc◀	●0338U	▶Oncology (solid tumor), circulating tumor cell selection, identification, morphological characterization, detection and enumeration based on differential EpCAM, cytokeratins 8, 18, and 19, and CD45 protein biomarkers, and quantification of HER2 protein biomarker–expressing cells, peripheral blood◀
▶SelectMDx® for Prostate Cancer, MDxHealth®, Inc, MDxHealth®, Inc◀	●0339U	▶Oncology (prostate), mRNA expression profiling of *HOXC6* and *DLX1*, reverse transcription polymerase chain reaction (RT-PCR), first-void urine following digital rectal examination, algorithm reported as probability of high-grade cancer◀
▶Signatera™, Natera, Inc, Natera, Inc◀	●0340U	▶Oncology (pan-cancer), analysis of minimal residual disease (MRD) from plasma, with assays personalized to each patient based on prior next-generation sequencing of the patient's tumor and germline DNA, reported as absence or presence of MRD, with disease-burden correlation, if appropriate◀
▶Single Cell Prenatal Diagnosis (SCPD) Test, Luna Genetics, Inc, Luna Genetics, Inc◀	●0341U	▶Fetal aneuploidy DNA sequencing comparative analysis, fetal DNA from products of conception, reported as normal (euploidy), monosomy, trisomy, or partial deletion/duplication, mosaicism, and segmental aneuploid◀
▶IMMray® PanCan-d, Immunovia, Inc, Immunovia, Inc◀	●0342U	▶Oncology (pancreatic cancer), multiplex immunoassay of C5, C4, cystatin C, factor B, osteoprotegerin (OPG), gelsolin, IGFBP3, CA125 and multiplex electrochemiluminescent immunoassay (ECLIA) for CA19-9, serum, diagnostic algorithm reported qualitatively as positive, negative, or borderline◀

(*Continued on page 300*)

▲=Revised code   ●=New code   ▶◀=Contains new or revised text   ✕=Duplicate PLA test   ⇅=Category I PLA   American Medical Association   **299**

Proprietary Name and Clinical Laboratory or Manufacturer	Alpha-Numeric Code	Code Descriptor
▶miR Sentinel™ Prostate Cancer Test, miR Scientific, LLC, miR Scientific, LLC◀	●0343U	▶Oncology (prostate), exosome-based analysis of 442 small noncoding RNAs (sncRNAs) by quantitative reverse transcription polymerase chain reaction (RT-qPCR), urine, reported as molecular evidence of no-, low-, intermediate- or high-risk of prostate cancer◀
▶OWLiver®, CIMA Sciences, LLC◀	●0344U	▶Hepatology (nonalcoholic fatty liver disease [NAFLD]), semiquantitative evaluation of 28 lipid markers by liquid chromatography with tandem mass spectrometry (LC-MS/MS), serum, reported as at-risk for nonalcoholic steatohepatitis (NASH) or not NASH◀
▶GeneSight® Psychotropic, Assurex Health, Inc, Myriad Genetics, Inc◀	●0345U	▶Psychiatry (eg, depression, anxiety, attention deficit hyperactivity disorder [ADHD]), genomic analysis panel, variant analysis of 15 genes, including deletion/duplication analysis of *CYP2D6*◀
▶QUEST AD-Detect™, Beta-Amyloid 42/40 Ratio, Plasma, Quest Diagnostics◀	●0346U	▶Beta amyloid, Aß40 and Aß42 by liquid chromatography with tandem mass spectrometry (LC-MS/MS), ratio, plasma◀
▶RightMed® PGx16 Test, OneOme®, OneOme®, LLC◀	●0347U	▶Drug metabolism or processing (multiple conditions), whole blood or buccal specimen, DNA analysis, 16 gene report, with variant analysis and reported phenotypes◀
▶RightMed® Comprehensive Test Exclude F2 and F5, OneOme®, OneOme®, LLC◀	●0348U	▶Drug metabolism or processing (multiple conditions), whole blood or buccal specimen, DNA analysis, 25 gene report, with variant analysis and reported phenotypes◀
▶RightMed® Comprehensive Test, OneOme®, OneOme®, LLC◀	●0349U	▶Drug metabolism or processing (multiple conditions), whole blood or buccal specimen, DNA analysis, 27 gene report, with variant analysis, including reported phenotypes and impacted gene-drug interactions◀
▶RightMed® Gene Report, OneOme®, OneOme®, LLC◀	●0350U	▶Drug metabolism or processing (multiple conditions), whole blood or buccal specimen, DNA analysis, 27 gene report, with variant analysis and reported phenotypes◀
▶MeMed BV®, MeMed Diagnostics, Ltd, MeMed Diagnostics, Ltd ◀	●0351U	▶Infectious disease (bacterial or viral), biochemical assays, tumor necrosis factor-related apoptosis-inducing ligand (TRAIL), interferon gamma-induced protein-10 (IP-10), and C-reactive protein, serum, algorithm reported as likelihood of bacterial infection◀
▶Xpert® Xpress MVP, Cepheid®◀	●0352U	▶Infectious disease (bacterial vaginosis and vaginitis), multiplex amplified probe technique, for detection of bacterial vaginosis–associated bacteria (BVAB-2, Atopobium vaginae, and Megasphera type 1), algorithm reported as detected or not detected and separate detection of Candida species (C. albicans, C. tropicalis, C. parapsilosis, C. dubliniensis), Candida glabrata/Candida krusei, and trichomonas vaginalis, vaginal-fluid specimen, each result reported as detected or not detected◀

★=Telemedicine   ◀=Audio-only   ✚=Add-on code   ⋀=FDA approval pending   #=Resequenced code   ⊘=Modifier 51 exempt

Proprietary Name and Clinical Laboratory or Manufacturer	Alpha-Numeric Code	Code Descriptor
▶Xpert® CT/NG, Cepheid®◀	●0353U	▶Infectious agent detection by nucleic acid (DNA), Chlamydia trachomatis and Neisseria gonorrhoeae, multiplex amplified probe technique, urine, vaginal, pharyngeal, or rectal, each pathogen reported as detected or not detected◀
▶PreTect HPV-Proofer`7, GenePace Laboratories, LLC, PreTech◀	●0354U	▶Human papilloma virus (HPV), high-risk types (ie, 16, 18, 31, 33, 45, 52 and 58) qualitative mRNA expression of E6/E7 by quantitative polymerase chain reaction (qPCR)◀

Rationale

A total of 70 new proprietary laboratory analyses (PLA) codes have been established for the CPT 2023 code set. PLA test codes are released and posted online at https://www.ama-assn.org/practice-management/cpt/cpt-pla codes on a quarterly basis (Fall, Winter, Spring, and Summer). New codes are effective the quarter following their publication online. Other changes include the deletion of seven codes (0012U-0014U, 0056U, 0097U, 0151U, 0208U), the revision of four codes (0022U, 0090U, 0229U, 0276U), the revision of test names only (0240U, 0241U), and the deletion of a laboratory name (0166U).

Code 0016M has been revised to identify 219 rather than 209 genes. The manufacturer name has also been updated. The correct identification of the number of genes will make clear that the code specifies the Decipher Bladder test.

Clinical Example (0016M)

A 69-year-old female is diagnosed with muscle invasive bladder cancer. A sample of tumor tissue is submitted for gene expression profiling to determine the tumor subtype and to help guide the patient's management.

Description of Procedure (0016M)

Extract RNA from a selected sample of formalin-fixed paraffin-embedded (FFPE) tumor tissue, purified, and reverse-transcribed into cDNA. Amplify, label, and hybridize the cDNA to an oligonucleotide microarray. Evaluate and analyze gene expression using an algorithm to generate a genomic classifier risk score for one of five molecular subtypes (luminal, infiltrated luminal, basal, basal claudin-low, or neuroendocrine-like). Send a report to the ordering clinician.

Notes

Appendix P

Summary of Additions, Deletions, and Revisions

The summary of changes shows the actual changes that have been made to the code descriptors.

New codes appear with a bullet (●) and are indicated as "Code added." Revised codes are preceded with a triangle (▲). Within revised codes, or if a code symbol has been deleted, the deleted language and code symbol appear with a ~~strikethrough~~, while new text appears <u>underlined</u>.

The ✗ symbol is used to identify codes for vaccines that are pending FDA approval. The # symbol is used to identify codes that have been resequenced. CPT add-on codes are annotated by the ✚ symbol. The ⊘ symbol is used to identify codes that are exempt from the use of modifier 51. The ★ symbol is used to identify codes that may be used for reporting telemedicine services. The ✖ symbol is used to identify a proprietary laboratory analyses (PLA) test that has an identical descriptor as another PLA test. A PLA code that satisfies Category I code criteria and has been accepted by the CPT Editorial Panel is annotated with the ↕ symbol. The ◀ symbol is used to identify codes that may be used to report audio-only telemedicine services when appended by modifier 93 (**see Appendix T**).

Code
<u>92507</u>
<u>92508</u>
<u>92521</u>
<u>92522</u>
<u>92523</u>
<u>92524</u>
<u>92526</u>
<u>92601</u>
<u>92602</u>
<u>92603</u>
<u>92604</u>
<u>96105</u>
<u>96125</u>
<u>99418</u>

Appendix P

CPT Codes That May Be Used For Synchronous Telemedicine Services

This listing is a summary of CPT codes that may be used for reporting synchronous (real-time) telemedicine services when appended by modifier 95. Procedures on this list involve electronic communication using interactive telecommunications equipment that includes, at a minimum, audio and video. The codes listed below are identified in CPT 2023 with the ★ symbol.

Rationale

The listing in Appendix P has been revised to include codes 92507, 92508, 92521-92524, 92526, 92601-92604, 96105, 96125, and 99418. These codes have been identified throughout the CPT code set with the ★ symbol.

To enable the reporting of additional telemedicine services, commercial and public payers continue to add CPT codes to their list of covered services that may be provided as telemedicine services. Note that the codes added for the CPT 2023 code set are services that have been included in the telemedicine coverage policies of at least one payer. As stated in the descriptor of modifier 95, Appendix P includes a list of CPT codes that describe services that are typically performed face-to-face but may be rendered via a real-time (synchronous) interactive audio and video telecommunications system.

90785	90968	97110	99231
90791	90969	97112	99232
90792	90970	97116	99233
90832	92227	97161	99242
90833	92228	97162	99243
90834	92507	97165	99244
90836	92508	97166	99245
90837	92521	97530	99252
90838	92522	97535	99253
90839	92523	97750	99254
90840	92524	97755	99255
90845	92526	97760	99307
90846	92601	97761	99308
90847	92602	97802	99309
90863	92603	97803	99310
90951	92604	97804	99406
90952	93228	98960	99407
90954	93229	98961	99408
90955	93268	98962	99409
90957	93270	99202	99417
90958	93271	99203	99418
90960	93272	99204	99495
90961	96040	99205	99496
90963	96105	99211	99497
90964	96116	99212	99498
90965	96125	99213	
90966	96160	99214	
90967	96161	99215	

★ = Telemedicine   ◀ = Audio-only   ✚ = Add-on code   ✒ = FDA approval pending   # = Resequenced code   ⊘ = Modifier 51 exempt

Appendix Q

Severe Acute Respiratory Syndrome Coronavirus 2 (SARS-CoV-2) (coronavirus disease [COVID-19]) Vaccines

▶This table links the individual severe acute respiratory syndrome coronavirus 2 (SARS-CoV-2) (coronavirus disease [COVID-19]) vaccine product codes (91300-91311) to their associated immunization administration codes (0001A, 0002A, 0003A, 0004A, 0011A, 0012A, 0013A, 0021A, 0022A, 0031A, 0034A, 0041A, 0042A, 0051A, 0052A, 0053A, 0054A, 0064A, 0071A, 0072A, 0073A, 0074A, 0081A, 0082A, 0083A, 0094A, 0104A, 0111A, 0112A), patient age, manufacturer name, vaccine name(s), 10- and 11-digit National Drug Code (NDC) Labeler Product ID, and interval between doses. These codes are also located in the **Medicine** section of the CPT code set.

Additional introductory and instructional information for codes 0001A, 0002A, 0003A, 0004A, 0011A, 0012A, 0013A, 0021A, 0022A, 0031A, 0034A, 0041A, 0042A, 0051A, 0052A, 0053A, 0054A, 0064A, 0071A, 0072A, 0073A, 0074A, 0081A, 0082A, 0083A, 0094A, 0104A, 0111A, 0112A and 91300-91311 can be found in the **Immunization Administration for Vaccines/Toxoids** and **Vaccines, Toxoids** guidelines in the **Medicine** section of the CPT code set.◀

Vaccine Code	Vaccine Administration Code(s)	▲Patient Age▼	Vaccine Manufacturer	Vaccine Name(s)	NDC 10/NDC 11 Labeler Product ID (Vial)	Dosing Interval
#91300 Severe acute respiratory syndrome coronavirus 2 (SARS-CoV-2) (coronavirus disease [COVID-19]) vaccine, mRNA-LNP, spike protein, preservative free, 30 mcg/0.3 mL dosage, diluent reconstituted, for intramuscular use	0001A (1st Dose) 0002A (2nd Dose) ●0003A (3rd Dose) ●0004A (Booster)	▲12 years and older▼	Pfizer, Inc	Pfizer-BioNTech COVID-19 Vaccine/Comirnaty	59267-1000-1 59267-1000-01	▲1st Dose to 2nd Dose: 21 Days 2nd Dose to 3rd Dose: 180 or More Days (CDC recommended population[s] [eg, immuno-compromised]): 28 or More Days Booster: Refer to FDA/CDC Guidance▼
#●91305 Severe acute respiratory syndrome coronavirus 2 (SARS-CoV-2) (coronavirus disease [COVID-19]) vaccine, mRNA-LNP, spike protein, preservative free, 30 mcg/0.3 mL dosage, tris-sucrose formulation, for intramuscular use	#●0051A (1st Dose) #●0052A (2nd Dose) #●0053A (3rd Dose) #●0054A (Booster)	▲12 years and older▼	▲Pfizer, Inc▼	▲Pfizer-BioNTech COVID-19 Vaccine/Comirnaty▼	▲59267-1025-1 59267-1025-01 00069-2025-1 00069-2025-01▼	▲1st Dose to 2nd Dose: 21 Days 2nd Dose to 3rd Dose (CDC recommended population[s] [eg, immunocompromised]): 28 or More Days Booster: Refer to FDA/CDC Guidance▼
#●91307 Severe acute respiratory syndrome coronavirus 2 (SARS-CoV-2) (coronavirus disease [COVID-19]) vaccine, mRNA-LNP, spike protein, preservative free, 10 mcg/0.2 mL dosage, diluent reconstituted, tris-sucrose formulation, for intramuscular use	#●0071A (1st Dose) #●0072A (2nd Dose) #●0073A (3rd Dose) #●0074A (Booster)	▲5 years through 11 years▼	▲Pfizer, Inc▼	▲Pfizer-BioNTech COVID-19 Vaccine▼	▲59267-1055-1 59267-1055-01▼	▲1st Dose to 2nd Dose: 21 Days 2nd Dose to 3rd Dose (CDC recommended population[s] [eg, immunocompromised]): 28 or More Days Booster: Refer to FDA/CDC Guidance▼
#●91308 Severe acute respiratory syndrome coronavirus 2 (SARS-CoV-2) (coronavirus disease [COVID-19]) vaccine, mRNA-LNP, spike protein, preservative free, 3 mcg/0.2 mL dosage, diluent reconstituted, tris-sucrose formulation, for intramuscular use	#●0081A (1st Dose) #●0082A (2nd Dose) #●0083A (3rd Dose)	▲6 months through 4 years▼	▲Pfizer, Inc▼	▲Pfizer-BioNTech COVID-19 Vaccine▼	▲59267-0078-1 59267-0078-01 59267-0078-4 59267-0078-04▼	▲1st Dose to 2nd Dose: 21 Days 2nd Dose to 3rd Dose: Refer to FDA/CDC Guidance▼
#91301 Severe acute respiratory syndrome coronavirus 2 (SARS-CoV-2) (coronavirus disease [COVID-19]) vaccine, mRNA-LNP, spike protein, preservative free, 100 mcg/0.5 mL dosage, for intramuscular use	0011A (1st Dose) 0012A (2nd Dose) ●0013A (3rd Dose)	▲12 years and older▼	Moderna, Inc	Moderna COVID-19 Vaccine	80777-273-10 80777-0273-10	▲1st Dose to 2nd Dose: 28 Days 2nd Dose to 3rd Dose (CDC recommended population[s] [eg, immunocompromised]): 28 or More Days▼
#●91306 Severe acute respiratory syndrome coronavirus 2 (SARS-CoV-2) (coronavirus disease [COVID-19]) vaccine, mRNA-LNP, spike protein, preservative free, 50 mcg/0.25 mL dosage, for intramuscular use	#●0064A (Booster)	▲18 years and older▼	▲Moderna, Inc▼	▲Moderna COVID-19 Vaccine▼	▲80777-273-10 80777-0273-10▼	▲Refer to FDA/CDC Guidance▼

★=Telemedicine ◀=Audio-only ✛=Add-on code ✗=FDA approval pending #=Resequenced code ⃠=Modifier 51 exempt

Vaccine Code	Vaccine Administration Code(s)	▲Patient Age▼	Vaccine Manufacturer	Vaccine Name(s)	NDC 10/NDC 11 Labeler Product ID (Vial)	Dosing Interval
#●91311 Severe acute respiratory syndrome coronavirus 2 (SARS-CoV-2) (coronavirus disease [COVID-19]) vaccine, mRNA-LNP, spike protein, preservative free, 25 mcg/0.25 mL dosage, for intramuscular use	●0111A (1st Dose) ●0112A (2nd Dose)	▲6 months through 5 years▼	▲Moderna, Inc▼	▲Moderna COVID-19 Vaccine▼	▲80777-279-05 80777-0279-05▼	▲1st Dose to 2nd Dose: 1 Month▼
#●91309 Severe acute respiratory syndrome coronavirus 2 (SARS-CoV-2) (coronavirus disease [COVID-19]) vaccine, mRNA-LNP, spike protein, preservative free, 50 mcg/0.5 mL dosage, for intramuscular use	#●●0094A (Booster)	▲18 years and older▼	▲Moderna, Inc▼	▲Moderna COVID-19 Vaccine▼	▲80777-275-05 80777-0275-05▼	▲Booster: Refer to FDA/CDC Guidance▼
#✗91302 Severe acute respiratory syndrome coronavirus 2 (SARS-CoV-2) (coronavirus disease [COVID-19]) vaccine, DNA, spike protein, chimpanzee adenovirus Oxford 1 (ChAdOx1) vector, preservative free, 5×10^{10} viral particles/0.5 mL dosage, for intramuscular use	0021A (1st Dose) 0022A (2nd Dose)	▲18 years and older▼	AstraZeneca, Plc	AstraZeneca COVID-19 Vaccine	0310-1222-10 00310-1222-10	28 Days
#91303 Severe acute respiratory syndrome coronavirus 2 (SARS-CoV-2) (coronavirus disease [COVID-19]) vaccine, DNA, spike protein, adenovirus type 26 (Ad26) vector, preservative free, 5×10^{10} viral particles/0.5 mL dosage, for intramuscular use	▲0031A (Single Dose) ●0034A (Booster)	▲18 years and older▼	Janssen	Janssen COVID-19 Vaccine	59676-580-05 59676-0580-05	▲Booster: Refer to FDA/CDC Guidance▼
#91304 Severe acute respiratory syndrome coronavirus 2 (SARS-CoV-2) (coronavirus disease [COVID-19]) vaccine, recombinant spike protein nanoparticle, saponin-based adjuvant, preservative free, 5 mcg/0.5 mL dosage, for intramuscular use	0041A (1st Dose) 0042A (2nd Dose)	▲18 years and older▼	Novavax, Inc	Novavax COVID-19 Vaccine	80631-100-01 80631-1000-01	21 Days
#✗●91310 Severe acute respiratory syndrome coronavirus 2 (SARS-CoV-2) (coronavirus disease [COVID-19]) vaccine, monovalent, preservative free, 5 mcg/0.5 mL dosage, adjuvant AS03 emulsion, for intramuscular use	●0104A (Booster)	▲18 years and older▼	▲Sanofi Pasteur▼	▲Sanofi Pasteur COVID-19 Vaccine, (Adjuvanted For Booster Immunization)▼	▲49281-618-20 49281-0618-20▼	▲Booster: Refer to FDA/CDC Guidance▼

Rationale

In accordance with the additions and revisions of codes for reporting severe acute respiratory syndrome coronavirus 2 (SARS-CoV-2) (coronavirus disease [COVID-19]) vaccine products and their administration, Appendix Q has been updated.

For CPT 2023, seven new codes for COVID vaccine products (91305-91311), as well as 20 COVID-19 vaccine administration codes (0003A, 0004A, 0013A, 0034A, 0051A-0054A, 0064A, 0071A-0074A, 0081A-0083A, 0094A, 0104A, 0111A, 0112A), have been added to the table in Appendix Q. The table was further modified for CPT 2023 with the addition of a new column to identify patient age. This new column shows the appropriate age ranges for each vaccine product and the associated vaccine administration codes to assist in providing clarity for the user.

Refer to the codebook and the Rationale for codes 0001A-0042A for a full discussion of these changes.

Appendix R

Digital Medicine–Services Taxonomy

Appendix R is a listing of digital medicine services described in the CPT code set. The digital medicine–services taxonomy table in this appendix classifies CPT codes that are related to digital medicine services into discrete categories of clinician-to-patient services (eg, visit), clinician-to-clinician services (eg, consultation), patient-monitoring services, and digital diagnostic services. The clinician-to-patient services and clinician-to-clinician services categories are differentiated by the nature of their services, ie, synchronous and asynchronous communication. The patient-monitoring services represent ongoing, extended monitoring that produces data that require physician assessment and interpretation and are further categorized into device/software set-up and education, data transfer, and data-interpretation services. The digital diagnostic services differentiate automated/autonomous, algorithmically enabled diagnostic-support services into patient-directed and image/specimen-directed services. The term "clinician" in the table represents a physician or other qualified health care professional (QHP) who may use the specific code(s).

This taxonomy is intended to support increased awareness and understanding of approaches to patient care through the multifaceted digital medicine services available for reporting in the CPT code set. The taxonomy is not intended to be a complete representation of all applicable digital medicine service codes in the CPT code set and does not supersede specific coding guidance listed in specific sections of the CPT code set. Furthermore, the table does not denote services that are currently payable through coverage policies by either public or commercial payers.

For purposes of this appendix, the following terms should be understood as:

- Digital medicine services represent the use of technologies for measurement and intervention in the service of patient health.

- Synchronous services represent real-time interactions between a distant-site physician or other QHP and a patient and/or family located at a remote originating site.

- Asynchronous services represent store-and-forward transmissions of health information over periods of time using a secure Web server, encrypted email, specially designed store-and-forward software, or electronic health record. Asynchronous services enable a patient to share health information for later review by the physician or other QHP. These services also allow a physician or other QHP to share a patient's medical history, images, physiologic/non-physiologic clinical data and/or pathology and laboratory reports with a specialist physician for diagnostic and treatment expertise.

Appendix R

▶ Digital Medicine—Services Taxonomy*

(*Note that the codes listed in this table are examples and not meant to be an exhaustive list) ▼

	Clinician*-to-Patient Services (Eg, visit)		Clinician-to-Clinician Services (Eg, consultation)		Patient Monitoring and/or Therapeutic Services			Digital Diagnostic Services	
	Synchronous	**Asynchronous**	**Synchronous**	**Asynchronous**	**Device/Software Set-Up and Education**	**Data Transfer**	**Data Interpretation**	**Patient Directed**	**Image/Specimen Directed**
Encounter Activity	Real-time audiovisual interaction	Store-and-forward digital communication	Real-time consultative communication between requesting and consulting clinicians	Store-and-forward consultative digital exchange of clinical information between requesting and consulting clinicians	In-person, virtual face-to-face, telephone, or other modalities of communication with patient to support device set-up education/supply	Acquisition of patient data with transfer to managing or interpreting physician/other QHP/clinical staff	Data review, interpretation, and patient management by clinical staff/physician/other QHP with associated patient communication	Automated and autonomous algorithmically enabled diagnostic support	Automated and autonomous algorithmically enabled diagnostic support
CPT Service	E/M performed as virtual face-to-face visit (*Use modifier 95*) / Telephone services (Audio only) (99441-99443)	Online digital evaluation & management (99421-99423) (98970-98972)	Interprofessional telephone/Internet/EHR consultation (Typically via telephone) (99446-99449, 99451) / If patient is present at originating site → transition to virtual face-to-face E/M consultation (*Use modifier 95*)	Interprofessional telephone/Internet/EHR consultation (99446-99449, 99451, 99452)	Remote physiologic monitoring initial set-up/education (99453)	Remote physiologic monitoring device supply (99454)	Physiologic data collection/interpretation by physician/other QHP (99091) / Remote physiologic monitoring treatment management by clinical staff/physician/other QHP (99457, 99458)	▲ Autonomous retinopathy screening (92229) ▼	Multianalyte assays with algorithmic analyses (MAAA)

★ = Telemedicine ◀ = Audio-only ✛ = Add-on code ⦅N⦆ = FDA approval pending # = Resequenced code ⊘ = Modifier 51 exempt

▲ Digital Medicine—Services Taxonomy* (cont'd) ▼

(*Note that the codes listed in this table are examples and not meant to be an exhaustive list) ▼

	Clinician*-to-Patient Services (Eg, visit)		Clinician-to-Clinician Services (Eg, consultation)		Patient Monitoring and/or Therapeutic Services			Digital Diagnostic Services	
CPT Service	Synchronous	Asynchronous	Synchronous	Asynchronous	Device/Software Set-Up and Education	Data Transfer	Data Interpretation	Patient Directed	Image/Specimen Directed
					Remote therapeutic monitoring initial set-up/education (98975)	Remote therapeutic monitoring device supply (98976 for respiratory system; 98977 for musculo-skeletal system)	Remote therapeutic monitoring treatment management by physician/other QHP (98980, 98981)		Computer-aided detection (CAD) imaging (77048, 77049, 77065-77067, 0042T, 0174T, 0175T)
					Remote pulmonary artery pressure sensor monitoring treatment management by physician/other QHP (93264)				
					Ambulatory continuous glucose monitoring hook-up, education, recording print-out (95250 for office-equipped; 95249 for patient-equipped)		Ambulatory continuous glucose monitoring analysis (95251)		
					External electrocardiographic recording (Recording, scanning analysis with report, review and interpretation) (93224, 93241, 93245)			External electrocardiographic recording (Autonomous algorithms used to analyze/create report) (93241-93243, 93245-93247)	
					External electrocardiographic recording (Recording) (93224, 93225, 93241, 93242, 93245, 93246)	External electrocardiographic recording (Scanning analysis with report only) (93226, 93241, 93243, 93247)	External electrocardiographic recording (Review and interpretation) (93224, 93227, 93241, 93244, 93248)		

(Continued on page 312)

Appendix R

▲ Digital Medicine–Services Taxonomy* (cont'd) ▼

(*Note that the codes listed in this table are examples and not meant to be an exhaustive list)

CPT Service	Clinician*-to-Patient Services (Eg, visit)		Clinician-to-Clinician Services (Eg, consultation)		Patient Monitoring and/or Therapeutic Services			Digital Diagnostic Services	
	Synchronous	Asynchronous	Synchronous	Asynchronous	Device/Software Set-Up and Education	Data Transfer	Data Interpretation	Patient Directed	Image/Specimen Directed
						External mobile cardiovascular telemetry technical support (93229)	External mobile cardiovascular telemetry review and interpretation (93228)		
						Digital amblyopia services (0704T for initial set-up/education; 0705T for surveillance center technical support, including data transmission)	Digital amblyopia services (Assessment of patient performance, program data) (0706T)		
					Automated analysis of CT study (Data preparation, interpretation and report) (0691T)				

*The term "clinician" in the table represents a physician or other qualified health care professional (QHP) by whom the specific code may be used.

★ = Telemedicine   ◀ = Audio-only   ✚ = Add-on code   ✗ = FDA approval pending   # = Resequenced code   ⊘ = Modifier 51 exempt

Rationale

A footnote has been added to the title of the table in Appendix R to indicate that the codes included within this table are examples only and not intended to be an exhaustive list. In addition, in accordance with the revisions to code 92229, the Appendix R table has been revised to specify that this code is for autonomous retinopathy screening.

Refer to the codebook and the Rationale for code 92229 for a full discussion of these changes.

Notes

▶Appendix S◀

▶Artificial Intelligence Taxonomy for Medical Services and Procedures◀

▶This taxonomy provides guidance for classifying various artificial intelligence (AI) applications (eg, expert systems, machine learning, algorithm-based services) for medical services and procedures into one of these three categories: assistive, augmentative, and autonomous. AI as applied to health care may differ from AI in other public and private sectors (eg, banking, energy, transportation). Note that there is no single product, procedure, or service for which the term "AI" is sufficient or necessary to describe its intended clinical use or utility; therefore, the term "AI" is not defined in the code set. In addition, the term "AI" is not intended to encompass or constrain the full scope of innovations that are characterized as "work done by machines." Classification of AI medical services and procedures as assistive, augmentative, and autonomous is based on the clinical procedure or service provided to the patient and the work performed by the machine on behalf of the physician or other qualified health care professional (QHP).

Assistive: The work performed by the machine for the physician or other QHP is assistive when the machine **detects** clinically relevant data without analysis or generated conclusions. Requires physician or other QHP interpretation and report.

Augmentative: The work performed by the machine for the physician or other QHP is augmentative when the machine **analyzes** and/or **quantifies** data in a clinically meaningful way. Requires physician or other QHP interpretation and report.

Autonomous: The work performed by the machine for the physician or other QHP is autonomous when the machine automatically **interprets** data and independently generates clinically meaningful conclusions without concurrent physician or other QHP involvement. Autonomous medical services and procedures include interrogating and analyzing data. The work of the algorithm may or may not include acquisition, preparation, and/or transmission of data. The clinically meaningful conclusion may be a characterization of data (eg, likelihood of pathophysiology) to be used to establish a diagnosis or to implement a therapeutic intervention. There are three levels of autonomous AI medical services and procedures with varying physician or other QHP professional involvement:

Level I. The autonomous AI draws conclusions and offers diagnosis and/or management options, which are contestable and require physician or other QHP action to implement.

Level II. The autonomous AI draws conclusions and initiates diagnosis and/or management options with alert/opportunity for override, which may require physician or other QHP action to implement.

Level III. The autonomous AI draws conclusions and initiates management, which require physician or other QHP action to contest.◀

▶Service Components	AI Category: Assistive	AI Category: Augmentative	AI Category: Autonomous
Primary objective	Detects clinically relevant data	Analyzes and/or quantifies data in a clinically meaningful way	Interprets data and independently generates clinically meaningful conclusions
Provides independent diagnosis and/or management decision	No	No	Yes
Analyzes data	No	Yes	Yes
Requires physician or other QHP interpretation and report	Yes	Yes	No
Examples in CPT code set	Computer-aided detection (CAD) imaging (77048, 77049, 77065-77067, 0042T, 0174T, 0175T)	Continuous glucose monitoring (CGM) (95251), external processing of imaging data sets	Retinal imaging (92229)◀

Rationale

Appendix S has been established to provide guidance for classifying various artificial intelligence (AI) applications. This Appendix is provided as guidance for the CPT Editorial Panel, potential applicants, and other CPT stakeholders who may want to engage with the CPT Editorial Panel process. It is designed to help shape and define CPT code-change applications (CCAs) that describe work associated with the use of AI-enabled medical services and/or procedures.

This taxonomy provides guidance for classifying various AI applications (eg, expert systems, machine learning, algorithm-based services) for medical services and procedures into one of three categories: assistive, augmentative, or autonomous.

★ = Telemedicine   ◀ = Audio-only   ✚ = Add-on code   ✖ = FDA approval pending   # = Resequenced code   ⊘ = Modifier 51 exempt

▶Appendix T◀

Summary of Additions, Deletions, and Revisions

The summary of changes shows the actual changes that have been made to the code descriptors.

New codes appear with a bullet (●) and are indicated as "Code added." Revised codes are preceded with a triangle (▲). Within revised codes, or if a code symbol has been deleted, the deleted language and code symbol appear with a ~~strikethrough~~, while new text appears <u>underlined</u>.

The ⊁ symbol is used to identify codes for vaccines that are pending FDA approval. The # symbol is used to identify codes that have been resequenced. CPT add-on codes are annotated by the ✚ symbol. The ⊘ symbol is used to identify codes that are exempt from the use of modifier 51. The ★ symbol is used to identify codes that may be used for reporting telemedicine services. The ⋇ symbol is used to identify a proprietary laboratory analyses (PLA) test that has an identical descriptor as another PLA test. A PLA code that satisfies Category I code criteria and has been accepted by the CPT Editorial Panel is annotated with the ⇅ symbol. The ◀ symbol is used to identify codes that may be used to report audio-only telemedicine services when appended by modifier 93.

Code
<u>90785</u>
<u>90791</u>
<u>90792</u>
<u>90832</u>
<u>90833</u>
<u>90834</u>
<u>90836</u>
<u>90837</u>
<u>90838</u>
<u>90839</u>
<u>90840</u>
<u>90845</u>
<u>90846</u>
<u>90847</u>
<u>92507</u>
<u>92508</u>
<u>92521</u>
<u>92522</u>
<u>92523</u>

Code
<u>92524</u>
<u>96040</u>
<u>96110</u>
<u>96116</u>
<u>96160</u>
<u>96161</u>
<u>97802</u>
<u>97803</u>
<u>97804</u>
99354
99355
99356
99357
<u>99406</u>
<u>99407</u>
<u>99408</u>
<u>99409</u>
<u>99497</u>
<u>99498</u>

★ = Telemedicine   ◀ = Audio-only   ✚ = Add-on code   ✗ = FDA approval pending   # = Resequenced code   ⊘ = Modifier 51 exempt

►Appendix T◄

►CPT Codes That May Be Used For Synchronous Real-Time Interactive Audio-Only Telemedicine Services◄

►This listing is a summary of CPT codes that may be used for reporting audio-only services when appended with modifier 93. Procedures on this list involve electronic communication using interactive telecommunications equipment that includes, at a minimum, audio. The codes listed below are identified in CPT 2023 with the ◀ symbol.◄

90785	90839	92523	97804
90791	90840	92524	99406
90792	90845	96040	99407
90832	90846	96110	99408
90833	90847	96116	99409
90834	92507	96160	99497
90836	92508	96161	99498
90837	92521	97802	
90838	92522	97803	

Rationale

The addition of modifier 93, *Synchronous Telemedicine Service Rendered Via Telephone or Other Real-Time Interactive Audio-Only Telecommunications Systems,* allows reporting of medical services that are provided via real-time interaction between the physician or other qualified health care professional and a patient through audio-only technology. The use of this modifier has been in effect since January 1, 2022, and was released to the American Medical Association (AMA) website at https://www.ama-assn.org/practice-management/cpt/cpt-appendix-t-and-modifier-93-audio-only-medical-services.

In addition, Appendix T was also released to the AMA website and has been effective since April 1, 2022. This appendix is a listing of CPT codes that may be used for reporting audio-only services when appended with modifier 93. Procedures on this list involve electronic communication using interactive telecommunications equipment that includes, at a minimum, audio. The codes listed in Appendix T have been identified with the ◀ symbol in the CPT 2023 code set.

Indexes

Instructions for the Use of the Changes Indexes

The Changes Indexes are not a substitute for the main text of *CPT Changes 2023* or the main text of the CPT codebook. The changes indexes consist of two types of content—coding changes and modifiers—all of which are intended to assist users in searching and locating information quickly within *CPT Changes 2023*.

Index of Coding Changes

The Index of Coding Changes list new, revised, and deleted codes, and/or some codes that may be affected by revised and/or new guidelines and parenthetical notes. This index enables users to quickly search and locate the codes within a page(s), in addition to discerning the status of a code (new, revised, deleted, or textually changed) because the status of each new, revised, or deleted code is noted in parentheses next to the code number:

0097U (deleted)..136, 151, 154, 256, 274, 301
36837 (new)..73, 94, 99, 128, 129, 131, 132

Index of Modifiers

The Index of Modifiers does not list all modifiers unless they are new, revised, or deleted, and/or if the modifier may be affected by revised and/or new codes, guidelines, and parenthetical notes. A limited Index of Modifiers, ie, limited to only those modifiers that appear in the Rationales and new or revised guidelines and/or parenthetical notes, is provided to help users quickly locate these modifiers and to know where in the book these modifiers are listed or mentioned.

50, Bilateral Procedure..2, 103, 112, 113, 119–121, 244, 245
51, Multiple Procedures 3, 80, 176, 177

★=Telemedicine ◀=Audio-only ✚=Add-on code ✗=FDA approval pending #=Resequenced code ⊘=Modifier 51 exempt

Index of Coding Changes

Codes in this index are in numerical order, with the four-digit alphanumeric codes first:

Category III changes (a four-digit code followed by the letter "T"); changes to administrative codes for multianalyte assays with algorithmic analyses (MAAA) (a four-digit code followed by the letter "M"); and changes to proprietary laboratory analysis (PLA) codes (a four-digit code followed by the letter "U"). Five-digit CPT codes follow.

0001A......................................169, 170, 172, 176, 177, 203, 305, 308
0002A 169, 170, 172, 176, 177, 203, 305, 308
0003A (new) 57, 58, 167, 169–172, 176–178, 203, 305, 306, 308
0004A (new) 58, 167, 169–172, 176, 177, 203, 305, 306, 308
0011A....................................169, 170, 172, 176, 177, 203, 305, 308
0012A....................................169, 170, 172, 176, 177, 203, 305, 308
0012U (deleted) 136, 151, 154, 255, 267, 301
0013A (new).............58, 167, 169–173, 176–178, 203, 305, 306, 308
0013U (deleted) 136, 151, 154, 255, 267, 301
0014U (deleted) 136, 151, 154, 255, 268, 301
0016M (revised)...255, 261, 301
0021A...169, 172, 176, 177, 203, 305, 308
0022A 169, 172, 176, 177, 203, 305, 308
0022U (revised) 136, 151, 154, 255, 268, 301
0031A (revised).........58, 167, 169, 171, 172, 176–178, 203, 305, 308
0034A (new) 58, 168, 169, 171–173, 176–178, 203, 305, 307, 308
0041A 169, 176, 177, 203, 308
0042A 169, 176, 177, 203, 308
0042T..315
0051A (new)..................58, 167, 169–173, 176, 177, 203, 305, 306
0052A 203
0052A (new) 58, 167, 169–171, 173, 176, 177, 203, 305, 306
0053A..203
0053A (new) 58, 167, 169–171, 173, 176, 177, 203, 305, 306
0054A 203
0054A (new) 58, 167, 169–172, 174, 176, 177, 203, 305, 306
0056U (deleted) 136, 151, 154, 256, 271, 301
0064A (new) 58, 167, 169–172, 174, 176–178, 203, 305, 306
0071A (new)............58, 167, 169–172, 174, 176, 177, 203, 305, 306
0072A (new) 58, 167, 169–171, 174, 176, 177, 203, 305, 306
0073A (new) 58, 167, 169–171, 174, 176, 177, 203, 305, 306
0074A (new)...................58, 167, 169–172, 174–177, 203, 305, 306
0081A (new).............58, 167, 169–172, 175–177, 203, 305, 306
0082A (new) 58, 167, 169–171, 175–177, 203, 305, 306
0083A (new) 58, 167, 169–172, 175–177, 203, 305, 306
0090U (revised) 136, 151, 154, 155, 256, 301
0094A (new) 58, 167, 169–172, 175–178, 203, 305, 307

0097U (deleted) 136, 151, 154, 256, 274, 301
00100-01999..241
0104A (new)............58, 168, 169, 171, 172, 175–178, 203, 305, 307
0111A (new) 58, 168, 169, 171, 172, 176–178, 203, 305, 307
0112A (new)............58, 168, 169, 171, 172, 176–178, 203, 305, 307
0151U (deleted) 136, 151, 154, 256, 280, 301
0163T (deleted)..81, 211, 215
0164T...215
0165T...215
0166U 154, 301
0174T...315
0175T...315
0208U (deleted) 136, 151, 154, 256, 285, 301
0212U 153
0213T...118, 131
0213U 153
0214T...118, 131
0215T...118, 131
0216T...118, 131
0217T...118, 131
0218T...118, 131
0229U (revised) 136, 151, 154, 256, 287, 301
0232T...131, 220, 221
0240U 154, 301
0241U 154, 301
0276U (revised)...........................136, 151, 154, 256, 292, 301
0278T...215, 239
0285U (new) 136, 151, 155, 256, 293
0286U (new) 136, 151, 155, 256, 293
0287U (new) 136, 151, 155, 256, 293
0288U (new) 136, 151, 155, 257, 293
0289U (new) 136, 151, 155, 257, 294
0290U (new) 136, 151, 155, 156, 257, 294
0291U (new)...................................136, 151, 156, 257, 294
0292U (new)...................................136, 151, 156, 257, 294
0293U (new)...................................136, 151, 156, 257, 294
0294U (new) 137, 151, 156, 257, 294

0295U (new) 137, 151, 156, 257, 294
0296U (new) 137, 151, 156, 257, 294
0297U (new) 137, 151, 156, 157, 257, 294
0298U (new) 137, 151, 157, 257, 294
0299U (new) 137, 151, 157, 257, 294
0300U (new) 137, 152, 157, 257, 295
0301U (new) 137, 152, 157, 257, 295
0302U (new) 137, 152, 157, 257, 295
0303U (new) 137, 152, 157, 158, 257, 295
0304U (new) 137, 152, 158, 257, 295
0305U (new) 137, 152, 158, 257, 295
0306U (new) 137, 152, 158, 257, 295
0307U (new) 137, 152, 158, 257, 295
0308U (new) 137, 152, 158, 257, 295
0309U (new) 137, 152, 158, 257, 295
0310U (new) 137, 152, 158, 159, 257, 295
0311U (new) 137, 152, 159, 257, 296
0312T (deleted) 211, 215
0312U (new) 137, 152, 159, 257, 296
0313T (deleted) 211, 215
0313U (new) 137, 152, 159, 257, 296
0314T (deleted) 211, 215
0314U (new) 137, 152, 159, 257, 296
0315T (deleted) 211, 215
0315U (new) 137, 152, 159, 257, 296
0316T (deleted) 211, 215
0316U (new) 137, 152, 159, 160, 257, 296
0317T (deleted) 211, 215
0317U (new) 137, 152, 160, 257, 296
0318U (new) 137, 152, 160, 257, 296
0319U (new) 137, 152, 160, 257, 296
0320U (new) 137, 152, 160, 257, 296
0321U (new) 137, 152, 160, 257, 297
0322U (new) 137, 152, 161, 257, 297
0323U (new) 137, 153, 161, 257, 297
0324U (new) 137, 153, 161, 257, 297
0325U (new) 137, 153, 161, 257, 297
0326U (new) 137, 153, 161, 257, 297
0327U (new) 138, 153, 161, 257, 297
0328U (new) 138, 153, 162, 257, 297
0329U (new) 138, 153, 162, 258, 297
0330U (new) 138, 153, 162, 258, 298
0331U (new) 138, 153, 162, 258, 298
0332U (new) 138, 153, 162, 258, 298
0333U (new) 138, 153, 162, 258, 298
0334U (new) 138, 153, 163, 258, 298
0335U (new) 138, 153, 163, 258, 298

0336U (new) 138, 153, 163, 258, 299
0337U (new) 138, 153, 163, 258, 299
0338U (new) 138, 153, 163, 258, 299
0339T 200, 215
0339U (new) 138, 153, 163, 258, 299
0340U (new) 138, 153, 163, 164, 258, 299
0341U (new) 138, 153, 164, 258, 299
0342U (new) 138, 154, 164, 258, 299
0343U (new) 138, 154, 164, 258, 300
0344U (new) 138, 154, 164, 258, 300
0345U (new) 138, 154, 164, 258, 300
0346U (new) 138, 154, 164, 165, 258, 300
0347U (new) 138, 154, 165, 258, 300
0348U (new) 138, 154, 165, 258, 300
0349U (new) 138, 154, 165, 258, 300
0350U (new) 138, 154, 165, 258, 300
0351U (new) 138, 154, 165, 258, 300
0352U (new) 138, 154, 165, 258, 300
0353U (new) 138, 154, 165, 166, 258, 301
0354U (new) 138, 154, 166, 258, 301
0362T 181, 202
0373T 181, 202
0402T 211
0402T (revised) 215, 216
0437T 217
0470T (deleted) 211, 217
0471T (deleted) 211, 217
0475T (deleted) 211, 217
0476T (deleted) 211, 217
0477T (deleted) 211, 217
0478T (deleted) 212, 217
0481T 131, 220, 221
0487T (deleted) 212, 217
0489T 220
0490T 221
0491T (deleted) 212, 217
0492T (deleted) 212, 217
0493T (deleted) 212, 217
0497T (deleted) 190, 212, 218
0498T (deleted) 190, 212, 218
0499T (deleted) 212, 218, 219
0514T (deleted) 212, 218
0554T 218, 219, 231
0555T 218, 219, 231
0556T 218, 219, 231
0557T 218, 219, 231
0558T 219

★ = Telemedicine   ◀ = Audio-only   ✚ = Add-on code   ✸ = FDA approval pending   # = Resequenced code   ⊘ = Modifier 51 exempt

0565T	220
0566T	221
0582T	131
0619T	219
0621T	219, 225, 226
0622T	219, 225, 226
0627T	132
0628T	132
0640T	217
0641T	217
0642T	217
0687T	184
0688T	184
0691T	219, 231
0702T (deleted)	212, 219
0703T (deleted)	212, 219
0714T (new)	211, 216, 220
0715T (new)	187–189, 212, 220
0716T (new)	212, 220
0717T (new)	212, 220, 221
0718T (new)	212, 220, 221
0719T (new)	212, 221
0720T (new)	212, 222
0721T (new)	212, 222, 223
0722T (new)	212, 222, 223
0723T (new)	212, 223, 224
0724T (new)	212, 223, 224
0725T (new)	125, 212, 224, 225
0726T (new)	212, 224, 225
0727T (new)	212, 224, 225
0728T (new)	186, 212, 224, 225
0729T (new)	186, 212, 224, 225
0730T (new)	121, 184, 185, 212, 219, 225, 226
0731T (new)	212, 226
0732T (new)	212, 226, 227
0733T	213
0733T (revised)	227
0734T	213
0734T (revised)	227
0735T (new)	213, 227, 228
0736T	213
0736T (new)	228
0737T	213
0737T (new)	83, 228, 229
0738T (new)	213, 229
0739T (new)	213, 229, 230
0740T (new)	213, 230
0741T (new)	213, 230
0742T (new)	133, 213, 230, 231, 234
0743T (new)	213, 218, 219, 231
0744T (new)	93, 213, 232
0745T (new)	197, 213, 233, 234
0746T (new)	213, 233, 234
0747T (new)	213, 233, 234
0748T (new)	213, 234
0749T (new)	213, 232, 234
0750T (new)	213, 232, 234
0751T (new)	146, 213, 235, 236
0752T (new)	147, 213, 235, 236
0753T (new)	148, 213, 235, 236
0754T (new)	148, 213, 235–237
0755T (new)	149, 213, 235–237
0756T (new)	149, 213, 235–237
0757T (new)	149, 213, 235, 237
0758T (new)	149, 150, 213, 235, 237
0759T (new)	150, 213, 235–237
0760T (new)	150, 213, 235–237
0761T (new)	150, 213, 235, 237
0762T (new)	150, 213, 235–238
0763T (new)	150, 151, 213, 235, 236, 238
0764T (new)	213, 238
0765T (new)	214, 238
0766T (new)	121, 182, 199, 200, 204, 214, 215, 239
0767T (new)	121, 182, 204, 214, 215, 239, 240
0768T (new)	121, 182, 199, 200, 204, 214, 215, 239, 240
0769T (new)	121, 182, 204, 214, 215, 239, 240
0770T (new)	214, 241
0771T (new)	214, 241–244
0772T (new)	214, 241–244
0773T (new)	214, 241–244
0774T (new)	214, 241–244
0775T (new)	82, 83, 214, 244, 245
0776T (new)	214, 245
0777T (new)	214, 245, 246
0778T (new)	214, 246, 247
0779T (new)	214, 247
0780T (new)	102, 214, 247, 248
0781T (new)	84, 214, 248
0782T (new)	84, 214, 248, 249
0783T (new)	214, 249
01996	116, 117
10004	131
10005	131
10006	131

Indexes

10021	131
10030	131
10160	132
15769	220
15771	220
15772	220
15773	220
15774	220
15778 (new)	76, 105, 216
15850 (deleted)	73, 77
15851 (revised)	77
15853 (new)	73, 77, 78
15854 (new)	73, 77, 78
15876	220
15877	220
15878	220
15879	220
17999	217
19083	131
19285	131
20100-69990	252
20206	132
20220	132
20225	132
20520	132
20525	132
20526	132
20550	132
20551	132
20552	118, 132
20553	118, 132
20555	132
20600	132
20604	131
20605	132
20606	131
20610	132, 220, 221
20611	131, 220, 221
20612	132
20615	132
21116	132
21550	132
22840	221
22853	215
22854	215
22857 (revised)	81, 215
22859	215
22860 (new)	73, 81, 82, 215
23350	132
24220	132
25246	132
27093	132
27095	132
27096	131
27279	244, 245
27280 (revised)	79, 82, 83, 244, 245
27299	244
27369	132
27415	228, 229
27416	228, 229
27648	132
30469 (new)	83, 84
31622- 31638	248
31640	248
31641	248
31643	248
31645	248
31646	248
31647	248
31648	248
31649	248
31651	248
31652	248
31653	248
31654	248
31660	248
31661	248
32400	132
32408	131
32553	132
32554	131
32555	131
32556	131
32557	131
33274	131
33275	131
33361	191, 192
33362	191, 192
33363	191, 192
33364	191, 192
33365	191, 192
33366	191, 192
33418	191, 192
33419	191, 192

★ = Telemedicine　◀ = Audio-only　✚ = Add-on code　✎ = FDA approval pending　# = Resequenced code　⊘ = Modifier 51 exempt

33477	191, 192
33741	191, 192
33745	191, 192
33894	191, 192
33895	191, 192
33900 (new)	87, 88, 191, 192
33901 (new)	87, 89, 191, 192
33902 (new)	87, 88, 90, 191, 192
33903 (new)	87, 88, 90, 191, 192
33904 (new)	73, 87, 88, 91, 191, 192
33957	132
33958	132
33959	132
33962	132
33963	132
33964	132
34501	232
34510	232
35883 (revised)	93
36002	132
36475	129
36476	129
36478	129
36479	129
36568	131, 132
36569	131, 132
36572	131, 132
36573	131, 132
36584	131, 132
36836 (new)	73, 94–99, 128, 129, 131, 132
36837 (new)	73, 94–99, 128, 129, 131, 132
37187	191, 192
37188	191, 192
37191	131
37192	131
37193	131
37211	129
37212	129
37213	129
37214	129
37236	191, 192
37237	191, 192
37238	191, 192
37241	129
37242	129
37243	129
37244	129

37246	191, 192
37248	191, 192
37760	131
37761	131
38220	132
38221	132
38222	132
38505	132
38794	132
41019	132
42400	132
42405	132
43232	131
43237	131
43242	131
43290 (new)	74, 100–102
43291 (new)	74, 100–102
44705	247, 248
44799	247, 248
45341	131
45342	131
45999	247, 248
46030	234
46940	234
46942	234
46948	131
47000	132
47001	132
48102	132
49010	215
49180	132
49411	132
49560 (deleted)	74, 76, 77, 103, 105, 217
49561 (deleted)	74, 103, 105, 217
49565 (deleted)	74, 103, 105, 217
49566 (deleted)	74, 103, 105, 217
49568 (deleted)	74, 103, 105, 217
49570 (deleted)	74, 103, 105, 217
49572 (deleted)	74, 103, 217
49580 (deleted)	74, 103, 217
49582 (deleted)	74, 103, 217
49585 (deleted)	74, 103, 217
49587 (deleted)	74, 103, 217
49590 (deleted)	74, 76, 77, 103, 105, 217
49591 (new)	76, 77, 103–105, 111, 216, 217
49592 (new)	103, 106, 216, 217
49593 (new)	103, 106, 216, 217

Indexes

49594 (new) 103, 106, 216, 217
49595 (new) 103, 105, 107, 216, 217
49596 (new) 103, 105, 107, 216, 217
49613 (new) 74, 103–105, 108, 111, 216, 217
49614 (new) 74, 103–105, 108, 111, 216, 217
49615 (new) 74, 103–105, 108, 111, 216, 217
49616 (new) 74, 103–105, 109, 111, 216, 217
49617 (new) 74, 103–105, 109, 111, 216, 217
49618 (new) 74, 77, 103–105, 110, 111, 216, 217
49621 (new) 74, 103–105, 110, 216, 217
49622 (new) 74, 76, 77, 103–105, 111, 216, 217
49623 (new) 74, 76, 77, 103–105, 111, 217
49652 (deleted) 74, 76, 77, 105, 111, 217
49653 (deleted) 74, 111, 217
49654 (deleted) 75, 111, 217
49655 (deleted) 75, 111, 217
49656 (deleted) 75, 111, 217
49657 (deleted) 75–77, 105, 111, 217
50080 (revised) 112–114, 129
50081 (revised) 112–114, 129
50200 132
50390 132
51100 132
51101 132
51102 132
51700 229
51702 229
52000 219
52441 219
52442 219
52450 219
52500 219
52601 219
52630 219
52640 219
52647 219
52648 219
52649 219
53850 219
53852 219
53854 219
53899 218
55700 132
55867 (new) 114, 115
55874 131
55876 132
58999 217

60100 132
61510 227
61512 227
61518 227
61519 227
61521 227
61645 129
61650 129
61651 129
62268 132
62269 132
62270 132
62272 132
62320 ....132, 245
62321 ....132, 245
62322 ....132, 245
62323 ....132, 245
62324 ....132, 245
62325 ....132, 245
62326 ....132, 245
62327 ....132, 245
62328 132
62329 132
63005 221
63012 221
63017 221
63030 221
63042 221
63047 221
63056 221
64400 ....116, 132
64400-64448 132
64405 ....116, 117, 132
64408 ....116, 117, 119, 132
64415 (revised) 116, 117, 119, 131, 132
64416 (revised) 116, 117, 119, 131, 132
64417 (revised) 116, 117, 119, 131, 132
64418 ....131, 132
64418-64435 119
64420 ....116, 117, 132
64421 ....116, 117, 132
64425 ....116, 117, 132
64430 ....116, 117, 132
64435 ....116, 117, 132
64445 (revised) 116–119, 131, 132
64446 (revised) 116–119, 131, 132
64447 (revised) 116, 118, 119, 131, 132

Indexes

64448 (revised) 116–119, 131, 132	69730 (new) 75, 122, 123, 125
64449 .... 116, 117, 119	69930 .... 125, 224
64450 .... 116, 119, 132	70450 222
64455 132	70460 222
64479 131	70470 222
64480 131	70480 222
64483 131	70481 222
64484 131	70482 222
64490 .... 118, 120, 121, 131	70486 222
64491 .... 118, 120, 131	70487 222
64492 .... 118, 120	70488 222
64493 .... 118, 120, 131	70490 222
64494 .... 118, 120, 121, 131	70491 222
64495 .... 118, 120, 131	70492 222
64505 132	71250 .... 219, 222
64566 .... 121, 239	71260 .... 219, 222
64600 132	71270 .... 219, 222
64605 132	71271 .... 219, 222
64999 215	71275 219
65850 .... 121, 225, 226	72125 .... 219, 222
65855 .... 121, 225, 226	72126 .... 219, 222
65860 121	72127 .... 219, 222
65865 121	72128 .... 219, 222
65870 121	72129 .... 219, 222
65875 121	72130 .... 219, 222
65880 121	72131 .... 219, 222
66174 (revised) 121	72132 .... 219, 222
66175 (revised) 121	72133 .... 219, 222
69209 122	72191 219
69210 122	72192 .... 219, 222, 229
69501 224	72193 .... 219, 222, 229
69501-69676 .... 122, 123	72194 .... 219, 222, 229
69502 224	72195 229
69505 224	72196 229
69511 224	72197 229
69601 224	73200 222
69602 224	73201 222
69603 224	73202 222
69604 224	73700 222
69714 123	73701 222
69716 (revised) 75, 122, 123	73702 222
69717 (revised) 75, 122, 123	74150 .... 219, 222
69719 (revised) 75, 122–124	74160 .... 219, 222
69726 (revised) 75, 122–124	74170 .... 219, 222
69727 (revised) 75, 122–124	74174 219
69728 (new) 75, 122–125	74175 219
69729 (new) 75, 122–125	74176 .... 219, 222, 229

74177 .... 219, 222, 229
74178 .... 219, 222, 229
74181 223
74182 223
74183 223
74261 .... 219, 222
74262 .... 219, 222
74263 .... 219, 222
74283 .... 247, 248
75571 .... 219, 222
75572 .... 219, 222
75573 .... 219, 222
75574 219
75635 219
75710 128
75716 128
75820 .... 128, 129
75822 129
75894 129
75898 129
76000 221
76376 223
76377 223
76496 221
76497 .... 222, 229
76498 229
76856 229
76857 229
76872 .... 219, 229
76873 229
76881 130
76882 (revised) 127, 130
76883 (new) 127, 130, 131
76937 131
76940 229
76942 .... 116, 117, 131, 220, 221, 229
76975 131
76998 .... 229, 232
76999 229
77001 132
77002 .... 116, 117, 132, 220, 221
77003 .... 116, 117, 132
77011 229
77012 229
77013 229
77021 229
77022 229

77048 315
77049 315
77065 315
77066 315
77067 315
77600 229
77605 229
77610 229
77615 229
77620 229
78434 .... 133, 231
78451 .... 133, 231
78452 .... 133, 231
78803 (revised) 127, 133, 134
78814 219
78815 219
78816 219
78830 (revised) 127, 133, 134
78831 (revised) 127, 134
78832 (revised) 127, 134
80503 139
80506 139
81418 (new) 135, 140
81425 153
81426 153
81441 (new) 135, 140, 141
81445 (revised) 135, 140–142
81449 (new) 135, 140–142
81450 (revised) 135, 140–142
81451 (new) 135, 140–142
81455 (revised) 135, 140–143
81456 (new) 135, 140–143
81479 139
84433 (new) 135, 143
87340 .... 143, 144
87467 (new) 135, 143, 144
87468 (new) 135, 144
87469 (new) 135, 144, 145
87471 144
87478 (new) 135, 144, 145
87484 (new) 135, 144, 145
87635 145
87636 145
87637 .... 145, 146
87913 (new) 136, 145, 146
88302 .... 146, 235, 236
88304 .... 147, 235, 236

★ = Telemedicine   ◀ = Audio-only   ✚ = Add-on code   ✗ = FDA approval pending   # = Resequenced code   ⊘ = Modifier 51 exempt

88305	148, 235, 236
88307	148, 235, 236
88309	149, 235, 236
88312	149, 235, 236
88313	149, 235, 236
88314	149, 235, 236
88319	150, 235, 236
88341	150, 235, 236
88342	150, 235, 236
88344	150, 235, 236
88360	150, 151, 235, 236
90460	169, 203
90460-90474	169, 172, 176, 177, 179, 180
90461	169, 203
90471	169, 203
90471-90474	169
90472	169, 203
90473	170
90474	170
90476-90759	169, 170, 172, 176, 177
90584 (new)	168, 179, 180
90678 (new)	168, 180
90739 (revised)	168, 180
90785	67, 180–182, 317, 319
90791	67, 181, 317, 319
90792	67, 181, 317, 319
90832	181, 182, 241, 317, 319
90833	54, 55, 181, 182, 241, 317, 319
90834	181, 182, 241, 317, 319
90836	54, 55, 181, 182, 241, 317, 319
90837	181, 182, 241, 317, 319
90838	54, 55, 181, 182, 241, 317, 319
90839	180, 181, 317, 319
90840	180, 181, 317, 319
90845	317, 319
90846	181, 317, 319
90847	181, 241, 317, 319
90849	241
90853	241
90863	182
90867	239
90868	239
90869	239
90870	180
90935	183
90937	183
90945	183
90947	183
91020	247
91022	247
91112	247
91117	247
91122	247
91132	247
91133	247
91300	169, 170, 172, 176, 177, 305
91301	169–172, 176–178, 305
91302	169, 170, 172, 176, 177, 305
91303	169–172, 176–178, 305
91304	169, 170, 172, 176, 177, 305
91305 (new)	168–172, 176–178, 305, 306
91306 (new)	168–172, 176–178, 305, 306
91307 (new)	168–170, 172, 176–179, 305, 306
91308 (new)	168–170, 172, 176, 177, 179, 305, 306
91309 (new)	168–172, 176–179, 305, 307
91310 (new)	168–172, 176–179, 305, 307
91311 (new)	58, 168–172, 176–179, 305, 307
92002-92014	185
92020	219
92065 (revised)	168, 184
92066 (new)	168, 184
92132	184, 185, 225, 226
92229 (revised)	168, 185, 310, 313, 315
92284 (revised)	168, 185, 186
92507	186, 241, 303, 304, 317, 319
92508	186, 241, 303, 304, 317, 319
92521	186, 303, 304, 317, 319
92522	186, 303, 304, 317, 319
92523	186, 303, 304, 317, 319
92524	186, 303, 304, 318, 319
92526	186, 303, 304
92532	186
92601	186, 224, 303, 304
92602	186, 224, 303, 304
92603	186, 224, 303, 304
92604	186, 224, 303, 304
92920	187, 189, 220, 252
92920-92944	191
92924	187, 189, 220
92928	187, 189, 220, 252
92933	187, 189, 220
92937	187, 189, 220
92941	187, 189, 220
92943	187, 189, 220

Indexes

92953 252
92960 252
92973 188
92974 188
92975 .... 187, 189, 191, 220
92977 191
92978 188
92979 188
92986 252
92987 252
92990 252
92997 .... 191, 192, 252
92998 .... 191, 192, 252
93000 238
93010 .... 190, 238
93224 190
93225 190
93226 190
93227 190
93228 190
93229 190
93241 190
93242 190
93243 190
93244 190
93245 190
93246 190
93247 190
93248 190
93268 190
93270 190
93271 190
93272 190
93296 208
93312 252
93313 252
93314 252
93315 252
93316 252
93317 252
93318 252
93451 .... 190–192, 195
93452 .... 190, 191, 252
93452-93462 128
93453 .... 191, 192
93454 195
93455 .... 191, 195

93456 .... 190–192, 195
93457 .... 190–192, 195
93458 .... 190, 191
93459 .... 190, 191
93460 190–192
93461 190–192
93503 193
93505 .... 192, 252
93563 .... 128, 191, 194–196, 252
93564 .... 128, 191, 194–196, 252
93565 .... 128, 190, 191, 194, 196
93566 .... 128, 190, 191, 194–196
93567 .... 128, 191, 195, 196
93568 .... 191, 194
93568 (revised) 85–87, 93, 128, 168, 191–196, 251, 252
93569 .... 191, 194
93569 (new) 85–87, 93, 128, 168, 191–196, 251, 252
93571 188
93572 188
93573 .... 191, 194
93573 (new) 85, 86, 93, 128, 168, 191–196, 251, 252
93574 .... 191, 194
93574 (new) 85, 86, 93, 128, 168, 191, 192, 194–196, 251, 252
93575 .... 191, 194
93575 (new) 85–87, 93, 128, 168, 191, 192, 194–196, 251, 252
93580 .... 191, 192, 252
93581 .... 191, 192, 252
93582 .... 191, 192, 195, 252
93583 .... 191, 192, 195
93590 252
93591 252
93592 252
93593 .... 128, 190–192, 195, 252
93594 .... 128, 190–192, 195, 252
93595 .... 128, 191, 192, 252
93596 .... 128, 190–192, 252
93597 .... 128, 190–192, 252
93598 .... 195, 252
93609 233
93613 197
93615 252
93616 252
93619 233
93620 233
93621 233
93622 .... 197, 233
93793 197

Indexes

★ = Telemedicine   ◄ = Audio-only   ✚ = Add-on code   � = FDA approval pending   # = Resequenced code   ⊘ = Modifier 51 exempt

93799 .... 217, 218	96402 203
93971 232	96409-96425 203
93998 217	96521-96523 203
94005 198	96999 217
94010-94799 198	97014 .... 204, 239
94760 208	97032 .... 204, 239
95249 230	97110 241
95250 .... 207, 230	97112 241
95251 .... 230, 315	97129 241
95885 .... 199, 239	97150 .... 204, 241
95886 .... 199, 200, 239	97151 .... 181, 202
95887 .... 199, 200, 239	97152 181
95905 .... 200, 239	97153 .... 181, 202, 241
95907 239	97154 .... 181, 202, 241
95907-95913 200	97155 .... 181, 202, 241
95908 239	97156 .... 181, 202
95909 239	97157 .... 181, 202
95910 239	97158 .... 181, 202, 241
95911 239	97530 241
95912 239	97533 241
95913 239	97535 241
95919 (new) 168, 200, 215	97537 241
96000 .... 246, 247	97545 204
96004 .... 246, 247	97546 204
96040 .... 201, 304, 318, 319	97802 .... 201, 206, 318, 319
96105 .... 303, 304	97803 .... 201, 318, 319
96110 .... 318, 319	97804 .... 201, 206, 318, 319
96116 .... 318, 319	98960 201
96125 .... 303, 304	98961 201
96156 201	98962 201
96158 .... 201, 241	98970 207
96159 .... 201, 241	98971 207
96160 .... 67, 318, 319	98972 207
96161 .... 67, 318, 319	98975 (revised) 61, 168, 201, 207, 208, 230, 246, 247, 311
96164 .... 201, 241	98976 (revised) 61, 168, 207, 208, 311
96165 .... 201, 241	98977 (revised) 61, 168, 207, 208, 246, 247, 311
96167 .... 201, 241	98978 (new) 61, 168, 201, 207–209, 219
96168 .... 201, 241	98980 .... 208, 209, 246, 247
96170 .... 201, 241	98981 .... 208, 246, 247
96171 .... 201, 241	99078 202
96202 (new) 168, 201–203	99091 .... 190, 207, 230
96203 (new) 168, 201–203	99151 241
96360-96379 203	99152 241
96360-96549 203	99153 241
96373 226	99155 241
96374 226	99156 241
96401 203	99157 241

Indexes

99184 245

99202 .... 197, 201, 203, 209

99202-99215 .... 29, 122, 169, 183, 185, 186, 199, 205, 206

99202-99255 .... 180, 182

99202-99285 180

99202-99316 181

99203 .... 197, 201, 203, 209

99204 .... 197, 201, 203, 209

99205 .... 197, 201, 203, 209

99211 .... 197, 201, 203, 209

99212 .... 197, 201, 203, 209

99213 .... 197, 201, 203, 209

99214 .... 197, 201, 203, 209

99215 .... 197, 201, 203, 209

99217 (deleted) 3, 31, 32, 72, 100, 102, 116,
122, 183, 184, 186, 199, 205, 207

99218 (deleted) 3, 31, 32, 93, 122, 183, 184, 186, 199, 205, 207

99218-99220 (deleted) 32

99219 (deleted) 3, 31, 72, 122, 183, 184, 186, 199, 205, 207

99220 (deleted) 4, 31, 32, 72, 93, 100, 102,
122, 183, 184, 186, 199, 205, 207

99221 (revised) ... 31, 33, 35, 42, 53, 61–63, 65, 66, 72, 92, 100, 102,
122, 180, 181, 183, 186, 197, 199, 201, 205, 206, 209

99221-99223 (revised) 32, 186, 199, 205

99221-99239 (revised) 31, 32

99222 (revised) 31–33, 35, 42, 53, 61, 62, 72, 92,
102, 122, 180, 181, 183, 197, 201, 206, 209

99223 (revised) 31–35, 42, 53–55, 61–63, 66, 72, 92, 100,
102, 122, 180, 181, 183, 186, 197, 199, 201, 205, 206, 209

99224 (deleted) 4, 31, 32, 72, 100, 102, 122,
183, 184, 186, 197, 199, 205–207

99224-99226 (deleted) 32, 122, 205

99225 (deleted) 4, 31, 122, 183, 184, 186, 197, 206, 207

99226 (deleted) 4, 31, 32, 72, 100, 102, 122,
183, 184, 186, 197, 199, 205–207

99231 (revised) 6, 31, 32, 34, 35, 37, 40, 42, 53,
61, 65, 66, 72, 92, 100, 102, 122,
180, 181, 183, 186, 197, 199, 201, 205, 206, 209

99231-99233 (revised) 186, 199, 205, 206

99232 (revised) 6, 31, 32, 34, 35, 37, 42, 53, 61, 72,
92, 102, 122, 180, 181, 183, 197, 201, 209

99233 (revised) 6, 31, 32, 34, 35, 37, 40, 42,
53–55, 61, 62, 65, 66, 72, 92, 102,
122, 180, 181, 183, 186, 197, 199, 201, 205, 206, 209

99234 (revised) 7, 31, 32, 35–37, 42, 45, 53,
72, 92, 183, 186, 201, 205, 206, 209

99235 (revised) 32, 35–37, 42, 45, 53, 72,
92, 183, 186, 201, 206, 209

99236 (revised) 7, 31, 32, 35–37, 42, 45, 53–55,
72, 92, 183, 186, 201, 205, 206, 209

99238 (revised) 31, 35, 37, 38, 42, 45, 72, 115, 122, 183

99239 (revised) 31, 32, 35, 37, 38, 42, 45, 72, 100, 115, 122, 183

99241 (deleted) 8, 32, 38, 58, 67, 72, 116, 122, 133,
139, 169, 183–186, 197–199, 203, 205–207

99241 (revised) 198

99242 (revised) 8, 32, 38, 39, 53, 58, 67, 72, 115, 122, 133,
139, 169, 183, 185, 186, 197–199, 201, 203, 205, 206

99243 (revised) 8, 38, 39, 53, 58, 67, 72, 115, 122, 133,
139, 169, 183, 185, 186, 197–199, 201, 203, 205, 206

99244 (revised) 8, 39, 40, 53, 58, 67, 72, 115, 122, 133, 139,
169, 183, 185, 186, 197, 199, 201, 203, 205, 206

99244 99241 198

99245 (revised) 9, 32, 39, 40, 53–55, 58, 67, 72, 115, 122, 133,
139, 169, 183, 185, 186, 197–199, 201, 203, 205, 206

99251 (deleted) 9, 32, 40, 62, 72, 133, 139, 205, 207, 209

99252 (revised) 9, 32, 40, 41, 45, 53, 61, 72, 122,
133, 139, 199, 201, 205, 206, 209

99252- 99255 (revised) 32

99253 (revised) 9, 32, 40, 41, 45, 53, 61, 72,
122, 133, 139, 199, 201, 205, 206, 209

99254 (revised) 10, 32, 40–42, 45, 53, 61, 72,
122, 133, 139, 199, 201, 205, 206, 209

99255 (revised) 10, 32, 40–42, 45, 53–55, 61, 72,
122, 133, 139, 180, 182, 199, 201, 205, 206, 209

99281 (revised) 20, 23, 25, 30, 31, 43, 53, 63, 72, 77,
115, 122, 169, 180, 182, 183, 198, 199, 201, 205, 206

99282 (revised) 43, 44, 53, 72, 77, 115, 122, 169,
180, 182, 183, 198, 199, 201, 205, 206

99283 (revised) 43, 44, 53, 72, 77, 115, 122, 169,
180, 182, 183, 198, 199, 201, 205, 206

99284 (revised) 43, 44, 53, 72, 77, 115, 122, 169,
180, 182, 183, 198, 199, 201, 205, 206

99285 (revised) 31, 43, 44, 53, 63, 72, 77, 115, 122,
169, 180, 182, 183, 198, 199, 201, 205, 206

99291 .... 183, 205

99292 .... 183, 205

99304 (revised) 45, 46, 53, 72, 122, 180,
182, 183, 186, 198, 199, 201, 205, 206

99304-99310 (revised) 186

99304-99316 (revised) 199

99305 (revised) 45, 46, 53, 72, 122, 180, 182, 183, 198, 201, 205

99306 (revised) 45, 46, 53–55, 72, 122,
180, 182, 183, 198, 201, 205

99307 (revised) 12, 40, 45–48, 53, 72, 122,
180, 182, 183, 198, 201, 205, 206

99308 (revised) 12, 45, 47, 48, 53, 72, 122,
180, 182, 183, 198, 201, 205, 206

99309 (revised) 13, 45, 47, 48, 53, 72, 122,
180, 182, 183, 198, 201, 205, 206

99310 (revised) 13, 40, 45–48, 53–55, 72,
122, 180, 182, 183, 198, 201, 205, 206

★ = Telemedicine   ◀ = Audio-only   ✛ = Add-on code   ⋏ = FDA approval pending   # = Resequenced code   ⊘ = Modifier 51 exempt

Indexes

99315 186
99315 (revised) 46, 48, 72, 122, 180, 183, 198, 201, 205
99316 186
99316 (revised) 46, 48, 72, 122, 180–183,
186, 198, 199, 201, 205, 206
99318 (deleted) 13, 46, 48, 72, 122,
181–184, 186, 198, 199, 205, 207
99324 (deleted) 13, 48, 49, 60, 62, 67, 72, 122,
181–184, 186, 198, 199, 205–207, 209
99325 (deleted) 14, 48, 122, 181–184, 186, 198, 205–207, 209
99326 (deleted) 14, 48, 122, 181–184, 186, 198, 205–207, 209
99327 (deleted) 14, 48, 122, 181–184, 186, 198, 205, 206, 209
99328 (deleted) 14, 48, 49, 60, 62, 67, 72,
122, 181–184, 186, 198, 205, 206, 209
99334 (deleted) 15, 48, 49, 60, 62, 67, 72, 122,
181–184, 186, 198, 205, 206, 209
99335 (deleted) 15, 48, 122, 181–184, 198, 205, 206, 209
99336 (deleted) 15, 48, 122, 181–184, 198, 205, 206, 209
99337 (deleted) 15, 48, 49, 60, 62, 67, 72, 122,
181–184, 186, 198, 199, 205–207, 209
99339 (deleted) 15, 49, 56–58, 60–62, 68–70, 198, 207
99340 (deleted) 16, 49, 56–58, 60–62, 68–70, 198, 207
99341 (revised) 48–50, 53, 61, 67, 71, 72, 77, 122,
180–183, 198, 199, 201, 205, 206, 209
99341-99350 (revised) 181, 183, 199, 205, 206
99342 (revised) 48–50, 53, 61, 67, 72, 77,
122, 180, 182, 183, 198, 201, 209
99343 (deleted) 16, 49, 62, 67, 72, 180, 183, 198, 209
99344 (revised) 48–50, 53, 61, 67, 72, 77,
122, 180, 182, 183, 198, 201, 209
99345 (revised) 48–50, 53–55, 61, 67, 72, 77,
122, 180, 182, 183, 198, 201, 209
99347 (revised) 38, 48, 49, 51, 53, 61, 67, 72, 77,
122, 180, 182, 183, 198, 201, 209
99348 (revised) 38, 48, 51, 53, 61, 67, 72, 77,
122, 180, 182, 183, 198, 201, 209
99349 (revised) 38, 48, 51, 53, 61, 67, 72, 77,
122, 180, 182, 183, 198, 201, 209
99350 (revised) 38, 48, 49, 51–55, 61, 67, 71, 72, 77,
122, 180–183, 198, 199, 201, 205, 206, 209
99354 (deleted) 18, 52, 55–57, 60, 84, 183, 184, 190, 203, 318
99355 (deleted) 18, 52, 183, 184, 190, 203, 318
99356 (deleted) 18, 52, 183, 184, 190, 193, 318
99357 (deleted) 18, 52, 55–57, 60, 183, 184, 190, 193, 318
99360 183
99366-99368 181
99374 207
99374-99378 198
99379 207
99380 207

99381-99429 .... 169, 199
99401 .... 201, 202
99401-99429 206
99401-99443 181
99402 .... 201, 202
99403 .... 201, 202
99404 .... 201, 202
99406 .... 57, 201, 202, 318, 319
99407 .... 57, 201, 202, 318, 319
99408 .... 57, 201, 202, 318, 319
99409 .... 57, 201, 202, 318, 319
99411 .... 201, 202
99412 .... 201, 202
99417 (revised) 18, 38, 39, 50–56, 58–60, 67
99418 (new) 18, 33, 34, 36, 40, 41, 46, 47,
52–56, 58–60, 189–191, 303, 304
99424 .... 198, 208
99425 .... 198, 208
99426 .... 207, 208
99427 .... 207, 208
99429 201
99437 .... 198, 207
99439 .... 207, 208
99446 (revised) 53, 59, 60, 310
99447 (revised) 53, 59, 60, 310
99448 (revised) 53, 59, 60, 310
99449 (revised) 53, 59, 60, 310
99451 (revised) 18, 53, 59, 60, 310
99453 .... 190, 191, 207, 208, 230
99454 .... 190, 191, 207, 208, 230
99466- 99480 183
99466-99480 .... 183, 205
99483 (revised) 53–55, 66, 67, 72
99484 208
99487 .... 207, 208
99489 .... 207, 208
99490 .... 207, 208
99491 .... 198, 207, 208
99492 .... 208, 209
99493 .... 208, 209
99494 .... 208, 209
99495 (revised) 19, 58, 61, 68, 70–72, 208, 304
99496 (revised) 19, 58, 61, 68, 70–72, 208, 304
99497 .... 67, 72, 304, 318, 319
99498 .... 67, 72, 304, 318, 319
99500-99600 209

Index of Modifiers

The modifiers in this Index of Modifiers is limited to only the modifiers that appear in the Rationales and in the new or revised guidelines and/or parenthetical notes.

Modifier, Descriptor

Page Numbers

25, Significant, Separately Identifiable Evaluation and Management Service by the Same Physician or Other Qualified Health Care Professional on the Same Day of the Procedure or Other Service 32, 45, 62, 100, 183, 199, 203, 205, 206

26, Professional Component 21

50, Bilateral Procedures 2, 103, 112, 113, 119–121, 244, 245

51, Multiple Procedures 3, 80, 176, 177

52, Reduced Services 80, 83, 100

59, Distinct Procedural Service 80, 100, 103, 104

63, Procedure Performed on Infants less than 4 kg 104, 251, 252

93, Synchronous Telemedicine Service Rendered Via Telephone or Other Real-Time Interactive Audio-Only Telecommunications System 2, 3, 73, 127, 135, 167, 211, 251, 252, 317, 319

95, Synchronous Telemedicine Service Rendered Via a Real-Time Interactive Audio and Video Telecommunications System 304

★ = Telemedicine   ◀ = Audio-only   ✚ = Add-on code   ✗ = FDA approval pending   # = Resequenced code   ⊘ = Modifier 51 exempt